500 TIME-TESTED
HOME REMEDIES
and the Science Behind Them

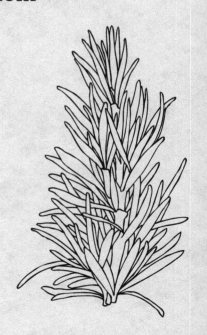

500 TIME-TESTED
HOME REMEDIES
and the Science Behind Them

Ease Aches, Pains, Ailments, and More
with Hundreds of Simple and Effective
At-Home Treatments

LINDA B. WHITE, M.D.

Barbara Brownell Grogan and Barbara H. Seeber

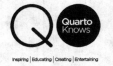

© 2014 Fair Winds Press
Text © 2014 Linda B. White, M.D., Barbara Brownell Grogan, and Barbara H. Seeber

First published in 2014 by Fair Winds Press, an imprint of The Quarto Group, 100 Cummings Center, Suite 265-D, Beverly, MA 01915, USA.
T (978) 282-9590 F (978) 283-2742
www.QuartoKnows.com

Fair Winds Press titles are also available at discount for retail, wholesale, promotional, and bulk purchase. For details, contact the Special Sales Manager by email at specialsales@quarto.com or by mail at The Quarto Group, Attn: Special Sales Manager, 401 Second Avenue North, Suite 310, Minneapolis, MN 55401, USA.

ISBN: 978-1-59233-575-6
Digital edition published in 2014
eISBN: 978-1-61058-857-7

Library of Congress Cataloging-in-Publication Data available

Cover design by Quayside Publishing Group
Cover images, Shutterstock.com
Book design by Kathie Alexander

The information in this book is for educational purposes only. It is not intended to replace the advice of a physician or medical practitioner. Please see your health care provider before beginning any new health program. The authors and publisher are not responsible for readers' misuse of these recipes and, as a result, any unintended effects.

Printed in USA

Dedicated to our families
and the good health of
our readers.

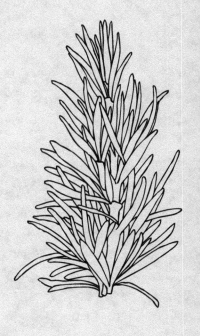

Contents

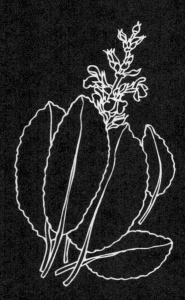

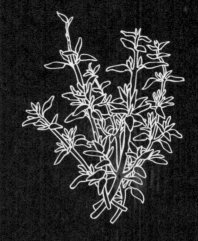

Introduction

In today's high-powered, health-conscious world, we're all smarter, more informed about our bodies, and preoccupied with ways to live long, healthy lives. We've accomplished half of that goal: living longer. But we're missing the "living healthier" part of the equation.

On December 15, 2012, the British medical journal *The Lancet* published data from the Global Burden of Disease Study 2010. Here are the key findings, starting with the good news: Around the world, longevity has increased. We're less likely to succumb prematurely to malaria and measles, but more likely to drop dead later in life from heart attack or stroke. The bad news is, we're more likely to spend our last years disabled by diseases—most of which are preventable.

Chronic illness has long dogged Americans. Now it's spreading to other countries. Where have we gone wrong? We have health-related facts and figures at our fingertips. We have expensive diagnostic tests, highly trained doctors, and cutting-edge treatments. The shelves in supermarkets groan under the weight of boxes, cans, and bags. Modern conveniences have reduced our need for physical labor. Computers give us up-to-date medical bulletins.

Despite these advances, and to some extent because of them, we've become fat, flabby, and frequently ill. We're too often hurried, harried, sleep-deprived, and socially disconnected. We eat in our cars, at our desks, in front of televisions—everywhere but at the dining room table in the company of others. We sit too much and move too little.

It turns out that health springs largely from old-fashioned behaviors—eating wholesome food, enjoying friends, relaxing, getting enough sleep, moving our bodies, and using natural remedies to heal.

The goal of this book is to help you get back to the basic lifestyle measures that point you toward a healthy, vibrant future.

In Part 1, we introduce six pillars of good health: a whole-foods diet, regular exercise, stress management, ample sleep, rich social connections, and spiritual health.

In Part 2, we provide lots of practical information on preventing and managing ailments. You'll find more than five hundred time-tested recipes and lifestyle tips—all designed to give you sometimes quick, always natural, ways to soothe a bee sting, eat for heart health, address that untimely cold, and help conquer those romance-killing bad breath microbes.

We hope you enjoy this book. May it enlighten you, guiding you along natural and simple paths to your healthy future.

Part

1

Building the Pillars of Good Health

Which factor do you think is most important in determining health and longevity?

A. Genetics

B. Medical care

C. Environmental factors and social circumstances

D. Personal behaviors (lifestyle)

Many people are surprised to learn the answer is D. Your lifestyle choices determine at least 40 percent of your health and longevity. Genetic predisposition contributes about 30 percent at best. Environmental factors (pollutants, toxins, and infectious agents) and social factors (social support, education, and income) account for 20 percent. Surprisingly, medical care determines a mere 10 percent.

We're not suggesting medical care is trivial and expendable—far from it. The message is that, to a large extent, you are the architect of your own health. That's great news.

Better still, most of those key personal behaviors are simple. Explorer Dan Buettner, author of the bestseller *The Blue Zones*, determined that several hotspots around the world harbor residents who consistently live to be one hundred years of age or more—and in vibrant good health. Their secret? Eat a traditional, whole-foods diet. Exercise daily. Get enough sleep. Manage stress. Enjoy friends and family. Engage in activities that

What everyone can have—no matter whether you're bothered by the occasional acute illness or are managing a condition—is **wellness**.

give your life meaning and purpose and that nurture your spirituality. Avoid tobacco in any form (including secondhand smoke); it's the number one preventable cause of death. Quitting is difficult, but well worth the sweat. Close rivals in premature death are inactivity and being overweight, two ills that are yoked together.

Is health the ultimate goal? We don't think so. No one is completely healthy all the time. You can pass your annual physical exam with flying colors, yet feel lonely and aimless.

What everyone can have—no matter whether you're bothered by the occasional acute illness or are managing a condition—is wellness. Wellness is not simply the absence of physical and mental illness. It includes feeling connected to other people, doing things you feel passionate about, feeling more joy than sorrow, and maintaining a sense of curiosity, wonder, and appreciation.

Wellness—and the elements that contribute to it—is nothing new. A key tenet is that the alchemy of the healthy body, mind, and spirit interact to produce our overall sense of wellness. Imbalance produces illness. Restoring balance allows the body to heal. This holistic approach to health has a long history. Ancient Greek physician Hippocrates practiced holistic medicine. Traditional healing practices around the world have used a holistic approach. Many of these concepts have been passed down from mothers and grandmothers to their children through the ages.

In a nutshell, there are six pillars of good health. They are as follows:

1. **Eat healing foods.**
2. **Move your body.**
3. **Manage stress.**
4. **Cherish sleep.**
5. **Go social.**
6. **Nourish your spirituality.**

The message is simple, though it often gets lost in the hustle and bustle of modern life. Don't worry: We've crafted the home remedies in this book to put them well within your grasp. Through its natural, time-tested home remedies, we hope this book will give you lots of ideas about positive lifestyle modifications. Remember that, though each new skill may seem modest, small changes add up to big results.

The First Pillar:
Eat Healing Foods

Although nutrition has become a science, you don't need a Ph.D. to know how to eat well. Ignore the ads on television urging you to buy processed food, designer beverages, or dietary supplements. None of them can replace a whole-foods diet, which both heals and promotes longevity. In this book, the simple, time-honored recipes show you how whole foods are also medicine.

What do we mean by "whole foods"? They're the things your great-grandparents recognized as food—fruits, vegetables, whole (unrefined) grains, nuts, seeds, meat, poultry, and seafood. Before the rise of the multibillion-dollar food industry, people instinctively ate food that provided all the needed nutrients. You could even trust toddlers to self-select a balanced diet. That was before the advent of processed foods.

Highly processed foods—edible items high in refined grains, added sugars and salt, and fat—pervert appetite. We're hardwired to seek out sweet, high-calorie foods. That predisposition once helped our species survive. However, the widespread availability of foods that were once rare treats has led us, as the English proverb goes, to dig our own graves with our teeth.

"Let food be thy **medicine** and thy medicine be food."

— HIPPOCRATES

Fast-food restaurants have ramped up our already busy lives. No time to cook? No problem. Just drive through and pick up a bag of greasy, inexpensive, high-calorie food. No time to sit at a dining room table? Gobble the burger and fries in your car, drop crumbles into your computer keyboard, or hunker down before the television and strap on a nosebag. Meantime, obesity rates have soared, along with its attendant chronic illnesses, such as heart disease and diabetes.

Recently, activists have taken a stand against what investigative journalist Eric Schlosser calls our "fast food nation." Take Slow Food, an international organization that raises consciousness about the personal and global impact of food choices, champions local food traditions, promotes sustainable agriculture, and advocates taking time to prepare and enjoy, ideally with friends, food that's both wholesome and aesthetically pleasing. Farmers' markets have made a comeback. Consumers increasingly support small, organic farmers, even though their food may cost more than the factory-produced fare at supermarkets. (Pay a little more now and you may pay less on future medical bills.)

Eating well is simple. Author Michael Pollan sums it up beautifully in his best-selling *In Defense of Food*, "Eat food. Not too much. Mostly plants." When he says "food," he means real, whole food, not what he calls "edible, food-like substances." If you stand by that mantra, you have a firm foundation for flourishing. Indeed, research indicates that plant-based diets, such as the traditional Mediterranean and Asian diets, decrease the risk of the chronic conditions so common in America today—obesity, heart disease, diabetes, some cancers, arthritis, and possibly Alzheimer's disease.

The Benefits of Plants

Edible plants promote our health for several reasons. For one, they provide sensory pleasures—colors, tastes, textures, and smells. For another, they're chock-full of macronutrients (protein, healthy fats, and carbohydrates, including fiber) and micronutrients (vitamins, minerals, and other beneficial chemicals). Many plant constituents are antioxidant and anti-inflammatory—properties that protect against many chronic illnesses. We'll get back to that theme in a minute.

We're not suggesting you become a vegetarian—unless you want to. We do, however, recommend you make plants the focus of each meal.

The recipes in this book guide you in that direction. Animal foods—red meat, pork, poultry, fish, eggs, and dairy—contain valuable nutrients, particularly proteins. But you don't need much of them. Most Americans meet or exceed recommended protein requirements. Plus, vegetarians consume plenty of protein from nuts, seeds, legumes, and whole grains.

No matter your philosophy about eating animals, what's important is the balance of plant to animal food. It's easy to shift from a meat-and-potatoes diet to a plant-based diet. Use your plate as a guide.

Rather than smother your plate with a steak, keep the meat the size of a pack of cards. Instead, cover half your plate with vegetables. The U.S. Department of Agriculture (USDA) recommends nine servings a day of fruits and vegetables—aim for about four servings of fruit and five of vegetables.

Whole grains can occupy one-quarter to one-third of your plate. You should get 25 grams, or two servings, of fiber a day. You don't need to measure. If you include plenty of whole grains, seeds, fruits, and vegetables in your diet, you'll consume enough. The fiber protects against heart disease, regulates blood sugar, prevents constipation, and may lower the risk of some cancers. You can also adopt the Asian pattern of chopping small portions of meat and poultry and blending it with all those vegetables. For more information on recommended servings of major food groups, visit the USDA's interactive website ChooseMyPlate.gov (www.choosemyplate.gov).

Speaking of plates, if you want to lose unhealthy pounds, try using smaller plates. That way you trick yourself into reasonable serving sizes. Research shows that people rely heavily on visual cues, mindlessly consuming everything they're served. Work that predilection to your advantage.

A Whole-Foods Guide

Many of the recipes in this book are whole-foods-centric. That means we rely on foods that are as close to their natural form as possible, with only minimal processing. Following are ways you can incorporate whole foods into your diet.

Become a savvy shopper. Work the grocery store's perimeter. Start in the produce section and stock up on vegetables and fruit. Buy nuts that are unsalted or low in salt. Next, select seafood and lean poultry and meat (organic, pasture-raised meat, if at all possible). If you eat dairy, that's your next stop. Keep cheese, which is high in fat, to a minimum.

With the exception of canned or dried legumes (peas, beans, lentils, and peanuts) and whole grains, stay out of the store's central aisles, which are where the processed foods are stocked. When selecting from the array of boxed and bagged items, scrutinize the food labels before adding them to your cart. If you see added sugar of any kind in the first three ingredients or hydrogenated (trans) fats, consider returning the item to the shelf.

When preparing foods, "simple" is the operative word. Sauté vegetables and sliced meat and poultry in a little olive oil. Add stock or water to keep the food moist. Bake meat. Avoid charbroiling, which creates cancer-causing substances. Pan-cook or poach fish. Dress salads lightly in olive oil and vinegar.

Make the switch to healthy snacks. Choose a baked sweet potato or sweet potato slices roasted in a little olive oil instead of a packet of French fries; grab a handful of almonds instead of a box of crackers; crunch on an apple rather than a candy bar. Smart choices can also help you regulate your weight.

Combating Oxidation and Inflammation with Food

You've probably heard of foods and supplements that contain antioxidants and anti-inflammatory substances. Foods and medicinal herbs rich in both these substances figure prominently in the book's recipes. They're important because oxidation and inflammation accelerate aging and underlie most chronic human diseases, including cardiovascular disease, diabetes, cancer, arthritis, cataracts, Parkinson's disease, and Alzheimer's disease.

The trouble starts with free radicals, which are atoms or groups of atoms with unpaired electrons. To stabilize themselves, free radicals steal electrons from other molecules, which can create a chain reaction of tissue-damaging electron raiding and what's called oxidative stress. Basically, the same process that turns apple slices brown and rusts iron occurs inside your body.

Normal cellular processes generate free radicals. Things that ramp up oxidative stress include infections, fever, high blood sugar (as happens in diabetes), extreme exercise, pollution, tobacco smoke, ultraviolet light, drugs, and consumption of unhealthy fats (trans fats and fats found in fried foods).

Oxidation also generates inflammation and vice versa. In the process of combating infection and injury, your immune system generates inflammation. Whereas acute inflammation is a normal and helpful response to injury and infection, chronic inflammation robs you of years and vitality.

To defend against oxidation and inflammation, your body makes antioxidants and anti-inflammatory substances. Antioxidant levels decline with age and may otherwise be insufficient to meet demands, particularly during illness.

To take up the slack, consume dietary antioxidants. Although animal food contains antioxidants, your richest sources are plants. To help them withstand the elements, plants make antioxidants, such as vitamins C and E, selenium, carotenoids, and flavonoids. Carotenoids and flavonoids double as plant pigments. You can easily recognize foods rich in them by their bright colors—blue, red, orange, yellow, and green. As long as you consume a variety of colorful plant foods, you'll receive a bounty of antioxidant and anti-inflammatory compounds. In this book, you'll find plenty of recipes whose ingredients include apricots, pumpkin, Brussels sprouts, papaya, strawberries, blueberries, carrots, red peppers, kale, and spinach, to name a few.

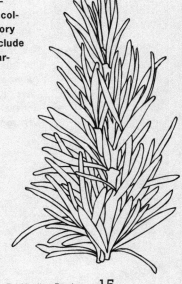

Good Fat Choices

Recipes in this book that use good fats will surprise and delight you in their deliciousness and healthful effects. Of all the macronutrients, fat is the most complicated. Carbohydrates and proteins are pretty straightforward. Favor the complex (unrefined) carbohydrates naturally present in fruits, vegetables, and whole grains. Eat animal foods, which are high in protein as well as fats, in moderation. Skip processed meats, such as bologna, ham, bacon, hot dogs, and deli meats. Among other additives, many preserved meats contain sodium nitrate and sodium nitrite, which increase the risk of cancer.

Fats, however, are another story. We've unfairly and categorically demonized them. Cookies, brownies, cakes, ice cream, and even granola boast labels proclaiming their low-fat or nonfat status. What many an unsuspecting dieter doesn't know, however, is that these foods are higher than ever in sugar, which is even worse for health, raising the risk for obesity, diabetes, and cardiovascular disease.

Although you don't need much in your diet, fats serve vital functions. They form your cell membranes, cushion your organs, insulate you from the cold, fill out the contours of your face, lubricate skin and hair, and help with absorption of fat-soluble vitamins (A, D, E, and K). Fats form much of your brain—a whopping 60 percent of that organ's dry weight. (Consider "fat head" a compliment.) Dietary fat also provides a sense of satiety, which is why adding a little olive oil to your salad greens satisfies appetite. That said, it helps to know which fats are good fats and how to use them.

Animal foods contain cholesterol and saturated fats. Despite the bad rap, cholesterol is vital to health. Your body makes plenty of it. If you consume cholesterol in your diet, your body compensates (to some extent) by making less. Saturated fats drive up levels of LDL (bad) cholesterol, which raises heart disease risk. Although they do increase HDL (good) cholesterol, it may not be a sufficient counterbalance. Limit your intake of saturated fat to 10 percent of daily calories. You can do that by buying low-fat or nonfat dairy, eating meat sparingly, and avoiding palm oil.

One fat to shun is trans fat. Although animal foods contain low amounts of trans fats, most of these dangerous fats in your diet are man-made through a process called hydrogenation, in which hydrogen atoms are added to polyunsaturated fatty acids. Hydrogenation increases the crispiness and shelf life of such products as crackers, chips, cakes, muffins, piecrusts, pizza dough, some breads (e.g., hamburger buns), popcorn, and cookies.

For several reasons, trans fats are disastrous for cardiovascular health. A mere 2 percent increase in calories from trans fats leads to a 23 percent increased risk of cardiovascular disease. Trans fats also increase inflammation and raise the risk of diabetes and cancer.

Note that the U.S. Food and Drug Administration (FDA) allows processed-foods manufacturers to label their products "trans-fat free" or "zero trans fats" if they contain less than 0.5 gram per serving. However, if you eat many processed foods, you may still exceed the 2-grams-a-day maximum recommended by the government. That's another reason to eat a whole-foods diet. Plus, if you shop for and prepare your food, you have a better idea what you're putting into your mouth.

So which fats should you chose? Unsaturated fats—monounsaturated and polyunsaturated—the kind that are found mainly in plants. These healthy fats fight LDL (bad) cholesterol and keep HDL (good) cholesterol levels high. And they add variety to your foods: canola, olive, sesame, and sunflower oils are a few examples. You'll find that our recipes in this book often tout unsaturated fats. We're particularly fond of heart-healthy olive oil (rich in monounsaturated fatty acids and other plant chemicals).

Fish and some plants contain omega-3 fatty acids, a type of polyunsaturated fatty acid that's anti-inflammatory and antioxidant. Plants particularly rich in the omega-3 fatty acid alpha-linoleic acid (ALA) include chia seeds, hemp seeds, sesame seeds (and therefore tahini and sesame seed oil), flaxseeds and flaxseed oil, canola oil, walnuts, purslane, edamame, and cruciferous vegetables, such as cauliflower, broccoli, and Brussels sprouts.

In very limited amounts, the body converts some of the ALA to other omega-3 fatty acids: eicosapentanoic acid (EPA) and docosahexaenoic acid (DHA). Because EPA and DHA are critical to health, especially nervous system health, many experts recommend eating rich sources such as fatty fish: for example, salmon, tuna, sardines, herring, and mackerel.

The omega 3s in fish lower triglyceride levels and blood pressure and also reduce the risk of clots forming within the arteries. EPA and DHA are essential for proper brain development. They may enhance cognitive function, reduce the risk of dementia (such as Alzheimer's disease), improve arthritis, and prevent and help manage depression and other mental health problems.

Hate fish? Don't worry. Our recipes provide you with plenty of vegetarian sources of the omega-3 fatty acid ALA.

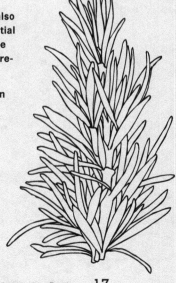

Sweet Alternatives

Sugar can foil any healthy diet. Americans consume about 22 teaspoons (about 90 grams) a day, adding a whopping 355 calories to their intake. These aren't the sugars that are found naturally in fruits, vegetables, and dairy products, but those that you add through sodas, cookies, and doughnuts. Eating too many sugars not only adds calories to your diet and crowds out nutritious foods, but it leads to unhealthy weight gain, diabetes, and heart disease. Many people seeking a heart-healthy diet don't realize that higher amounts of sugar and refined carbohydrates in the diet increase LDL cholesterol and triglycerides and decrease HDL cholesterol.

In limited amounts, sugar is fine. Save the sweet stuff for small servings of dessert. Eliminate from your diet sugar-sweetened beverages—sodas, sports drinks, energy drinks, coffee drinks, and most juices.

The recipes in this book show you how to enjoy the inherent sweetness in many whole foods and use natural sweeteners sparingly. For instance, we use honey, agave nectar, or stevia, a plant-based sweetener that has zero calories and is multiple times sweeter than table sugar (a pinch goes a long way). Feel free to try the recipe first without the sweetener and then add only as much as you need.

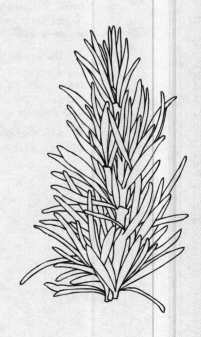

Organic Options

In 1961, Polyface Farm in central Virginia was bought by Joel Salatin in a run-down condition. Using his own version of TLC—natural practices, such as planting trees, building compost piles, and moving his animals to continually green pastures—he turned the farm into today's gold standard for organic, nonindustrial food production. Although his farm focuses on producing organic meats, he is an example for every farmer who produces environmentally enhanced meats, fruits, and vegetables. And he is dedicated to selling locally so that the foods, which are not chemical-laden, can be enjoyed fresh and whole, in surrounding counties.

Each recipe in this book will be even better for your lasting health if you use organic ingredients. What does that "certified organic" label mean? Organic crops are grown without the use of synthetic pesticides, fertilizers, sewage sludge, ionizing radiation, or genetic modifications; animals aren't fed nontherapeutic antibiotics and growth hormones.

How do you "go organic"? Read labels. You can also support local organic farmers who don't get the big government subsidies doled out to large operations. Frequent farmers' markets. Ask questions. Or read labels on foods at your grocery store. Request organic products at the store and in restaurants.

If you're on a tight budget, save your money for organic animal foods. Pesticides and other toxins concentrate in animal fat. If you have room in your heart, consider the conditions in which the animals were raised. Look for pastured, grass-fed beef, free-range chickens, and sustainably harvested fish. Your health, along with the health of animals and the environment, will benefit. For instance, compared to grain-fed beef, grass-fed beef is leaner and higher in omega-3 fatty acids.

If you have money left over for organic fruits and vegetables, check out the Dirty Dozen and Clean Fifteen charts, which list the most and least contaminated produce. The Environmental Working Group, in collaboration with the FDA and the USDA, created the list. You can use it as a buying companion.

The Dirty Dozen, in order of most contaminated:

1. Apples
2. Celery
3. Strawberries
4. Peaches
5. Spinach
6. Nectarines (imported)
7. Grapes (imported)
8. Sweet bell peppers
9. Potatoes
10. Blueberries (domestic)
11. Lettuce
12. Kale/collard greens

The Clean Fifteen, in order of least contaminated:

1. Onions
2. Corn
3. Pineapple
4. Avocadoes
5. Asparagus
6. Sweet peas
7. Mangoes
8. Eggplant
9. Cantaloupe
10. Kiwi
11. Cabbage
12. Watermelon
13. Sweet potatoes
14. Grapefruit
15. Mushrooms

We hope you can take time to appreciate the sensuality of purchasing (or growing), preparing, and consuming these foods. Savor the sights, textures, smells, and tastes. That mindful awareness will enhance the healing experience.

Chapter
2

The Second Pillar: Move Your Body

If there's a fountain of youth, it's exercise. The human genome evolved under conditions of high physical activity. We're designed to move. Inactivity signals our bodies that it's time to pack up the tents. Bones demineralize. Muscles atrophy. As a result, strength, endurance, and flexibility tank, and the risk of falls and bone fractures rises. Appetite is less keen, which may not reduce eating. Sleep is less satisfying. Mood deteriorates, and mental skills waver. Quality of life erodes. The risk of obesity and a number of chronic diseases rises.

On the other hand, regular physical activity increases longevity, and decreases the risk of many chronic illnesses, including the big killers in America: heart disease, stroke, cancer, and diabetes.

The benefits of regular exercise are so far-reaching that it's difficult to think of a bodily system that doesn't benefit. (The urinary system nearly qualifies, although the kidneys reap the benefits of increased circulation and certain exercises prevent bladder incontinence.) In the cardiovascular system, resting heart rate and blood pressure decline, LDL (lousy) cholesterol falls and HDL (good) cholesterol rises, and the delivery of fresh oxygen and nutrients becomes more efficient. Respiratory mucus clears. The immune system functions better. The bowels are more regular. Bones become denser. Joints are less likely to deteriorate. Muscles strengthen. Extra muscle mass raises metabolic rate, which burns more calories, which in turn fends off fat. Flexibility, endurance, strength, and agility reduce fall risk. Hormones, such as insulin, work more efficiently. Libido sashays. The nervous system sparkles, with enhancements in learning and memory.

Exercise relieves stress, improves sleep, and buoys mood. It lowers the likelihood of anxiety and depression and can augment conventional treatment of these conditions. Some research suggests exercise may reduce the risk of degenerative brain conditions, such as Alzheimer's disease and Parkinson's.

How much do you need and what types of exercise should you do? The most important activity is cardiorespiratory exercise, also called aerobic exercise. It engages several large muscle groups with enough vigor to make talking challenging but not impossible. Examples include brisk walking, jogging, swimming, cycling, skating, and cross-country skiing. The government recommends at least 150 minutes a week (30 minutes five days a week).

Resistance training involves loading muscles with more weight than they're accustomed to. You lift weights (jugs of water or milk work fine) or work against elastic bands or rubber tubes. Such exercise builds muscle and bone. Weight-bearing aerobic exercise (e.g., walking and jogging—no need to carry weights while you do so) also stimulates bone to deposit more minerals, which combats osteoporosis (brittle bones). The government recommends resistance training two times a week. Each time, work out all the major muscle groups—your arms, legs, shoulders, back, abdomen, and buttocks. (You can also work out fewer groups on any given day, as long as you get through the series twice.)

Flexibility training keeps you limber, making it possible to tie your own shoes and other useful skills. Stretch your joints through their full range of motion, two to three days a week. The older you get, the more you may welcome a series of stretches each morning. Throughout this book, we recommend a number of stretches to keep your joints warmed up and flexible.

We'd also like to dispel some basic myths:

1. *If you can't exercise for the recommended minimum of 30 minutes a day, you shouldn't bother.* No way. Get off the couch. You don't have to get the 30 minutes in one fell swoop. Ten-minute chunks will do. Some activity is better than none.

2. *Exercise must be intense for it to count.* Wrong. A brisk walk can be just as beneficial. In fact, running a marathon counts as a physical stressor.

3. *Exercise has to happen at a gym or on a court.* Nope. Raking leaves, pruning bushes, dusting, vacuuming, strolling, dancing, or skipping— any physical activity counts.

4. *Exercise will accelerate joint degeneration.* Au contraire. A recent study found that arthritis was more likely among sedentary folk and those who engaged in intense, prolonged workouts. Moderate exercisers protect their joints.

5. *If you already have arthritis, you should not exercise.* Actually, exercise helps maintain muscles that support joints and flexibility. People with severe arthritis should discuss exercise with their doctor. Physicians often recommend physical therapy.

6. *If you have heart disease, diabetes, asthma, etc., you should not exercise.* Wrong again. Physical activity improves most chronic conditions and overall quality of life. That said, medical clearance is recommended.

7. *If you want a flat stomach, you should do lots of crunches.* That statement is wrong for three reasons. For one, you need to become more physically active and modify your diet if you want to lose abdominal fat. Two, it's more important to tone your entire core (muscles in the trunk). (Simply holding a plank position—the top of a pushup—will strengthen the entire core.) Three, people with osteoporosis in their vertebrae or disk injuries shouldn't do crunches or sit-ups.

Many people have good intentions about physical activity, but don't follow through. That's why it helps to examine barriers. Common reasons for not exercising are fear of looking flabby in workout clothes, fatigue, lack of time, and concerns of physical discomfort. To all of that we say, "Nonsense." Other people are too self-absorbed to notice. You'll feel more energetic and sleep better afterward. Really? You don't have even 10 minutes? You're busier than the president? Start slow and build up. If it hurts, dial back. If it still hurts, talk to your doctor and consider working with a professional trainer.

You have many options for incorporating activity into your daily routine. When you travel, park farther from your destination; commute on a bike; take the bus and walk to your destination. At the airport, sidestep the people-moving conveyor belt and stroll. Whenever possible, take the stairs rather than the elevator. If you work at a desk, stop every 40 minutes to stretch, turn on some tunes and dance, or do a couple of pushups. Find an exercise buddy. Make social gatherings active: walk together, toss a ball or Frisbee, play Ping-Pong, or bowl.

The most important thing of all is to find activities you enjoy and look forward to doing. If you do, you'll soon find that you plan your day to include them and feel less vibrant when you can't.

You can find valuable resources on the Internet. For instance, the American College of Sports Medicine and the American Medical Association joined forces to create Exercise Is Medicine. Basically, the idea is that doctors should be prescribing exercise to their patients. The website, http://exerciseismedicine.org/public. htm, helps you to create an exercise routine and provides training videos. You can also find helpful information, including videos, on the Centers for Disease Control and Prevention website at www. cdc.gov/physicalactivity/everyone/guidelines/ adults.html.

Chapter
3

The Third Pillar: Manage Stress

Stress overload fuels most of diseases afflicting modern humans. Roughly one-third of American adults feel routinely overwhelmed by stress. Children and teens aren't immune. The authors of the American Psychological Association's 2011 *Stress in America* survey noted that "the nation is on the verge of a stress-induced public health crisis."

Before we go further, we need to define terms. The word stress has many connotations. Originally an engineering term, stress referred to the force applied to an object such that the object becomes deformed (squeezed, stretched, or bent). Researcher Hans Selye applied that term to human stress. A stressor is anything that activates a person's stress response. Selye's research showed that, regardless of the nature of the stressor (excessive heat, cold, pain, physical exhaustion, or social upheaval), organisms responded in a fairly predictable fashion.

During the stress response, the autonomic (mainly automatic and involuntary) nervous system shifts from the parasympathetic nervous system (rest and digest) to the sympathetic nervous system (fight or flight). As a result, respiratory rate, heart rate, blood pressure, and blood sugar rise. The pupils of the eyes dilate. Senses sharpen. The mouth dries. Skin becomes paler and cooler. Blood flow diminishes to nonessential organ systems (reproductive, urinary, and gastrointestinal). The goal is to deliver sugar and oxygen to organs critical for survival: the brain, heart, and skeletal muscles. When acutely stressed, you think and move quickly.

One of the sympathetic nervous system's tasks is to release epinephrine (adrenaline) from the adrenal gland. That happens swiftly. After a delay, a hormone from the brain's pituitary gland reaches the adrenal gland, triggering the release of cortisol. Cortisol's main job is to keep blood sugar high (even if it means dismantling carbohydrate, fat, and protein stores). It also reduces inflammation and regulates the immune system. This hormone lingers longer in the system than epinephrine does.

Our stress response has survival advantages. Because our ancestors faced mainly physical stressors, the stress response was beautifully designed to help us perform impressive physical feats—fight, flee, and endure famines.

While we continue to face physical challenges, many of our modern stressors are psychological. If you're stuck in traffic, it does you no good—in fact, it can do much harm—to mount a stress response.

Worse, humans, unlike other animals, don't always live in the moment. Our big brains are capable of rumination (mulling over past events) and anticipation. We relive past failures and embarrassments and fret over events in the distant future. Once you've learned from past events, let them go. Planning and preparation have merits. We save for a rainy day, study for exams, and prepare for meetings. Worrying, especially about things you have no control over, is useless and corrodes well-being.

We often reward a harried, overworked lifestyle and regard the low-grade, chronic stress that comes with it as normal, even admirable.

The truth is, however, that chronic stress overload can shorten your life and ruin your health. It strains every organ system, contributing to many diseases and aggravating others. It reveals the vulnerabilities to diseases. (Stress finds your Achilles' heel.) Coping with stress in maladaptive ways, such as skipping meals, abusing alcohol, and becoming a workaholic, accelerates the downward spiral.

Here's an incomplete list of the potential downsides of chronic stress:

- increased appetite (more people overeat than undereat when stressed), with a tendency to select sugary, fatty food

- weight gain (preferential deposition of fat in the abdomen, which raises the risk of a number of diseases)

- increased inflammation

- depressed immune function (often manifesting as more colds and faster progression of HIV infection)

- insomnia (which further drives up stress hormones)

- irritability, moodiness, and, eventually, apathy

- impaired learning, concentration, and memory

- increased sensitivity to pain

- fatigue

- dampened libido (sex drive), impaired erectile function, lower sperm counts, and irregular menstrual cycles

- increased risk or aggravation of chronic diseases

- high blood pressure

- heart disease

- diabetes

- metabolic syndrome (a constellation of signs indicating risk for cardiovascular disease and diabetes)

- peptic ulcers (stress contributes but doesn't directly cause them)

- irritable bowel syndrome

- gastroesophageal reflux disease (heartburn)

- anxiety

- depression

- allergic and autoimmune condition (stress contributes to inappropriate immune system responses)

The point is not to avoid stress altogether. One, it's impossible. Two, a bland, uneventful life would be boring, which isn't good for your health, either. Three, some stressors are fabulous—landing a great job, getting married, or traveling to foreign lands.

Identify the "bad" stressors in your life. Common examples include job instability, financial insecurity, concerns about personal safety, witnessing or experiencing violence, dysfunctional interpersonal relationships, taking care of chronically ill family members, social isolation, loss of a loved one, and severe injury or illness. Less recognized stressors include excessive noise, lack of exposure to sunlight and open spaces, pollution, sleep deprivation, insufficient time for relaxation, sedentary lifestyle, junk-food diets, information overload, and "technostress" (becoming a slave to your electronic devices).

Your next step depends upon the nature of the stressor. If it's odious and you can eliminate it, do so. That may mean curtailing relationships that only make you unhappy. Others can't be easily eliminated or avoided.

However, you can always change your attitude. For instance, losing your job can be devastating. But it also opens the door for new opportunities. There are people who've had to sell their cars to make ends meet—only to feel surprisingly liberated by that loss (and lose weight and gain muscle after cycling to work or school). Some have gone into entirely new professions and discovered new passions.

Here's an interesting fact about how the brain responds to a potential threat. Information from the senses quickly alerts primitive brain centers. Those brain centers kick-start the sympathetic nervous system. But then loftier brain centers (the prefrontal cortex) have a chance to evaluate the situation. Take advantage of that. Ask yourself, "Is this situation a serious threat to my health and well-being?"

Let's go back to the traffic jam. Maybe you're going to be late to an important meeting. That's not good. Maybe next time you need to leave earlier (learning opportunity). Will the sluggish movement of cars physically harm you? Probably not—unless you start darting in and out of lanes, honking, and angering other motorists. What can you do to soothe yourself? Maybe (if it's safe to do so), you phone to say you'll be late. Perhaps you turn on relaxing music or an audio book. You take some slow, deep breaths. You tell yourself, "All is well." You wave and smile at motorists. You might even start a chain reaction of goodwill.

Changing the way you think about a situation is what psychologists call "cognitive reframing." It's a powerful tool. View change as interesting challenges and opportunities for personal growth. Notice how you're getting stronger and wiser because of them. As Winston Churchill said, "Kites rise highest against the wind, not with it."

Spend more time in the present moment. Usually any given moment isn't that bad, though our predictions of doom and gloom make it so. If you pay close attention, you may become aware of how many things are beautiful and amazing—right now. Ask yourself what's great about your life. Of course, some moments contain pain and sorrow. But they don't go on forever. It's when we worry that life seems worse than it actually is. We lose sight of our blessings.

In Part 2, we'll discuss remedies for stress overload. In addition, here are some tips for restoring your equanimity right now.

• Make a list of what's going right.

• Write down three sources of stress you're able and willing to change.

• Identify ways you have reasonable control over those situations. If the commute to work makes you feel hassled, would you feel more relaxed on public transportation? What if you left earlier or later? Can you work at home some days?

• Check in with your thoughts. Are they contributing needlessly to your sense of stress? How can you put a positive, but realistic, spin on them? If the inner chatter sounds like, "I'm so stressed. I can't handle this. I'm freaking out," stop. Try, "I have a lot to do. It will take time, but I can do it. Right now, I'm going to do this one task."

• Exercise every day. Physical activity is a great way to let off steam. Solutions that eluded you at work or home may suddenly become clear.

• Learn to say no. For some of us that's not easy. You may need to figure out why you feel so responsible. Give someone else a chance to rise to the occasion.

• Schedule time to unwind and to play. That's not the same as television time. Learn to relax and enjoy yourself. You'll be a better person for it.

- Sleep eight hours a night. If you don't, you'll add to your stress load. See the next chapter for tips.

- Treat yourself. Get a massage, practice yoga, take a dance class, and soak in a hot tub. If co-workers, friends, or others try to schedule things during those times, tell them you have an appointment.

- Get enough sleep. Sleep deprivation activates the stress response.

- Eat a whole-foods diet. Junk food activates the stress response. Take time to leisurely prepare and savor a meal. Put flowers on the dinner table. Notice how much better this approach feels than gobbling a sandwich in the car or at your desk.

- Seek social support. Hug someone. When you do, you release an antistress, bonding hormone called oxytocin.

- Spend time in nature. You needn't drive to a national park. City gardens and parks do just fine. Put a plant on your desk. Watch trees, birds, and squirrels outside your window. Gaze at the stars. Jump in a pile of leaves. Make a snow angel. Natural environments reduce stress and enhance overall well-being. Ready access to green spaces can buffer the negative health effects of stressful life events.

- Pet a friendly animal. Science shows it reduces stress.

- Manipulate your senses. Soften the lighting. Listen to soothing music. Wear fabrics that comfort you. Surround yourself with peaceful colors—green, blue, and pink. Infuse the air with calming plant essential oils (lavender, orange, jasmine, or any other scent that makes you feel relaxed and happy).

- Learn to meditate. Try mindfulness meditation (paying attention to the present moment) and recitation of a mantra (a repeated sound). Numerous studies show that regular meditation reduces perceptions of stress, decreases stress hormones, reduces the risk of many stress-related diseases, and helps people become less reactive to potential stressors. You'll find short meditation exercises throughout the book.

- Breathe. Slow, deep breathing immediately turns up your parasympathetic nervous system and dials down the sympathetic nervous system. Even though the autonomic nervous system is also called the involuntary nervous system, you do have some control over it.

- Stay optimistic. Believe that things will improve. Make that possible.

Chapter

4

The Fourth Pillar: Cherish Sleep

Sleep is mysterious. Scientists don't fully understand why all animals must sleep, despite the inherent vulnerability of the act. You're never fully aware of the moment your brain shuts off. And, to a certain extent, you can't control the process. If you're exhausted, you may fall asleep at inconvenient and even dangerous moments, such as when driving—despite your best efforts to remain alert. Perversely, you may have trouble sleeping when you most desire it.

We do know that sleep is vital to health. Unfortunately, many Americans are chronically sleep-deprived. The National Sleep Foundation's 2011 Sleep in America Poll revealed that 43 percent of Americans aged thirteen to sixty-four rarely or never got enough sleep on week-days. Even infants and children don't get enough sleep.

Most people don't recognize the potential adverse effects on personal health and public safety. They struggle through the day, unaware that sleeping more might erase their persistent fatigue and malaise. It doesn't help that relatively few doctors ask their patients about the quality and quantity of their sleep.

Many people also cling to the myth that they can train themselves to get by on less sleep or to work at night and sleep by day. Not so. The brain tightly orchestrates our sleep-wake cycle, as well as other daily, or circadian, rhythms. Humans are diurnal. Light syncs our nervous and hormonal systems. Few of us can fully adapt to working the night shift.

After you lie down at night, your brain repeatedly cycles through five stages. Stages 1 through 4 take you from the lightest to deepest and most restorative sleep. Your most vivid dreams occur during rapid eye movement (REM) sleep, during which time your brain is active and your skeletal muscles are paralyzed to prevent you from acting out your dreams. Although the cycle repeats about every 90 minutes, you have more deep sleep earlier in the night and more REM toward the morning.

Age affects the architecture of sleep stages. Compared to young adults, elders have relatively less stage 3 and 4 and REM sleep. That leaves more stage 1 and 2, from which you're more easily awakened. Also, circadian rhythms shift. Teens and young adults don't feel sleepy until later at night. Elders become larks, falling asleep earlier in the night and awakening early in the morning.

Now for the most important point: Like a banker counting coins, your brain keeps track of how much you sleep. Children need 10 hours of sleep a night. Teens and young adults need 8.5 to 9.5 hours. Most adults feel rested after 8 hours, though the exact need varies. If you instead limp along on 7 hours a night, by week's end your brain has totaled 7 hours of sleep debt. You feel as though you missed an entire night's sleep.

How do you know if you're getting enough sleep? You awaken feeling refreshed. A good time to figure out your sleep needs is on a relaxing vacation—one without schedules and alarm clocks. The first few nights, you may sleep a lot as you catch up on missed sleep. After that, you should fall into a rhythm.

The perils of sleep deprivation are serious and include the following:

- excessive daytime sleepiness (your main warning sign you're not getting enough sleep)

- impaired mental function—spotty attention, concentration, memory, and alertness

- impaired physical function—clumsiness, diminished reaction times, and diminished agility

- accidents—due to impaired mental and physical function and falling asleep during a task (about 5 percent of Americans doze off while driving each month)

- inability to deal with stress and a sleep-deprivation-induced rise in stress hormones

- more pain, including tension headaches

- more inflammation, which can aggravate inflammatory conditions, such as asthma and arthritis

- flagging social skills

- irritability

- increased risk of work burnout, depression, and anxiety

- reduced alcohol tolerance (plus, sleep deprivation can impair your skills on par with alcohol intoxication)

- weight gain (due to hormonal shifts and changes in behavior)

- poor blood sugar control; increased risk of diabetes and cardiovascular disease

- diminished quality of life

What can you do to feel more rested? Make sure you allow plenty of time to sleep. Keep in mind that it often takes 15 to 30 minutes to fall asleep. If you need 8 hours of sleep to feel good, allow yourself at least 8.5 hours in bed. Otherwise adopt what's known as good "sleep hygiene." This sort of housekeeping entails the following practices:

- Establish regular hours to go to bed and wake up—seven days a week.

- Keep naptimes short (no more than 30 minutes) and limit them to once a day.

- Exercise daily, but avoid vigorous late-night exercise (stretching is fine).

- Eat a light dinner, but consider a bedtime snack if you notice low blood sugar jolts you awake in the night.

- Avoid excessive amounts of alcohol and stop drinking entirely within a few hours of bedtime. (Alcohol may make it easier to fall asleep, but disrupts sleep later in the night.)

- Skip caffeine in the late afternoon and evening. (It takes an average of five hours to clear half of the caffeine from the blood.)

- Nix the nicotine. (It's a central nervous system stimulant.)

- Use your bed only for sleep and sex (no working, bill-paying, or arguing).

- Create a cozy sleep environment—quiet room, comfortable mattress, good pillows, enough covers to keep you warm but not sweaty, shades to block street lights and dark cloths over digital clocks, charging electronic devices, LED lights.

- Establish a soothing bedtime routine (a warm bath, candlelight, music, pleasure reading, stretching, breathing exercises, meditation, or prayer).

If you feel irresistibly sleepy during the day, close your eyes. Research shows that power naps improve productivity. If you can't, exercise briefly. A brisk walk outdoors can temporarily refresh you. Inhale a plant essential oil that's associated with brain alertness, such as peppermint, eucalyptus, lemon, or rosemary. Caffeine definitely increases alertness. Choose beverages that naturally contain caffeine (green tea, black tea, or coffee), rather than sodas or energy drinks. To avoid insomnia, resist consuming them in the late afternoon or evening (and also refrain from adding sugar to them). (More sensitive people have to curtail caffeine intake after lunch.) We'll cover insomnia in Part 2.

If you become drowsy while driving, get off the road. Drowsiness is the last sign that your brain is poised to switch into sleep mode. Take a nap. Chewing gum, opening the window, and turning up the radio will not keep you awake. Caffeine takes about 30 minutes to kick in. Nodding off for a second is all it takes to cause a serious accident.

If you routinely suffer from persistent daytime sleepiness or have any concerns about the quality or quantity of your sleep, make an appointment with your doctor.

You may need to spend a night in a sleep clinic to determine whether you have a sleep disorder, such as sleepwalking, periodic limb movement disorder (recurrent, rhythmic jerking of the limbs during sleep), restless legs syndrome (unpleasant sensations in the limbs temporarily relieved by movement), narcolepsy (poor nighttime sleep with daytime sleep attacks), or obstructive sleep apnea (repeated episodes of snoring and breath-holding). Obstructive sleep apnea, which is a potentially life-threatening condition, has become increasingly common, affecting about 4 percent of Americans. The good news is that treatments exist for all these conditions.

The Fifth Pillar: Go Social

At the Institute for Integrative Nutrition, a school devoted to holistic nutrition, director Joshua Rosenthal holds that the key to health lies in balancing primary and secondary foods. Primary foods, he says—the foods you must have to thrive—are not the healthy vegetables, grains, and protein that you put on your plate. Those are secondary. Primary for healthy and long life are relationships and love, physical activity, spirituality, and love of the work you do each day. These are the key to joy; and joyful people thrive. Without these elements, all the broccoli, apples, and spirulina in the world won't matter.

Friendship Is Golden. There is nothing like a friend, with whom you can share confidences, grow in depth, and remain connected for years.

On the other hand, feeling socially disconnected takes a serious toll on health. Socially isolated people tend to cope poorly with stress and have higher blood pressure in response to daily hassles. They do not sleep as well and exhibit slower wound healing. Loneliness raises vulnerability to mental illness, substance abuse, eating disorders, and premature death. It also worsens physical health and elevates the risk for heart attack, stroke, cancer, and diabetes.

In contrast, people with bounteous social support enjoy buffers against minor illnesses, such as the common cold, as well as major diseases, such as heart disease, depression, and dementia. And serious conditions, such as HIV and cancer, often have better outcomes. Recovery from alcohol and other addictions improves with social and emotional support from such groups as Alcoholics or Narcotics Anonymous. In a 2012 study, researchers polled people from 142 countries and found that high levels of social support and social trust (having someone you can count on) increased life satisfaction, heightened positive feelings, and reduced negative emotions.

A huge benefit of friendships is that they give you positive emotional support in times of stress or a lifeline during crisis. For years, the stress response was characterized by fight-or-flight behavior. In 2000, Shelley Taylor, Ph.D., and colleagues at the University of California, Los Angeles published a paper proposing that, when stressed, women are more likely to "tend and befriend," thus activating oxytocin, also called the "bonding hormone." Perhaps she noticed that if her latest experiment hit a roadblock, she'd go to her friend's office for a hug and a chat and feel the better for it. There's some evolutionary sense to that dichotomy. In the face of a physical threat, the men fought and the women rounded up and guarded the children.

Here theory holds true. Intimate relationships increase oxytocin, which, in turn, reinforces social attachments and increases empathy and feelings of trust. This hormone also decreases depression and anxiety, counteracts aggression and the stress response, decreases pain sensation, reduces inflammation, and favorably alters heart rate. No wonder infants fail to thrive without tender loving care. Our interactions with adoring animals offer similar benefits.

There are other reasons why close relationships benefit us. Positive social interactions can release natural pain relievers such as endorphins, those chemicals famed for creating the runner's high, and dopamine, a brain chemical involved in the pleasure-reward system. Furthermore, good friends look out for us, bring us food when we're ill, comfort us when we're sad, and confront us if we've strayed into unhealthy lifestyles.

FRIENDSHIP: (fren[d]-ship). The emotion or conduct of friends; the state of being friends.

— MERRIAM-WEBSTER

Avoid Cyber-seclusion

In this cyber-centric world we share, it is easy to live in isolation. People are glued to television screens and cell phones; they wear headphones delivering nonstop music and tune out the world as they walk, drive, and pursue daunting workdays. It is easier to send a text message than to pick up the phone and hear a human voice. Even though electronic communications are supposed to connect us, frequent users can paradoxically end up feeling lonelier and more at risk for depression.

Sadly, a close-knit extended family in America is rare, and young people move halfway across the world to pursue exciting careers. Others are on the go, living in airports and hotels, rarely seeing their families for dinner or reading to their children at bedtime.

Many of the remedies in this book remind you to stop and renew your connections with others. Social connection is a powerful healing source: instilling hope, bringing relaxation, giving inspiration, and underscoring your self-worth as a human being.

When you trust a friend or other loved one, you feel safe to let down your guard and be yourself. True friends support your commitment to growing in a healthy lifestyle. On the other hand, it's natural to seek alone time, and to thrive on it. For some, energy comes from solitude; then they go forth and conquer the world.

In this book, we provide remedies to suit any personality type. You may be an introvert, whose renewal comes from being alone, writing in a journal or meditating, rather than spending time with a close friend. You may be an extrovert, constantly on the go and in touch with a wide circle of friends and acquaintances; your nourishment comes from being around people and sharing their spheres and energies.

Knowing which you are will help you find the right balance of social interaction and seek the circle of friends who bring you support and add purpose and depth to your life. Appreciate who you are and build around it.

There is nothing like a good friend who is always there with a willing ear and the right words. That person "gets you." Here are a few tips on friendship:

- Seek friends who reflect your lifestyle and passion for healthy living and whose habits and goals you admire. If you are a vegetarian who loves yoga and meditation, your best match is likely not a party person who drinks and smokes. At the same time, stay open to meeting new people whose company you find stimulating whether or not you share all the same values.

- Welcome change. You may be holding on to friends who have not evolved as you have. That's okay. Take time to reassess and think about what that friendship means to you. Are you enriching one another's lives, or are you the only one who truly gives? If it's the latter, find a way to gradually move away and fill that empty space with those who will bring a healthy, meaningful synergy.

- Take a chance. You've probably heard of the dating service It's Just Lunch. Singles meet their potential Mr. or Ms. Right by spending about an hour together over a midday meal. You can do the same thing to jump-start a new friendship. Is there an acquaintance you want to know better? Invite that person to lunch or coffee. An hour of connection could lead to a long relationship of talk and trust. If the person says no, or if you discover there's no connection, just chalk it up to experience. Your desire to make new friends will lead you to other new and meaningful opportunities.

- Give back. This can be through invitations for a bike ride or dinner at your home. It can be simply through listening. Becoming a good listener is one of the highest respects you can pay a person; and it is a way that you can help a friend through crises large and small. Give your full attention. While the other person speaks, hold your tongue, except to offer occasional verbal cues. You'll be surprised how you can help people solve their own problems by speaking only a few phrases. You'll be praised for your powers as a conversationalist!

- In his book *The Blue Zones*, Dan Buettner steps into the life of Seventh Day Adventists in Loma Linda, California—where many seniors thrive into their hundreds. One octogenarian noted that whenever she feels down, giving back becomes a priority. Going out to help someone else gives her a sense of purpose and makes all the difference in her attitude. Try it: You'll see the infectious power of giving to others.

- Keep a secret: Learn the power of keeping confidences. Building trust is the key to long-standing relationships of any kind. A friend offers you heart and soul in an unwritten pact and expects you to keep him or her safe. You do the same. Remember the Golden Rule: Do unto others as you'd have them do unto you.

- Be there: Whether your pal is stressing out over a wretched work day or family crisis, make time. You are one another's lifeline. Take that job seriously.

A family can be the one you're born with or one you create with a new mate or a circle of dedicated friends. In the five thriving communities he studies in *The Blue Zones*, Dan Buettner notes that each one puts family first. In Ikaria, Greece, and Sardinia, Italy, they enjoy traditional, big-dinner family gatherings. In Okinawa, the *moai*, or circle of long-standing friends, becomes a family. They meet almost daily, and their closeness, support, and contentment may account for so many thriving centenarians on the island. In a *moai*, someone is always there to step in, for reasons ranging from sadness to financial crisis.

"Home is the place where, when you have to go there, they have to take you in," wrote poet Robert Frost. The confidence of deep friendships and family connections has this immediate benefit: There is always someone to open the door. But the lasting benefits are what really reveal the truth. Studies show that such meaningful connections provide an ongoing lifeline that guards us against heart disease, depression, and dementia, among other ailments.

The Healing Power of Touch

Touch is the key to socialization. Babies who are hugged, bounced, and cuddled grow into more adaptable human beings than those who are not. Studies show that they tend to grow up secure and loved, better poised to form healthy relationships later in life. Gentle massage helps premature babies in neonatal intensive care units gain weight more readily and gives babies withdrawing from the drugs of an addicted mother a greater chance of survival and a healthy future.

Throughout life, touch is central to the primary food experience touted by the Institute for Integrative Nutrition. You may come home after a trying day at work or a bad date and want to run to the refrigerator to grab a box of ice cream or a cold beer. If a hug from a loved one intercepts you on the way, you may be less likely to go for the unhealthy response and more likely to feel better.

Enduring intimate relationships derail unhappiness, heal on deep levels, and build a platform for security and joy. Person-to-person massage is an easy and long-lasting way to connect. Ask a friend or family member to rub your neck for just 5 minutes. Offer to do the same. The sense of well-being will linger.

Deeper professional massage can have multiple benefits. It improves local blood circulation, relieves pain, eases stress, and boosts oxytocin and endorphins.

Mirth Has Worth

At the end of the day, laughter between friends just may be the best medicine. Author Barbara Brownell Grogan's large and spontaneous family devoured the popular "Laughter Is the Best Medicine" column in the monthly *Reader's Digest* and even sent in a few of their own anecdotes. Laughter connected them as a family, and today they have only to say a phrase or give a certain cross-eyed look to send one another into peals of healing, love-building laughter.

Laughter is fun and infectious—and it goes deeper than a moment's release. Scientific evidence for its healing effects is gaining ground. Doctors actually use the term "laughter therapy." Humor relaxes people, lifts mood, promotes overall well-being, aids in coping with stress, and actually reduces stress hormones. Laughter benefits the immune system, improves some measures of heart function, and reduces pain perception. The benefits of 1 minute of laughter have been compared to 10 minutes on the rowing machine.

During Barbara's integrative nutrition studies, she and co-students were directed in one lecture to let down their guard and laugh. At the beginning it was forced and tentative; pretty soon the guffaws and belly laughs were authentic and hard to stop. And everyone felt better for it.

Psychologist and laugh therapist Steve Wilson notes that laughter and exercise have similar effects. He recommends laughing and waving your arms as just one effective way to ramp up your heart rate.

What we do know is that laughing together builds vital social connections. And those social connections lead us all to thrive.

Chapter
6

The Sixth Pillar:
Nourish Your Spirituality

Through the ages, humans have engaged in spiritual practices. Worldwide, traditional healers have treated body, mind, and spirit to restore health. They prescribed yoga, qigong, meditation, limpias (cleansings), sweats, fasting, chanting, and singing. Although modern Western medicine focuses on the physical body, researchers have begun investigating the health effects of religious and spiritual practices.

In fact, some scientists believe our brains are hardwired for religion and spirituality. It seems that yearning for transcendence is human nature.

Before we go further, let's define *spirituality* and *religion*. The two differ but intertwine. Spirituality involves having an inner path for personal growth, self-discovery, and an interest beyond the material. It's a personalized belief that need not involve higher powers.

Religion, on the other hand, usually represents an organized belief system. Rituals and sermons glorify deities and establish cultural traditions that take place around holidays, births, deaths, and other important events. Most religions incorporate spiritual practices, such as prayer, meditation, and contemplation.

Participation in organized religion has some documented health benefits. Clearly defined moral values can reduce risky behaviors. For instance, religious people are less likely to succumb to addictions, depression, anxiety, and suicide. On the other hand, religious dogma can also create guilt and inner conflict. Religions that embrace individual differences, promote kindness and compassion, and encourage members to care for the sick and needy do much good for public health. Those that teach intolerance can ultimately do harm.

Participation in religious services and spiritual practices can provide a sense of community, which contributes to social health. Both give people a sense of meaning and purpose. Spiritual practices such as prayer and meditation relieve stress. Faith can promote optimism and resilience in the face of hardship.

At this point, we're going to focus on spirituality. It's available to everyone—from the atheist to the devoutly religious. You don't need to move to a cave, meditate and fast, study philosophy, become a Buddhist, work with a shaman, or wear a hair shirt. Small acts can nourish your spirit. Simply paying attention to the here and now can fill you with wonder and gratitude. According to the Dalai Lama, "There is no need for temples; no need for complicated philosophy. Our own brain, our own heart is our temple; the philosophy is kindness."

The challenge is remaining open to appreciation when distractions cram our daily lives. We dash from one event to the next and struggle to stay afloat on a torrent of e-mails, phone calls, and texts. In the face of nearly instantaneous communications, we feel obligated to respond quickly and immediately. Boundaries between work and home blur. Too often, we mistakenly equate multitasking and overwork with success. The mental chatter interferes with relaxation, sleep, attentive social interactions, and quiet contemplation.

Despite our modern conveniences, many of us feel short on time and leisure, long on worry, and overwhelmed by all the challenges we face. We become stressed, disconnected, and ill.

Can spirituality help to restore balance to our lives? Yes. Some forward-thinking doctors have provided scientific proof of that. Meditation, a practice that trains and quiets the mind, is an area of hot research. After studying Zen Buddhism, Jon Kabat-Zinn, Ph.D., founded the Center for Mindfulness in Medicine, Health Care, and Society, as well as the Stress Reduction Clinic, at the University of Massachusetts Medical School. His stress-reduction program teaches mindfulness meditation. Mindfulness involves purposeful attention to and acceptance of the present moment. It sounds deceptively simple. Most Westerners need lots of practice. Throughout the book, you'll find mindfulness exercises.

Does mindfulness help? Absolutely. Multiple studies show that mindfulness meditation reduces stress, emotional reactivity, anxiety, depression, pain, and inflammation. It helps chronically ill people cope and improves mood and quality of life. It's even been successfully incorporated into the treatment of eating disorders.

Scientists have also amassed research support for Transcendental Meditation (TM). TM is a type of mantra meditation, which means you sit quietly while repeating a mantra, a sound, syllable, word, or phrase. TM teachers give students individual mantras and instruct them to sit while repeating the mantra for 15 to 20 minutes morning and evening. Studies show that TM reduces stress, blood pressure, and symptoms of angina pectoris (chest discomfort due to coronary artery disease). It also helps people kick alcohol and tobacco habits. Several types of meditation seem to improve attention and also increase the thickness of the brain's gray matter.

The ancient Indian practice of yoga also has astounding health benefits. Although there are many types of yoga, Western practices typically include a combination of asanas (physical poses), pranaymas (breathing techniques), and meditation. In that way, yoga addresses body, mind, and spirit. It increases relaxation, muscle strength, and flexibility. It reduces blood pressure, blood levels of sugar and cholesterol, and body weight. It decreases pain and improves function in arthritis. Mood improves and anxiety diminishes.

Another meditation style is called loving-kindness meditation. Loving kindness forms the cornerstone of many world religions. The focus shifts from the self to the safety, peace, health, and well-being of others. A 2012 British study showed that this kind of nonverbal style of a physician toward his or her patient has biological effects. The volunteers had no idea of the doctors' intent. In fact, for part of the experiment, the doctors appeared to be reading. Practitioners and volunteers wore heart monitors. Heart rates declined in both groups when doctors silently meditated on loving kindness. Volunteers reported feeling more relaxed and peaceful.

Tai chi and qigong (pronounced *chee gung*) are two ancient Chinese moving meditations. *Qi*, or *chi*, roughly translates to "the animating life force." In theory, blocks or imbalances in qi produce disease. Traditional Chinese medicine uses tai chi, qigong, acupuncture, and other techniques to restore qi. Tai chi evolved from the martial arts, though the practice is fluid and nonviolent. In qigong, slow and rhythmic movements flow with the breath. Both practices help people maintain balance, strength, flexibility, and agility into old age. Tai chi reduces stress and pain and improves function in arthritis. It's been used to restore physical function and improve quality of life in people with Parkinson's disease and those who've suffered a stroke. Qigong has been shown to help manage high blood pressure and diabetes, improve asthma, and reduce side effects of cancer treatment.

So far, these therapies require a certain level of training and commitment. However, even simpler behaviors nourish the spirit. A sense of appreciation for blessings small and large is one. Repeated studies have shown that gratitude engenders positive emotions and decreases symptoms of depression. In one study, researchers instructed three groups of college students to keep a journal for ten weeks. Each day, group one described five things that made them feel grateful. Group two noted five hassles. Group three listed any five events of their choosing. The results: Gratitude led to significant increases in optimism, well-being, and physical activity. The gratitude group also experienced fewer illnesses.

Counting your blessings is a great way to end your day. If you express your thanks, you'll double the benefits—making you and the recipients of your appreciation feel better. Write thank-you notes (or at least send electronic thanks). Leave notes of appreciation under the pillows of family members. Acknowledging your colleagues' work fosters collegiality. Reward even the smallest acts of kindness. If someone holds the door for you, say thank you. Thank the people who cook and serve your food. Notice their response. Notice how you feel.

Reciprocity also feeds your spirit. Give. Small acts of kindness and compassion can float your spiritual boat as effectively as grand ones. As ancient philosopher and author of the *Tao Te Ching*, Lao-tzu, wrote, "Great acts are made up of small deeds." Let someone on the bus before you. Honor a friend's birthday in a thoughtful, personal way. Buy a coffee for the person behind you in line. Pop a quarter in an expiring parking meter.

Service can also express spirit in modest ways: taking up an elderly neighbor's trash bins or raking her leaves, bringing soup to a sick friend, listening to a friend or co-worker who's sad, planting a tree, or volunteering to help clean up a storm-stricken neighborhood. All these acts express and sustain the spiritual you.

We believe that all of the other elements of health discussed in this chapter have a relationship to spirituality. Take nutrition. Spirituality enters when you grow your own vegetables, fruits, and herbs. The farmers' market engages all your senses. You might hear live music and the banter of local farmers, smell roasting chile peppers and sweet apples, see tables overflowing with fresh produce and flowers, or sample local cheese. If you take time to prepare, savor, and share meals from whole foods, the sensory experience can make you downright giddy with joy.

We already discussed the merits of physical activity for physical and mental health. Any sport you play goes better when you're in the present moment, or as athletes say, the flow. Take that activity outside and—voilà—you're connecting with nature. If you're aware and appreciative of those natural surroundings, you might experience an elevation of your spirits.

Spirituality is all about connection—connection with self, others (including animals), nature, and the great unknown. Our intimate social relationships speed our personal growth because of that sublime opportunity to connect, give and receive, and practice patience, empathy, kindness, and compassion. Sometimes it's the nettlesome relationships that teach us the most. Through them, we learn the power of forgiveness and love.

Relationships with animals bring solace. Even the most socially awkward among us can bond with animals. Pets provide companionship and unconditional love. The healing effects are so well documented that pet-assisted therapy has become a bona fide treatment. Pay attention to how you feel when a dog returns your gaze, a cat allows you to stroke its silky fur, or a horse nuzzles you with its warm nose.

Take time to savor the moment. Honor your rest. Relax, play, and connect with the world around you. Create rituals that allow you to be still and thoughtful. Preparing your morning coffee can become a spiritual act if you make it one. If you're tied to your computer for the day, take breaks to watch trees, squirrels, and birds outside your window. Take four deep breaths that you feel from your collarbones to your belly. Think of someone you love and feel the emotion in your heart. In that instant, you changed your bodily functions for the better. Keep it up and you can change your world.

Preventing and Managing Everyday Ailments

Disease-causing microorganisms, accidental injuries, wear and tear, daily hassles, worries, and the occasional hard knock—life is full of things that can set us back. Fortunately, humans are resilient and possessed of innate healing abilities that allow us to get back on our feet soon. We also have the means to prevent injury and illness and to access natural remedies that enhance healing. This part is devoted to giving you the tools to do just that.

For each ailment, you'll find the following:

- **Introduction:** A brief look at what the ailment is and what's happening when your body gets out of whack, including information about factors that increase the risk of the illness, as well as those that defend against it.

- **History:** The ailments—and many of their remedies—have been around since humans first roamed the planet. We'll provide a snapshot of those early effective treatments that endure today and the wacky remedies that thankfully do not!

- **Remedies:** For each ailment, we provide five to ten recipe-based remedies. The ingredients are common and easy to prepare and use.

- **Ingredient Lists:** Our recipes use ingredients from the kitchen pantry, bathroom cabinet, spice rack, and refrigerator, with a healthy addition of herbs from your health food store or garden. In Part 1, you'll find key charts that guide you to find, buy, or grow these simple and effective resources.

- **How it Works:** Ending every recipe, this short, science-based insight tells you how the remedy—or elements of it—can help turn around the ailment.

- **Lifestyle Tips:** Five or more of these tips throughout the chapter give you ways to jump-start your new health regime.

- **Fact or Myth?** These will surprise you and debunk falsehoods many of us have heard for years. You'll learn whether popping a pimple is OK, wet hair causes you to catch cold, and stress can lead to ulcers.

- **When Simple Doesn't Work:** This important entry at the end of the chapter reminds you that home remedies are only one way to approach an ailment. In this part, you'll read about treatments a bit more sophisticated than those you can cook up in your kitchen.

- **When to Call the Doctor:** This vital ending to every chapter drives home this point: *Never take a chance.* If home remedies don't make you feel better, you develop severe symptoms, or have any questions about your health, contact your doctor. Sometimes dialing 911 is the only thing to do. Also, keep your doctor informed of any home remedies you use or plan to use. Please do not use this book to substitute for professional medical care or advice. It is vital that your physician guide your medical care and serve as your primary source of medical information. If you have medical concerns or questions, always seek advice from a health-care professional. The main purpose of this book is to further your knowledge about personal health and responsible home treatment. To the best of our knowledge, the information provided is accurate, as of the time of publication.

- **Spotlights:** Scattered throughout the book, spotlights on specific healing foods, herbs, and practices will give insights into how they work and what their short- and long-term benefits might be. Although many of these deserve full books of their own, these concise introductions show you how you can use them in simple recipes to begin reaping their healing powers.

Moving Forward

We've kept the recipes simple. Most of the ingredients you can't find at home are readily available in supermarkets and pharmacies. For some, you may need a trip to the natural food store (or to order from an online retailer). You may want to grow some of the herbs we refer to frequently—lavender, sage, thyme, oregano, mint, and aloe. Most grow well in indoor pots.

We've also included some must-have essential oils. These natural oils are distilled from plants. They are strong and when used in small amounts can have restorative properties. The recipes here call for only a few drops. Take care when using them. Dilute them in oils or lotions when applying directly. Such carrier oils include olive, almond, apricot, grape seed, jojoba, and unscented lotion. Don't take them by mouth, keep them away from small children, and use extra dilution during pregnancy.

In addition, many of the recipes require nothing other than your inner resources. You'll learn about breathing exercises, meditations, journal activities, yoga postures, and other simple exercises that will keep your life in balance.

Useful Shopping Lists

Use these charts for your shopping list:

Top pantry/bath cabinet items

- Baking soda
- Tea: *chamomile, peppermint, and green tea*
- Apple cider vinegar
- Spices: *cinnamon, clove, curry, turmeric, ginger, cardamom, fennel, anise, and cayenne*
- Salt
- Culinary herbs: *thyme, oregano, rosemary, sage, and basil*
- Hydrogen peroxide
- Honey
- Witch hazel
- *Aloe vera* gel
- Olive oil and coconut oil
- Oats and bran

Top grocery items

- Fruit: *apples, berries, lemons, and avocados*
- Yogurt and kefir (with live bacterial cultures)
- Nuts: *almonds, walnuts, Brazil nuts*
- Nondairy milk made from almonds, soy, oats, or flax
- Olives
- Vegetables: *leafy greens; carrots, squash, and others rich in carotene*
- Fish: *salmon, tuna, and sardines*

Top health food store items

- Seeds: *psyllium seed husks, flaxseeds, chia seeds, and hemp seeds*
- Herbs: *peppermint, and chamomile*
- Essential oils: *peppermint, lavender, eucalyptus, tea tree, and German chamomile*

Essential oils	Properties
Peppermint	*Decongestant, analgesic, mentally stimulating*
Lavender	*Calming, anti-inflammatory*
Eucalyptus	*Expectorant, decongesting, antimicrobial*
Tea tree	*Antimicrobial, anti-inflammatory*
German chamomile	*Anti-inflammatory, calming, antianxiety, antiseptic*

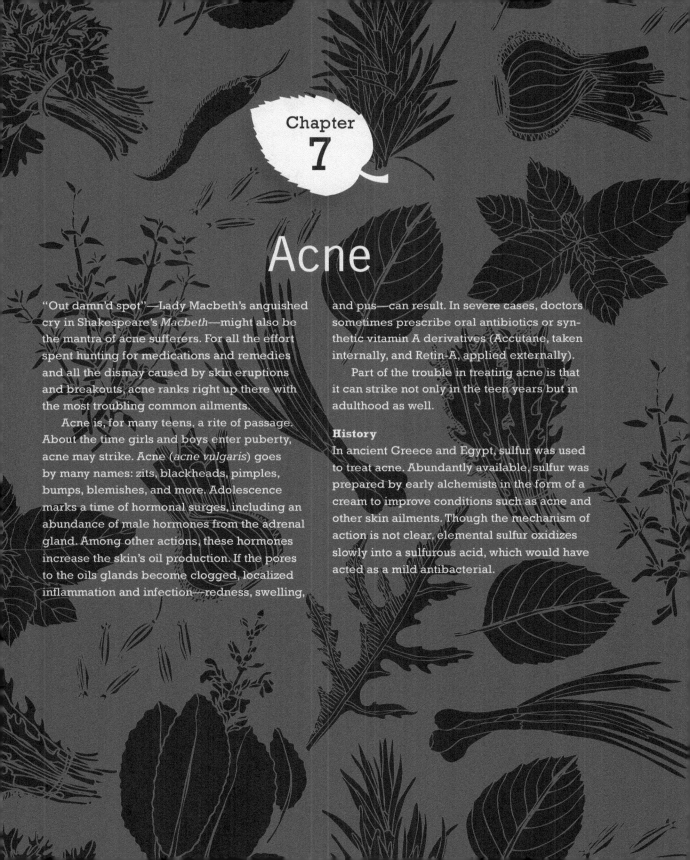

Chapter 7

Acne

"Out damn'd spot"—Lady Macbeth's anguished cry in Shakespeare's *Macbeth*—might also be the mantra of acne sufferers. For all the effort spent hunting for medications and remedies and all the dismay caused by skin eruptions and breakouts, acne ranks right up there with the most troubling common ailments.

Acne is, for many teens, a rite of passage. About the time girls and boys enter puberty, acne may strike. Acne (*acne vulgaris*) goes by many names: zits, blackheads, pimples, bumps, blemishes, and more. Adolescence marks a time of hormonal surges, including an abundance of male hormones from the adrenal gland. Among other actions, these hormones increase the skin's oil production. If the pores to the oils glands become clogged, localized inflammation and infection—redness, swelling,

and pus—can result. In severe cases, doctors sometimes prescribe oral antibiotics or synthetic vitamin A derivatives (Accutane, taken internally, and Retin-A, applied externally).

Part of the trouble in treating acne is that it can strike not only in the teen years but in adulthood as well.

History

In ancient Greece and Egypt, sulfur was used to treat acne. Abundantly available, sulfur was prepared by early alchemists in the form of a cream to improve conditions such as acne and other skin ailments. Though the mechanism of action is not clear, elemental sulfur oxidizes slowly into a sulfurous acid, which would have acted as a mild antibacterial.

Green Tea Wash

1 green tea bag

PREPARATION AND USE:
Brew a cup or small bowl of green tea. Let cool to the touch. Apply to the affected area with a clean cloth.

YIELD: 1 APPLICATION

❓ How it works: *Tea is astringent, anti-inflammatory, and antibacterial. One study found that a 2 percent green tea lotion reduced acne.*

Essential Oil Lotion

"I've had my kids apply these essential oils directly to acne. Aloe adds a soothing element." ~LBW

2 drops pure tea tree or lavender essential oil
1 teaspoon (5 g) *Aloe vera* gel

PREPARATION AND USE:
Blend the tea tree essential oil with the aloe gel. Dot the mixture on blemishes using a cotton swab or clean finger.

YIELD: 1 APPLICATION

❓ How it works: *Tea tree and lavender are both anti-inflammatory and antimicrobial. Lavender smells nicer and can be applied without dilution. Aloe vera is also anti-inflammatory and antimicrobial. In addition, it reduces discomfort and speeds healing. Topical applications of 5 percent tea tree oil gel have been proven as effective as benzoyl peroxide (Oxy-5) and other commercially available products.*

Essential Oil Face Spritzer

This is a soothing and reviving elixir.

½ cup (120 ml) witch hazel
½ cup (115 g) *Aloe vera* gel
20 drops lavender essential oil

PREPARATION AND USE:
Place the ingredients in a clean spray bottle and shake until combined. Mist over your face.

YIELD: 1 WEEK OF TWICE-DAILY APPLICATIONS

❓ How it works: *Witch hazel extract, which you can find in most drugstores, is an astringent. It can be used alone to gently clean the skin. It also tones the skin and decreases inflammation. This mixture stays good for one week.*

Fact or Myth?

MASTURBATION CAUSES ACNE.

It doesn't. Neither does how much or how little sex you have. A 2006 article in *Australian Family Physician* says that people continue to have misconceptions about outbreaks. Another is that acne vanishes at the end of adolescence. Although that's true for many people, blemishes continue for some people into middle age. Another myth is that poor hygiene causes acne. That belief can drive people to scrub their face repeatedly, which only further irritates the skin.

Apple Cider Vinegar Wash

Some people apply vinegar undiluted, but we recommend cutting it with water. You can always build back up to full strength.

½ cup (120 ml) water
2 tablespoons (28 ml) apple cider vinegar

PREPARATION AND USE:
Pour the water and vinegar into a small, clean bowl. Stir to combine.

With a cotton swab or cotton ball, dab the diluted vinegar on each blemish. (Use one swab or ball per blemish to keep infection from spreading.) The application may briefly sting, but that should soon stop. Apply nightly for best results.

YIELD: 1 APPLICATION

❷ **How it works:** *Vinegar contains acetic acid, which is an antiseptic and helps regulate skin acidity.*

❶ **Warning:** *Because undiluted vinegar may irritate the skin, always start with a 1:8 dilution of vinegar to water (e.g., 2 tablespoons [28 ml] of vinegar to 1 cup [235 ml] of water) and build up to 1:4 and, if possible, to vinegar only.*

Yogurt Honey Mask

¼ cup (60 g) plain yogurt
1 tablespoon (20 g) honey
2 strawberries

PREPARATION AND USE:
In a small bowl, blend the yogurt and honey. Mash the strawberries and fold into the yogurt mixture.

Pull back your hair and wash your face with warm water. Use a cotton ball to spread the mask onto your face. Recline for 10 minutes while the fruit and milk acids do their work. Wash with cool water and pat dry with a clean towel.

YIELD: 1 APPLICATION

❷ **How it works:** *Yogurt contains lactic acid and strawberries contain several fruit acids, primarily citric acid. These acids help remove dead skin cells and unclog pores. Honey is antibacterial, anti-inflammatory, and antioxidant.*

Note: Alternatively, dab on straight honey, allow it to dry, and then rinse.

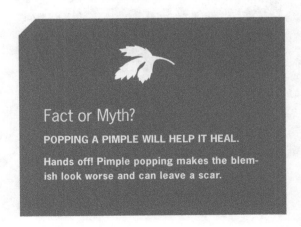

Fact or Myth?

POPPING A PIMPLE WILL HELP IT HEAL.

Hands off! Pimple popping makes the blemish look worse and can leave a scar.

Pineapple Refresh

1 fresh pineapple

PREPARATION AND USE:
Slice away the sides of the pineapple, separating the fruit from the rind. Set the fruit aside in a bowl. Rub the inside of the rind on your face. Mash a single slice of pineapple and rub it onto your face. Let the pineapple juices work for about 15 minutes—while you enjoy eating the fruit. Wash your face and pat it dry with a clean towel. Repeat weekly as needed.

YIELD: 1 APPLICATION

 How it works: *Pineapple contains an anti-inflammatory enzyme called bromelain and fruit acids (mainly citric acid), which gently exfoliate the skin, unblock pores, and dry excess skin oil. (A number of over-the-counter anti-acne products contain a type of fruit acid called alpha-hydroxy acid.) One study found that a commercially prepared fruit acid product, applied to the face every two weeks for six months, decreased the number of pimples.*

Warning: *Do not apply pineapple to your skin if you're allergic to it. If you develop any redness or irritation, stop.*

Bitter Greens Salad

Be creative with this natural cleanser by trying greens you've never used before.

½ cup (28 g) fresh dandelion greens
½ cup (10 g) arugula
½ cup (20 g) radicchio
½ cup (25 g) endive
½ cup (150 g) fresh or canned artichoke hearts

PREPARATION AND USE:

Tear the greens into bite-size pieces. Slice the artichoke hearts. Mix all the ingredients together in a salad. Add other favorite vegetables but avoid adding ingredients with sugars, which may cause skin flare-ups.

YIELD: 2 SERVINGS

 How it works: *Bitter foods stimulate the liver, the organ that breaks down hormones and many other chemicals so they can more easily be cleared from the body.*

Herbal Steam Bag

This herbal remedy can also be used as a soothing facial anytime you need it.

1 quart (946 ml) water
1 tablespoon (2 g) crushed dried calendula (also called pot marigold) flowers
1 tablespoon (2 g) dried elderflowers
3 drops lavender essential oil

PREPARATION AND USE:

Bring water to a boil in a kettle. Put the calendula flowers and elderflowers in a large, heatproof bowl and add the water, covering the flowers.

Add the lavender oil and stir to combine. Lower your head over the bowl and cover it completely with a towel. Allow the steam to work for 15 minutes or until it abates. Rinse your face with cool water.

YIELD: 1 APPLICATION

 How it works: *Calendula and elderflower have anti-inflammatory and antiseptic properties.*

Note: You'll find dried herbal flowers in bulk at most health food stores. Also, although calendula (*Calendula officinalis*) also goes by the common name of pot marigold, it is not the same as marigold (*Tagetes erecta, T. patula*, and other species).

When Simple Doesn't Work

- First, check your stress level. Severe acne is associated with psychological stress, though it's hard to distinguish chicken from egg because acne can generate distress. It is known, however, and that taking medicine derived from the stress hormone cortisol (e.g., cortisone and prednisone) can trigger acne.

- Second, most doctors say diet has little bearing on acne. A few studies and anecdotal reports, however, link pimples with drinking milk and eating fried foods, potato chips, and sweets. To that reason, we recommend you eliminate junk foods, minimize dairy, and emphasize vegetables, fruits, and fish. Stick to lean cuts of poultry and meat. Notice whether a more wholesome diet improves your complexion.

- Third, if you're a woman, you might like to know that some studies show that extracts of chaste tree berries reduce premenstrual acne. You can find herbal extracts at natural food stores.

If the above gentle treatments don't work, see your doctor.

Chapter 8

Allergic Skin Reactions

The skin is the body's largest organ. A number of things can trigger local skin inflammation, or dermatitis, in sensitive people. In contact dermatitis, the offending agents come into direct contact with the skin. Examples include poison ivy, nickel jewelry, sheep's lanolin, topical antibiotics, and ingredients in detergents and body-care products. Radiation administered to cancer patients can also cause dermatitis.

Some people have eczema, also called atopic dermatitis, a condition that tends to run in families, along with hay fever and asthma. Affected patches of skin are red, itchy, scaly, and thickened, and in some cases oozing and crusty. Allergens that provoke the inflammation may be difficult or impossible to identify.

Hives is another skin condition often caused by an allergic reaction. Red, raised itchy patches of skin appear suddenly and may disappear as quickly as they came. Caused by a release of histamine in response to an allergen, hives can be triggered by just about anything—food, sun, dust mites, stress, medication, and more.

Treatment for any of these conditions depends upon the underlying cause. If your watch's nickel backing left a red, crusty patch on your wrist, you'll need to replace it. If you're allergic to the antibiotic you're taking, you may need to switch medications and remember to never take that antibiotic again (as the reaction could be more severe next time around). If you're allergic to bee venom and are stung, you'll need an epinephrine injection. If you are prone to hives, a simple antihistamine can often calm the allergic reaction. If you have eczema, your doctor will probably advise switching to hypoallergenic personal care products and laundry detergent, keeping your skin hydrated, and prescription anti-inflammatory creams for flare-ups.

History

In ancient China, healers considered eczema "asthma of the skin," as many who suffered skin outbreaks also suffered asthma. Allergies were treated through acupuncture, herbs, and most important, by modifying the diet to increase foods that cool the body (fresh fruits and vegetables and green tea) and to reduce foods that heat the body (pumpkin, squash, onion, garlic, chiles, and ginger). In India, healers saw dermatitis as a mild form of leprosy and balanced three treatments: reducing stress, abstaining from dairy and fish, and using massage to increase circulation. Many of these treatments are still in use today.

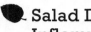 Salad Dressing to Foil Inflammation

1 part olive oil
1 part flaxseed oil
1 part balsamic vinegar
1 part apple cider vinegar

PREPARATION AND USE:
Combine all the ingredients in a dressing shaker and shake vigorously ten times. Pour over salad and toss.

YIELD: 4 TO 6 SERVINGS

❓ **How it works:** *You may think that eating oil will cause your skin to break out; in fact, oil is an anti-inflammatory. The omega-3 fatty acids in fish oil are especially effective in retarding inflammatory reactions in cells.*

Fact or Myth?
MOST U.S. RESIDENTS WILL SUFFER SOME FORM OF DERMATITIS DURING THEIR LIFETIME.

Yes! From diaper rash to psoriasis, up to 90 percent of the population will have allergic skin outbreaks in their lifetime.

Lifestyle Tip

For an extra jolt of good-for-you oils, never consume cod liver oil. It contains too much vitamin A for your system and can even cause a bleeding disorder. Instead, opt for other sources of healthy oils. Add walnuts and avocados to salad. Add hemp seeds to cereal and smoothies. Eat oily fish (salmon, mackerel, sardines, etc.) at least once a week. Or take a daily EPA/DHA capsule.

Colloidal Oatmeal Bath

2 to 3 cups (160 to 240 g) regular
   or colloidal oats

PREPARATION AND USE:
If using regular oats, pour them into a food processor, coffee grinder, or blender and blend to a powder. This turns them into colloidal oats. Pour the oats into warm, running bathwater. Disperse oats with your hand. (Alternatively, pour the oats into a sock, bag, or bandana to contain the particles and help with cleanup and place the sock in the bathwater.) Climb in and soak for at least 15 minutes. (Avoid using soap, which only dries and further irritates the skin.) After leaving the bath, pat your skin dry with a clean towel.

YIELD: 1 APPLICATION

❓ **How it works:** *Oats have antioxidant and anti-inflammatory activity. Applied topically, oats moisturize the skin and decrease itching. The gooeyness you feel when you squeeze the sock is caused by the complex carbohydrates in the oats.*

Note: You can make a large batch of colloidal oats and store in a tightly sealed jar or tin in a cool, dry place.

Afterbath Natural Moisturizer

¼ cup (55 ml) *Aloe vera* gel
¼ cup (60 ml) high-quality oil (olive, almond, coconut, apricot, or grapeseed)
12 drops German chamomile essential oil

PREPARATION AND USE:

In a clean bowl, whisk together the aloe gel and oil. Blend in the German chamomile oil.

Immediately after bathing or showering, while your skin is still damp, apply a generous amount to your skin with clean fingers. Allow a couple of minutes for the moisturizer to absorb before getting dressed.

YIELD: MULTIPLE APPLICATIONS

❷ How it works:

- Aloe vera gel *is anti-inflammatory, soothing, and hydrating. Lab studies indicate that aloe can promote healing and may reduce inflammation in eczema.*

- *German chamomile* (Matricaria recutita) *has chemicals that reduce inflammation and allergies. More specifically, the flavonoids quercetin and apigenin inhibit the release of histamine from immune cells called mast cells. Lab studies indicate that it improves eczema-like skin conditions. Essential oil of chamomile looks blue, due to a potent anti-inflammatory chemical called* chamazulene.

Note: Store leftover moisturizer in a clean, dry jar and throw it away after two weeks when it's time for a fresh recipe.

Soothing Oat Paste

1 tablespoon (5 g) colloidal oatmeal
1 teaspoon (5 g) baking soda
Drops of water, as needed

PREPARATION AND USE:

In a small bowl, stir together the colloidal oatmeal and baking soda until blended. Gradually add just enough water to form a paste. Apply to irritated areas with clean fingers. Once dry, rinse it off with warm water.

YIELD: 1 APPLICATION

❷ How it works: *The antioxidant and anti-inflammatory activities in oatmeal relieve itching. Baking soda neutralizes the acids that promote itchy skin.*

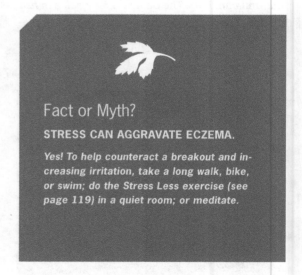

Fact or Myth?

STRESS CAN AGGRAVATE ECZEMA.

Yes! To help counteract a breakout and increasing irritation, take a long walk, bike, or swim; do the Stress Less exercise (see page 119) in a quiet room; or meditate.

🦠 Poison Ivy (or Oak) Potion

This is an effective, time-honored recipe for the rash caused by poison ivy and poison oak.

1 part calamine lotion
1 part *Aloe vera* gel

PREPARATION AND USE:
Mix the lotion and aloe gel in a clean bowl. Apply to affected areas with clean fingers, cotton swabs, or cotton balls. Allow the mixture to dry and then rinse off.

YIELD: 1 APPLICATION

❓ **How it works:** *The zinc oxide and ferric oxide in calamine lotion are antipruritic, or anti-itch, agents. Aloe vera gel feels cool and adds anti-inflammatory relief.*

Fact or Myth?

ALL CHAMOMILES HAVE THE SAME HEALING PROPERTIES.

No! Roman chamomile (Chamaemelum nobile) is a different species and chemically distinct. Although it has benefits of its own, it lacks German chamomile's anti-inflammatory impact.

Lifestyle Tip

Brew a fresh pot of coffee and take a handful of the wet grounds. Rubbing them on your hands will soothe them and relieve inflammation.

🦠 Jewelweed Rub

Jewelweed (Impatiens capensis) is a tall, stemmed plant with orange and yellow trumpet-shaped flowers, usually found growing wild near streams and in deep shade in the woods. My family keeps a batch of this handy during poison ivy season. (Jewelweed can sometimes be found at nurseries, but don't confuse it with the shade-tolerant garden annual Impatiens walleriana, also known as "Busy Lizzy." That one will not help your poison ivy.) ~ BHS

1 quart (946 ml) water (or more if you have lots of jewelweed)
Armful of jewelweed

PREPARATION AND USE:
Bring the water to a boil in a big pot. Turn off the heat. Put the jewelweed in the pot, cover it, and let it steep for at least 30 minutes. Pour the mixture (a deep brown tea) into a gallon jar or into icecube trays and freeze. Rub on the poison ivy rash as soon as you experience the first signs of itching.

YIELD: ENOUGH FOR DOZENS OF APPLICATIONS

❓ **How it works:** *Urushiol, an oily resin in the sap of poison ivy, poison oak, and poison sumac, causes an allergic reaction in those who are sensitive to it. Jewelweed has strong anti-inflammatory properties. It acts on urushiol to relieve the itching and blisters and halt the spread of the rash.*

Scalp Therapy Oil

½ cup (120 ml) olive or vegetable oil
3 drops lavender essential oil

PREPARATION AND USE:
Before bedtime, warm the oil in a saucepan until it feels soothing to the touch.

Apply to your scalp. Put an old cloth or towel over your pillow and sleep. In the morning, use a mild shampoo to wash away the remaining oil.

YIELD: 1 APPLICATION

? How it works: *This natural moisturizer soothes the affected scalp.*

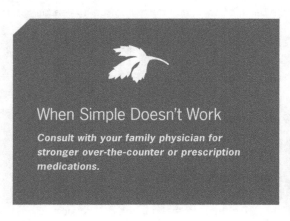

When Simple Doesn't Work

Consult with your family physician for stronger over-the-counter or prescription medications.

Sage Skin Wash

1 cup (235 ml) water
1 tablespoon (2 g) dried sage

PREPARATION AND USE:
In a small pot, bring the water to a boil and then pour into a cup. Add the dried sage, cover, and let steep for at least 15 minutes. Strain and allow to cool to room temperature.

Apply to the affected area with a clean cloth. Allow the skin to dry before getting dressed. Do not rinse off the sage mixture.

YIELD: 1 APPLICATION

? How it works: *In a 2011 study in Japan, researchers used sage and rosemary, among other herbal extracts, on dermatitis lesions on mice and found that repeated applications significantly healed the skin lesions.*

When to Call the Doctor

- *You develop a rash around your eyes, mouth, genitals, or over much of your body from poison ivy or poison oak.*

- *Skin inflammation worsens or becomes infected, as evidenced by increased redness, heat, and pus.*

- *Fever or other signs of more serious illness accompany skin inflammation.*

Chapter 9

Asthma

Each day, nine Americans die during an asthma attack. Unfortunately, an increasing number of Americans have asthma. The current count is about 25 million people. Asthma has become the most common chronic disease in childhood. Theories about the rise in asthma include changes in dietary habits, environmental pollutants, indoor lifestyles, and an increase in obesity.

This inflammatory condition usually begins in childhood. African-American and Puerto Rican children are at particularly high risk. Symptoms include a cough that's typically worse at night and in the early morning, chest tightness, wheezing, shortness of breath, and increased respiratory rate. The airways become inflamed, swollen, constricted, and congested with excess mucus. It's like trying to breathe through a straw.

A combination of genetic predisposition and environmental factors causes asthma. Part of the treatment involves identifying and avoiding (or preparing for) triggers. Triggers for an attack vary and include the following:

- respiratory infections
- airway irritants (e.g., perfume, dust, air pollution, and smoke from tobacco, marijuana, or wood burning)
- allergies (e.g., food, pollen, dander, mold, dust mites, and cockroaches)
- weather (e.g., cold air or a drop in barometric pressure)
- exercise
- strong emotions (e.g., anger)
- gastroesophageal reflux (e.g., heartburn)

Medications don't cure asthma; rather, they help keep the condition under control. The drug regimen depends upon whether the symptoms are intermittent or persistent. Inhaled bronchodilators open the airway to nip an attack in the bud. For persistent asthma, inhaled anti-inflammatory medications are taken daily. It's important to follow the treatment plan. That said, a number of foods and exercises can gently and safely support lung health.

Natural asthma remedies include acupuncture, chiropractic treatments, massage therapy, biofeedback, homeopathy, dietary improvements, and dietary supplements, such as herbs, vitamins, and minerals. Research supporting these therapies is preliminary at best. Science has yet to discover a cure for asthma—natural or otherwise. Kids sometimes grow out of it—that is, stop being symptomatic as their lungs grow bigger.

Such remedies as deep abdominal breathing, progressive muscle relaxation, guided imagery, biofeedback, and regular massage can help relieve emotional stress, which can aggravate asthma. Dietary changes are important for avoiding known food triggers and maximizing intake of natural antioxidants.

History

Some 3,500 years ago, the ancient Egyptians treated asthma by heating herbs on bricks and having asthmatics inhale the fumes to breathe easier. A thousand years later, Greek physician Hippocrates described asthma as excess phlegm in the lungs caused by an imbalance in the bodily humors. The recommended treatment was purging and bleeding. In the 1600s, asthmatics were bled, purged, and also treated with the dung of stallions, powdered millipedes, and volatile salts. Not until the nineteenth century did physician Henry Hyde Salter realize that triggers, such as hay and animals, could set off an asthmatic attack. He recommended strong black coffee (still suggested today) and belladonna (to block airway spasms and coughing, despite significant toxicity). Today, asthma sufferers have an arsenal of medications that more specifically and safely address underlying biological problems.

Lifestyle Tip

Eat a handful of baby carrots every day for a carotenoid boost—to help keep respiratory linings strong and counter inflammation. But don't overdo it. Your skin can turn yellow from too much of a good thing.

RECIPES TO TREAT ASTHMA

 ## Omega-Packed Salmon Fillets

Don't overdo the baking time, or your fish will be dry and unappealing. If you keep it pink in the center and cook it until it just flakes at the touch of a fork, this omega-3 powerhouse is divine.

2 salmon fillets (6 to 8 ounces, or 170 to 225 g each)
2 teaspoons (10 ml) olive oil
1 to 2 tablespoons (14 g) bread crumbs
½ teaspoon dried tarragon
1 tablespoon (15 g) Dijon mustard
Pinch of paprika
Lemon slices, for garnish

PREPARATION AND USE:
Preheat the oven to 450°F (230°C, or gas mark 8). Rinse the salmon fillets and pat them dry. Lightly grease a glass baking dish with the olive oil. Place the fish skin side down in the dish. Mix the tarragon into the mustard and spread over the fish. Sprinkle each fillet with the bread crumbs and paprika. Bake for 10 to 15 minutes until just past pink in the center. Top with the lemon slices and serve.

YIELD: 2 SERVINGS

❓ How it works: *The omega-3 fatty acids in high-oil fish, such as salmon, sardines, tuna, and mackerel, are anti-inflammatory. Studies suggest that diets higher in the omega-3 fatty acids found in fish oil may improve asthma.*

Antioxidant-Rich Waldorf Salad

We like this recipe because it's refreshing, easy to make, and contains a number of ingredients that promote lung health.

6 tablespoons (75 g) plain Greek yogurt
2 tablespoons (28 ml) fresh lemon juice
⅛ teaspoon each sea salt and freshly ground
  black pepper
1 cup (100 g) chopped celery
1 cup (150 g) sliced seedless red grapes
2 large red sweet apples, peeled, cored,
  and chopped
1 cup (100 g) walnuts
Pinch of paprika
Celery leaves, for garnish

PREPARATION AND USE:
In a large bowl, whip the yogurt and lemon juice together. Stir in the salt and pepper. In a separate bowl, mix the celery, grapes, apple, and walnuts. Pour the yogurt mixture over the fruit mixture until fully covered. Stir to combine. Add a pinch of paprika to each serving. Garnish with the celery leaves.

YIELD: 4 SERVINGS

 How it works: *Apples, grapes, and celery leaves are high in flavonoids (water-soluble plant pigments that benefit health) and vitamin C. Both are antioxidant. People with chronic lung conditions, such as asthma, often have low levels of antioxidants, perhaps because this inflammatory condition depletes them. One study found that vitamin C supplementation helped protect against exercise-induced asthma. Others studies have shown that more fresh fruit in the diet improves asthma. Also, the beneficial bacteria in yogurt promote gut health. Research increasingly suggests that abnormal resident "flora," or bacteria, predispose people to asthma and other allergic conditions. Preliminary research suggests that some probiotic supplements improve airway responses. Whether eating yogurt improves asthma isn't yet known, but it does seem to fortify immune function.*

Carotene Booster

Autumn is the perfect time of year to enjoy those colorful, carotene-rich pumpkins, which are members of the squash family.

1 pumpkin (3 pounds, or 1.36 kg) washed, cut
  in half, and seeded
⅓ cup (80 ml) olive oil
2 tablespoons (28 ml) balsamic vinegar
1 teaspoon (2 g) ground cinnamon
1 teaspoon (7 g) honey
1 tablespoon (14 g) unsalted butter

PREPARATION AND USE:
Preheat the oven to 425°F (220°C, or gas mark 7). Cut the pumpkin into ten wedges. Put the wedges on a baking sheet. Mix the olive oil and vinegar together, pour over the pumpkin, and toss until the pumpkin is covered. Spread the wedges in a single layer across the sheet. Sprinkle each

(Continued)

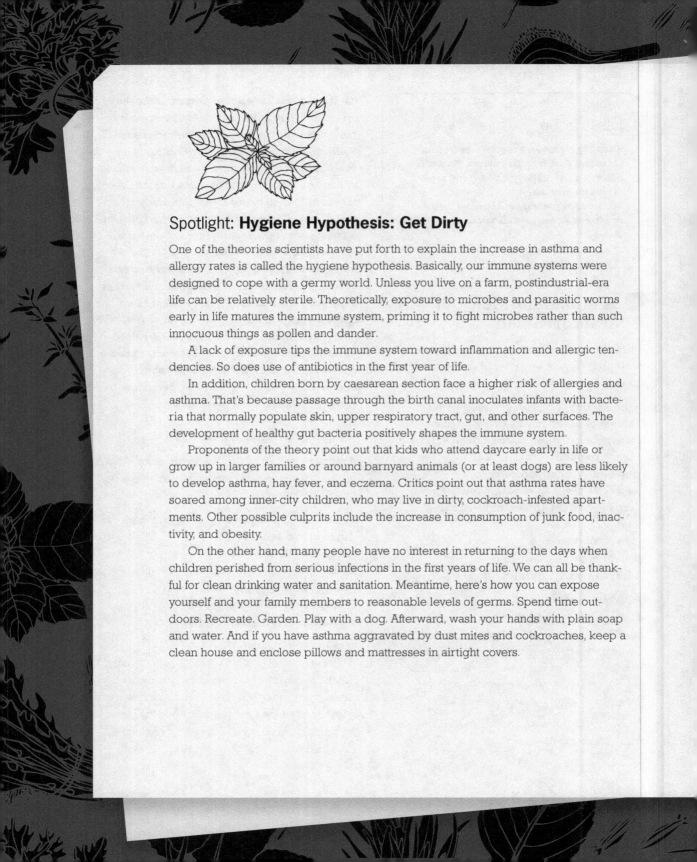

Spotlight: **Hygiene Hypothesis: Get Dirty**

One of the theories scientists have put forth to explain the increase in asthma and allergy rates is called the hygiene hypothesis. Basically, our immune systems were designed to cope with a germy world. Unless you live on a farm, postindustrial-era life can be relatively sterile. Theoretically, exposure to microbes and parasitic worms early in life matures the immune system, priming it to fight microbes rather than such innocuous things as pollen and dander.

A lack of exposure tips the immune system toward inflammation and allergic tendencies. So does use of antibiotics in the first year of life.

In addition, children born by caesarean section face a higher risk of allergies and asthma. That's because passage through the birth canal inoculates infants with bacteria that normally populate skin, upper respiratory tract, gut, and other surfaces. The development of healthy gut bacteria positively shapes the immune system.

Proponents of the theory point out that kids who attend daycare early in life or grow up in larger families or around barnyard animals (or at least dogs) are less likely to develop asthma, hay fever, and eczema. Critics point out that asthma rates have soared among inner-city children, who may live in dirty, cockroach-infested apartments. Other possible culprits include the increase in consumption of junk food, inactivity, and obesity.

On the other hand, many people have no interest in returning to the days when children perished from serious infections in the first years of life. We can all be thankful for clean drinking water and sanitation. Meantime, here's how you can expose yourself and your family members to reasonable levels of germs. Spend time outdoors. Recreate. Garden. Play with a dog. Afterward, wash your hands with plain soap and water. And if you have asthma aggravated by dust mites and cockroaches, keep a clean house and enclose pillows and mattresses in airtight covers.

wedge with cinnamon. Roast for about 40 minutes. Remove from the oven and top the inside of each wedge with a tiny pat of butter. Enjoy the pumpkin by scooping it out of the skin.

YIELD: 4 TO 6 SERVINGS

? How it works: *Pumpkins, yellow squash, carrots, bell peppers, and other orange-hued vegetables and fruits get their pigment from carotenoids, powerful antioxidants that reduce inflammation, support the immune system, and maintain respiratory linings. One study found that a supplement containing a mixture of carotenes helped to prevent exercise-induced asthma.*

Lifestyle Tip

Breathe clean air. Steer clear of smoke-filled rooms or of strong odors from perfume, air fresheners, or paint. On days of heavy pollen or outdoor pollution, stay indoors, close windows, and use air-conditioning as necessary.

◖ Iced Coffee Pick-Me-Up

We love this drink for a late morning boost; try to enjoy it before noon, especially if caffeine keeps you awake at night.

2 cups (475 ml) water
¼ cup (55 g) ground dark roast coffee
¼ cup (78 g) sweetened condensed milk, divided
8 ice cubes

Fact or Myth?

PEOPLE WITH ASTHMA SHOULD NOT EXERCISE.

Myth. Physical activity conditions the lungs, heart, muscle, bones, and brain. Enjoyable exercise is a great stress buster. Swimming is thought to be a good exercise for people with asthma because of the breathing patterns typical of that sport. If you have exercise-induced asthma, you may need to use your inhaler before you start. Check with your doctor about that. Cold, dry air can also aggravate asthma. In that case, indoor activities may be the ticket.

PREPARATION AND USE:

Brew the coffee. Pour half of the condensed milk into each of two mugs. Divide the hot coffee between the mugs. Stir until the milk is dissolved. Fill two tall glasses with four ice cubes each. Gradually pour each portion of hot coffee over the ice and stir to chill (for a thinner, cooler drink, add more cubes). Enjoy!

YIELD: 2 SERVINGS

Recipe Variation: On chilly days, try this coffee hot—just leave out the ice cubes and add a pinch of ground cinnamon.

? How it works: *Several studies have shown that caffeine modestly improves lung function for up to 4 hours in people with asthma. Avoid late afternoon or evening intake, which could interfere with a good night's sleep. Caffeine is related to theophylline, an asthma medication that helps open airways, reducing breathlessness.*

Eucalyptus Chest Rub

The smell alone of this soothing rub brings respiratory relief.

1 tablespoon (15 ml) unscented lotion, olive oil, or (15 g) petroleum jelly
2 drops eucalyptus essential oil

PREPARATION AND USE:

Blend the lotion and essential oil in a small, clean jar. Rub the mixture onto your chest: Start with a small amount to see how you respond to eucalyptus. Inhale deeply as you work. You're drawing some of those aromatic, medicinal oils into your lungs. Wash your hands thoroughly before touching your eyes, nose, or other sensitive mucous membranes. If you have any remaining rub, store it in the jar and cap tightly.

YIELD: 1 RUB

❓ How it works: *Eucalyptus has anti-inflammatory, expectorant effects. It may also help open the airways by relaxing the encircling muscles. One study found that a special preparation taken internally eased asthma symptoms and reduced the need for medications. However, it is not safe to take eucalyptus essential oil by mouth. Plant essential oils are highly concentrated. Many are toxic when taken internally.*

Lifestyle Tip

Check out your allergic reactions. Eighty percent of people who suffer asthma attacks are allergic to airborne particles that come from mold, pollen, trees and grasses, animal dander, and cockroach droppings.

Beneficial Tuna with Brazil Nuts

Once you've enjoyed this dish hot from the oven, keep up your omega-3s by putting the leftovers in tuna salad sandwiches (mix with plain yogurt and a little lemon instead of mayonnaise).

4 tuna medallions (4 ounces, or 115 g each)
2 teaspoons (10 ml) olive oil
¼ teaspoon sea salt
Freshly ground black pepper, to taste
¼ cup (33 g) crushed Brazil nuts
Lemon wedges, for garnish

PREPARATION AND USE:

Preheat the oven to 425°F (220°C, or gas mark 7). Rinse the tuna medallions and pat dry. Brush each side with olive oil and sprinkle with salt and pepper. Roll the medallions in the crushed nuts. Coat a glass baking dish with vegetable oil spray. Bake the tuna for 15 to 20 minutes until the center is just past pink.

YIELD: 4 SERVINGS

❓ How it works: *Brazil nuts and seafood are excellent sources of selenium, an antioxidant that works against inflammation. At least two studies have shown that people who consumed selenium in their diet were less likely to have asthma than were those who did not. Tuna is a good source of omega-3 fatty acids, which help reduce inflammation in airways. One survey showed that families that ate oily fish high in omega-3s, such as tuna, sardines, and salmon, had a nearly three times' lower percentage of children with asthma than families that did not.*

Yoga Relaxer: Puppy Pose

Yoga poses can swiftly calm, ground, and bring you into your body. This particular pose stretches your spine, giving your lungs a chance to fill and empty to their full capacity.

You
A clean mat or rug

PREPARATION AND USE:
Start on your hands and knees. Align your body so that your shoulders are directly above your wrists and your hips are above your knees. Breathe in slowly and deeply. Breathe out slowly, expelling as much air as possible.

Move your hands forward a few inches (centimeters) along the floor. Move your buttocks halfway back toward your heels while your hands remain in the same place. Drop your forehead down to the floor and relax your neck. Push your hands forward, fully stretching your arms. At the same time, move your hips back to hover just above your heels (this stretches the spine). Breathe normally, feeling your spine stretch. Maintain the pose for 30 seconds to 1 minute. Bring your buttocks down to rest on your heels. Relax.

YIELD: 1 SESSION

? How it works: *Yoga may help in several ways. For one, it reduces stress, which can aggravate asthma. For another, it emphasizes breath control. Last, the exercise helps condition the heart and lungs. Some studies show yoga and progressive muscle relaxation (see the insomnia exercise on page 357) improve asthma.*

! Warning: *If you have knee problems or feel any pain during this pose, stop.*

Take a Breather

Anyone who's had an asthma attack knows how frightening shortness of breath can feel. Anxiety can make things worse. Create a habit of literally finding your breath, which immediately calms your nervous, heart, and respiratory systems. Practice allows you to access that state—even in a crisis.

You
A comfortable chair

PREPARATION AND USE:
Sit comfortably with your hands relaxed in your lap. While counting slowly to four, inhale slowly and deeply. Hold your breath for the same number of seconds. Exhale for the same number of seconds. Try to steadily increase your times, but without causing discomfort.

YIELD: 1 SESSION

? How it works: *Stress aggravates asthma. One of the most immediate ways to reduce stress is to breathe deeply. Deep breaths send a message to your brain to relax, and the brain sends that message to the rest of your body. In 1952, Russian physiologist Konstantin Buteyko designed a breathing technique to help asthma patients. The basic idea is that, when you hold your breath, carbon dioxide levels rise in the lungs, which stimulates airways to dilate. The Buteyko breathing technique teaches people to have controlled pauses in their breathing. It's akin to the breathing pattern used while swimming. This method isn't well researched, but a couple of studies do show benefits.*

🍂 Lifestyle Journal Exercise

We find that keeping a journal helps us see patterns and release emotions. In this case, you're looking for patterns linked to your asthma.

A journal
A pen

PREPARATION AND USE:

Keep a daily journal for six weeks, noting the foods you eat, your daily schedule, stress levels, and exercise. In it, note respiratory symptoms that occur.

Look for patterns. For instance, you may notice a relationship between asthma symptoms and certain emotions, exercise, foods, and perfume scents. When you have asthma symptoms, what thoughts and emotions occur?

You're trying to find patterns that make you feel better and those that make you feel worse. Your goal is to have more of the former and less of the latter.

When you close your journal each day, how do you feel? Does writing in the journal give you a sense of perspective?

YIELD: 1 JOURNAL SESSION PER DAY

❓ **How it works:** *Some studies show that people who wrote in a journal most days of the week about their asthma had a reduction of symptoms and less need for rescue medication.*

🍂 Turmeric Toddy

Enjoy this soothing beverage throughout the day, especially before bed.

1 cup (235 ml) milk
1 teaspoon (2 g) ground turmeric

PREPARATION AND USE:

Heat the milk to your desired warmth, but do not boil it. Stir in the turmeric. Drink this mixture up to three times daily.

YIELD: 1 SERVING

❓ **How it works:** *This Indian spice is a potent anti-inflammatory agent. Preliminary research suggests that concentrated extracts of turmeric and other anti-inflammatory herbs can improve some aspects of asthma. The fat in milk can improve intestinal absorption of curcumin, the active ingredient in turmeric.*

When Simple Doesn't Work

Preliminary research suggests that standardized, concentrated extracts of some herbs may hold modest benefits for people with asthma. They include ginkgo, coleus, long pepper, curcumin (an active ingredient in turmeric), and pycnogenol (from French maritime pine). Herbalists often recommend horehound and mullein as general lung tonics. However, check with your health provider before taking any herbs or other dietary supplements.

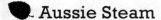 **Aussie Steam**

Eucalyptus trees are native to Australia and have long been used to manage coughs and asthma.

1 quart (946 ml) water

1 to 2 drops eucalyptus essential oil, or ¼ cup (6 g) crushed, dried eucalyptus leaves

PREPARATION AND USE:

Boil the water. Turn off the heat.

If using eucalyptus essential oil, remove the pot from the burner. First try inhaling the steam. If steam alone doesn't trigger asthmatic coughing, add 1 drop of eucalyptus oil. Lean in gradually. If the eucalyptus vapors don't trigger coughing, you can add the second drop of essential oil. Cover your head with a clean towel to entrap the steam. Breathe through your mouth slowly and deeply for 1 to 2 minutes.

If using dried eucalyptus leaves, add them to the pot, cover, and steep for 10 to 15 minutes. Remove the lid. If you no longer have steam, heat the liquid again—just to the boiling point—and remove from the burner. Lean over the steam and cover your head with a clean towel. Breathe slowly and deeply. If the steam triggers coughing or seems to worsen your asthma in any way, stop.

YIELD: 1 APPLICATION

❓ How it works: *Inhaling steam helps to relax airways, increase circulation, and thin respiratory mucus, which makes it easier to expel. The eucalyptus is antioxidant, anti-inflammatory, and expectorant. A 2003 study found that an oral preparation of a key chemical in eucalyptus (eucalyptol) had an anti-inflammatory effect in people with asthma and reduced the need for steroids. (Plant essential oils, including eucalyptus essential oil, however, should not be taken by mouth.)*

Note: For some people with asthma, essential oil vapors trigger coughing.

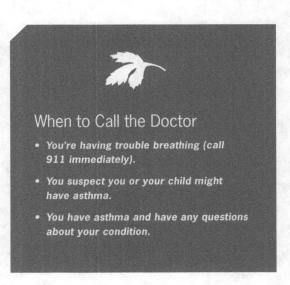

When to Call the Doctor

- *You're having trouble breathing (call 911 immediately).*

- *You suspect you or your child might have asthma.*

- *You have asthma and have any questions about your condition.*

Athlete's Foot

Athlete's foot, or *tinea pedis* in medical lingo, is a fungal infection of the top layers of the skin. The species of fungi infecting the skin go by the collective name of *dermatophytes*. Like most fungi, these thrive in damp, warm places. Other vulnerable areas are the groin (jock itch, or *tinea cruris*), and the head (ringworm, or *tinea capitis*).

The fungi that cause athlete's foot can also infect the nails. Usually trauma (a nick in the nail or crush injury) occurs, giving the fungi an entry point. The nail yellows and thickens. Diagnosis is usually made by inspection, plus or minus microscopic examination of scrapings from under the nail.

These infections are contagious. In the case of athlete's foot, you pick up the fungi when the soles of your feet come in contact with dead skin cells shed from an infected person. The sign of athlete's foot is red, flaky, itchy skin on the soles and heels. The toe webs may be involved. The skin may also blister and crack.

The main treatment for fungal skin infections is application of an over-the-counter antifungal cream, such as miconazole or clotrimazole. It can take up to a month for skin to heal. Fungal nail infections, however, are more difficult to clear. Because topical antifungal creams often aren't enough, doctors usually prescribe antifungal drugs taken by mouth.

History

The first reported case of *tinea pedis*, or athlete's foot, in the United States was in Birmingham, Alabama, in the 1920s. But the fungi that caused it—endemic to regions of Southeast Asia and Africa and Australia—doubtlessly had been afflicting humans for centuries. In 1925, Australian scientist Arthur Penfold showed that oil from the Australian tea tree (*Melaleuca alternifolia*) was antimicrobial. Science confirmed what Australian Aborigines had long known: Tea tree oil was good for treating a number of ills, including athlete's foot and other fungal and skin infections. Although tea tree oil's use waned in the midtwentieth century, by the 1980s it had made a comeback. A number of studies have confirmed that a relatively strong solution of tea tree oil inhibits the fungi that cause athlete's foot.

Tea for Two Feet

Tea tree oil can be powerful stuff, so take care in mixing and applying this remedy as noted below.

1 tablespoon (15 ml) unscented body lotion
1 teaspoon (5 ml) tea tree oil

PREPARATION AND USE:

Blend the lotion and tea tree oil in a small, clean jar or bowl. Apply to affected areas on the feet. Wash your hands afterward.

YIELD: 1 APPLICATION

❓ **How it works:** *At least two studies have shown creams containing between 10 and 50 percent tea tree oil help resolve athlete's foot. In the more recent study, which lasted four weeks, 25- and 50-percent solutions were similarly effective when compared to a placebo cream. A few of the volunteers did, however, develop skin irritation. If that happens to you, stop using tea tree oil.*

❗ **Warning:** *Keep your bottle of tea tree oil out of the reach of children. Internal use can be toxic.*

Thyme and Oregano Footbath

While it fights athlete's foot, this footbath delivers delicious relaxation.

1 quart (946 ml) water
2 tablespoons (5 g) dried thyme leaves
2 tablespoons (6 g) dried oregano leaves
¼ cup (72 g) salt

PREPARATION AND USE:

Boil the water in a saucepan. Turn off the heat, add the herbs, cover, and steep for 20 minutes. Stir in the salt. Reheat over low heat until the water feels warm but not scalding. Strain into a basin big enough for your feet. Soak your feet for 15 to 20 minutes until the water is no longer warm. Dry your feet, including between your toes, with a clean towel. Then put the towel in the laundry to wash (do not reuse without laundering).

YIELD: 1 APPLICATION

❓ **How it works:** *A lab experiment compared the fungicidal (fungus-killing) power of several essential oils. In order from highest to lowest fungicidal activity were oregano, thyme, cinnamon, lemongrass, clove, palmarosa, peppermint, lavender, geranium, and tea tree. Adding salt and heat to the essential oil solution amplified the fungicidal power.*

Note: Alternatively, you can put hot-to-tolerance water and salt in the foot basin. Stir in 5 drops of essential oil of oregano. You can use thyme essential oil instead, but only if you select the linalool type. The others are irritating to skin and mucous membranes. Other alternatives include peppermint and lavender oil.

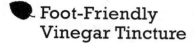

Foot-Friendly Vinegar Tincture

¼ cup (60 ml) white, distilled, or apple
   cider vinegar
5 drops tea tree essential oil
5 drops peppermint essential oil
2 to 3 drops eucalyptus essential oil

PREPARATION AND USE:

Combine all the ingredients in a jar and shake.
Soak cotton balls in the mixture and apply, covering the affected area. If you have any solution left
over, cap the jar tightly to prevent the evaporation
of the plant essential oils.

YIELD: 1 APPLICATION FOR EACH RECIPE/VARIATION

❓ **How it works:** *Vinegar contains acetic acid,
which discourages fungal growth. Consistent
application has often been met with success in
clearing up fungal infection. It may take several
weeks, even months, but many people swear by
it. Adding the plant essential oils, all of which
have direct antifungal activity, may accelerate
the process.*

Recipe Variations:

- Pour enough vinegar into a small tub to
immerse your toes or feet. Mix in the essential
oils above. Soak for 2 minutes. Then rinse your
toes and dry thoroughly with a clean towel.
(Do not reuse the towel without laundering
it.) Apply twice daily until the itch disappears.
Then continue application for one additional
week.

- Because vinegar is acidic, it may irritate the
skin. In that case, dilute the vinegar, using one
part vinegar to three parts water. Mix in the
essential oils. Soak for 15 minutes three times a
week. When finished, rinse and dry as above.

- Some people are also sensitive to plant essential oils. If you have sensitive skin, try the vinegar or diluted vinegar solution alone. If you
have no reaction, try one essential oil at a time.
Don't combine the three until you know your
skin can tolerate it.

Garlic Fungal Chaser

*Be sure to test this strong antidote on a patch of
skin before covering your feet with it.*

1 garlic clove
1 to 2 teaspoons (5 to 10 ml) olive oil

PREPARATION AND USE:

Mash the garlic and olive oil together into a paste.
Apply to the infected area. Remove after 1 hour.

YIELD: 1 APPLICATION

❓ **How it works:** *Vampires merely ran at the
sight of garlic, but microbes have less chance
for a clean getaway. Garlic is a microbe-slayer.
Its action includes antifungal power. Two studies have shown that ajoene, a compound found
in garlic, heals athlete's foot. One of the studies,
which lasted sixty days, showed that, in nearly
fifty Venezuelan soldiers with athlete's foot,
cream containing 1 percent ajoene had a 100
percent cure rate versus 94 percent for a cream
containing 1 percent of the conventional antifungal terbinafine. The other study, conducted by
the same research group, only followed the volunteers for two weeks. However, they reported
a 79 percent cure by seven days, and a 100 percent cure after fourteen days of topical ajoene.*

❗ **Warning:** *Don't use the garlic alone, as this
strong herb can irritate the skin. The olive oil
creates a protective coating. Most people can
tolerate 1 hour. Remove sooner if you have sensitive skin or the application causes discomfort.*

Note: Yes, your feet will smell a bit like garlic. (The plant wasn't dubbed "the stinking rose" for nothing.) But most people aren't going to sniff your feet.

Here's a fun experiment: The antimicrobial chemicals in garlic contain sulfur. Some of them absorb across your skin, into the bloodstream, and across the air sacs in your lungs. See whether a friend can smell garlic on your breath after the hour is up. If you dislike that smell (or others do), chew parsley leaves or fennel seeds or try other remedies in Chapter 11 on bad breath.

Probiotic Foot Fix

This simple and soothing treatment comes out of your refrigerator and onto your feet. There is no odor to worry about, as with the garlic treatment above.

2 to 3 tablespoons (30 to 45 g) plain yogurt (Make sure it has live cultures of acidophilus.)

PREPARATION AND USE:
Apply to the infected areas—toe webs, heels, and so on—for 15 to 20 minutes. Rinse off and dry feet thoroughly before putting on socks and shoes.

YIELD: 1 APPLICATION

 How it works: *Yogurt's live ingredient, acidophilus, makes lactic acid, which helps fight fungus. Daily application can soothe and help heal the infected area.*

Lifestyle Tip

To prevent athlete's foot, practice good hygiene:

- **Keep your feet dry. If your feet sweat, change your socks. Put talcum powder or cornstarch in your shoes.**

- **Wear socks that absorb and wick away moisture. Although many doctors recommend cotton, a good alternative is wool, which you can now find in all styles and thicknesses.**

- **In hot weather, wear sandals or other shoes with good ventilation.**

- **Air out shoes after each use.**

- **Don't share socks, shoes, towels, or nail clippers with someone with athlete's foot or a fungal nail infection.**

Clove and Cinnamon Soother

The essential oil versions of these holiday spices are helpful healers when diluted in a soothing olive oil mixture and applied to your feet.

¼ teaspoon cinnamon or clove essential oil
2½ teaspoons (13 ml) olive oil

PREPARATION AND USE:
Mix together the essential oil and olive oil. Test a little on a patch of skin before doing full-blown foot therapy.

YIELD: 1 APPLICATION

How it works: *Studies show that these two pantry spices have antifungal properties that help foil common skin infections.*

Tea Bags for Happy Toes

Use this quick and easy treatment to soothe athlete's foot burn and boost the healing process.

1 quart (946 ml) water
6 black tea bags

PREPARATION AND USE:
Boil the water and steep the tea bags in it. Pour the water and tea bags into a small tub. When tea has cooled enough to be comfortable, immerse your feet. Soak for 15 to 20 minutes. Rinse your feet after soaking and dry thoroughly before putting on your socks.

YIELD: 1 APPLICATION

❷ How it works: *Black tea contains tannic acid, which is antifungal. It helps fight the infection.*

Cornstarch = Dry Feet

You'll love the drying effect of this starchy flour made from corn; it's usually used in cooking to thicken sauces.

½ cup (64 g) cornstarch

PREPARATION AND USE:
Preheat the oven to 325°F (170°C, or gas mark 3).

Spread the cornstarch across the bottom of a clean glass baking dish. Bake for 3 to 5 minutes until just browned on top. Remove from the oven and let cool. Rub onto affected areas before putting on your socks and shoes.

YIELD: 1 APPLICATION

❷ How it works: *Cornstarch absorbs foot moisture that can help launch fungal infections. Cornstarch right from the box is a good start; but a quick browning in the oven removes its moisture, allowing it to take in more moisture from your feet.*

Note: Shake a teaspoon (3 g) of the toasted cornstarch into your shoes to coat the insides—another way to absorb moisture.

Coconut Fungal Fighter

¼ cup (56 g) coconut oil
1 teaspoon (2 g) ground turmeric

PREPARATION AND USE:

Over low heat, melt the oil in a pan. It happens in a matter of seconds. Whisk in the turmeric. Turn off the heat. Pour the mixture into a clean dish. When cool, spread on the affected area. Allow to soak in for 15 to 20 minutes. Rinse off and dry the area thoroughly.

YIELD: 1 APPLICATION

❷ **How it works:** *African studies show that virgin coconut oil, a folk remedy for treating such fungal skin infections as athlete's foot and ringworm, has antifungal properties. Likewise, turmeric is an antifungal agent.*

Note: Turmeric is traditionally used to dye fabrics yellow. It will temporarily stain your skin and permanently stain clothing.

When Simple Doesn't Work

A traditional Mexican treatment for athlete's foot involves the topical use of a plant called Ageratina pichinchensis (commonly known as snakeroot and previous classified as Eupatorium pichinchense or E. aschenbornianum). Studies have shown that topical applications of a special extract from this plant worked as well as the antifungal drug ketoconazole. Extracts have also been shown to be therapeutic in fungal nail infections. Unfortunately, products containing this extract are not yet available for sale in the United States.

If home remedies aren't working for you, you can try antifungal creams available over the counter at drugstores and supermarkets: terbinafine (Lamisil AT), tolnaftate (Tinactin), clotrimazole (Lotrimin AF), and miconazole (Micatin).

Vicks-en Toenail Treatment

My husband and I used this for nearly a year to clear up long-standing toenail fungus. It worked—my sexy toes are back! And we saved plenty in over-the-counter medications. ~ BBG

Hydrogen peroxide
Vicks VapoRub

PREPARATION AND USE:

In the evening, shower and wash your toes carefully or soak and wash your toes in a small tub of warm water. Dry them thoroughly with a clean towel (launder the towel after each use).

Wet a cotton ball with hydrogen peroxide and apply to each toenail, using a fresh cotton ball for each nail so as not to spread infection. Let your toes air dry or pat them dry after the peroxide foaming subsides.

Make sure they are thoroughly dry, and then coat each toenail with Vicks. Cover your feet with cotton socks (which you must wash after wearing); this keeps the Vicks working on your toes and off your sheets.

YIELD: 1 APPLICATION

❷ How it works: *Hydrogen peroxide is antifungal. Vicks VapoRub contains essential oils from plants with antifungal activity, specifically thymol from thyme, menthol from peppermint, eucalyptol from eucalyptus, and camphor from a relative of cinnamon (Cinnamomum camphora).*

When to Call the Doctor

- *You can't clear the infection after two weeks of using home remedies or over-the-counter antifungal creams. It may be time to try a prescription antifungal medication.*

- *The fungal infection is spreading.*

- *The soles of your feet begin to blister.*

- *Your skin becomes cracked, reddened, swollen, and painful.*

- *You see pus or red streaks extending from the infected area.*

- *You develop a fever.*

- *You have diabetes and have any sign of infection on your feet.*

Chapter 11

Bad Breath

Bad breath affects an estimated 25 to 30 percent of the world's population. About 2.4 percent of adults have chronic halitosis. The majority of the time, the origin is in the mouth. Examples include gum disease, dental cavities, coated tongue (sometimes a white or yellow layer blankets the tongue, usually due to inflammation), and poor oral hygiene. Beneficial microorganisms normally line our entire intestinal tract, peacefully coexisting with us. However, oral diseases involve proliferation of certain microorganisms that produce sulfurous smells.

Smokers have bad breath. Food and drink, such as onions, garlic, coffee, and alcohol, can temporarily taint breath. Other peoples' reactions are tempered by whether they have also indulged in the same food or drink and whether they happen to dislike that smell. Some say vegetarians have sweeter breath than meat eaters. That difference has to do with how mouth microbes act on amino acids (the building blocks in protein) and digestive processes deeper in the intestinal tract.

Because saliva has an antimicrobial effect, having a dry mouth sours breath. Advanced age, stress, depression, mouth breathing, alcohol abuse, certain medications, diabetes, and Sjögren syndrome (an autoimmune disease wherein white blood cells attack glands that make saliva and tears) diminish saliva. Reduced nighttime saliva production also causes morning breath.

In addition, malnutrition contributes to overall ill health and bad breath. Insufficient consumption of carbohydrates or severe caloric restriction leaves your body no choice but to break down fat, which gives your breath a telltale fruity odor. Uncontrolled diabetes also creates disturbances in oral health.

Such infections as sore throat and sinusitis cause halitosis. So do stomach and intestinal disorders, such as heartburn, stomach inflammation and ulcers, and lactose intolerance.

Treatment involves correcting the underlying disorder.

History
As early as 2700 BCE, the Chinese advocated mouth rinsing to treat bad breath. Ayurvedic medicine, the traditional Hindu system, recommended chewing areca nut wrapped in betel leaves (later found to be harmful). Courtesans in the Renaissance used sweet wine mixed with herbs to sweeten their breath. In the twentieth century, a host of mouthwashes and breath mints have been marketed to fight bad breath—many of them containing alcohol and other substances that exacerbate the problem.

Freshen Up

You're on a big date and have had a dinner rich in garlic. Pop a sprig of parsley or other garnish in your mouth and pucker up.

Fresh sprig of parsley, basil, mint, or cilantro

PREPARATION AND USE:

Place a sprig of any of these leaves in your mouth, chew, and swallow.

YIELD: 1 APPLICATION

❓ How it works: *All green plants contain chlorophyll, which neutralizes odors. Also, aromatic herbs contain essential oils that freshen breath.*

Lemon Breath Lift

Lemon and pomegranate taste and smell fresh.

1 cup (235 ml) water
2 tablespoons (28 ml) fresh lemon juice
1 tablespoon (15 ml) pomegranate juice
1 packet (1 g) stevia, or to taste

PREPARATION AND USE:

Pour the water and pomegranate juice into a glass and stir in the lemon juice. Add the stevia. Drink in the morning (after your daily cuppa joe).

YIELD: 1 SERVING

❓ How it works: *Lemon contains essential oils that create the characteristic zesty (or citrus) scent. It's long been used to reduce unpleasant odors. Both lemon and pomegranate contain flavonoids that help strengthen connective tissues, such as those in the gums. Pomegranate also has a mild antibacterial effect.*

Citrus Fresh Breath

The rind tastes bitter at first bite, but chewing it gives your mouth a natural, refreshing zing.

1 organic lemon or orange

PREPARATION AND USE:

Wash the rind thoroughly and tear off a piece. Chew for a flavorful, mouth-freshening burst.

YIELD: 1 APPLICATION

❓ How it works: *Citric acid will stimulate the salivary glands to create saliva, which is a natural breath freshener.*

Minty Mouth-Freshening Tea

2 tablespoons (12 g) loose green tea, or 2 tea bags
1 teaspoon (2 g) crushed fresh mint leaves
1 cinnamon stick
2 cups (475 ml) boiled water

PREPARATION AND USE:

Add the tea, mint leaves, and cinnamon to the boiled water. Steep for 5 minutes. Remove the tea bags, if using, and strain out the herbs. Sip and enjoy!

YIELD: 1 LARGE OR 2 SMALL SERVINGS

❓ How it works: *Green tea has antibacterial compounds. Cinnamon is antimicrobial and aromatic. The oils in mint fight mouth bacteria that cause halitosis.*

Crunch It

1 cup (150 g) apple chunks
1 cup (110 g) grated carrot
1 cup (120 g) diced celery
½ cup (60 g) dried cranberries
½ cup (60 g) crushed walnuts
3 to 5 tablespoons (45 to 75 g) plain
  nonfat yogurt
Ground cinnamon

PREPARATION AND USE:

Mix the apple, carrot, celery, cranberries, and walnuts together in a large bowl. Add the yogurt by the tablespoon (15 g) to moisten the mixture and hold it together slightly. Divide between two plates, sprinkle with cinnamon, and serve.

YIELD: 2 SERVINGS

❷ **How it works:** *Raw, crunchy foods clean the teeth. Apples contain pectin, which helps control food odors. It also promotes saliva, which cleanses breath. Cinnamon is antimicrobial. Yogurt contains the type of bacteria you want in your intestinal tract. Studies show that the active bacteria and cultures in yogurt help reduce odor-causing bacteria in the mouth.*

Tongue Scrape

A coated tongue is a prominent factor behind bad breath. Although you can use a toothbrush, a tongue scraper works better. You can buy one at most pharmacies. In a pinch, use a spoon.

Tongue scraper or spoon

PREPARATION AND USE:

Each morning, gently scrape your tongue. It helps to hold the tip of the tongue with a piece of gauze or a clean cloth so that you can pull it forward to better clean the back of the tongue (and reduce the chance of stimulating your gag reflex).

YIELD: 1 SESSION EVERY MORNING

❷ **How it works:** *The coating on the tongue contains some mixture of dead tongue cells, bacteria, and fungi that become trapped between the small projections (papillae) on the tongue's surface. Daily tongue scraping and brushing decreases this material carpeting the tongue and improves mouth odor.*

Peroxide Swish

Hydrogen peroxide is a versatile cleansing agent, in the right doses. Be sure to cut it with water before using.

2 tablespoons (30 ml) hydrogen peroxide
2 tablespoons (30 ml) water

PREPARATION AND USE:

Mix the hydrogen peroxide and water in a clean glass. Swish in your mouth for 30 seconds and then spit out. Rinse twice a day, once in the morning and once in the evening.

YIELD: 1 APPLICATION

❓ How it works: *Hydrogen peroxide's oxygen content kills the bacteria in your mouth that cause bad breath.*

Lifestyle Tip

When nothing else is available, swish fresh, cool water around in your mouth. Water freshens breath and makes you feel better in general.

Mouthwash in a Minute

We love the fresh and natural taste of this mouthwash—and it's alcohol-free, unlike so many off-the-shelf products. Do not swallow it!

1 cup (235 ml) water
1 teaspoon (5 g) baking soda
3 drops peppermint essential oil

PREPARATION AND USE:

Mix together all the ingredients. Pour into a clean glass jar with a tight-fitting lid, cap, and shake. Use a small amount to rinse your mouth for about 30 seconds. Spit out—do not swallow.

YIELD: SEVERAL RINSES; MAKE A FRESH BATCH AFTER A FEW DAYS, OR ALTER THE RECIPE TO MAKE A LITTLE AT A TIME.

❓ How it works: *Peppermint is antimicrobial. Baking soda changes the pH (acid) levels in the mouth, creating an antiodor environment.*

Lifestyle Tip

Practice good oral health regularly:

- **Brush your teeth after every meal.**

- **Be gentle on your gums.**

- **Floss at least once a day, preferably twice, before you brush.**

- **If you can't brush after a meal, drink water, swish, and spit to remove residual food particles.**

- **Replace your toothbrush every two to three months.**

- **Keep up with regular dental checkups, including cleanings. Ask your dentist how often you should come.**

Yogurt Breath Blaster

1 cup (230 g) vanilla yogurt
1 cup (170 g) sliced strawberries
¼ cup (30 g) chopped walnuts
Sprigs of mint

PREPARATION AND USE:

Combine the yogurt, strawberries, and walnuts in a small bowl. Top with mint sprigs and serve.

YIELD: 1 SERVING

❷ How it works: *Studies say that yogurt's active bacteria may help control the mouth bacteria that release malodorous chemicals, such as hydrogen sulfide. In one study, researchers found that eating 6 ounces (170 g) of yogurt a day reduced levels of this gas.*

Fresh Chew

Handful of fennel seeds, cloves, or aniseeds

PREPARATION AND USE:

Pop your spice of choice into your mouth. Chew the seeds, savoring the release of their fresh and spicy, odor-fighting tastes.

YIELD: 1 SERVING

❷ How it works: *These spices all have antiseptic qualities that help fight halitosis-causing bacteria and sweeten your breath.*

When to Call the Doctor

- *Halitosis persists despite improved oral hygiene.*

- *You notice your tongue often looks coated.*

- *Your mouth is often dry.*

- *You have sores in your mouth, painful gums, or tooth pain (for example, when drinking cold liquids or chewing).*

- *You have diabetes or another chronic condition and notice a change in your breath.*

- *You feel ill. (Infection of the tongue, throat, and gums, oral cancer, and many other illnesses affect the breath.)*

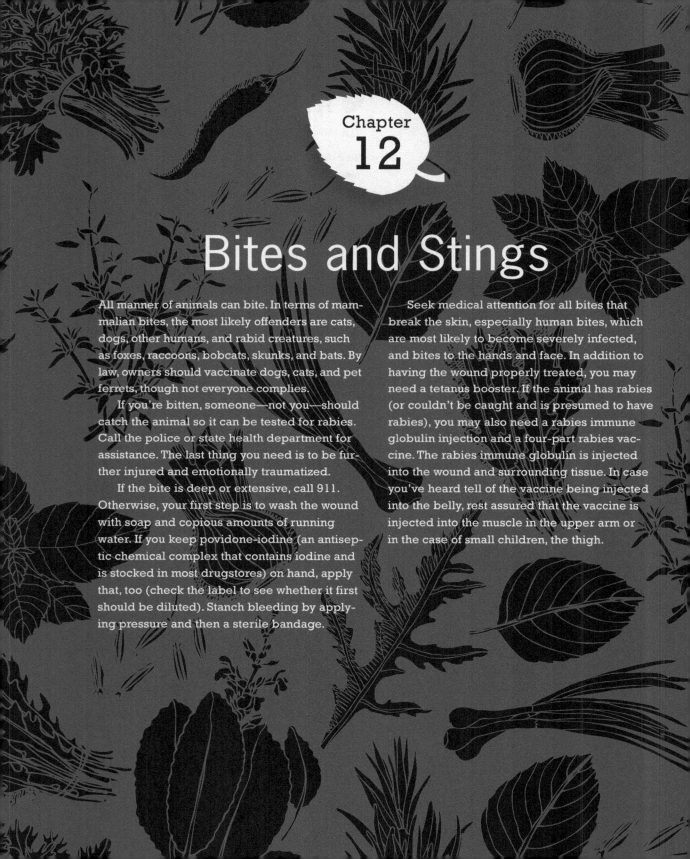

Chapter 12

Bites and Stings

All manner of animals can bite. In terms of mammalian bites, the most likely offenders are cats, dogs, other humans, and rabid creatures, such as foxes, raccoons, bobcats, skunks, and bats. By law, owners should vaccinate dogs, cats, and pet ferrets, though not everyone complies.

If you're bitten, someone—not you—should catch the animal so it can be tested for rabies. Call the police or state health department for assistance. The last thing you need is to be further injured and emotionally traumatized.

If the bite is deep or extensive, call 911. Otherwise, your first step is to wash the wound with soap and copious amounts of running water. If you keep povidone-iodine (an antiseptic chemical complex that contains iodine and is stocked in most drugstores) on hand, apply that, too (check the label to see whether it first should be diluted). Stanch bleeding by applying pressure and then a sterile bandage.

Seek medical attention for all bites that break the skin, especially human bites, which are most likely to become severely infected, and bites to the hands and face. In addition to having the wound properly treated, you may need a tetanus booster. If the animal has rabies (or couldn't be caught and is presumed to have rabies), you may also need a rabies immune globulin injection and a four-part rabies vaccine. The rabies immune globulin is injected into the wound and surrounding tissue. In case you've heard tell of the vaccine being injected into the belly, rest assured that the vaccine is injected into the muscle in the upper arm or in the case of small children, the thigh.

To prevent getting bitten, follow these guidelines:

- Any wild animal that approaches you is behaving aberrantly. Do not lapse into Disney-esque romanticism and try to pet it.

- Teach children how to behave around domesticated animals. Those rules include the following:
  - Don't try to touch strange pets unless the owner offers assurance that the animal is friendly.
  - Don't stick your hand over neighbors' fences and into car windows to pet a dog. That dog may feel territorial of its space.
  - Handle cats gently. Don't try to restrain them.
  - Don't pet dogs that are eating, sleeping, or tending puppies—not unless you know that the dog doesn't mind.
  - Let dogs new to you sniff your hand before you try to pet them.
  - Teach children not to run up to dogs, then run away screaming.
  - If an aggressive-looking dog (wild or domestic) approaches, avoid eye contact and stand still. If the dog knocks you down, curl into a ball to protect your face and belly.

Animal Bites

Tick bites are another problem because they can carry disease-causing bacteria. If you live in the Northeast, Midwest, or Southeast and have a tick bite, contact your doctor about prophylactic antibiotics against Lyme disease. If you live in the Rocky Mountains or eastern United States, look for signs of Rocky Mountain spotted fever (fever, muscle pain, headache, abdominal pain, and rash). For more information about ticks, go to the Centers for Disease Control and Prevention website at www.cdc.gov/ticks/.

The bites of venomous snakes are among the more feared as the consequences can be serious. (Before antivenom was developed, one in ten people bitten by coral snakes died.) However, all snakes play useful roles in nature, and many aren't venomous. Most of the time, bites occur because humans (or their dogs) have startled, handled, or harassed the animals. The trick is to avoid inadvertently threatening a snake because you simply didn't see it—an easy mistake to make when snakes blend into the landscape. If you're hiking in venomous snake habitat, wear boots and pants. The pants won't stop the fangs, but the snake may bite the fabric rather than you.

If you're bitten, call 911. Lie calm and still. Remember that few people die of venomous snakebites. (Children and elders are most at risk.) Immobilize the bitten limb and try to keep it below the level of the heart to slow the spread of venom through your circulatory system. Remove jewelry. Do not apply ice or a tourniquet, incise the bite, or attempt to suck out the venom. Those techniques aren't effective and can cause tissue damage. At the hospital, you may be given antivenom, depending upon the type of snake.

Note: Attempting to capture a venomous snake can put you or others at risk. It's usually enough to describe the snake to hospital staff.

Despite their small size, venomous spiders can cause a surprising amount of suffering. In fact, the venom of a female black widow is fifteen times more potent than that from a rattlesnake. Fatalities, however, are rare. As with snakebites, small children and elders are most at risk for adverse outcomes. And as with snakes, most spiders are benign and beneficial to the environment. Two venomous spiders common in the United States are black widow spiders (black with a red hourglass shape on the underside of the abdomen) and brown recluse spiders (brown with a violin shape on the top of the thorax).

Spiders don't hunt humans. They bite when you disturb them. Symptoms of black widow bites include a sharp pain and redness at the site of the bite, followed by sweating, weakness, muscle cramps (especially in the abdominal wall), chest tightness, nausea, and vomiting.

Lifestyle Tip

To avoid bee stings, don't wear brightly colored or pastel clothing and avoid wearing perfumes. (You don't want to look or smell like a flower.) When cooking outdoors, watch out for yellow jackets; they're especially attracted by the smells.

Brown recluse spider bites sting. The area first turns red. Pain intensifies and itching becomes severe. Subsequent symptoms include fever, chills, nausea, vomiting, joint pain, a rash, and possibly blood in the urine. Sometimes the bite area blisters and ulcerates. One case was reported of the victim developing heart problems after being infected by the venom.

If you can safely capture the spider, do so. A specimen will ensure positive identification at the hospital. Right after being bitten, wash with soap and cool (not hot) water, apply ice, elevate the area above the heart, lie still, and have someone take you to the doctor or emergency room. Treatment may include pain medication, tetanus immunization, and antihistamines (for the itching of a brown recluse spider). Brown recluse spider bites may necessitate follow-up appointments for wound care.

Insect Stings

In the United States, scorpions inhabit the Southwestern desert. A scorpion's stinger lies at the end of its tail, which it flicks over its head. Most species aren't dangerous to humans, but some (for example, the bark scorpion) have venom strong enough to make you ill. Symptoms include local pain, swelling, itching, and changes in the skin's color, hives, as well as sweating, nausea, vomiting, diarrhea, stomach pain, anxiety, drowsiness, faintness, muscle twitching, blurred vision, numbness of the tongue, drooling, rapid heart rate, seizures, and unconsciousness.

If you are stung, call your doctor. Home treatment is the same as for spider bites. Severe symptoms require a visit to the emergency room. Children are most at risk for severe reactions. Antivenin exists for particular scorpion species.

Bees don't sting unless threatened, probably because they die after they do. Wasps (which include paper wasps, hornets, and yellow jackets) may require only minimal provocation. Fire ants also sting.

Symptoms are usually relatively mild and include pain, redness, local swelling, itching, and burning. Multiple stings can cause fever and drowsiness. For people allergic to bee venom, an anaphylactic reaction can ensue. This life-threatening allergic reaction leads to hives; nausea, vomiting, and dizziness; swelling of lips, mouth, and respiratory linings; runny nose, wheezing, respiratory distress, and, potentially, loss of consciousness.

Your first (and typically instinctive) step is to move away from the bees, wasps, or ants. Only honeybees leave behind their stinger. Immediately, scrape or flick off the stinger with your nail or a credit card. Some say to avoid squeezing the base, which releases more venom. Other experts say speed is more important.

People allergic to bee venom should carry an epinephrine auto-injector (EpiPen) and use it immediately. If an EpiPen isn't available, call 911. Don't wait for symptoms to develop. If you have an antihistamine on hand, take it. People with multiple stings may also need emergency treatment, especially if stung inside the mouth.

History

Legends abound in the lore of bites and stings: Cleopatra died from the bite of an asp; scorpion bites are fatal; tarantulas' eyes turn red before they leap up to attack you; and sidewinder rattlesnakes can sidewind faster than a human can run. All are untrue. (An asp *probably* was not the cause of Cleopatra's death, according to a 2010 biography by Stacy Schiff.)

But, of course, bites and stings are real—and humans have applied various remedies down through the ages. First-century Greek physician Dioscorides and Roman naturalist Pliny the Elder recommended lemon balm *(Melissa officinalis)* for the bites of "venomous beasts" and "the stings of scorpions." Calendula *(C. officinalis)* was also used medicinally in ancient Rome to treat scorpion bites. The Plains Indians used purple coneflower *(Echinacea purpurea, E. angustifolia, E. pallida)* as a universal application for the bites and stings of many creeping, crawling, and leaping bugs. The Dakota and Winnebago peoples applied the crushed bulbs of wild onions *(Allium spp.)* and garlic *(Allium sativum)*.

Today, herbalists still recommend calendula lotions and creams for bites and stings and echinacea to treat wounds. Most bites are not serious, but many require medical attention and sometimes even emergency care. Read on for remedies, tips, and when to call the doctor.

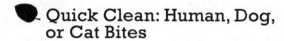

Quick Clean: Human, Dog, or Cat Bites

When you're bitten, cleaning is just part of the care; follow all the important steps below.

Warm water
Soap
Antibacterial ointment

PREPARATION AND USE:

With a clean cloth, apply direct pressure to stop the bleeding. Once the bleeding slows, rinse the wound with running water (by holding the area under the tap). Then dip a second clean cloth into the warm water, rub with soap, and clean the wound thoroughly. Rinse again. Pat dry.

Apply an antibacterial ointment and cover the wound with a sterile bandage. Clean the wound and change the bandage every day—sooner if it gets dirty, wet, or bloody.

Next, call your doctor's office to find out whether your injury warrants prompt medical treatment. Cat bites count as puncture wounds, which means they're at higher risk for becoming infected. You also want to check that your tetanus shot is up to date. If any wound is deep (or 10 to 15 minutes of steady pressure doesn't stop the bleeding), proceed to the emergency room. In the event of severe injury, call 911.

YIELD: 1 APPLICATION

❓ How it works: *Running water flushes out microbes. Washing with soap and water and applying an antibacterial ointment further reduce the risk of subsequent infection.*

Unstick the Tick

Make a thorough body search after a summer walk in the woods—and have the items below handy. If bitten, follow the instructions.

Soap and water
Antibiotic ointment

PREPARATION AND USE:

With tweezers, carefully grasp the tick as close to your skin as possible. Gently pull until the tick comes free (do not twist or jerk, as the head may break off and remain embedded). Wash thoroughly, pat dry, and apply the antibiotic ointment. Save the tick in a resealable plastic bag and place in the freezer, in case medical staff later request it for identification. If mouthparts remain behind, see your doctor.

Wash your hands well and clean the tweezers to disinfect from the tick.

YIELD: 1 APPLICATION

❓ How it works: *Careful removal of the tick, immediate cleansing, and application of antibiotic ointment will prevent topical infection. Prompt removal of the tick can reduce the risk of transmission of such diseases as Lyme disease.*

Bee Stinger Removal

Don't let that venom sink in!

Ice cube
Warm water
Soap

PREPARATION AND USE:
As quickly as possible, remove the stinger by gently scraping it off with your fingernail, a credit card, or another stiff object. Grasp an ice cube and rub it briskly over the stung area for a full minute. Wash with warm water and soap. If you're stung on the arm, remove rings and bracelets before swelling occurs.

YIELD: 1 APPLICATION

❷ How it works: *A bee usually leaves behind a sac of venom and a stinger. Removing it immediately stops more venom from entering. Cleansing the site wards off infection. Keep the area clean during the healing process, which may take up to five days.*

❶ Warning: *Do not pinch or pull the stinger; this can inject more venom.*

◖ Fight the Swelling

Use this method for any insect sting; it applies to more than a bee or wasp sting. Before using, remove the stinger and cleanse the area with soap and water.

Crushed ice

PREPARATION AND USE:
Fill a resealable plastic bag with the ice and wrap it in a clean cloth. Apply to the site and then elevate the area. Remove the ice pack after 15 to 20 minutes. Repeat hourly as needed.

YIELD: 1 APPLICATION

❷ How it works: *Ice numbs the area and arrests inflammation caused by the poison.*

Lifestyle Tip

For bites from fire ants, try a dab of Vicks VapoRub on the sting area to relieve pain and itching.

Bee-lieve the Relief

College student Candice McCay keeps bees in Denver. She and her husband find this recipe helpful in relieving pain and swelling.

Water
5 drops lavender essential oil

PREPARATION AND USE:
Wet a washcloth with water and wring out the excess moisture. Dot on the lavender essential oil. Seal the washcloth in a resealable freezer bag and store in the freezer at the beginning of bee season. It will be good for the summer months. Replace it with a fresh one when it's used.

If you're stung, remove the cloth from the bag and apply it directly to the area.

YIELD: 1 APPLICATION

❷ How it works: *Ice reduces swelling and relieves pain. Lavender is anti-inflammatory, analgesic, and calming.*

De-Itcher

This remedy is a quick and easy fix for bee and fire ant stings.

1 teaspoon (4.6 g) baking soda
3 drops lavender essential oil
Water

PREPARATION AND USE:
Put the baking soda in your palm. Add the lavender essential oil and enough water to form a paste. Plaster the paste over the sting site, covering the swelling. After 30 minutes, rinse off the paste. Reapply as needed.

YIELD: 1 APPLICATION

❷ How it works: *Bee and fire ant stings are acidic, though the venom contains other chemicals at well. The baking soda paste may help neutralize the acidic venom. As noted above, lavender decreases inflammation, pain, and anxiety.*

Sting Relief

1 teaspoon (5 ml) vinegar or fresh lemon juice

PREPARATION AND USE:
Soak a cotton ball with the vinegar and apply to the sting area or drip lemon juice directly onto the area.

YIELD: 1 APPLICATION

❷ How it works: *Venom contains a mix of chemicals. Wasp stings are primarily alkaline. Theoretically, you can neutralize the venom with an acidic solution, such as apple cider vinegar or lemon juice. Some experts, however, doubt the efficacy. It may be worth a try. If the lemon juice makes the area sting more, wash it away.*

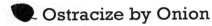 ## Ostracize by Onion

1 teaspoon (3 g) chopped onion

PREPARATION AND USE:

After removing the stinger, carefully place the chopped onion on the affected area. Cover the onion with gauze and secure with tape. Keep it in place from 20 minutes to an hour or more until the pain and swelling subside. Rinse thoroughly after you remove it.

YIELD: 1 APPLICATION

❓ **How it works:** *Freshly cut onions contain enzymes that help break down inflammation-causing compounds in a sting. Onion is anti-septic. The onion should not sting but instead alleviate the pain. If it does sting, remove it immediately.*

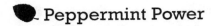 ## Peppermint Power

1 drop peppermint essential oil

PREPARATION AND USE:

Let the peppermint essential oil fall onto the area of an ant bite or wasp or bee sting. (For bee stings, remove the stinger first.) Gently massage into the skin.

YIELD: 1 APPLICATION

❓ **How it works:** *Peppermint oil is cooling and analgesic.*

Honey Fix for Stings or Bites

This remedy is appropriate for any bite or sting that doesn't require emergency medical attention.

1 teaspoon (7 g) honey

PREPARATION AND USE:

Apply the honey to the bite site so it is fully covered. Leave in place for 30 minutes and then rinse. Reapply as needed.

YIELD: 1 APPLICATION

❓ **How it works:** *Honey is an ancient wound healer that has recently garnered scientific support for its antibacterial and anti-inflammatory effects. Studies show it improves the healing of cuts, scrapes, burns, and other wounds.*

Lifestyle Tip

To ward off spiders and insects:

- **Clear away debris and clutter from around your house.**
- **Take care when gathering wood and rummaging in crawl spaces, sheds, and other outbuildings.**
- **Seal cracks and crevices in your house.**
- **Put up screens.**

🫚 Plantain the Pain

Herbalists swear by fresh leaf poultices for relieving insect stings and bites and superficial wounds. They call the plant "backyard Band-Aid." This recipe uses the leaves of a plantain (Plantago species), a weed found in most fields.

5 to 10 plantain leaves

PREPARATION AND USE:
Tear the leaves in half and mash them between your fingers to create a pulp and release the tannin juices. Apply the pulp and juice to the sting area for about 30 seconds. Repeat as needed.

YIELD: 1 APPLICATION

❷ How it works: *The leaf provides an immediate outdoor remedy. It contains substances that are soothing, pain-relieving, and astringent. A 2012 test-tube study showed that leaf extracts help heal scratches in a layer of cells taken from the mouth. (This test, called a scratch assay, mimics wound closure.)*

🫚 Stingray Detox

Just off the shore of Cozumel in the Caribbean, my husband met a small stingray. A quick stab left his hand inflamed and swollen. Fortunately, the stinger did not break off. This remedy helped—the swelling went down within an hour and gradually subsided completely, leaving only a small red mark. ~ BBG

Soap and water, for cleansing
Hot tap water

PREPARATION AND USE:
If the sting is on the hand, immediately remove any rings that can become stuck by the swelling. Wash the area thoroughly with soap and water, and then immerse the poisoned body part in tap water that is as hot as you can stand it without burning the skin. Soak for 30 to 90 minutes until the swelling begins to recede. Reheat the water to the highest temperature endurable when it begins to cool.

YIELD: 1 APPLICATION

❷ How it works: *Researchers studying the effects of marine creature stings have found that immersion in hot water helps relieve the pain. Some reports suggest that marine venoms consist of proteins and enzymes that may become deactivated at temperatures above 122°F (50°C).*

❶ Warning: *This wound came from a small stingray. Stingray envenomation is rarely fatal. However, some stinging water creatures do deliver life-threatening venom.*

Note: This recipe is for a small, barely bleeding sting that does not have a broken stinger in it. If a stinger remains in the wound, only attempt to remove it carefully with tweezers; otherwise, the poison may spread. If it is bleeding profusely, apply pressure. Seek medical attention immediately.

When to Call the Doctor

CALL 911 IF:

- *You sustain a severe animal bite.*

- *A venomous snake bites you.*

- *You receive a bee sting and know you're allergic. Carry your EpiPen (epinephrine auto-injector) everywhere. After you use it, call 911 anyway, in case you need further treatment. If your EpiPen isn't available, call 911 immediately. Don't wait for symptoms to occur.*

- *Signs of anaphylaxis (a potentially life-threatening allergic reaction) develop as evidenced by:*

  - *difficulty breathing or wheezing*
  - *swollen tongue*
  - *throat tightness, hoarseness, or trouble speaking*
  - *wheezing or difficulty breathing*
  - *nausea, abdominal pain, or vomiting*
  - *rapid pulse*
  - *hives and itching*
  - *anxiety or dizziness*
  - *loss of consciousness*

CALL YOUR DOCTOR IF:

- *A human or nonhuman animal bite breaks the skin.*

- *You develop fever, pain, muscle cramps, stomach upset, or other severe symptoms after a spider bite.*

- *A scorpion stings you.*

- *A tick bites you in a Lyme disease region.*

- *You can't remove all of the tick.*

- *You develop a rash, headache, fever, or joint and muscle aches after a tick bite. (Symptoms of Rocky Mountain spotted fever typically develop within five to ten days of a bite. Symptoms of Lyme disease usually develop within three to fourteen days, though in some cases may not occur for months. Keep in mind that many people are not aware of ever having a tick bite.)*

- *You receive multiple bee or wasp stings, especially if stings occur inside your mouth.*

- *A bite or sting becomes infected, as evidenced by redness, warmth, swelling, and drainage of pus from the area, as well as fever.*

Chapter 13

Bladder Health

If you're a woman, chances are fifty-fifty that you've had at least one episode of cystitis, better known as a bladder infection. Urinary tract infections, or UTIs (infection anywhere along the urinary system from the kidney to the urethra), are the most common bacterial infections in women. Within the category of UTIs, bladder infections top the list—so much so that people use UTI and bladder infection interchangeably.

The reason such infections are predominantly a female affliction has to do with relative shortness of the urethra (the tube that transports fluids from the kidneys to the genitals for removal). Bowel bacteria such as *E. coli*, the usual cause of UTIs, simply don't need to travel far to reach the bladder. And bacteria are, the most common cause of acute bladder infections.

Classic symptoms include burning with urination, increased frequency of urination, an urgent need to urinate (even if the bladder isn't very full), nighttime urination, and discomfort above the pubic bone. The urine may be cloudy and foul smelling. Previously toilet-trained children may have "accidents." Young children may have only nonspecific symptoms, such as a mild fever, irritability, poor feeding, and restless sleep.

At the doctor's office, you'll be asked to provide a clean midstream urine sample. Because small children can't usually provide an uncontaminated urine sample, doctors typically insert a catheter into their bladder or a needle through the skin of the lower abdomen into the bladder. A urine sample is taken and then analyzed. If bacteria are present, oral antibiotics are prescribed.

Antibiotics not only quickly stamp out the infection but prevent the bacteria from ascending to the kidneys. Kidney infection (pyelonephritis) is serious. Symptoms include flank pain, fever, and chills. It can scar the kidneys, leading to problems such as high blood pressure and kidney failure. Treatment often requires hospitalization, with intravenous fluids and antibiotics.

After a bladder infection, your doctor will probably ask you to return for a repeat urine culture to make sure no bacteria survived. Boys younger than twelve months of age with a first-time infection and little girls with more than one infection usually undergo tests to check for anatomical abnormalities that would lead to repeated infection and kidney damage.

If you have recurrent bladder infections, you can do a number of things to reduce your risk of recurrence. For example:

- Drink lots of water—drink at least eight glasses a day, more if you live in a dry or hot environment or have been exercising. Thirst is a sign you need more fluid. Obey that urge.

- Urinate whenever you feel the urge; don't "hold it." Urination helps flush out any bacteria before they have a chance to stick to the bladder lining.

- Always wipe from front to back. Teach your children to do the same.

- Avoid constipation because it can trigger a UTI.

- Avoid irritants to the genital area, such as bubble baths, scented soaps, and deodorizing sprays. Such agents can inflame the urethra and vagina, creating symptoms that mimic a bladder infection.

- Don't douche. In general, douching undermines vaginal health. It also increases the risk of UTIs.

- Urinate after having sex. (Intercourse can facilitate the movement of bacteria into the urethra and bladder.)

- If you're using spermicidal gels with or without a diaphragm, ask your doctor whether a different contraceptive might be a better choice for you.

History

As early as 1550 BCE, the Egyptians described the inflammation of urinary tract infections as "sending forth heat from the bladder." From then until the 1930s, when antibiotics became available, bleeding (both through leeches and cupping—a Chinese medicine procedure that applies suction to the skin without actual blood loss), bed rest, and herbs were prescribed to treat UTIs.

One of the most effective of the herbal treatments was the use of uva ursi, or bearberry (*Arctostaphylos uva-ursi*). A Welsh herbalist from the 1200s recommended the use of uva ursi for kidney and bladder problems. Native Americans also used uva ursi leaves to treat inflammation of the bladder and urinary tract. In modern herbal treatment, uva ursi is still used for its antibacterial properties. Goldenseal (*Hydrastis canadensis*) and buchu (*Agathosma betulina*, synonym *Barosma betulina*) have also been used historically to combat bladder infections. Although none of these herbs are appropriate for long-term use to prevent infection, herbalists often recommend such herbs to nip beginning bladder infections in the bud.

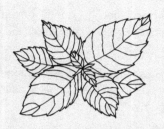

Spotlight: **Cranberries and Cousins**

Many beautiful, tasty, health-promoting berries are in the *Vaccinium* genus, including cranberry, blueberry, bilberry, lingonberry, and huckleberry. These shrubby, acidic-soil-loving plants belong to the heath family. Their berries contain a number of chemicals, including *polysaccharides* (complex sugars) and *anthocyanidins*, which are a type of flavonoid responsible for the berries' deep blue and red hues.

Cranberry is most famous for its ability to reduce recurrent bladder infections. An analysis of ten studies found that juice or concentrated extracts lower the likelihood of women's urinary tract infections by 35 percent. Chemical constituents in cranberries wrap around *Escherichia coli (E. coli)*, the bacterium most often infecting the bladder. This coating prevents the bacteria from binding to the bladder's lining. Urination flushes out those feckless bugs. However, if bacteria have already attached themselves to bladder cells, cranberry doesn't kill them. That's why the juice prevents but doesn't seem effective in treating such infections.

Preliminary research suggests that the same mechanism may help prevent gum and stomach infections involving *Helicobacter pylori* (the bacterium that also causes ulcers). Cranberry's chemicals are anti-inflammatory, antioxidant, antiplatelet (to prevent clotting within blood vessels), and anticancer.

European native bilberry extracts improve eye damage (retinopathy) caused by diabetes and high blood pressure. Other flavonoids, aside from anthocyanidins, include resveratrol (a substance trumpeted as contributing to the benefits of red wine and red grape juice) and quercetin. A recent study showed that bilberry improved ulcerative colitis.

Whereas bilberry is blue all the way through, blueberry's inner fruit is white. Blueberry is native to North America. It's also rich in anthocyanidins, resveratrol, quercetin, and other flavonoids, as well as fiber and vitamin C. The berries are anti-inflammatory and antioxidant. Blueberry has a number of antidiabetes actions and improves the response of tissues to insulin. The berries also protect the cardiovascular system. Blueberry discourages food-borne disease-causing bacteria such as *E. coli* and *Salmonella*. A study showed that blueberries may improve arterial function. In fact, all of these berries protect and strengthen arteries and veins.

❗ *Before recommending recipes for bladder health, we'd like to stress the importance of proper medical treatment of UTIs. These remedies are not intended as a replacement for antibiotic treatment. They may, however, help prevent recurrent infections.*

🍷 Cranberry Mocktail

1 cup (235 ml) unsweetened cranberry juice
¾ cup (175 ml) carbonated (sparkling) water
2 lemon slices
2 teaspoons (14 g) honey

PREPARATION AND USE:
Mix together all the ingredients. Aim to drink both servings of this cocktail in one day.

YIELD: 2 SERVINGS

Recipe Variation: Substitute apple juice or sparkling cider for the carbonated water and omit the honey.

❓ How it works: *Research studies show that cranberry juice and concentrated cranberry tablets reduce UTI recurrences. Also, the tannins that create the characteristic mouth-puckering effect of cranberries are also astringent in the urinary system. (Astringents tighten tissues and are thought to reduce surface irritation and inflammation. Cranberry is acidic, but it takes a lot of volume to acidify the urine enough to kill bacteria.)*

Note: The daily volume of cranberry juice used in studies ranges from 2 tablespoons (30 ml) to 1 cup (235 ml) of pure cranberry juice. Higher doses can loosen stools. If you find you can't stomach cranberry juice, try taking concentrated cranberry in capsule form as directed on the label. Be aware that commercially prepared cranberry juice drinks contain added water and sugar.

Do not combine cranberry with the blood-thinning medication warfarin (Coumadin) without first discussing with your doctor. Case reports suggest cranberry may augment the effect of Coumadin, further reducing the ability of blood to clot. However, the problem has not been detected in clinical trials.

🫐 Beneficial Blueberry Smoothie

1 cup (230 g) plain yogurt
½ cup (75 g) blueberries
½ cup (120 ml) "crabapple" juice (cranberry juice and apple juice combined)

PREPARATION AND USE:
Mix all the ingredients in a blender. Enjoy.

YIELD: 1 SERVING

❓ How it works: *Blueberries belong to the same plant family as cranberries. They, too, contain flavonoids that inhibit the adhesion of bacteria to bodily surfaces. The yogurt contains beneficial bacteria (probiotics) that can help restore normal bowel bacteria if you've taken antibiotics to treat a UTI. However, the research is inconclusive as to whether probiotics (taken by mouth or used intravaginally) help prevent recurrent cystitis.*

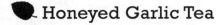 Honeyed Garlic Tea

2 cups (475 ml) water
4 garlic cloves
1 to 2 teaspoons (7 to 14 g) honey

PREPARATION AND USE:

Bring the water to a boil in a saucepan.
Crush the garlic cloves and put in a mug (consider placing the crushed garlic inside a muslin bag or mesh tea ball). Pour the boiled water over the garlic. Cover the mug with a saucer. Let it steep for 10 to 15 minutes. Remove the garlic, add the honey, and drink.

YIELD: 1 SERVING

❓ **How it works:** *Garlic is active against* E. coli *and other bacteria that can cause UTIs.*

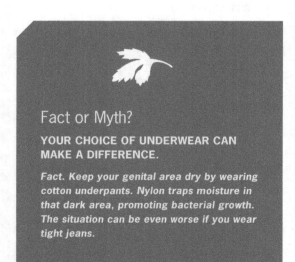

Fact or Myth?

YOUR CHOICE OF UNDERWEAR CAN MAKE A DIFFERENCE.

Fact. Keep your genital area dry by wearing cotton underpants. Nylon traps moisture in that dark area, promoting bacterial growth. The situation can be even worse if you wear tight jeans.

Nutrient-Rich Dandelion Tea

If in season, pick spring dandelion leaves—as long as they're not exposed to pesticides or growing near a road. Bundle and hang to dry in a warm, dim place. Once dry to the touch, crumble the leaves; place in a clean, dry jar; and store in the cupboard. You may also be able to find them dried or fresh at a natural food store.

1 quart (946 ml) water
3 tablespoons (4.5 g) dried, chopped dandelion leaves
1 teaspoon (0.5 g) chopped dried peppermint leaves, or 2 teaspoons (4 g) fresh, chopped
Honey, as needed

PREPARATION AND USE:

Bring the water to a boil in a saucepan. Turn off the heat and add the dandelion and peppermint. Cover and steep for 20 minutes. Strain. Sweeten with honey to taste. Drink throughout the day.

YIELD: 4 SERVINGS

❓ **How it works:** *Dandelion is nutrient-rich and gently increases urine output. You can also enjoy the tender greens in salads, steamed, or sautéed. Peppermint is antispasmodic and also tastes pleasant.*

Lifestyle Tip

Use warmth. Fill a hot water bottle or turn on a heating pad and place it over your lower abdomen. Heat improves blood flow, relaxes muscles, and helps relieve discomfort from a bladder infection.

Yogurt-Berry Ice

This delicious dessert is smooth and creamy and delivers friendly bacteria to your system. For a drinkable smoothie version, see the variation below.

2 cups (about 200 g) frozen mixed berries, or ⅔ bag (16-ounces, or 455 g)
½ cup (115 g) plain yogurt
3 tablespoons (60 g) honey
⅛ teaspoon almond extract

PREPARATION AND USE:

Allow the berries to thaw for 7 to 10 minutes. Pour into a blender or processor and grind until the fruit pieces look like shaved ice. While the blender is running, add the yogurt, honey, and almond extract. Continue blending until the mixture is creamy.

Eat immediately, as the texture will change when refrozen.

YIELD: 4 SERVINGS

Recipe Variation: For drinkable smoothies, add ½ cup (120 ml) of almond milk.

❷ How it works: *Antibiotics effectively treat UTIs. However, they also kill some of the normal, friendly bacteria in the bowel. Probiotics, taken in supplement form, help recolonize normal bacteria and prevent side effects such as diarrhea. Yogurt and other fermented foods, which contain beneficial bacteria, may also help.*

Lifestyle Tip

Try employing essential oils for relief from UTIs. Massage a couple drops of lavender essential oil into the skin above the pubic bone and then apply warmth to help relieve any discomfort.

When Simple Doesn't Work

If you have recurring infections, you may want to see a urologist. He or she may prescribe antibiotics for a specific event, or a low dose of antibiotics over an extended time period, which can help avoid repeat infections. Also, you may want to purchase an over-the-counter, in-home test kit that can help you determine whether you need to call the doctor.

Soothing Sitz Bath

If using oats for this recipe, be sure to put them in a coffee mill and grind them to a powder; otherwise, they'll clog the drain.

2 to 3 cups (576 to 864 g) salt(442 to 663 g), baking soda, or (160 to 240 g)colloidal oatmeal

PREPARATION AND USE:

Fill your bathtub with water as warm as you can stand it. Pour in the salt, baking soda, or oatmeal and disperse. Soak for at least 30 minutes.

YIELD: 1 APPLICATION

Recipe Variation: You can also use 2 to 3 cups (475 to 700 ml) of vinegar, but don't combine it with baking soda, or you'll have a fizzy reaction.

❷ **How it works:** *The warmth of the water with the soothing ingredients helps relax the urethra. Baking soda and salt can soothe irritated membranes. Oatmeal has anti-inflammatory properties and promotes wound healing. Vinegar, which you can also add, is mildly acidic and helps relieve irritation of the vagina and urethra.*

Note: Clean your feet before sitting in the tub so you do not introduce new bacteria.

Encourage children who have trouble urinating because of pain to go ahead and squat in the water and let it go. Then have them step out of the tub immediately.

When to Call the Doctor

Call during office hours if:

- *Your symptoms are consistent with a bladder infection.*

- *Antibiotics haven't brought relief after twenty-four hours.*

Seek urgent medical care if:

- *You're pregnant and think you have a UTI.*

- *You have blood in your urine.*

- *You develop additional symptoms, such as flank pain, fever, chills, nausea, and vomiting.*

- *You have diabetes or an immune deficiency syndrome (e.g., AIDS) with new signs of a UTI.*

Chapter 14

Body Odor

Aromatic appeal is, to some extent, subjective. The sense of smell is primal, mysterious, and deeply personal. Compared to that of most other mammals, our olfactory perception is dull. Yet, it remains important for survival. It helps us detect smoke, identify whether food has gone bad, and determine whether we or our clothes need washing.

Odor receptors in the nose connect swiftly to deep and ancient parts of the brain, including those involved in strong emotions and memory formation and retrieval. Mothers and babies of all mammalian species recognize one another by scent. Scent figures in our choice of a mate. In fact, body odors provide subconscious information about a potential mate's genetic compatibility, social status, and reproductive vigor. Fluctuations in female hormones temper a woman's olfactory sensitivity.

What creates a person's signature aroma? A lot of things: diet, overall state of health, age, emotional state, levels of certain hormones, hygiene, and some medications. Some diseases create characteristic chemicals detectable on skin and in breath. Examples of illnesses that alter skin smells include infectious diseases (for example, tuberculosis and scarlet fever), scurvy (vitamin C deficiency), and schizophrenia.

Americans tend to be particularly preoccupied with body odor. The armpits are the usual source. Armpit sweat, which is richer in proteins and fats than secretions from the sweat glands covering most of your skin, doesn't stink until bacteria that normally colonize your skin break down chemicals in sweat into acids. What can you do?

- Bathe regularly, paying special attention to your armpits and bottom. You don't need to use harsh antibacterial soaps. In fact, some of the antibacterial chemicals (e.g., triclosan) aren't good for you or the environment. Use a mild soap with a natural (plant-derived) fragrance.

- Wear natural fabrics. These allow your sweat to evaporate freely. It's when your armpits are hot, sweaty, and lacking in oxygen that odor-causing bacteria thrive. In winter, you can't beat wool for warm and wicking action.

- Eat more fruits and vegetables. Vegetarians are said to smell sweeter than people who eat a lot of meat.

- Harness the antibacterial and aromatic properties of plant essential oils. See the recipes throughout this chapter.

History

Once upon a time, we lived in caves and didn't worry about body odor. In fact, anthropologists think our smelly selves might have protected us from animals who didn't fancy a really stinky dinner. Fast-forward a few eons and the ancient Egyptians were figuring out how to mask bodily odors. Cleopatra and her countrymen took perfumed baths and used incense, carob, and porridge as deodorants. Egyptian women even put scented wax in their hair—its perfume releasing slowly as the wax melted.

The Romans perfumed not only themselves and their clothes but their horses and pets as well. The Elizabethans were more creative: Lovers exchanged love apples. "A woman would keep a peeled apple in her armpit until it was saturated with her sweat and then give it to her sweetheart," according to *The Naked Woman* by Desmond Morris. At the same time, all of Christendom dating back to about the fourth century up through the Puritans deemed bathing bad—because you had to get naked to take a bath.

So, except for the privileged few who could afford perfumes, most people exuded their own particular odors until the late nineteenth century, when Mum, the first trademarked deodorant, went on the market. A few centuries later, Madison Avenue still controls our perception that we must deodorize ourselves. Contrary to the sensual examples of Elizabethan love apples and a few cultures that sniff each other in greeting, most Americans use deodorant.

Lifestyle Tip

Fill an empty box of your favorite scented powder with baking soda, a natural odor eliminator. Use the puff to apply the newly scented baking soda to underarms.

RECIPES TO REDUCE BODY ODOR

 ### Take a Powder

Using just two pantry ingredients, this recipe is quick, easy, and effective. Essential oils add sweetness to this natural remedy.

¼ **cup (55 g) baking soda**
¼ **cup (32 g) cornstarch**

PREPARATION AND USE:
Mix the baking soda and cornstarch together in a small glass dish. Apply to underarms with a clean makeup pad. Apply to feet and the insides of shoes to sop up foot odors.

YIELD: MULTIPLE APPLICATIONS

Recipe Variation: Add 10 to 12 drops of lavender or another favorite essential oil per ½ cup (87 g) of the mixture. Drop the oil into a bowl, pour the powder mixture into a sieve, and shake it into the oil, gradually mixing the two to blend.

❓ How it works: *Baking soda is a natural odor eliminator. Cornstarch absorbs excess moisture.*

❗ Warning: *Be careful not to inhale the particles.*

Coconut Tea Tree Deodorizer

This recipe, used with permission from Rachel Hoff of Dog Island Farm, an urban farm northeast of San Francisco, is easy to make and safe for you and the environment.

2 tablespoons (28 g) virgin coconut oil
1 tablespoon (14 g) grated beeswax
8 drops tea tree essential oil
2 tablespoons (28 g) baking soda
2 tablespoons (16 g) cornstarch

PREPARATION AND USE:

In a saucepan over low heat, melt the coconut oil and beeswax. (Alternatively, you can use the double-boiler method to make sure you don't burn the oil.) Once melted, remove from the heat. Immediately add the essential oil, baking soda, and cornstarch and stir to combine. (If you wait, the cooling beeswax will harden the oil, making it difficult to mix in the dry ingredients.)

Pour the mixture into a clean, dry, empty push-style deodorant container (recycle a used one). Use a spatula or butter knife to pack in the mixture and smooth over the top.

YIELD: ENOUGH FOR 1 MEDIUM-SIZE DEODORANT CONTAINER

❓ How it works: *Virgin coconut oil is antibacterial and an emollient. Tea tree oil is antimicrobial. Beeswax holds the mixture together, smells pleasant, and soothes irritated skin.*

Note: Alternatively, buy beeswax pastilles (pellet-size pieces of beeswax). If you bought a 1-ounce (28 g) piece of beeswax, simply cut it in half. Save the other half for later.

Lavender-Apple Cider Vinegar Wash

A refreshing spray of this underarm elixir has post-shower power.

¼ cup (60 ml) apple cider vinegar
6 drops lavender essential oil

PREPARATION AND USE:

Place the ingredients in a small, clean spray bottle, cap, and shake. Spritz on underarms after a shower or bath.

YIELD: MULTIPLE APPLICATIONS

❓ How it works: *Apple cider vinegar lowers the pH level of the skin (that is, makes the skin more acidic), discouraging bacteria that turn body sweat into body odor. Lavender discourages bacterial growth and adds a scent-ual lift.*

Lifestyle Tip

If you don't do so already, consider shaving your underarms. Hair holds the bacteria that mix with sweat to create body odor. However, we recommend that if you use aluminum-containing antiperspirants, you shave at night and hold off on using the antiperspirant till morning, giving your body overnight to heal tiny nicks. Underarm shaving is a cultural matter and personal decision. More important is to shower at least once a day to wash away bacteria that collect on your skin, as well as on pubic and underarm hair.

◗ Sage Therapy

This freshening agent can be grown year-round in your backyard. Be sure to chop or crush the sage—you want the plants in small pieces to increase their surface area of exposure to the solvent, in this case vinegar.

2 tablespoons (5 g) crushed or chopped
   fresh sage
¼ cup (60 ml) apple cider vinegar

PREPARATION AND USE:

Combine the sage and vinegar in the small, clean jar. Cap and shake the mixture until the sage is thoroughly soaked. Place the mixture in the pantry or cabinet for about a week. (This allows the vinegar to extract the essence of the sage.) When the vinegar smells strongly of sage, the potion is ready.

Strain the mixture through cheesecloth and pour it into a small, clean spray bottle. Spritz your underarms, feet, or other body parts prone to odor.

YIELD: MULTIPLE APPLICATIONS

❷ **How it works:** *Sage has a drying effect and is antimicrobial. Combined with the pH-reducing apple cider vinegar, it makes a perfect elixir for reducing perspiration and body odor.*

◗ Vinegar Spritz

Use your favorite scent or make a new one by trying different essential oils together.

¼ cup (60 ml) white vinegar
12 drops favorite essential oil (eucalyptus,
   rosemary, lemon, lavender, or tea tree)

PREPARATION AND USE:

Mix the vinegar and essential oil(s) of your choice. Pour the mixture into a clean spray bottle, cap it tightly, and shake. Spritz your underarms and all over your body.

YIELD: MULTIPLE APPLICATIONS

❷ **How it works:** *Vinegar is acidic, which inhibits bacterial growth. Essential oils (such as rosemary, eucalyptus, tea tree oil, lemon, and lavender) are antibacterial.*

◗ Essentially Yours

Essential oils not only fight bacteria and microbes, keeping you at your freshest, but they infuse your home with soothing scent.

¼ cup (60 ml) witch hazel
1 tablespoon (15 ml) vodka
10 drops tea tree oil
10 drops lavender essential oil
5 drops eucalyptus essential oil
5 drops sage essential oil

PREPARATION AND USE:

In a clean spray bottle, mix the witch hazel and vodka. Add all the essential oils. Cap and shake the bottle until the ingredients are completely blended. Spritz away at those odiferous body parts.

YIELD: MULTIPLE APPLICATIONS

❷ **How it works:** *Witch hazel is astringent and antiseptic; vodka is antibacterial. Lavender, eucalyptus, and sage essential oils are antibacterial, while tea tree oil is antimicrobial. Sage also has drying properties.*

Aloe Zest

¼ cup (115 g) *Aloe vera* gel
6 drops eucalyptus essential oil
6 drops lavender essential oil

PREPARATION AND USE:

In a small, clean jar, mix the aloe gel with the essential oils, and then shake the jar vigorously until the ingredients are fully blended. With a clean pad or cloth, dab the mixture onto your armpits after showering for a zesty feel and deodorizing action.

YIELD: 4 TO 6 APPLICATIONS

❷ How it works: Aloe vera *is antiseptic and soothing. The essential oils are antibacterial.*

Hydro Solution

1 cup (235 ml) water
1 teaspoon (5 ml) hydrogen peroxide
  (3 percent solution)

PREPARATION AND USE:

Mix the water and hydrogen peroxide. Using a clean washcloth or pad, wipe the solution on your underarms, feet, or groin and feel refreshed.

YIELD: 1 APPLICATION

❷ How it works: *Hydrogen peroxide is antibacterial.*

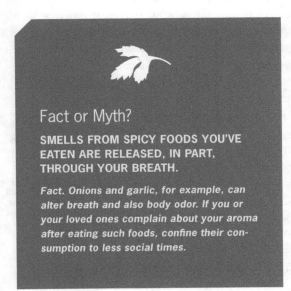

Fact or Myth?

SMELLS FROM SPICY FOODS YOU'VE EATEN ARE RELEASED, IN PART, THROUGH YOUR BREATH.

Fact. Onions and garlic, for example, can alter breath and also body odor. If you or your loved ones complain about your aroma after eating such foods, confine their consumption to less social times.

Lifestyle Tip

Manage stress. As if there weren't already enough reasons to tame stress, now we can add an obscure fact: A person's psychological state affects his or her body odor. You may have noticed that, when nervous, not only do you sweat more, but you also smell worse than after a carefree run on a tropical beach.

In a 2011 study published in the *Journal of Chemical Senses*, researchers had thirteen male volunteers do a benign workout on an exercise machine and participate in a "high rope course." The latter entailed climbing a 21-foot (6.4 m) pole and standing atop this pole. Because the men couldn't see the securing device attached to their back, they literally felt "out on a limb." Next, female volunteers smelled the men's armpit pads. Interestingly, the pads drenched with the sweat during the anxiety of the high rope course induced anxiety in the female sniffers. Sweat from a routine workout had no such effect.

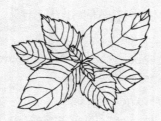

Spotlight: **Antiperspirants**

Underarm antiperspirants contain aluminum salts, which temporarily block sweat gland ducts. Aluminum is also used in the manufacturing of many products (for example, paper, dyes, paints, textiles, cosmetics, and medications). Our bodies absorb the aluminum. Scientists and the public have raised concerns that women who nick their underarms shaving may absorb even more. Aluminum can alter DNA and the binding of estrogen to breast cells. Test-tube studies indicate possible cancer-causing effects.

Some studies have correlated higher levels of aluminum in fluid from the breasts of women with cancer compared to those without it. Others, however, have not found a difference in aluminum between cancerous breast and normal breast tissue.

Further, antiperspirants, deodorants (which mask the stink but don't stop perspiration), and many other personal care products may contain parabens, compounds used as preservatives that have weak estrogen-like effects. (Estrogen stimulates cell division in the breast and other sensitive tissues, raising the risk for cancer.)

However, a review of fifty-nine studies on the link between antiperspirants, deodorants, and breast cancer came up empty. For one, many underarm products didn't contain parabens. For another, analysis of the data didn't show a significant association between aluminum and breast cancer. The American Cancer Society echoes that conclusion. A 2013 study noted that there isn't yet enough evidence to link aluminum exposure to breast cancer, although research will continue to explore the issue. For more information, go to the American Cancer Society website, www.cancer.org, and search for "antiperspirants and cancer."

Aluminum has also been linked to Alzheimer's disease. The metal is a nerve toxin and is found in the amyloid plaques that are characteristic of the disease. However, studies don't correlate aluminum-containing deodorants with Alzheimer's. Plus, these products negligibly raise body levels of aluminum, especially when compared to amounts of the metal in drinking water, toothpaste, antacids, and beverages in aluminum cans. (By the way, crystal deodorants also contain aluminum.)

If you're concerned, a safe bet is to switch to a deodorant (rather than an antiperspirant) that contains plant-derived fragrances. As noted in our recipes, many plant essential oils (which produce these natural fragrances) have antibacterial effects.

Refreshing Bath Fizzie

This recipe comes from one of the staff at a Denver herb store called Apothecary Tinctura. It leaves you smelling clean and feeling refreshed.

¼ to ½ cup (60 to 120 ml) witch hazel
½ cup (115 g) citric acid
1 cup (220 g) baking soda
15 drops eucalyptus essential oil
10 drops bay laurel essential oil

PREPARATION AND USE:

Pour the witch hazel into a small, clean spray bottle. In a small bowl, combine the citric acid and baking soda. Add the essential oils to the powder one drop at a time, stirring constantly to distribute evenly. Pick up the mixture in your hands and spritz two times with witch hazel. Keep shaping and spritzing the material with your hands until you have a ball that's moist but not soggy. Press into muffin tins, filling halfway. Once dry, pop out the fizzies and store in a tightly capped jar. Add one fizzie to a warm bath.

YIELD: 6 REFRESHING BATH FIZZIES

❓ **How it works:** *The citric acid and baking soda are delivery systems for the refreshing aromatic essential oils. Eucalyptus and bay laurel essential oils are antibacterial agents that help counter odor-causing skin bacteria.*

When to Call the Doctor

If you are staying clean, practicing good hygiene, eating well, and still experiencing body odor, make an appointment with your doctor. Some medical conditions and medications alter body smells. Also, a condition called hyperhidrosis leads to excessive sweating. Prescription antiperspirants are one possible remedy.

Also see your doctor if you notice unusual vaginal odors or discharge. Refrain from using commercially sold vaginal sprays and douches. These products can upset the acid-base balance and kill resident microbes that defend against infection-causing microbes. Plus, if you do have an infection, the pressure of douching can cause the "bad" microbes to ascend into your pelvic organs.

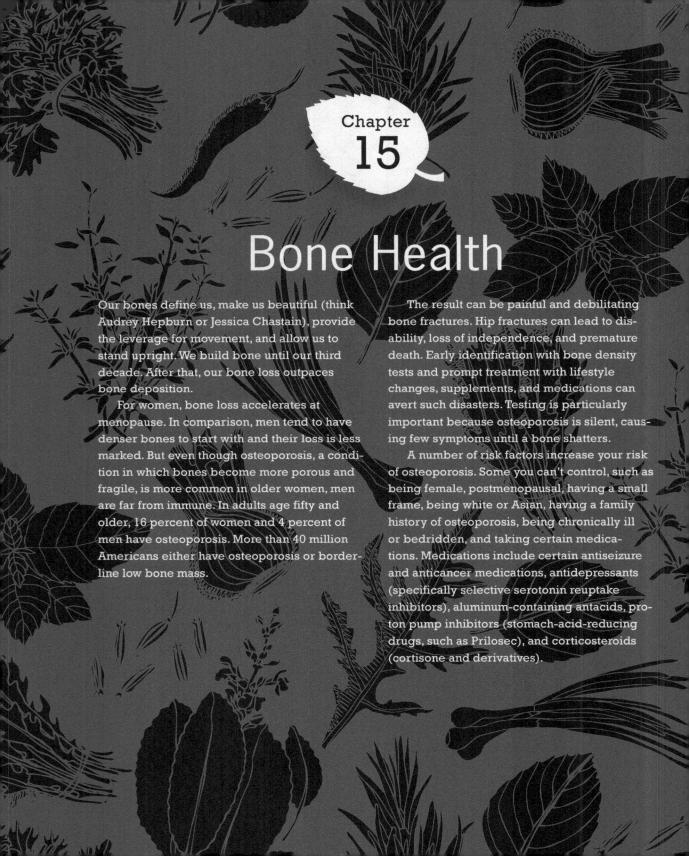

Chapter 15

Bone Health

Our bones define us, make us beautiful (think Audrey Hepburn or Jessica Chastain), provide the leverage for movement, and allow us to stand upright. We build bone until our third decade. After that, our bone loss outpaces bone deposition.

For women, bone loss accelerates at menopause. In comparison, men tend to have denser bones to start with and their loss is less marked. But even though osteoporosis, a condition in which bones become more porous and fragile, is more common in older women, men are far from immune. In adults age fifty and older, 16 percent of women and 4 percent of men have osteoporosis. More than 40 million Americans either have osteoporosis or borderline low bone mass.

The result can be painful and debilitating bone fractures. Hip fractures can lead to disability, loss of independence, and premature death. Early identification with bone density tests and prompt treatment with lifestyle changes, supplements, and medications can avert such disasters. Testing is particularly important because osteoporosis is silent, causing few symptoms until a bone shatters.

A number of risk factors increase your risk of osteoporosis. Some you can't control, such as being female, postmenopausal, having a small frame, being white or Asian, having a family history of osteoporosis, being chronically ill or bedridden, and taking certain medications. Medications include certain antiseizure and anticancer medications, antidepressants (specifically selective serotonin reuptake inhibitors), aluminum-containing antacids, proton pump inhibitors (stomach-acid-reducing drugs, such as Prilosec), and corticosteroids (cortisone and derivatives).

Here's what you can do to save your bones:

- **Don't smoke.** That includes breathing second-hand smoke.

- **Keep alcohol intake under control.** Women should have no more than one drink a day and men no more than two a day.

- **Exercise each day.** The best activities are those that stress your bones: weight-bearing exercise (jogging, walking, dancing, etc.) and resistance training (working against weights). Cycling and swimming build aerobic capacity, but they don't force your bones to bear weight, which helps bones maintain healthy density.

- **Eat well.** Consume plenty of mineral-rich vegetables, fruits, nuts, and seeds. Many Americans consume dairy products to fulfill their calcium needs, others are lactose intolerant. Further, some research disputes that dairy is the best bone-building food.

- **Catch some rays.** Ultraviolet light stimulates vitamin D production in the skin, and is essential for calcium absorption from the intestines. Sunscreen interferes with this process. Because few foods contain vitamin D, many people have insufficient levels. During the summer, fair-skinned people need 10 to 15 minutes of sun exposure to generate plenty of vitamin D. Dark-skinned people, who are more at risk for vitamin D insufficiency, need longer exposure. Wear a hat to protect your face. After your sun-bath, slop on the sunscreen, cover up, or seek shade.

- **Avoid the calcium-stealers.** In addition to alcohol, excessive intake of protein, sodium, caffeine, and sodas (which contain phosphoric acid) lead to calcium loss in urine.

History

Osteoporosis is not new. Long before we had a name for it, osteoporosis appeared in the stooped postures and so-called dowager's hump of older women. In the early nineteenth century, French pathologist Jean Lobstein coined the term *osteoporosis*, or porous bone, to describe the condition in which bones were riddled with larger than normal holes.

A century later, researchers established a connection between osteoporosis and the loss of estrogen in postmenopausal women. Not until the 1960s were devices for detecting bone density and bone loss developed, allowing early detection of osteoporosis (and osteopenia, reduced bone density that's not low enough to meet criteria for osteoporosis). At about the same time, compounds known as bisphophonates were discovered. These powerful medications (Boniva, Fosamax, and others) stem bone loss and resorption, though not without side effects. Whether they actually prevent fractures—which often become life-changing events—is still a matter of debate.

Lifestyle Tip

Go whole. Stay away from processed foods. They are missing the vital natural nutrients in whole foods. Read labels carefully on bread and cereal packages: "Whole grain" is the operative phrase.

Artichoke Heart Salad

¼ red onion, sliced thinly
2 tablespoons (30 ml) fresh lemon juice
1 pound (455 g) asparagus
1 tablespoon (15 ml) olive oil
1 jar (13 ounces, or 365 g) artichoke hearts, sliced in half
½ pint (225 g) cherry tomatoes, sliced in half
½ teaspoon garlic powder

PREPARATION AND USE:
Preheat the oven to 400°F (200°C, or gas mark 6). Cover the onion slices with the lemon juice and set aside to soak. Spray a glass baking dish with a light coating of olive oil.

Slice off the ends of the asparagus and line up the spears in the dish. Drizzle the olive oil over the asparagus and toss to coat. Roast for about 10 minutes.

Remove the asparagus from the oven and cut each spear into thirds. In a medium-size bowl, toss together the asparagus, artichoke hearts, and cherry tomatoes. Stir in the onion slices and their lemony marinating liquid. Sprinkle the salad with the garlic powder and toss.

YIELD: 4 SERVINGS

❷ **How it works:** *Packed with 135 milligrams of calcium, a medium-size artichoke is a bone support system.*

Super Green Sauté

2 tablespoons (28 ml) olive oil
4 garlic cloves, minced
¼ cup (28 g) diced pecans
¼ cup (35 g) raisins
4 cups (144 g) collards, chopped, stems removed
4 cups (220 g) turnip greens, chopped
½ cup (120 ml) water
Salt and freshly ground black pepper
Sprigs of parsley, for garnish

PREPARATION AND USE:
Heat the olive oil in a large skillet over medium heat. Add the garlic and sauté for about a minute. Add the pecans, raisins, and greens and sauté for 4 to 5 minutes until the greens wilt. Pour in the water and then let it boil away. Remove from the heat, transfer to plates, add salt and pepper to taste, and garnish with parsley.

YIELD: 2 SERVINGS

❷ **How it works:** *These leafy greens contain a powerful calcium punch. One-half cup (95 g) of cooked collards or (72 g) turnip greens provides about 100 milligrams of calcium. Parsley, pecans, and raisins contain lesser amounts of calcium, as well as other bone-friendly nutrients. Further, leafy greens and raisins are alkaline. That's important because bones release calcium salts to neutralize excess acid in the body.*

Note: Alternatively, add or substitute your favorite greens: Chinese cabbage, kale, mustard greens, dandelion greens, or purslane. Consider adding seaweed, which is rich in a healthy amount of calcium, magnesium, and potassium.

Bone-Boosting Tahini

Use this Middle Eastern staple to make hummus, add to a calcium-rich legume soup, or use in the Taratoor with Crudités (at right).

2½ cups (360 g) sesame seeds
¾ cup (175 ml) olive oil, plus more if needed

PREPARATION AND USE:
Preheat the oven to 350°F (180°C, or gas mark 4). Spread the sesame seeds on a baking sheet and toast the seeds for about 10 minutes, tossing several times to prevent scorching. Remove the seeds from the oven and let cool for 15 minutes. Place the sesame seeds and olive oil in a food processor. Blend for about 2 minutes to gain a thick but pourable consistency, adding more oil if needed.

Store in an airtight container for up to three weeks.

YIELD: 2 CUPS (480 G)

❓ How it works: *One ounce (28 g) of roasted sesame seeds contains about 280 milligrams of calcium. Sesame seeds are high in calcium and other nutrients.*

Lifestyle Tip

Drink green tea. People who regularly consume green and black tea (*Camellia sinensis*) have a reduced osteoporosis risk. Research suggests that tea enhances bone mineral density, increases the activity of bone cells, producing more bone, and inhibits cells that break down bone.

Taratoor with Crudités

Sesame seeds run on the acidic side. Temper that effect by spreading taratoor on carrots, celery sticks, sugar snap peas, and other vegetables. This traditional Middle Eastern dip combines sesame seed paste (tahini) with garlic, lemon, and water.

For the *taratoor*:
1 cup (240 g) Bone-Boosting Tahini (at left)
1 garlic clove, crushed
Juice of 2 lemons, plus more as needed
¼ cup (60 ml) water, plus more as needed
1 teaspoon (6 g) salt
¼ cup (15 g) chopped fresh parsley

For the crudités:
1 broccoli crown, steamed and cooled
1 cup (128 g) baby carrots
2 celery stalks, chopped
1 cup (75 g) sugar snap peas

PREPARATION AND USE:
Blend all the *taratoor* ingredients in a blender until smooth. Add more lemon, as needed, to reach the tangy flavor desired, and more water as needed for the desired consistency. Serve with the crudités.

YIELD: 4 APPETIZER SERVINGS OF *TARATOOR* AND VEGGIES

❓ How it works: *With veggies, this Mediterranean dip will nourish your bones. Sesame is a calcium king and broccoli alone has 178 milligrams of calcium in 1 cup (71 g).*

◗ Soy-ful Dip

This edamame recipe is a guacamole look-alike, with its own great taste; edamame also delivers way more calcium than guacamole's avocados. It's a recipe for happy bones.

1½ teaspoons (7.5 ml) olive oil
¼ teaspoon ground cumin
1 garlic clove, minced
¾ cup (113 g) shelled edamame
1½ tablespoons (25 g) Bone-Boosting
    Tahini (page 103)
1½ tablespoons (25 ml) water
¼ cup (15 g) chopped fresh parsley
Juice of 1 lemon, plus more as needed
Salt

PREPARATION AND USE:

In a blender, combine the olive oil, cumin, and garlic. Add the edamame, tahini, water, parsley, and lemon juice and blend completely. Add more lemon as desired for tangier flavor and thinner consistency. Stir in the salt to taste.

Serve with crudités (see page 103).

YIELD: 4 SERVINGS

❓ **How it works:** *Edamame are immature soybeans. Among other beneficial chemicals (protein and calcium), soy contains isoflavones. (The isoflavone content for edamame, however, is not as high as for mature soybeans.) Test-tube and animal studies show that soy isoflavones (compounds that weakly mimic estrogen) inhibit osteoclasts (bone-dissolving cells) and stimulate osteoblasts (bone-adding cells). Rather than consume isolated isoflavones, consider adding tofu, tempeh, or cooked soybeans to meals. One-half cup (124 g) of firm tofu has 258 milligrams of calcium.*

◗ Edamame-Spinach Omelet

Most studies of women going through menopause or past menopause show the beneficial effects of soy on bone health.

1 tablespoon (15 ml) milk
1 tablespoon (5 g) grated Parmesan cheese
⅛ teaspoon ground nutmeg
Salt and freshly ground black pepper
1 cup (30 g) torn and rinsed baby spinach
    leaves, packed
½ cup (75 g) shelled edamame,
    frozen or thawed
¼ cup (37.5 g) finely chopped and seeded
    red bell pepper
½ teaspoon minced onion

PREPARATION AND USE:

In a medium-size bowl, whisk together the eggs, milk, cheese, nutmeg, salt, and black pepper and set aside.

Spray a skillet with olive or canola oil cooking spray and place over medium heat. Add the spinach, edamame, bell pepper, and onion and sauté for about 2 minutes. Pour in the egg mixture.

Cook for 2 to 3 minutes until the egg mixture sets. Fold in half, flip with a spatula, and cook for an additional 2 to 3 minutes. Reduce the heat to low and cook for another 2 to 3 minutes, to the desired consistency.

YIELD: 2 SERVINGS

❓ **How it works:** *Edamame contains isoflavones. Just ½ cup (80 g) a day also significantly increases the fiber, protein, and vitamins your healthy diet needs. In addition, spinach packs its own calcium punch, with 146 milligrams in ½ cup (90 g) of the cooked greens (the daily recommended calcium dose is 1,000 to 1,200 milligrams).*

Soy Snack

Enjoy this dish for lunch or as an afternoon snack.

1 large apple, cored and cut into chunks
½ cup (75 g) golden raisins
½ cup (50 g) crushed almonds
1 cup (230 g) vanilla soy yogurt
Pinch of ground cinnamon

PREPARATION AND USE:

In a medium-size bowl, mix together the apple, raisins, and almonds. Blend in the yogurt and sprinkle with the cinnamon. Enjoy.

YIELD: 1 LARGE OR 2 SMALL SERVINGS

❓ How it works: *Raisins and almonds contain calcium. In fact, 1 ounce (28 g) of almonds (20 to 25 nuts) has as much calcium as ¼ cup (60 ml) of milk. Apples and especially raisins are alkalinizing, helping bones retain calcium and reducing the risk of osteoporosis.*

Pom-Tan-Chia

1 tablespoon (13 g) chia seeds
1 cup (235 ml) pomegranate juice
1 cup (235 ml) calcium-fortified tangerine juice

PREPARATION AND USE:

Place the chia seeds in a clean, wide-mouthed pint-size (475 ml) jar, pour in the juices, and stir. Cap the jar and shake until completely blended. Leave in the refrigerator for about 2 hours and then serve.

YIELD: 2 SERVINGS

❓ How it works: *One tablespoon (13 g) of chia seeds contains 65 milligrams of calcium, as well as magnesium and potassium. And pomegranate juice is a major source of antioxidants, making this a healthy anytime drink.*

When to See the Doctor

- *Keep up with annual exams, especially as you crest age 50.*

- *Talk to your doctor about his or her assessment of your risk for osteoporosis. Most physicians recommend that women get a bone density test at age 65. Women considered at higher risk may need the screening test sooner. Risk factors include family history of osteoporosis, small frame, premature menopause, hyperthyroidism, anorexia nervosa, and long-term use of corticosteroid medications.*

- *Make an appointment if you notice you've lost height, have become slumped or hunched in your upper back, or develop the sudden onset of back pain (which could signify an osteoporotic vertebra collapsed).*

Chapter 16

Brain Health

A 2013 study showed that women who've crossed the menopause threshold experience subtle declines in cognitive function. These skills include learning, remembering, problem-solving, and paying attention. Before you beg your doctor for a prescription for hormones, know that (1) the early menopause brain fog is transient; (2) the long-term effects of menopause on mental function are negligible; and (3) hormone replacement doesn't seem to help and may, in fact, worsen cognitive performance.

For men and women, rates of dementia rise with age. According to the Centers for Disease Control and Prevention, the risk of Alzheimer's disease (the most common type of dementia) doubles every five years for people over age sixty-five. By age eighty-five, between 25 and 50 percent of people have signs of the disease.

Does that mean that if you live long enough, you're destined to develop dementia? Certainly not! Dementia is a disease, not a normal age change. It's marked by the progressive deterioration of memory, other intellectual functions, and the ability to perform daily tasks. The other most common type of dementia is vascular dementia (also called multi-infarct dementia), a condition that occurs when blood clots in brain arteries destroy small areas of tissue.

How do you know if memory loss is normal? Some degree of age-related forgetfulness happens to almost everyone. Whereas long-term memory (the names of your loved ones, significant events from your past) is normally well preserved, short-term memory gets a bit fuzzier. For instance, you may remember exactly what you were doing when you learned about the terrorist attacks on September 11, 2001, but forget where you put your car keys, why you walked into a room, or the name of the actor in the movie you saw last week. People with dementia forget big things: the names of close friends, how to balance a checkbook, or how to navigate from home to grocery store.

Research has shown that some two-thirds of memory-zapping aging can be attributed to lifestyle. This means there's a lot you can do to "head" it off! See the following list.

- Pay attention. Often, we forget mundane things (especially things we can do automatically) out of distraction. The drawback is that we may later forget, say, where we parked the car or whether we turned off the stove. Stay, as much as possible, in the present moment. Life is often more enjoyable when we are fully aware.

- Develop routines. Store the keys (and glasses, checkbooks, cell phones, etc.) in the same place. That way, you know where to find them.

- Stay organized. Calendars and to-do lists can act as peripheral brains. The simple act of writing things down (the people you met at last night's party, or the title of the book you heard about) helps lay down memory tracks.

- Protect your cardiovascular system. Arterial disease raises the risk for Alzheimer's, vascular dementia, and stroke.

- Manage your blood sugar. People with type-2 diabetes or even borderline high blood sugar have problems with insulin, the hormone that ushers glucose from the blood into the cells. Specifically, tissues don't respond well to insulin (a condition called *insulin resistance*), which causes the pancreas to churn out more insulin. Insulin resistance has been linked to an increased risk of Alzheimer's disease. Possible reasons include alterations in neurotransmitters (chemicals used to communicate nerve impulses) and increases in inflammation, glucose, and beta-amyloid (misfolded protein that's toxic to brain cells). In addition, diabetes greatly increases the risk of stroke, primarily because high glucose damages arteries. If you have diabetes, work closely with your physician to keep your blood sugar within the normal range.

- Exercise. Studies show that regular physical activity maintains brain health. A 2012 study of seniors with mild cognitive impairment found their condition was less likely to progress if they stayed active. Another study showed that an aerobic training program for older adults increased the size of the hippocampus (a brain region critical to memory that shrinks with advancing age and more dramatically in those with Alzheimer's) and improved spatial

memory. Why is exercise so protective? The reasons include increased blood flow to the brain, reduced risk of cardiovascular disease and stroke, stress relief, social and mental stimulation, and a boost in chemicals that protect brain cells.

- Eat plants. Diets high in saturated fat increase dementia risk, but, those full of vegetables and fish lower it. The Mediterranean diet, which emphasizes fruits, vegetables, fish, nuts, and olive oil, serves as a stellar example. It seems to protect against Alzheimer's disease and slows the rate of age-related cognitive decline. It fends off cardiovascular disease and diabetes, both dementia risk factors. It's replete with antioxidants, anti-inflammatory fatty acids, and other brain-friendly nutrients. Inflammation and oxidation place stress on the brain and are correlated with Alzheimer's disease.

- Limit servings of meat and whole-fat dairy products.

- Limit servings of meat, butter, and full-fat dairy. These foods contain protein and other nutrients, but they're also high in saturated fats, which are linked with a risk of dementia.

- Avoid junk food which is low in valuable nutrients and high in simple sugars and unhealthy fats such as trans fatty acids. High intake of junk foods can, over time, promote disease of the blood vessels that supply the brain with nutrients and oxygen. Studies indicate that trans fatty acids increase beta-amyloid in the brain.

- Shake off salt. Excessive intake increases blood pressure, raises the risk of stroke, and possibly impairs cognitive function. Don't worry that you won't get enough. Many foods naturally contain salt. Plus, whenever you eat prepared foods, you're getting an ample dose.

- Shun tobacco smoke. It's a source of inflammation and a factor in cardiovascular disease and stroke which are, risk factors for dementia.

- Enjoy small amounts of alcohol. Moderate alcohol intake (one glass a day for women and two for men—each glass consisting of 5 ounces [150 ml] of wine, 12 ounces [355 ml] of beer, or 1.5 ounces [42 ml] of 80-proof distilled spirits) provides some degree of dementia protection. Red wine, thanks to its resveratrol (an antioxidant, anti-inflammatory polyphenol) may have an added benefit. Keep a lid on it. High intake of alcohol damages the brain.

- Stress less. Chronic, serious stress damages the hippocampus, an area involved in forming and retrieving memories.

- Sleep deep. You consolidate (gel) recently acquired memories during sleep. Sleep deprivation undermines cognitive skills. In mice, sleep deprivation increases brain levels of damaging beta-amyloid.

- Stay socially connected. Robust relationships protect health in many ways. A recent study found that feeling lonely (which is different from being alone) correlated with an increased risk of dementia.

- Use your intellect. Read, work, attend lectures, listen to the news, solve crossword puzzles, or play music. These activities build cognitive reserve, the equivalent of a savings account. This reserve is thought to explain why up to a third of cognitively normal people have, upon their death, tissue signs of Alzheimer's disease. A recent study found that continued intellectual activity delayed the onset of symptoms of Alzheimer's, even when brain scans suggested tissue changes associated with that disease.

- Keep learning. Lean a new language, sport, or activity, expand your vocabulary, try tango lessons, or take up a musical instrument. It's never too late. Older people sometimes take a bit longer to learn new skills. That's fine. What's the rush, anyway?

- Meditate. A regular meditation practice improves cognitive function.

In addition to dementia, another feared brain calamity is stroke. Most of the time what happens is akin to a heart attack. In this case, a blood clot obstructs blood flow in arteries that supply the brain rather than the heart. Less often, a weakened artery bleeds into the brain. The loss of function depends upon the size of the damage.

History

"There's rosemary, that's for remembrance. Pray you, love, remember." This line, spoken by Ophelia in Shakespeare's *Hamlet*, has sparked literary debate for centuries. But there's no question that rosemary (*Rosmarinus officinalis*) has long been associated with memory and concentration. As early as 500 BCE, Greek scholars wore sprigs of rosemary in their hair during examinations to improve their mental performance.

Recent research supports that tradition. A 2003 study in the *International Journal of Neuroscience* showed that inhaling the smell of rosemary essential oil improved memory and alertness. Inhaling the aroma of lavender essential oil, on the other hand, relaxed people and slowed speed of memory. A 2012 study published in the *Journal of Medicinal Food* showed that relatively low doses of rosemary leaf (equivalent to the amount you might consume with a rosemary-seasoned meal) improved cognitive performance in seniors, whereas a high dose actually worsened mental function.

Simple Salmon

If you remember to eat just this fish, you may find the adage, "Seafood is brain food" may turn out to be true.

1 pound (455 g) salmon fillet, or 4 fillets
   (4 ounces, or 115 g each)
Freshly ground black pepper (optional)
1 tablespoon (15 ml) olive oil
1 teaspoon (1 g) crushed fresh oregano
1 lemon, cut into wedges

PREPARATION AND USE:

Preheat the oven to 450°F (230°C, or gas mark 8). Wash the fillet(s) and pat dry. Place the fish skin down on a baking sheet. Sprinkle with pepper, if using.

In a small bowl, mix the olive oil and oregano. Brush this mixture onto the salmon. Bake for 10 to 15 minutes until flaky. Serve with the lemon wedges.

YIELD: 4 SERVINGS

❓ How it works: *People who eat more cold-water fish, which is rich in the brain-friendly fatty acid docosahexaenoic acid (DHA), reduce their risk of cognitive decline and dementia. Fatty fish is also one of the few food sources of vitamin D, a vitamin with multiple functions, including proper brain function and nerve protection. Many Americans have insufficient blood levels of this vitamin. Unfortunately, low levels correlate with dementia.*

🌶 Spicy Milk

I learned about this remedy while interviewing a National Institutes of Health pharmacologist for a story on herbs that protect against dementia. ~ LBW

1 teaspoon (2 g) ground turmeric
½ teaspoon freshly ground black pepper
1 cup (235 ml) whole milk

PREPARATION AND USE:

Mix the turmeric and pepper into the milk. Drink one serving twice daily—morning and evening.

YIELD: 1 SERVING

❓ How it works: *The key ingredient in curry is turmeric. It contains the potent anti-inflammatory and antioxidant agent curcumin, which may help to counter the inflammation and oxidation that promotes nerve-degenerating conditions such as dementia. Furthermore, curcumin inhibits the formation of beta-amyloid and improves its clearance. However, curcumin isn't well absorbed from the intestine. Consuming it with fat (as in full-fat milk, butter, or oil) and pepper improves absorption.*

Lifestyle Tip

Eat breakfast. Nights are long. The brain demands a constant supply of glucose (blood sugar) to function well. Studies show that a nutritionally balanced breakfast each morning will help improve mood and keep energy and cognitive performance on an even keel.

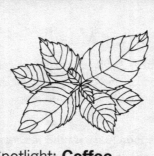

Spotlight: **Coffee**

For years, doctors fretted that coffee wasn't good for us and tried to get us to quit or switch to decaf. However, recent studies show coffee's bright side. Like most medicinal plants, it's chemically complex, includes a group of powerful polyphenols, and has multiple benefits. A large thirteen-year study linked drinking two to three cups of coffee a day with a 10 percent decreased risk of death. (Note that one cup measures 8 ounces [235 ml]—a smaller amount than what fills most mugs.)

Chief among coffee's specific benefits is protection of the nervous system. In addition to keeping us alert, regular coffee consumption reduces the risk of stroke, depression, dementia, and Parkinson's disease. When people with mild cognitive impairment (a condition of loss of memory and other mental functions less severe than outright dementia) drank three to five (8-ounce [235 ml]) cups a day, they cut their risk of progressing to dementia.

Ingestion of pure caffeine, which we don't recommend, temporarily increases blood pressure. And unfiltered coffee can raise cholesterol levels. Nevertheless, coffee's overall effect is to shield against cardiovascular disease. Furthermore, regular coffee consumption lowers the risk of type-2 diabetes and may also help with weight loss. Both being overweight and having diabetes elevate cardiovascular disease risk.

Coffee reduces the risk for some cancers, including colon, prostate, uterine, skin (basal cell carcinoma), and head and neck cancer. It also benefits the liver and reduces the risk of gallstones. Because caffeine relaxes smooth muscle encircling the airways, it was a traditional remedy for asthma. Effects on muscle can enhance strength and endurance.

Enjoy your coffee in the early half of the day and keep intake moderate. Most of the side effects of high doses are caused by caffeine. They include jitteriness, restlessness, anxiety, hand tremors, insomnia, and increased blood pressure. It takes five hours for your body to eliminate half of the caffeine circulating in your blood—double that time in women who are pregnant or on oral hormonal contraceptives.

Note: Decaffeinated coffee still has some caffeine. Whereas an 8-ounce (235 ml) cup of coffee contains 100 to 200 milligrams of caffeine, an 8-ounce (235 ml) cup of decaf contains 2 to 12 milligrams.

🫐 Berry Strong Brain

This sweet dessert salad will not disappoint your taste buds or brain cells.

1 cup (150 g) halved red grapes
1 cup (160 g) halved strawberries
1 cup (145 g) blackberries or blueberries
½ cup (87 g) pomegranate arils (sometimes called seeds)
½ cup (87 g) dark chocolate chips (optional)
Plain or honey-flavored Greek yogurt, for topping

PREPARATION AND USE:

Mix the grapes and berries in a large bowl. Stir in the pomegranate arils. Fold in the chocolate chips, if using. Divide among four dessert plates. Top each serving with a dab of yogurt.

YIELD: 4 SERVINGS

❷ How it works: *Berries, red grapes, pomegranate, and chocolate are rich in chemicals called polyphenols, which are antioxidant and anti-inflammatory. Regular consumption of berries is associated with a reduced risk of Parkinson's disease, which can cause dementia. In the cellular equivalent of housekeeping, extracts of strawberries and blueberries help the brain cells clean up toxic debris. In rats, a diet high in extracts of strawberries, blueberries, and blackberries reverses age-related deficits in learning and memory. Grape polyphenols reduce production of beta amyloid, inhibit its tendency to clump, protect the brain cells from its toxic effects, and curb inflammatory activity.*

Note: To peel and remove the arils from a pomegranate, see http://mideastfood.about.com/od/tipsandtechniques/ss/deseedpomegrana_2.htm.

Also, for a superfast, nonwater removal, go to http://vimeo.com/39205407.

🫐 Moroccan Sage Tea

This traditional drink is popular in Morocco in the winter months. It gives brain-healthy benefits throughout the year.

1 teaspoon (2 g) green tea leaves
1 teaspoon (1 g) dried sage
2 cups (475 ml) boiling water
Stevia, to taste

PREPARATION AND USE:

Place the tea leaves and sage in a teapot. Pour the boiling water over the mixture. Steep for 5 minutes. Gently stir the tea and strain into two cups. Add stevia.

YIELD: 2 SERVINGS

❷ How it works: *Lab experiments show green tea polyphenols are antioxidant and nerve protectant and inhibit beta-amyloid–induced nerve damage. Populations that drink more green tea have been found to have a lower rate of cognitive impairment.*

Chemicals in garden sage are anti-inflammatory and antioxidant, help preserve the brain's acetylcholine (a brain chemical decreased in Alzheimer's), and protect neurons from beta-amyloid's toxic effects. Several studies demonstrate memory enhancement with oral consumption of either dried leaf extracts or small amounts of diluted essential oil in healthy people, both old and young. At least one study shows that inhalation of the essential oil improves memory and mood.

Mind-Enhancing Hot Chocolate

Throw out that instant hot chocolate and rediscover the wonders in the cocoa powder your mom used.

1 cup (235 ml) almond milk
2 tablespoons (10 g) unsweetened cocoa powder
½ teaspoon vanilla extract
Pinch of salt
Stevia (we use ½ packet [0.5 g]), equivalent to 1 teaspoon [4 g] sugar)
Pinch of ground cinnamon

PREPARATION AND USE:

In a medium-size saucepan, mix together the almond milk, cocoa powder, vanilla extract, and salt. Warm over low heat. Add stevia to taste. Whisk as the mixture warms until it is frothy and steaming. Pour into a cup and top with the cinnamon. If it's too thick for your taste, try adding up to ½ cup (120 ml) of water.

YIELD: 1 SERVING

❓ **How it works:** *Consumption of another polyphenol-rich food, chocolate, has been shown to reduce the risk of stroke. A dose of cocoa increased blood flow to the brain's gray matter while healthy volunteers took a cognitive test. In one study, 90 seniors with mild cognitive impairment drank cocoa with varying amounts of flavanols (a polyphenol) for eight weeks. Those with the higher amounts in their drink tested with improved attention and other mental skills.*

When Simple Doesn't Work

So far, no dietary supplement has been convincingly shown to prevent dementia. Ginkgo (Ginkgo biloba) extracts do seem to reduce symptoms of dementia and may improve mild memory impairment in elders. The Ayurvedic herb bacopa (Bacopa monnieri) has lately gained scientific traction for improving learning and memory in healthy adults.

Several studies show that consumption of extracts made from the leaves of common garden sage (Salvia officinalis and S. lavandulifolia) enhance memory in healthy people and improve mental function in people with Alzheimer's disease. One study found that inhalation of the aroma of essential oil improves memory and mood. Lemon balm (Melissa officinalis) also appears to improve mood and cognitive performance and promote calmness.

Mental Focus
Aromatherapy
(or, Think Sharp Scents)

This delightfully scented remedy enhances memory.

1 drop sage essential oil
2 drops rosemary essential oil
3 drops peppermint essential oil

PREPARATION AND USE:

In a small, clean jar, blend the sage, rosemary, and peppermint oils. Drop a cotton ball into the jar. Apply the essential oils to the cotton ball. Cap tightly. Open the jar and sniff daily.

YIELD: A WEEK'S WORTH OF SNIFF SESSIONS

❓ **How it works:** *Studies show that among essential oils, sage, rosemary, and peppermint all enhance memory.*

Fact or Myth?

DRINKING WINE IS GOOD FOR THE BRAIN.

Maybe. Moderate drinking has cardiovascular benefits. And healthy arteries promote healthy brain function. Studies have indeed linked light and moderate alcohol consumption with a lower risk of Alzheimer's disease. However, alcohol in excess is toxic to nerves. Alcoholism is a cause of dementia.

Lifestyle Tip

Crack open a Brazil nut. Brazil nuts are rich in selenium, a mineral that acts as an antioxidant and contributes to normal brain functions. Scientists have linked higher selenium levels in the body with a lower risk of depression. Preliminary research suggests that low selenium is a risk factor for cognitive decline. Brown rice, oatmeal, and whole-grain breads are other good sources of selenium.

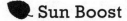 Sun Boost

A few minutes without sunscreen can make a difference in your vitamin D levels.

Sunny day
You, without sunscreen

PREPARATION AND USE:
Sit in the sun for 15 minutes. If you plan to be outdoors after that, apply sunscreen.

YIELD: 1 SESSION

❷ **How it works:** *Low vitamin D is linked with poor cognitive function and dementia. Few foods contain this vitamin; it is found in fatty fish, such as salmon and mackerel; egg yolks; beef liver; cheese; and some fortified foods, such as orange juice or soy milk. However, our skin generates vitamin D when exposed to ultraviolet light. A study in older women found that higher dietary intake of vitamin D lowered the risk of developing Alzheimer's disease.*

Note: If you have sensitive skin or skin cancer, talk to your doctor first before using this remedy.

Riddle Me This

Mentally stimulating leisure activities, such as doing crossword puzzles, seem to help keep the brain sharp.

1 crossword or Sudoku puzzle
A pencil

PREPARATION AND USE:
Complete a puzzle per day.

YIELD: 1 CHALLENGE DAILY

❷ **How it works:** *Studies show that activities that flex your mental power may delay mental decline with age, possibly by building the brain's reserve capacity. In a 2011 study, researchers compared seniors who regularly worked crossword puzzles ("puzzlers") to those who didn't (the "nonpuzzlers"). The puzzlers delayed the onset of accelerated memory loss (a sign of dementia) by an average of 2.54 years. In 2009, the same research group found that greater participation in a variety of mentally stimulating activities—puzzles, writing, playing board or card games, playing music, and participating in group discussions—delayed memory decline.*

A Fast Walk to Clear Your Head

Do this every day to heighten awareness, take in vitamin D, and boost brain health.

1 pair walking shoes
You

PREPARATION AND USE:
Walk daily outside for 30 minutes. Identify a safe route and let yourself go; you'll find you are solving problems and thinking creatively as you become healthy and fit. For a vitamin D boost, walk 15 minutes without sunscreen and then slather it on your face, neck, and arms for the second half of your walk.

YIELD: 1 SESSION DAILY

❓ **How it works:** *Repeated studies show that regular exercise enhances learning and memory, improves vascular function, and helps prevent diseases such as diabetes and heart disease, both of which negatively affect the brain. Furthermore, physical activity lessens the impact of aging on the brain, as well as all other organ systems. It's never too late to start. A 2013 study published in the* Journal of Aging Research *demonstrated that, in seniors who already had mild cognitive impairment (a condition that's less severe than outright dementia), twice-weekly exercise—particularly aerobic exercise— improved memory. Walking halfway without sunscreen adds a vitamin D boost.*

When to See the Doctor

- *Make an appointment if you have any concerns about your brain function.*

- *If your friends or family express concerns about your memory, take them seriously.*

- *Call 911 if you or someone else notices a sudden change in your mental function— slurred words, confusion, or memory blackout. Other emergency signs for stroke are sudden numbness, tingling, weakness, or unsteady gait.*

Chapter 17

Breast Tenderness

A number of things can cause *mastalgia*, the medical name for breast pain. Hormonal shifts cause cyclic breast discomfort. The onset of puberty renders a girl's breasts more sensitive. Many teenage girls and women experience heaviness and soreness just before menstruation, a symptom that may be part of the great constellation of premenstrual syndrome.

Breasts enlarge during pregnancy—more so just after the birth. Before nipples toughen, breastfeeding can initially cause soreness. During that time, women are vulnerable to breast infection, called mastitis.

Sometimes the discomfort has nothing to do with hormones. Obviously, surgery and accidental trauma will hurt. If you're bustier, the sheer weight can be uncomfortable—especially when exercising.

Further, many women develop fibrocystic breast changes. Fibrous tissue and cysts (fluid-filled sacs) cause the breasts to feel lumpy. Premenstrual hormonal shifts can enlarge the cysts and may lead to tenderness. Fibrocystic changes do not increase a woman's cancer risk, though they can make screening tests more difficult to interpret.

Speaking of breast cancer, it usually does not cause pain. Neither do benign (noncancerous) enlargements called fibroadenomas.

You should see your doctor immediately if you detect a new lump, regardless of whether it's tender. A biopsy may be needed to determine whether the mass is benign.

History

Time-honored remedies for breast tenderness included castor oil packs and warm compresses, often augmented by such herbs as calendula, cleavers, burdock, and yarrow. Herbs were taken internally, too.

Herbalists traditionally combined several medicinal plants: chaste tree berries (*Vitex agnus castus*); dandelion (*Taraxacum officinale*), which acts as a gentle diuretic; cleavers (*Galium aparine*), which promotes lymphatic circulation; and black cohosh (*Actaea racemosa*) and dong quai (*Angelica sinensis*), both of which reduce inflammation and help regulate female hormones. Chaste tree berries—once believed to suppress sexual desire and promote chastity—do nothing of the kind. But modern research shows that the herb regulates menstrual cycles and relieves breast tenderness and other unpleasant premenstrual symptoms.

Natural healers also recommended women increase the intake of anti-inflammatory plant oils. Initial studies of flaxseed show promise in relieving cyclic breast pain.

🍂 Monthly Breast Exam

This recipe comes from the American Cancer Society. Practice it once a month. If you notice any changes, such as a lump, thickening, dimpling, discoloration, or nipple discharge, contact your doctor immediately.

You
A mirror
A shower
A bed

PREPARATION AND USE:

In the mirror: Look carefully at your breasts to see whether there is any difference in their position, shape, or size or if there is any skin discoloration. Note anything unusual, such as dimpling or sores. Are your nipples peeling, or is there a change in their direction?

Review the outer parts of your breasts: Place your hands on your hips and press down to tighten your chest muscles. Inspect your breasts as you turn side to side to look for unusual changes as mentioned above. Roll your shoulders and elbows forward to tighten your chest muscles. As your breasts fall forward, look for any changes in their "forward" shape, as well as in coloration or skin consistency from the last mirror exam.

Look carefully at the area underneath your breasts, lifting each breast with your hands to examine it. Place your thumb and forefinger on the tissue around each nipple and pull out, toward the nipple's tip. Look for fluid discharge.

In the shower: Check for any lumps or thickening in your underarm area. Place one hand on your hip. With your other hand, check for lumps or thickening in the opposite armpit. Check both sides. Feel for lumps or thickening above and below your collarbone.

Lift one arm behind your head to spread your breast tissue. With the fingers from the other hand, press gently into the breast in an up-and-down motion, moving from bra line to collarbone, over the full breast. Repeat on the other side.

In bed: Lie flat and place a small pillow under your right shoulder. Put your right hand behind your head. Place your left hand on the upper portion of your right breast with your fingers together and flat.

Think of your breast as the face on a clock and start at the top, or twelve o'clock. In small, circular motions, move toward one o'clock. Continue around the entire circle until you reach twelve o'clock again. Your fingers should be flat and always in contact with your breast. Next, complete another similar circle around the nipple. Then, feel the upper outer areas that extend into your armpit. Finally, place your fingers flat and directly on top of your nipple, feeling for changes under the nipple. Press your nipple inward. It should move easily.

YIELD: MONTHLY APPLICATION

❷ **How it works:** *Examine your breasts regularly at the same time each month. In that way, you know their normal texture and can better recognize changes. To learn more, ask your doctor or check online sources, such as the National Breast Cancer Foundation, the American Cancer Society, and BreastCancer.org.*

Hot-Cold Compresses

This soothing remedy helps relieve PMS symptoms and inflammation from nursing.

1 bowl of hot water (should be a soothing
   temperature)
6 ice cubes, crushed

PREPARATION AND USE:
Immerse a washcloth in the hot water, wring out, and form a compress. Hold on the inflamed breast for 5 minutes. Fill a resealable plastic bag with the crushed ice and wrap in another wash-cloth. Apply the cold compress to the same area for 5 minutes. Repeat the process for the total timeof 30 minutes.

YIELD: 1 APPLICATION

❷ **How it works:** *Alternating warmth and cold will soothe inflamed breast tissue to give relief while nursing.*

❶ **Warning:** *If nursing, don't apply cold just before feeding your baby, as doing so can slow your milk letdown.*

 ## Tame the Tenderness

Warm water improves circulation, which helps clear local inflammation, and promotes tranquility.

2 cups (480 g) Epsom salts
10 drops lavender or other favorite
   essential oil

PREPARATION AND USE:
While running warm bath water, stir in and dis-solve the Epsom salts. Add the lavender drops and swirl with your hand to mix. Enjoy!

YIELD: 1 APPLICATION

❷ **How it works:** *Warm water relaxes the body and stimulates circulation. Lavender is a relax-ing and anti-inflammatory agent. Although the medicinal properties of Epsom salts have not been confirmed, they do contain magnesium, which also helps relax muscles. People also use magnesium-containing compresses to manage tissue infections.*

Note: Although it feels wonderful, bathing can also lead to nipple dryness, so moisturize your nipple area right after bathing to seal in moisture. A sim-ple nonfragrant, lanolin-based cream will work. You can also use a little coconut or jojoba oil.

Soothing Baby-Safe Nipple Cream

These natural ingredients will soothe and seal in moisture. This cream can be used before or after nursing without harming your baby.

1¼ cup (281 g) coconut oil
¼ cup (55 g) shea butter
¼ cup (55 g) cocoa butter

PREPARATION AND USE:
In a small bowl, mix together all the ingredients. If too hard to mix, place in a heatproof bowl and immerse in a pan of hot water on the stove top until softened (a tempered glass measuring cup works well here; hang it on the side of the pot by its handle). For a creamy texture, mix the ingredients together in a blender.

Put mixture into a clean bottle with a cap. Store in a cool, dry place. Apply after each nursing, taking a small amount and warming it in your palms before spreading it on the nipple.

YIELD: ABOUT ¾ CUP (165 G) FOR MULTIPLE APPLICATIONS

❓ **How it works:** *Coconut oil, shea oil, and cocoa butter are soothing and emollient. This mixture prevents cracks, which are painful and through which bacteria can enter to cause infection.*

Stress Less

This short exercise is vital if you're experiencing premenstrual tension or are pregnant or nursing.

A quiet place
You

PREPARATION AND USE:
Close your eyes. Breathe deeply, counting in four counts. Hold your breath for seven counts. Expel your breath for eight counts, exhaling longer if you can. Repeat three more times. Practice daily, once in the morning and once in the evening.

YIELD: 1 APPLICATION

❓ **How it works:** *Many women notice that stress worsens premenstrual breast tenderness. One possible reason is that stress increases a hormone called prolactin (the same one that enlarges breasts and increases milk production when a woman breastfeeds). Mindful breathing reduces stress and creates a feeling of well-being. In the evening, it calms you and helps promote sleep.*

Lifestyle Tip

When you are nursing, feed your baby often. This helps empty your breasts and make them more comfortable. After a nursing session, air-dry your nipples. This will help prevent cracking and itching.

Avocado-Walnut "Good Fat" Salad

Eating the right kind of fats helps control breast discomfort. That means more EFAs and fewer fats from meat, dairy, and processed foods.

For the salad:
2 teaspoons (10 ml) fresh lime juice
1 avocado, peeled, pitted, and sliced
2 ears corn, with husks
2 cups (110 g) chopped Bibb lettuce
½ cup (60 g) crushed walnuts
½ cup (50 g) chopped black olives
¼ cup (58 g) thinly sliced radishes

For the dressing:
½ cup (120 ml) olive oil
¼ cup (60 ml) white wine vinegar
Sea salt

PREPARATION AND USE:
To make the salad: Preheat the oven to 450°F (230°C, or gas mark 8).

In a small bowl, pour the lime juice over the avocado slices and toss lightly to coat. Set aside.

Place the corn on a baking sheet and roast for 15 to 20 minutes. Remove the corn from the oven, let cool, husk, and cut the kernels from the cob.

In a large bowl, combine the corn kernels, lettuce, walnuts, black olives, and radishes. Fold in the avocado mix and toss.

To make the dressing: Blend the oil and vinegar in a blender for 12 seconds and whisk together. Add sea salt to taste.

Divide the salad among four plates, if serving at once. Serve the dressing on the side.

YIELD: 4 SERVINGS

❷ How it works: *The good fats found in avocados and walnuts, as well as in seeds, vegetables, and fish, reduce inflammation. In addition, walnuts are rich in magnesium, which may relieve premenstrual fluid retention, and in alpha-linoleic acid, an anti-inflammatory essential fatty acid.*

Flax and Raisin Muffins in a Mug

There's no excuse for going flax-less. You can whip these up in just a few minutes.

For the dry ingredients:
½ cup (55 g) flaxseed meal
1 teaspoon (5 g) baking powder
1 teaspoon (2 g) ground cinnamon
1 teaspoon (¼ packet [0.5 g]) stevia

For the wet ingredients:
2 large eggs
2 teaspoons (10 ml) vegetable oil
2 tablespoons (18 g) golden raisins
A dollop of Greek yogurt (optional)
A drizzle of honey (optional)

PREPARATION AND USE:
Mix all the dry ingredients in a small bowl. Stir in the wet ingredients. Fold in the raisins.

Spoon the mixture into two microwave-safe mugs. Microwave each on HIGH for 1 minute.

Enjoy with Greek yogurt or honey, straight from the mug.

YIELD: 2 SERVINGS

❷ How it works: *Clinical research shows that eating a muffin containing 25 grams of flaxseed meal daily for three months significantly reduces symptoms of severe cyclic breast tenderness.*

When Simple Doesn't Work

Over-the-counter pain relievers can help relieve breast pain: aspirin (but not for women under the age of twenty or breast-feeding mothers), acetaminophen (Tylenol), ibuprofen (Motrin, Advil), and naproxen (Naprosyn, Alleve). Take as directed.

Hormonal contraceptives (for example, birth control pills) can reduce cyclic breast tenderness. However, for some women hormonal contraceptives cause breast tenderness.

A half-dozen studies show that extracts from the berries of chaste tree (Vitex agnus castus), taken for three continuous months, reduce premenstrual symptoms, including breast tenderness. Doses vary, depending upon how the herb is prepared. Follow the package instructions. The usual daily dose is 2 droppersful (½ teaspoon, or 2.5 ml) of tincture diluted in water, or 20 to 40 milligrams of a concentrated solid extract. Take in the morning. These extracts are not recommended for women who are pregnant or long-term in women who are nursing or taking hormonal contraceptives.

Evening primrose oil, taken as a supplement, may also help. The oil contains gamma linolenic acid, an essential fatty acid. One study found that supplemental vitamin E and/or evening primrose oil brought relief to study participants.

Beneficial Black Bean Salad

This magnesium-rich recipe works toward reducing PMS symptoms, including breast tenderness.

1½ cups (355 ml) water
¾ cup (146 g) uncooked brown rice
1 can (14 ounces, or 400 g) black beans, drained and rinsed
1 cup (164 g) cooked corn kernels
4 scallions, chopped
1 jalapeño pepper, seeded and minced
1 red bell pepper, seeded and diced
1 medium-size tomato, seeded and chopped
2 tablespoons (28 ml) olive oil
2 tablespoons (28 ml) lime juice
1 teaspoon (1 g) dried oregano
½ cup (8 g) fresh cilantro
1 avocado

PREPARATION AND USE:

Combine the water and rice in a small saucepan and bring to a boil. Lower the heat to a simmer and cook until tender, about 30 minutes.

Combine the beans, corn kernels, scallions, peppers, and tomato in a large bowl. In a smaller bowl, whisk together the olive oil, lime juice, and oregano. Drizzle this into the large bowl and mix. Refrigerate for 2 hours.

When ready to serve, toss in the cilantro. Peel, pit, and slice the avocado and arrange on top of the salad before serving.

YIELD: 8 SERVINGS

❷ How it works: *Some studies show that magnesium supplementation reduces premenstrual syndrome symptoms, such as water retention and breast tenderness. The recommended daily intake is 310 milligrams for women. Beans and lentils are rich in magnesium. Other good sources include wheat bran (89 milligrams per ¼ cup [25 g]), almonds (80 milligrams per ounce [28 g]), cooked spinach (78 milligrams per ½ cup [90 g]), cashews (74 milligrams per ounce [28 g]), and peanuts (50 milligrams per ounce [28 g]).*

◖ Simply Good Broccoli

This easy nondairy recipe delivers important calcium and magnesium, which helps guard against premenstrual breast pain.

1 broccoli crown, broken into 8 or so florets
2 garlic cloves, thinly sliced
2 tablespoons (30 ml) olive oil
¼ cup (25 g) crushed almonds
Sea salt

PREPARATION AND USE:

Wash and slice the broccoli florets. Combine the broccoli and garlic in a skillet. Cover with the olive oil and toss. Place the skillet over high heat and stir-fry the broccoli mixture continuously for about 2 minutes. Remove from the heat and then toss in the crushed almonds and sea salt to taste.

Serve while steaming hot.

YIELD: 2 SERVINGS

❷ How it works: *Broccoli and almonds both provide calcium and magnesium. Studies show that calcium supplements (1,000 to 1,200 grams a day) have decreased premenstrual symptoms, including pain. Magnesium supplements are often recommended for treating PMS symptoms.*

When to Call the Doctor

Keep up with yearly breast exams by a doctor, nurse, or other qualified health practitioner. Ask whether he or she recommends you get a mammogram. There's currently some controversy about the timing and frequency of this screening test. Call your doctor's office if you notice anything new or unusual, such as:

- *a new lump, regardless of whether it's tender, in your breast or armpit*
- *nipple discharge (unrelated to breast-feeding an infant)*
- *pain*
- *puckering, dimpling, thickening, or discoloration of the skin*

If you're breastfeeding a baby and have any problems, including a suspected breast infection, call. More serious cases of mastitis may require antibiotic treatment.

Lifestyle Tip

Get support. Wear a sports bra when exercising. Also give your breasts some time outside the harness so that blood and lymph can freely circulate.

Chapter 18

Bruises

Life is full of bumps and bruises. When we learn to crawl, walk, ride a bike, stand on our hands, or skate—anytime we push the envelope of our physical capabilities, we risk falling. It's how we learn and gain new skills.

Of course, we also bruise ourselves in embarrassing ways. When hurried, harried, and distracted, your own house can become a minefield. Bruises can result from surgical procedures and accidental injuries—slips on icy walks, car crashes, and so forth.

No matter how you sustain one, a bruise (also called a contusion) represents soft tissue trauma. Skin turns plum-colored because burst blood vessels have spilled red blood cells into the surrounding tissue. Later, breakdown products from those cells create green and yellow hues. Extra fluid in the tissues causes swelling. And, unfortunately, there's some degree of tenderness. Deeper bruising of muscle and the lining of bones may be particularly painful.

If you bump your head, you can end up with an "egg." That bump indicates that a blood vessel tore under the scalp. You can also bruise your brain. Although both stem from physical trauma, brain contusions aren't the same as brain concussions. The former involves

a localized bruising. Concussions affect the brain more globally and microscopically. For instance, if someone rear-ends your car, the forward and backward motion of your head causes your brain to bobble, striking the inside of the skull as it does.

History

Down through the ages many herbal remedies—from catnip to evening primrose—have been applied to bruises. A few have stood the test of time.

Ancient Greek and Roman physicians, along with the Crusaders, dressed bruises and battle wounds with St. John's wort (*Hypericum perforatum*). Later, the 1597 first edition of *Gerard's Herbal* recommended the oil of St. John's wort (*wort* is the old English word for "plant") for a bruise. Soaked in olive oil, the bright yellow flowers were placed in the sun for several weeks (to infuse the oil), then applied externally. Known as "red oil," for the blood-red liquid hypericin released from the petals, the preparation was still available in pharmacies in the twentieth century. Recent studies confirm that creams and gels containing St. John's wort, applied to bruises, have significant anti-inflammatory effects.

Arnica *(Arnica montana)* has been used in Europe, at least since the 1500s, also to treat bruising, inflammation, and swelling. Mountain climbers used the fresh plant to relieve aching muscles and for bruises from falls. Some studies indicate it may reduce bruising after injuries. The European Scientific Commission on Phytotherapy also endorses its topical use in gels, ointments, salves, or creams on unbroken skin, but notes (unless taken as a highly diluted homeopathic product) that arnica should never be used internally.

RECIPES TO TREAT BRUISES

Cold Pack

6 ice cubes, crushed

PREPARATION AND USE:
Place the ice in a resealable plastic bag. Wrap in a clean cloth. Apply to the bruised area for 15 to 20 minutes. Repeat at least three times a day.

YIELD: 1 APPLICATION

❷ How it works: *Immediate application of an ice pack can help slow, or even prevent, swelling from a bruise.*

Lifestyle Tip

Peas, please. Keep a pack of frozen peas in the fridge. It's a good alternative for the ice pack above. Apply for 10 to 15 minutes when a bruise starts to burgeon.

❧ Elevation Salvation

This is for serious bruising. Minor bruises, from bumping into a chair or table, for example, don't cause much swelling.

3 pillows
Your bruised area
An ice pack (see Cold Pack, at left)

PREPARATION AND USE:
Sit or lie in a comfortable position. Pile up the pillows in a strategic place. Rest the bruised arm, leg, foot, or head against the pillows so that the area is above heart level. Apply the ice pack. Practice this as often as possible when injury first occurs.

YIELD: 1 APPLICATION

❷ How it works: *Keeping the bruised area above your heart level and applying ice will help minimize swelling.*

Fact or Myth?

EVEN THOUGH IT HASN'T BROKEN THE SKIN, BRUISING AFTER A SERIOUS INJURY STILL REQUIRES AS CAREFUL ATTENTION AS A CUT.

Fact. The injury may in fact be deeper, and immediate care is as essential as for broken skin.

Aloe Vera Gel

2 tablespoons (28 g) *Aloe vera* gel
1 tablespoon (6.8) ground turmeric
1 teaspoon ground ginger
2 drops peppermint essential oil

PREPARATION AND USE:

In a small bowl, blend all the ingredients to form a paste. Apply to the skin, covering the bruise. Cover the paste with gauze or a clean cloth. Rest for 15 to 30 minutes. Remove the gauze and paste.

YIELD: 1 APPLICATION

❓ **How it works:** *Turmeric and ginger are both anti-inflammatory and analgesic. Peppermint reduces pain. Aloe vera is anti-inflammatory and speeds wound healing. Because aloe is readily absorbed into the skin, it may help drag other chemical ingredients along with it.*

❗ **Warning:** *Take care not to get this mixture on your clothes, as it will stain. Also, avoid contact with your eyes. The turmeric will temporarily turn your skin yellow.*

Lifestyle Tip

Apply gentle pressure. Whenever you have bleeding, even if it's under the skin, compressing the spot for at least 2 minutes helps a clot form. You can also wrap a bruised extremity—just make sure it's loose enough to slide a finger underneath. Later, gentle massage can help relieve pain and encourage blood flow.

Kale and Blueberry Salad

1 bunch kale, thinly sliced, minus stems
1 cup (145 g) blueberries
¼ red onion, sliced
1 cup (110 g) finely chopped pecans or (120 g) walnuts
1 tablespoon (15 g) fresh lime juice
1 tablespoon (15 g) fresh lemon juice
¼ cup (30 g) blue cheese

PREPARATION AND USE:

Toss the kale, blueberries, onion, and nuts in a large bowl.

Mix the lemon and lime juice and add to the salad, coating all the pieces. Let the salad sit for about 10 minutes as the kale wilts. Toss in the blue cheese and serve.

YIELD: 4 MAIN COURSE SERVINGS, OR 8 SIDE DISH SERVINGS

❓ **How it works:** *Vitamin K is essential for blood clotting. Good sources include leafy greens, such as kale, spinach, collard, and turnip greens, as well as asparagus. Vitamin C and flavonoids are needed for the production of collagen, a protein that keeps skin and blood vessels strong. All fresh fruits and vegetables contain them and blueberries in particular are an excellent source.*

Lifestyle Tip

Act quickly! Ice, elevate, and rest the bruised area, unless the bruise is minor. Always assess a bruise for further injury.

Pineapple Press

Cut open a fresh pineapple. Because canned pineapple undergoes pasteurization, which involves heat, the beneficial enzyme bromelain is lost.

1 fresh pineapple

PREPARATION AND USE:
Slice a piece of pineapple and apply the flesh to the bruise. Hold in place for 15 minutes. Meantime, eat as much pineapple as you like.

YIELD: 1 APPLICATION

❓ How it works: *Pineapple contains the enzyme bromelain, which reduces inflammation. In one study, bromelain (taken internally as a supplement) reduced pain and swelling after blunt trauma.*

❗ Warning: *If pineapple irritates your skin, don't use it.*

Note: Alternatively, apply fresh pineapple juice to a clean cloth or piece of gauze and apply to the area for 5 to 10 minutes.

 ## Witch to the Rescue

Witch hazel

PREPARATION AND USE:
Soak a clean cloth in witch hazel and apply directly to the bruise. Hold for 15 to 20 minutes, allowing the elixir to soak into the skin.

YIELD: 1 APPLICATION

❓ How it works: *Witch hazel is an astringent, meaning it contracts tissue to reduce bleeding and swelling.*

When Simple Doesn't Work

If you have pain unrelieved by ice and rest, take acetaminophen (Tylenol), ibuprofen (Advil, Motrin), or naproxen (Naprosyn, Aleve). Keep in mind, however, that non-steroidal anti-inflammatory drugs (ibuprofen, naproxen, or aspirin) taken in higher amounts impair clotting and can make you more susceptible to bruising and spontaneous bleeding.

Many people swear by homeopathic Arnica montana used internally and externally to prevent swelling and bruising after trauma. (In homeopathy, the active substances are highly diluted.) Research is inconclusive, though some studies have shown that a homeopathic arnica gel, applied topically, may help.

Topical applications of the herb comfrey (Symphytum officinale) have been shown to reduce bruising, swelling, and pain after trauma. You can find comfrey-containing salves in natural food stores.

Lifestyle Tip

Don't smoke! Smoking decreases blood circulation and retards wound healing.

🫐 Folic "No Folly" Salad

Folic acid is a bruise defender. Because your body stores only a small amount, try to maintain adequate levels by regularly eating the following foods—whether in this salad or in their own tasty combos.

4 cups (120 g) spinach, rinsed and drained

½ cup (150 g) artichoke hearts

6 cherry tomatoes, halved

1 mandarin or regular orange, peeled, seeded, and sectioned

1 tablespoon (15 ml) olive oil

½ cup (80 g) chopped onion

½ red bell pepper, seeded and sliced

16 asparagus spears, woody bottoms chopped off

½ block (about 7 ounces, or 200 g) firm tofu, cut into squares

1 tablespoon (11 g) low-sodium honey mustard

1 tablespoon (7 g) sliced almonds

PREPARATION AND USE:

Mix the spinach, artichoke hearts, tomatoes, and orange. Divide between two or among four plates.

Pour the oil into a large skillet over medium-high heat. Add the onion and red pepper and stir-fry for about 2 minutes until lightly browned. Add the asparagus and tofu and lower the heat to medium. Cook for another 3 minutes. Mix in the mustard and stir for another 30 seconds to 1 minute. Top the salads with this delicious folic-rich combo.

YIELD: 2 LARGE SALADS OR 4 SIDE SALADS

❓ **How it works:** *Spinach, asparagus, oranges, artichokes, red peppers, and tofu are high in the B vitamin folic acid. Folic acid boosts production of red and white blood cells and platelets. Deficiency of folic acid, as well as of the vitamins C, K, or B_{12}, can impair blood clotting and increase the risk of bruising. Dark leafy greens also contain vitamins C and K.*

When to Call the Doctor

- *You're taking a blood thinner or have a blood-clotting disorder and sustain more than a minor bruise, especially if the affected area is a joint.*

- *You notice that you have bruises not associated with significant trauma.*

- *You have significant pain.*

- *The injury has reduced the mobility at a joint.*

- *You're unable to bear weight or walk.*

- *A bruise is still apparent after two weeks.*

- *Skin infection or other symptoms begin to develop.*

- *After striking your head, you:*
    - *fall more than a few feet*
    - *lose consciousness, however briefly*
    - *vomit more than once*
    - *become confused, sleepy, or have trouble walking*
    - *have a prolonged, severe headache*
    - *notice your neck hurts*

Note: For suspected concussions and fractures, have someone drive you to the emergency room. If you suspect you injured your neck, don't move. Have someone else call 911.

Chapter 19

Burns

Most anyone who spends much time in the kitchen or out in the sun has experienced a burn. Causes of burns include ultraviolet light, hot liquids, fire, electricity, and chemicals. Although the skin is normally involved, hot liquids can burn the mouth and throat; inhalation of smoke and some chemicals can burn the lungs.

Burns come in three varieties:

- First-degree burns affect the epidermis, the outermost layer of skin. They cause redness and pain, and, after a couple of days, peeling skin.

- Second-degree burns extend into the dermis, the bottom layer of skin. In addition to redness, pain, and swelling, they raise blisters.

- Third-degree burns, also called full-thickness burns, destroy the skin and damage underlying tissues. Because nerves are damaged, the area may be numb. Other signs include white or charred skin.

If a first- or second-degree burn occurs, swiftly remove the skin from the source of heat. Plunge the area into cool water for five minutes. If clothing can't be quickly removed (or is stuck to the skin), thrust it into the water, too. Afterward, wash the area with mild soap and water and cover with sterile gauze. Remove any constricting jewelry from the area. If arms or legs are involved, elevate to about the level of the heart.

Once the injury has occurred, it can take twenty-four to forty-eight hours for the burn to stop progressing. Redness, blisters, and peeling will steadily evolve.

We'll discuss indications for physician treatment at the end. More severe burns can lead to dehydration, infection, scarring, and even death.

History
The ancients used the plant and animal sources available to them to treat burns. Animal "curatives" included cow dung, beeswax, bear fat, lard, milk, butter, eggs, and honey. Except for honey, these animal sources were usually harmful because they retained heat or were contaminated with bacteria.

Plants were also used with tea leaves and *Aloe vera* gel proving helpful for first- and second-degree burns. During the Renaissance, physicians treated burns from gunpowder by cleansing them with boiling oil! The use of carbolic acid in the nineteenth century seems barbaric by today's standards of care. However, the use of maggots—also used in the past to debride burns—has made a recent comeback. Without damaging healthy tissue, maggots remove dead tissue, which otherwise would delay healing and possibly become infected.

The discovery of sulfa drugs and antibiotics, such as penicillin, to treat infection in acute burns led to drastic changes. The emphasis on adequate fluids, along with skin grafts, compressive dressings, and antibiotics, revolutionized treatment for serious burns. However, many burn victims still die of infection, a leading cause of death for millennia. Today, infection is often the result of antibiotic resistance, the worst being from methicillin-resistant *Staphylococcus aureus* (MRSA).

Interestingly, the use of honey—used by the Egyptians in 2000 BCE—has come full circle and is once again being applied to burns to ward off the infections that threaten burn victims. Manuka honey, made by bees that pollinate a particular New Zealand plant, has antibacterial effects.

Lifestyle Tip

Once a burn has cooled down and begins to heal, cover it with an herbal salve to help reduce dryness and promote healing. Don't apply it too soon. If the burn is still warm, the salve will lock in heat and could increase damage to the skin.

 Burn Response 101

Burn victim

PREPARATION AND USE:
Pull the victim away from the fire, boiling liquid, or steam.

If the victim is on fire, push him or her to the ground and roll his or her body to smother the flames. Pull away smoking material or charred clothing from victim. If clothing sticks to the skin, cut or tear around it. Immediately remove any jewelry, tight clothing, and restrictive accessories, such as belts, to prevent swelling.

To treat a first-degree burn (which affects only the top layer of skin): Hold the skin under cool water until the pain is relieved or apply cool compresses. Cover with a sterile, nonstick bandage or clean cloth and do not apply ointment. Whereas cool water dispels heat, the old-fashioned treatment with butter (a simple type of ointment) can actually hold in heat. Once the wound has cooled, antibacterial ointment or healing herbal salve is fine.

To treat a second-degree burn (which affects the top two layers of skin): Immerse the burn area in cool water for 10 to 15 minutes or apply cool compresses. Do not apply ice or submerge in an ice bath, as prolonged exposure to cold temperatures will further damage tissue. Cover loosely with a sterile, nonstick bandage and do not apply ointment.

If the second-degree burn covers a large part of the body, also: Lay the person flat. Elevate his or her feet by about 12 inches (30 cm). Raise the burn area above the heart level. Drape the victim with a blanket or warm clothing. Call the doctor immediately.

(Continued)

To treat a third-degree burn (which damages all layers of skin and may extend even deeper): Call 911. Cover the area with a sterile, nonstick bandage, a sheet for larger areas, or any clean material that will not leave cloth in the wound. Separate the victim's fingers and toes with sterile cloth. Do not apply water or ointments.

YIELD: DIFFERENT FOR EACH CIRCUMSTANCE

❓ How it works: *Burns require immediate attention. Assess the situation and act as set out above. Never take a chance. See a doctor immediately for second-degree burns. Dial 911 when a fire or other life-threatening situation causes third-degree burns.*

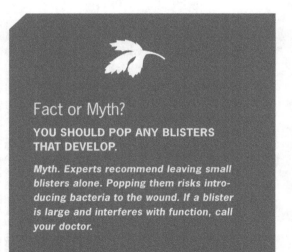

Fact or Myth?

YOU SHOULD POP ANY BLISTERS THAT DEVELOP.

Myth. Experts recommend leaving small blisters alone. Popping them risks introducing bacteria to the wound. If a blister is large and interferes with function, call your doctor.

🌵 Aloe-ah Burns

1 tablespoon (15 g) *Aloe vera* gel (Look for a product that's at least 90 percent aloe.)
10 drops lavender essential oil

PREPARATION AND USE:

Blend the aloe gel and essential oil to make a paste. Apply the paste as needed to the burn.

YIELD: SEVERAL APPLICATIONS FOR A SMALL BURN

❓ How it works: Aloe vera *gel inhibits pain-producing substances. It is anti-inflammatory, promotes circulation, and inhibits bacteria and fungi. Studies show that it speeds healing of burns and wounds, improves psoriasis, and enhances tissue survival after frostbite. Although not all studies have been positive, cumulative research does indicate that topical aloe gel benefits first- and second-degree burns. Lavender essential oil is anti-inflammatory, pain-relieving, antibacterial, and antifungal.*

Lifestyle Tip

For sunburns, try a cream or gel with menthol or camphor. Either will help take the sting away.

🍯 Sweet Soother

Honey (a fresh, uncontaminated jar)

PREPARATION AND USE:

With a clean butter knife, spread the honey on a piece of sterile gauze large enough to cover the burn. Tape the edges of the gauze in place so that the bandage is comfortable—not too tight across the burn. Every 6 hours, gently wash the skin and change the dressing.

YIELD: 1 APPLICATION

❓ How it works: *Honey is an ancient wound healer. Scientific studies show it's antibacterial and speeds healing of burns on par with the more conventional burn dressings containing silver sulfadiazine.*

Note: Manuka honey is especially effective if you are concerned about skin infection. (It is available at health food stores and is expensive.)

Alternatively, mix a teaspoon of honey with a teaspoon of *Aloe vera* gel and apply to the gauze. You'll get double the healing action.

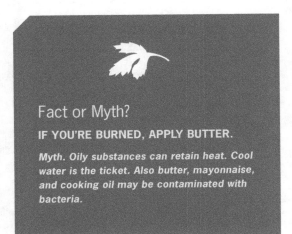

Fact or Myth?

IF YOU'RE BURNED, APPLY BUTTER.

Myth. Oily substances can retain heat. Cool water is the ticket. Also butter, mayonnaise, and cooking oil may be contaminated with bacteria.

🍵 Tea-Total Compress

½ cup (120 ml) boiling water
Green or black tea bag (chamomile is
   a favorite)

PREPARATION AND USE:

Pour the boiling water into a cup. Dunk your tea bag of choice. Steep and let cool to room temperature. Dip the clean cloth into the tea and apply to the burn.

YIELD: 1 APPLICATION

❓ How it works: *Tea compresses are a time-honored treatment for sunburns. Tea (Camellia sinensis) is anti-inflammatory, antioxidant, antibacterial, and astringent (contracts the skin). Green tea has captured more of the research than has black tea (which is darker due to further processing).*

Relative to black tea, green tea has stronger antioxidant and antibacterial effects. Experiments show green tea extracts applied to the skin provide some protection against the detrimental effects of ultraviolet light. Consuming green tea does, too. Although it protects against skin damage from solar radiation, topical green tea extract appears to be more effective when applied before, rather than after, sunburn. German chamomile (Matricaria recutita) is antioxidant, anti-inflammatory, antimicrobial, and wound healing. Lab experiments show it improved healing of burns and other wounds.

Note: Alternatively, apply the cooled tea bag directly to the irritated skin.

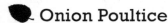 Lavender Soothe-sayer

This recipe is suitable only for small burns, no greater than 2 inches (5 cm) in diameter.

2 drops lavender essential oil

PREPARATION AND USE:
Smooth the essential oil over the burned area.

YIELD: 1 APPLICATION

❷ **How it works:** *The essential oil made from the lavender flower relieves discomfort and reduces inflammation. Studies also show improved healing of surgical wounds.*

Note: Essential oils are not true oils. Do not apply true oils, such as olive, almond, or vegetable oils to burned skin until the burn has fully resolved.

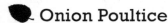 Onion Poultice

½ freshly cut onion, diced
⅛ teaspoon salt

PREPARATION AND USE:
Mash the onion pieces with the salt or blend in a food processor. Apply the mixture directly to the burn, and then wrap with clean muslin.

YIELD: 1 APPLICATION

❷ **How it works:** *The juice of an onion is a disinfectant. The coolness of an onion slice can also draw out heat. Raw, cool potato slices have been used to relieve burned skin, but there is no evidence-based research to support why.*

Note: As a quick alternative, apply a slice of freshly cut onion or potato directly to the burned area for 15 minutes to draw out the heat.

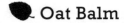 Oat Balm

6 tablespoons (30 g) rolled oats
¾ cup (175 ml) water

PREPARATION AND USE:
Combine the oats and water in a microwave-safe bowl. Microwave on high for 2 minutes or until cooked. Let cool. Cover the burned area with the cooled oat mixture. Wrap in clean muslin or gauze and keep it in place for 30 minutes to an hour.

YIELD: 1 APPLICATION

❷ **How it works:** *Oatmeal is soothing to burned skin. The gooeyness comes from a polysaccharide (complex sugar) called beta-glucan. It helps protect and hold water in the skin. Other compounds called phenols have antioxidant and anti-inflammatory activity.*

Note: Alternatively, in coffee mill or food processor, grind ½ cup (40 g) of rolled oats to a powder and add to a tepid bath. If you don't want to grind the oats, put them in a sock and tie the top to avoid clogging your drain. Swish the sock around for 5 minutes before you step into the bathtub.

Lifestyle Tip

After a sunburn, use a moisturizer to lubricate areas where the burn will rub against skin or clothes.

Calendula Tincture

2 teaspoons (1 g) dried calendula flowers (also
called pot marigold, available at a natural
food store)
1 cup (235 ml) boiling water

PREPARATION AND USE:

Steep the calendula flowers in the boiling water
for 10 minutes. Strain and let cool. Apply to
the burn with a clean cloth. Repeat as often as
possible.

YIELD: 1 OR MORE APPLICATIONS

❓ How it works: *The calendula flower is antiseptic and helps heal wounds. It is also anti-
inflammatory and cooling, which soothes a burn.*

Fact or Myth?

IF YOU'RE BURNED, APPLY ICE.

*Myth. Prolonged contact with ice and ice
water can further injure tissues and also
may lead to hypothermia (abnormally low
body temperature). If, on the other hand,
you burn your hand in the kitchen, dunking
it for 1 to 5 minutes into a cup of ice water
is fine.*

Green Tea Cocktail

*Burned skin loses its barrier function, allowing
water to escape. Be sure to drink extra fluids after
being burned.*

2 cups (275 ml) boiled water
2 teaspoons (4 g) green tea leaves
2 teaspoons (4 g) chopped fresh spearmint
1 teaspoon (14 g) honey
2 tablespoons (28 ml) fresh lime juice

PREPARATION AND USE:

Put the tea leaves in the boiled water to steep. Stir
in the spearmint. Continue to steep for 15 minutes. Strain the tea and stir in the honey until dissolved. Chill the remaining liquid. Stir in the lime
juice and serve.

YIELD: 2 SERVINGS

❓ How it works: *As noted earlier, science touts
green tea for its antibacterial, antioxidant, and
anti-inflammatory properties. Although it can
be topically applied to help guard skin from the
sun's damaging rays, consuming green tea also
helps provide protection against the detrimental
effects of ultraviolet light.*

When Simple Doesn't Work

- *Take acetaminophen (Tylenol), ibuprofen (Motrin, Advil), or naproxen (Aleve,
  Naprosyn) for pain.*

- *Over-the-counter anesthetic creams and
  sprays can reduce discomfort.*

● Burn-out (Delicious Roasted) Chicken

Your body needs extra protein to heal wounds. Unless the burned area is small, be sure to consume enough during the process.

1 teaspoon (1 g) freshly ground black pepper
½ teaspoon sea salt
¼ cup (7 g) crushed fresh rosemary
1 whole chicken, (4 pounds, or 1.8 kg), thoroughly washed, with skin
2 sprigs of rosemary

PREPARATION AND USE:
Preheat the oven to 350°F (180°C, or gas mark 4). Crush together the pepper, salt, and rosemary. Lifting up the chicken skin, rub the dry mixture directly onto the flesh. Re-cover the chicken with the skin. Place the rosemary sprigs inside the chicken cavity. Place the chicken on a rack in a baking pan. Roast uncovered for 20 minutes per pound, plus an extra 15 minutes. A meat thermometer should read 165°F (74°C). Remove from the oven and cover with aluminum foil for about 10 minutes. Slice and serve.

YIELD: 6 SERVINGS

❓ How it works: *When you have a wound of significant size, your body needs extra protein for healing. Chicken—white and dark meat— provides ample protein. When you've plucked the bones clean, use them to make delicious bone soup.*

When to Call the Doctor

Call 911 for third-degree burns, lightning strikes, or electrical burns (from being electrocuted). While awaiting help, cover the area with a sterile bandage or clean sheet. Do not submerse in cool water. Elevate burned limbs above the heart.

Call poison control (the US National Poison Hotline is 800-222-1222) for chemical burns.

Proceed to the emergency room if:

- *A chemical burned your eye.*

- *The burn involves your face, hands, feet, genitals, throat, or a joint. (If minor sunburn affects the face, hands, or feet, you can probably manage with home care.)*

- *A second-degree burn is larger than the size of your hand.*

- *Smoke was inhaled.*

- *You otherwise suspect the burn is serious.*

- *The burn victim is an infant.*

Visit the doctor or clinic if:

- *Your tetanus shot is out of date.*

- *Pain continues for longer than forty-eight hours.*

- *You're concerned the wound might be becoming infected (as evidenced by purulent discharge, swollen lymph nodes in the area, or increased redness and pain).*

- *The wound is not healing. First-degree burns should heal within three to six days. Second-degree burns can take two weeks.*

Chapter 20

Cancer Prevention

The big C. The crab. The crustacean that scuttles in and out of nightmares. Too many of us know the touch of its claw. Cancer is the second-leading cause of death in the United States, accounting for one in four deaths. Annually, an estimated 1.6 million Americans receive a cancer diagnosis—a number that excludes skin cancers, which are so common they're not reported to cancer registries. The most common cancers involve the lung, colon, breast, and prostate; combined they cause half of all cancer deaths.

Many types of cancer are either preventable or easily treatable. In terms of lifestyle factors, scientists attribute one-third of cancers to tobacco use, one-third to diet, and one-third to environmental exposures (infectious microorganisms, ultraviolet light, radiation, pollutants, and other toxins). Physical inactivity, obesity, insufficient sleep, and alcohol are also linked to some cancers. Genetics play a significant role in only a few cancers.

Keep in mind that twenty to thirty years often elapse between the microscopic start of cancer and diagnosis of a tumor. A host of events can conspire to initiate and propagate a tumor. Furthermore, we can't completely control environmental exposures and have zero control over past exposures. What we can all do is to start now to reduce our modifiable risks. A number of organizations provide information on how to do just that: Prevent Cancer (http://preventcancer.org), the American Cancer Society (http://www.cancer.org), and the National Cancer Institute (www.cancer. gov). Authorities agree that the four most important things you can do to prevent cancer are to avoid tobacco, eat a healthy diet, exercise regularly, and get recommended screening tests. For more details, read on.

History

As early as 168 BCE, Roman physician Galen made the association of an unhealthy diet with cancer. It took until the eighteenth century, however, to recognize the link between tobacco use and cancer (and until 1950 to confirm it). Chemicals, such as arsenic and aromatic amines, were added to a list of environmental risk factors in the nineteenth century. In the twentieth century, the list of tumor-inducing factors grew longer: X-rays, viruses, and coal tar. But cancer prevention research was still extremely limited.

A corner was turned in 1939 with the establishment of the National Cancer Institute. Not until the 1960s, however, did environmental and lifestyle causes of cancer begin to receive more attention. About this time, screening tests for breast cancer and colorectal cancer were also introduced. By the 1980s, the American Institute for Cancer Research was looking into the roles of diet, physical activity, and obesity in cancer prevention. At the end of the century, moderating exposure to solar UV radiation was added to the skin cancer prevention guidelines.

Clinical trials and research studies in the twenty-first century continue to add to our body of knowledge on cancer prevention. In one example, human papillomavirus (HPV) clinical trials have shown that the HPV vaccine effectively prevents cervical cancer as well as HPV. In another, secondhand smoke has been classified as carcinogenic to humans.

Lifestyle Tip

Protect your skin. Ultraviolet light ages the skin and increases the risk of skin cancer. On the other hand, it generates vitamin D, which has anticancer properties. One solution is to allow yourself brief sunbaths. Exposing unsunscreened arms and legs to 10 to 15 minutes of sunshine generates plenty of vitamin D. Otherwise, cover up or seek shade. And definitely skip the hazards of the tanning salon.

 ## Go Greek Salad

1 teaspoon (5 g) fresh lemon juice
4 teaspoons (20 ml) olive oil, divided
Sea salt and freshly ground black pepper
6 ounces (170 g) salmon
2 tablespoons (30 ml) red wine vinegar
1 garlic clove, crushed
3 cups (141 g) torn romaine lettuce
½ medium-size cucumber, peeled and diced
1 Roma tomato, diced
¼ cup (35 g) pitted and sliced black olives
¼ cup (40 g) diced red onion
¼ cup (38 g) crumbled feta cheese

PREPARATION AND USE:
Preheat the oven to 450°F (230°C, or gas mark 8).

In a small bowl, mix together the lemon juice, 1 teaspoon (5 ml) of the olive oil, and a pinch of salt and pepper. Baste the salmon in the mixture, transfer to a roasting pan, and roast for 10 minutes.

Meanwhile, in a large bowl, whisk together remaining 3 teaspoons (15 ml) of olive oil, and the vinegar, crushed garlic, and additional salt and pepper to taste. Toss in the lettuce, cucumber, tomato, olives, and onion. Fold in the feta. Divide between two plates. Top each with 3 ounces (85 g) of roasted salmon.

YIELD: 2 SERVINGS

❓ **How it works:** *The Mediterranean diet is associated with a reduced risk of cancer. It's rich in a number of foods thought to protect against cancer: vegetables, fruits, grains, legumes, and olive oil, and fish as well as a moderate amount of red wine (which contains resveratrol, an anticancer substance). Plant-based diets seem to shield us from cancer.*

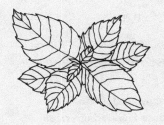

Spotlight: **Turmeric**

Doctors of Ayurvedic and Chinese medicine have long used turmeric to treat multiple ailments, including cancer, age-related disease, arthritis and musculoskeletal pain, liver distress, and indigestion. Current science supports its effectiveness, especially its main active ingredient, curcumin—sometimes called "cure-cumin." According to laboratory studies, the curcumin in turmeric appears to discourage the development of tumors and if tumors do take root, it inhibits their growth, particularly colon cancer.

And that's not all. Turmeric counters multiple other diseases:

- **Chronic, age-related ailments:** India's low rate of Alzheimer's disease and other types of dementia has long intrigued researchers. Lab studies show that curcumin inhibits the growth of beta-amyloid (an abnormal protein that develops in the brains of Alzheimer's sufferers) and also helps to clear it. Note, however, that another study on patients already suffering from Alzheimer's showed that curcumin supplements did not help reverse the symptoms.
- **Infection:** Turmeric's antimicrobial powers counter bacteria, parasites, and fungi. And it can be used as a topical antiseptic for scrapes, cuts, and burns.
- **Osteoarthritis pain:** The curcumin in turmeric acts as a powerful anti-inflammatory. Turmeric was found in one study to treat pain similarly to ibuprofen. Early research also shows that curcumin improves rheumatoid arthritis symptoms.
- **Gastrointestinal concerns:** Turmeric has been shown to protect the liver, relieve indigestion, and help prevent ulcers or relieve existing ones. It also shows promise for Crohn's disease, ulcerative colitis, and other inflammatory bowel diseases.

Absorbing turmeric into the system can be a challenge. When taking it internally, look for top-quality supplements that have absorption capability. Or add oil and pepper when cooking. Although consuming turmeric as a cooking spice is safe, pregnant women should not take concentrated products until they're proven safe. Also, people suffering from gallstones or bile duct obstruction should not ingest concentrated turmeric products. Like many bitter foods and spices, turmeric stimulates the gallbladder to empty itself of bile, causing pain if stones are obstructing the outlet.

Color Guard

Berries, cherries, and grapes make great snack foods. Add them to smoothies or top cereal, salads, and yogurt with them.

1 cup (145 g) blueberries
1 cup (155 g) pitted, sliced cherries
1 cup (150 g) grapes
1 cup (200 g) plain nonfat Greek yogurt
Drizzle of honey
¼ cup (28 g) crushed pecans or almonds

PREPARATION AND USE:
Combine the blueberries, cherries, and grapes in a large bowl. Fold in the yogurt. Drizzle with honey. Sprinkle with the nuts. Luscious!

YIELD: 4 SERVINGS

❷ How it works: *Berries, cherries, and grapes: these tasty, nutrient-dense packets owe their red, blue, and purple color to flavonoids, such as anthocyanins and proanthocyanins, which pack potent antioxidant, anti-inflammatory, and anti-cancer effects. Red grapes contain resveratrol, a well-known anticancer substance.*

Pom Balm

All parts of the pomegranate fruit—rind, pith, and juicy seeds (arils)—have valuable chemicals. Because commercially sold juices use the whole fruit, you can consume them all. The seeds also taste delicious alone, in salads, and atop yogurt.

1 pomegranate
Water
Honey

PREPARATION AND USE:
Wash the skin of the pomegranate and cut off the top and bottom. Cut it in half and then score the skin. Submerge the pomegranate in a large bowl of water. Underwater, remove the arils (fruity seeds) from the whitish membrane—they'll drop to the bottom. (Throw out or compost the membrane and peel.) Strain out the water and pour the arils into a blender or food processor. Blend the arils until they liquefy; they will still have pulp. Pour the pulpy mixture through a strainer into the now-empty bowl, pressing down against the pulp to push the optimal amount of juice through the strainer into the bowl. (You should get 2 ounces [¼ cup, or 60 ml] of pomegranate juice.) Pour the juice from the bowl into an 8-ounce (235 ml) glass. Add water to fill the glass. Stir in honey to taste.

YIELD: 1 SERVING

❷ How it works: *Pomegranate shows promise as an anticancer agent. Pomegranate extracts inhibit the growth of breast, prostate, colon, and lung cancers in cell cultures and animals studies. Extracts also protect against ultraviolet light–induced skin cancer. In men with prostate cancer, drinking 8 ounces (235 ml) of pomegranate juice a day significantly slowed the rise in blood levels of prostate-specific antigen, a protein used to track benign and cancerous prostate conditions.*

Note: You can see how to cut a pomegranate at http://mideastfood.about.com/od/tipsandtechniques/ss/deseedpomegrana_2.htm.

Also, for a quick, nonwater removal, go to www.vimeo.com/39205407.

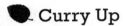 **Curry Up**

2 tablespoons (30 ml) olive oil

Juice of 1 lemon

2 tablespoons (13 g) curry powder

1 teaspoon (3 g) paprika

1 head cauliflower, cut into florets

1 medium-size onion, cut into quarters

PREPARATION AND USE:

Preheat the oven to 425°F (220°C, or gas mark 7).

In a large bowl, whisk together the olive oil, lemon juice, curry powder, and paprika. Add the cauliflower and onion and toss, coating the vegetables with the oil mix.

Spray a baking sheet with olive oil spray. Spread the curried vegetables in a single layer across the baking sheet. Roast for 25 minutes, turning the cauliflower frequently to fully brown. They should be tender in the center when pierced with a fork.

YIELD: SERVES 4

? **How it works:** *The plant family of cruciferous vegetables—broccoli, cauliflower, cabbage, rapini, mung beans, alfalfa sprouts, and Brussels sprouts, among others—contains glucosinolates, which the body breaks down into anticancer substances. Animal and population studies link increased consumption of cruciferous vegetables with reduced cancer risk. Broccoli is particularly famous for its anticancer power.*

Among other spices, curry contains turmeric (Curcuma longa) and ginger (Zingiber offinalis). Both contain potent anti-inflammatory and antioxidant substances. Curcumin, a key chemical in turmeric, inhibits cancer cell growth and migration, blocks the creation of blood vessels to the cancer, and induces cancer cells to die. The optimal dose for supplemental curcumin isn't clear, though doses up to 8 grams a day seem to be safe. Bioavailability is low, so some supplement manufacturers get around that limitation by combining curcumin with bromelain (an enzyme in pineapple), piperine from pepper, or phosphatidyl choline to increase absorption. Curried foods contain pepper and oil, which also improve curcumin's absorption.

Fact or Myth?

SLEEP HAS NOTHING TO DO WITH GETTING THE BIG C.

Myth. Several theories explain the link between sleep deprivation and night-shift work and cancer. They include hormonal shifts that favor obesity and diabetes, disruption in the sleep-regulating (and anticancer) hormone melatonin, and immune suppression. Likewise, chronic stress overload and depression alter hormonal rhythms and suppress immune function.

 # Gingered Carrots

1 tablespoon (15 ml) olive oil
3 large carrots, grated
1 teaspoon (2 g) minced fresh ginger
¼ cup (60 ml) fresh orange juice
¼ cup (35 g) golden raisins
Sea salt
Zest of ½ orange
Freshly ground black pepper

PREPARATION AND USE:

In a skillet, heat the oil over medium heat. Add the carrots. Stir in the ginger and cook for about 2 minutes. Add the juice, raisins, and salt to taste. Simmer for about 2 minutes until the carrots are tender and the juice has evaporated. Stir in the zest. Sprinkle with pepper to taste.

YIELD: 2 TO 3 SERVINGS

How it works: *Ginger is in the same plant family as turmeric. The anticancer research on it is less extensive, but preliminary data look promising. It reduces nausea and vomiting from many causes. Some studies show it may help people going through chemotherapy.*

Garlic Shiitake Greens

2 tablespoons (30 ml) olive oil
⅔ cup (93 g) stemmed and sliced shiitake
  mushrooms
1½ cups (100 g) torn kale leaves
¼ cup (27 g) torn dandelion greens
1 garlic clove, minced
1 teaspoon (5 ml) sesame oil
3 tablespoons (45 ml) soy sauce
Salt and freshly ground black pepper

PREPARATION AND USE:

In a skillet over medium heat, heat the olive oil.
Add the mushroom pieces and heat for 2 to 3
minutes, stirring continuously. Reduce the heat
to low. Add the kale, dandelion greens, garlic,
sesame oil, and soy sauce. Cook for about 2 more
minutes until the kale is just wilted. Sprinkle with
salt and pepper to taste. Serve.

YIELD: 2 SERVINGS

Lifestyle Tip

Drink tea. Population studies link higher
tea consumption with a reduced risk of
gastrointestinal, pancreatic, bladder, prostate, ovarian, uterine, and breast cancer.
Black, green, and oolong tea all come
from the same plant *(Camellia sinensis)*.
Green tea is particularly rich in a polyphenol called epigallocatechin gallate. In lab
research, it inhibits cancer cell formation,
proliferation, invasiveness, and metastasis
and provokes cancer cell death. Animal
studies show protection against many cancers, including skin cancer.

? How it works: *Kale, collards, mustard
greens, bok choy, arugula, watercress, and maca
belong to the cruciferous family. They're natural
sources of minerals such as calcium and magnesium, both of which protect against colon cancer. Women who eat more leafy greens enjoy a
reduced risk of breast cancer.*

*Dandelion (Taraxacum officinale) and sting-
ing nettle (Urtica dioica), though not crucifers,
brim with vitamins and minerals. Preliminary
research suggests they also have anticancer
activity. (Consider allowing dandelion to grow in
a patch of your yard. Harvest before the plants
flower. Avoid wild greens that may have been
sprayed with pesticides.)*

*Population studies and lab research show
that garlic (Allium sativum) has cancer-
protective effects. Garlic enhances enzymes in
our body that detoxify carcinogens, quenches
oxidation, inhibits proliferation of cancer cells,
induces cancer cell death, and boosts immunity.
Heat deactivates some of garlic's key ingredients. To maximize benefits, add raw, minced
garlic to dressings, dips, soups, and sauces.
Alternatively, crush garlic, let it sit for 10 minutes (which allows time for critical enzymatic
changes), and then add it to the cook pot.*

*Mushrooms contain polysaccharides and
other ingredients that both enhance immunity
and have anticancer properties. Most of
the research has been done on more exotic
mushrooms such as shiitake, maitake, and
reishi. However, all edible mushrooms have
benefits. Even the pedestrian button mushrooms
(Agaricus bisporus), more commonly eaten in
America, enhance immune cell functions and
fight cancer. Women who regularly eat mushrooms have a reduced risk of breast cancer.*

Good for You Garlic Dip

1 tablespoon (15 ml) olive oil
1 teaspoon (5 ml) fresh lemon juice
1 cup (200 g) plain Greek yogurt
3 to 4 garlic cloves, minced
3 tablespoons (18 g) chopped fresh mint

PREPARATION AND USE:

Whisk together the olive oil and lemon juice in a small bowl or measuring cup.

Place the yogurt in a medium-size bowl. Fold the oil mixture into the yogurt and mix thoroughly. Stir in the garlic and mint. Refrigerate and serve.

YIELD: 4 APPETIZER SERVINGS AS A DIP

❓ **How it works:** *As noted earlier, garlic has several actions that defend against cancer.*

Lifestyle Tip

Limit your alcohol intake. Heavy drinking increases the risk of cancer of the mouth, throat, gastrointestinal tract, liver, pancreas, uterus, and elsewhere. Even light and moderate drinking, regardless of the type of alcoholic beverage, can raise the risk of breast cancer. Scientists attribute 20 percent of breast cancer cases to drinking two or more alcoholic drinks a day.

Go for the Gold

1 acorn squash, cut in half and seeded
1 teaspoon (7 g) honey
1 tablespoon (16 g) mango chutney
1 teaspoon (5 ml) fresh lemon juice
1 teaspoon (5 ml) soy sauce
1 tablespoon (15 ml) olive oil
Salt and freshly ground black pepper

PREPARATION AND USE:

Preheat the oven to 375°F (190°C, or gas mark 5).

Place the squash halves on a baking sheet cut side up and bake for 15 minutes. While the squash bakes, mix together the honey, chutney, lemon juice, soy sauce, and olive oil. Brush the mixture over the half-baked squash. Bake for another 15 to 20 minutes, until succulent.

YIELD: 2 SERVINGS

❓ **How it works:** *Orange fruits and vegetables are rich in plant pigments called carotenoids. These substances protect against cancer, including prostate, breast, cervical, ovarian, lung, gastrointestinal, and pancreatic cancers. Non–vitamin A carotenoids (lycopene, lutein, astaxanthin, and zeaxanthin) protect against DNA damage. Good sources of carotenoids are orange vegetables (carrots, pumpkin, sweet potatoes, and winter squash), orange fruits (cantaloupe, mangoes, apricots, guava, goji berries), and dark green leafy vegetables.*

Tomato Garlic Bake

2 tomatoes, quartered
2 tablespoons (30 ml) olive oil
1 teaspoon (1 g) crushed fresh basil
2 garlic cloves, pressed, divided
Salt and freshly ground black pepper

PREPARATION AND USE:

Preheat the oven to 450°F (230°C, or gas mark 8).

Spread the tomatoes across a baking sheet. Mix the olive oil, basil, and 1 crushed garlic clove in a small bowl or measuring cup. Baste the tomatoes with the sauce. Lightly sprinkle the tomatoes with salt and pepper. Roast for 25 minutes until tender. Top with the other pressed garlic clove.

YIELD: 2 SERVINGS

❓ How it works: *In the United States, tomatoes are a major source of dietary carotenoids. They owe their red color to lycopene. Research associates regular consumption of tomatoes and tomato products with a reduced risk of prostate cancer and possibly breast cancer. Even a single daily serving of a tomato or tomato product may help protect DNA from damage. Whether lycopene supplements protect against prostate cancer is controversial.*

❗ Warning: *When using canned tomatoes in any recipe, look for "BPA-free" on the label. Cans are often lined with BPA, a chemical found in hard plastics that disrupts normal hormone function and may increase the risk of some cancers. Tomatoes, which are acidic, increase the release of BPA.*

Fact or Myth?

YOU CAN GET A VACCINE TO WARD OFF CANCER.

Fact—in some cases. Certain strains of human papillomavirus (HPV) cause cancer of the cervix, vagina, vulva, anus, penis, mouth, and throat. Hepatitis B can cause liver cancer. Vaccines, which are available for HPV and hepatitis B, need to be given before exposure.

Lifestyle Tip

Although better known as an herb that supports the liver, milk thistle (*Silybum marianum*) also has protective effects against cancer. It contains an antioxidant, anti-inflammatory flavonoid complex called silymarin. Research shows that it promotes repair of DNA, blocks angiogenesis, and suppresses proliferation and metastasis of a variety of cancers. Milk thistle is available as a tincture or standardized extract. You can also make the ground seeds into tea or sprinkle them atop foods. Milk thistle's delicious relative, the artichoke (*Cynara scolymus*), also contains polyphenols. Steam and enjoy.

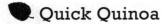 ## Quick Quinoa

1 cup (235 ml) almond milk
Pinch of salt
1 cup (173 g) uncooked quinoa
1 teaspoon (2 g) ground cinnamon
2 tablespoons (18 g) golden raisins
2 tablespoons (19 g) blueberries
1 tablespoon (20 g) honey
1 tablespoon (15 g) yogurt
2 tablespoons (15 g) crushed walnuts

PREPARATION AND USE:

Pour the almond milk into a saucepan and stir in the salt, quinoa, and cinnamon. Heat the quinoa mixture over medium-low heat, stirring in the raisins and blueberries. Continue stirring until the grain has soaked up the liquid and the raisins and blueberries plump up, about 10 minutes. Add the honey. Divide between two bowls, topped with the yogurt and crushed walnuts.

YIELD: 2 SERVINGS

❓ **How it works:** *In addition to providing vitamins and minerals, quinoa (which is a seed) and whole grains are high in complex carbohydrates, which provide fiber and release their sugars relatively slowly into the bloodstream. Refined carbohydrates lack fiber and lead to spikes in blood sugar, insulin, and insulinlike growth factors, which can stimulate tumor growth. Fiber-rich diets seem to protect against colon cancer. Fiber may help bind to potentially cancer-causing substances in the bowel, thus preventing their absorption into the bloodstream. Breakdown products of fiber also support a healthy population of gut microorganisms, which, in turn, contribute to immune function.*

When Simple Doesn't Work

Following a healthy lifestyle does not make you immune from cancer. You can't control everything, such as your genetic composition and past environmental exposures.

Keep appointments for annual examinations and be sure to get recommended screening tests for common cancers. Ask your doctor about screening guidelines for these cancers, particular those of the skin, skin, breast, cervix, prostate, colon, and lung. Or check with the American Cancer Society at www.cancer.org/ or Memorial Sloan-Kettering Cancer Center at www.mskcc.org/cancer-care/screening-guidelines.

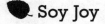 Soy Joy

1 package (8 to 10 ounces, or 225 to 280 g)
   frozen edamame, thawed for 1 hour
2 tablespoons (30 ml) olive or sesame oil
½ teaspoon chili powder
¼ teaspoon curry powder
⅛ teaspoon paprika

PREPARATION AND USE:
Preheat the oven to 375°F (190°C, or gas mark 5).
   Strain and pat dry the thawed edamame. Pour
the edamame into a medium-size bowl. In a small
bowl, stir together the oil, chili and curry powders, and paprika. Drizzle the mixture over the
edamame and toss. Spread the edamame across
a baking sheet and place the sheet on the middle
rack of the oven. Roast for 15 to 20 minutes until
just browned. Serve warm and delectable.

YIELD: 4 SERVINGS

Fact or Myth?

**MICROWAVING FOODS AND
BEVERAGES IN A PLASTIC CONTAINER
IS DANGEROUS.**

*Fact! Plastics marked on the bottom with
"7" or "PC" (for polycarbonate) contain BPA,
a hormone disruptor that contributes to
cancer and other ills. Cans are often lined
with BPA-containing epoxy. Drink beverages
from glass, steel, or ceramic vessels. Store
food in glass containers. Do not microwave
food in plastic containers.*

❷ How it works: *In addition to being fiber-
rich, legumes contain phytoestrogens (plant
estrogens). Soybeans are a particularly rich
source of phytoestrogens called isoflavones.
Estrogen has been implicated in the development of breast and uterine cancers. Like all
hormones, estrogen has to bind to cell receptors
(the equivalent of docking stations) to have an
effect. Phytoestrogens compete with our estrogen at this receptor sites, but have much weaker
effects. In other words, phytoestrogens undermine the potency of estrogen in the body.*

*Population studies link higher consumption
of soy foods with a reduced incidence of breast,
uterine, ovarian, prostate, and colon cancers.*

*A concern has been whether isoflavones
present a risk for breast cancer survivors.
Reassuringly, a study of Chinese and American
women found that soy food consumption correlated with a reduced risk of recurrence. Although
soy foods seem to be safe, some experts discourage
against supplementing with soy protein (which
contains isoflavones) or soy isoflavones. The
concern is that large amounts of phytoestrogens
might stimulate estrogen receptors, thereby
increasing the risk of breast cancer. If you're at
risk for breast cancer, consult your doctor.*

Nutty Flax Breakfast

½ cup (56 g) flaxseed meal
½ cup (120 ml) almond milk
¼ cup (38 g) diced apple
¼ cup (30 g) crushed walnuts
1 tablespoon (15 g) Greek yogurt
Pinch of ground cinnamon

PREPARATION AND USE:

Mix together the flaxseeds, almond milk, apple, and walnuts in a microwave-safe glass bowl. Microwave on high for 30 seconds, stir, and heat for 30 seconds more. Remove from the microwave. Top with the yogurt and cinnamon.

YIELD: 1 TO 2 SERVINGS

? **How it works:** *Seeds and nuts contain vitamins, minerals, healthy fats, and fiber. Greater consumption correlates with a reduced risk of certain cancers, particularly colon cancer. Flaxseeds, sesame seeds, sunflower seeds, and pumpkin contain lignans, which our intestinal bacteria can convert into phytoestrogens. Flaxseeds, the richest source of lignans, inhibit the growth of breast, colon, and prostate cancer. Regular consumption of pumpkin and sunflower seeds has been linked with a reduced risk of breast cancer. Walnuts also inhibit colon and breast cancer.*

When to Call the Doctor

In addition to keeping up with routine exams, make an appointment immediately if you notice any new bumps, lumps, or unusual symptoms.

Lifestyle Tip

Eat a healthy diet. Research shows that plant-based diets protect against many cancers. Based on a thorough research review, the American Institute of Cancer Research urges people to eat 5 servings of vegetables and fruit at day. Emphasize nonstarchy vegetables, such as leafy greens, zucchini, broccoli, cabbage, Brussels sprouts, mushrooms, and peppers. Avoid sugary drinks, fried foods, fast foods, smoked foods, processed meats, and grilled or barbecued animal foods.

Chapter 21

Cholesterol Management

Cholesterol gets a bad rap. You know—the stuff that gums up the arteries and causes heart disease. But this waxy, much-maligned molecule is also essential. Our body requires cholesterol to form the outer layer of cells, make vitamin D, and produce hormones, such as estrogen, progesterone, and testosterone. It's so important that our livers manufacture plenty of it, regardless of whether we get it in such foods as meat, poultry, fish, eggs, and dairy.

But, yes, too much cholesterol is harmful. High cholesterol is a big risk factor for atherosclerosis, a disease in which cholesterol, fat, calcium, and other substances narrow and harden the arteries and lead to reduced blood flow. The result is heart attack, stroke, and vascular disease. Atherosclerosis is the leading cause of death in people over age forty-five. For most Americans, it takes root in childhood and progresses with each passing year. Genetics influence blood levels. Some people, no matter how healthy their lifestyle, have elevated levels.

Cholesterol travels in a package called a lipoprotein. These little protein-cholesterol tugboats transport several types of cholesterol, including low-density, high-density, very

low-density, and other fats, through the blood. The lower the density, the greater the fatty freight. That's why low-density lipoprotein (LDL) and very-low-density lipoprotein (VLDL) are "bad," and high-density lipoprotein (HDL), which can pick up excess cholesterol and carry it to the liver for elimination, is "good." Further, LDL cholesterol becomes toxic to our cells when oxidized, a process akin to butter going rancid. Oxidized cholesterol causes free radical damage and promotes atherosclerosis. So your goals are to keep VLDL and LDL cholesterol within normal limits. Fortunately, nature provides a host of plants that do just that.

History

Not until the 1950s did scientists work out how the body makes cholesterol. In the 1960s, guidelines were established by the American Heart Association recommending not only reducing cholesterol but also maintaining principles of good nutrition and sound eating habits. In 1976, a Japanese scientist discovered how to block cholesterol synthesis—leading to the development of statin drugs commonly used today to control cholesterol levels.

RECIPES TO SUPPORT HEALTHY CHOLESTEROL LEVELS

Cuppa Tea

1 green tea bag
1 cup (235 ml) boiling water
Honey or other sweetener, such as stevia
    (optional)

PREPARATION AND USE:
Drop the tea bag into the cup of hot water. Add your sweetener of choice, if desired. Enjoy.

YIELD: 1 SERVING

❓ **How it works:** *Green tea protects arteries from atherosclerosis. Tea drinkers seem to enjoy a reduced risk of heart attack. Some studies show it lowers cholesterol.*

❗ **Warning:** *Green tea contains caffeine. If you are on a noncaffeinated diet, check with your doctor about herbal alternatives.*

Lifestyle Tip

Keep a bowl of red grapes handy. They contain resveratrol, a potent antioxidant with cardiovascular benefits.

Lifestyle Tip

Drink a glass of cranberry juice every day or pop a handful of blueberries. Both contain polyphenols, which help increase the resistance of LDL to oxidation, thus playing a part in protecting the arteries and reducing blood pressure and heart disease.

Mom's Oatmeal

1 cup (235 ml) water
½ cup (40 g) regular or quick-cooking
    (not instant) rolled oats
Pinch of salt
½ cup (75 g) diced apple
2 tablespoons (15 g) sliced or chopped walnuts
Honey (optional)
1 teaspoon (2 g) ground cinnamon

PREPARATION AND USE:
Combine the water, oats, and salt in a microwave-safe bowl. Microwave on high for 1 minute and then stir in the apple, walnuts, and cinnamon. Microwave for another minute. Remove from the microwave. Taste it before adding honey. (The apple provides natural sweetness.) Enjoy while still piping hot.

YIELD: 1 SERVING

❓ **How it works:** *Oatmeal contains soluble fiber, which reduces the absorption of dietary cholesterol from the intestines into the blood. Some research shows that cinnamon can reduce cholesterol. Apples contain pectin and flavonoids that both lower cholesterol. Walnuts also lower cholesterol.*

Fab Flax Smoothie

1 cup (230 g) nonfat yogurt
6 strawberries, halved
2 tablespoons (14 g) flaxseed meal

PREPARATION AND USE:

Place the yogurt, strawberries, and flaxseeds in a blender and process until combined.

YIELD: 1 TO 2 SERVINGS

❷ **How it works:** *Scientists believe that the fiber in the coat of the flaxseed binds with cholesterol in the intestine to inhibit absorption into the bloodstream. Strawberries also contain soluble plant fibers and plant stanols that block cholesterol absorption.*

Fact or Myth?

A DIET HIGH IN PLANTS IS AN EFFECTIVE CHOLESTEROL MEDICATION.

In a recent study, researchers asked thirty-four people with high cholesterol to try three diets. The first was low in saturated fat; the second was the same diet, only adding the cholesterol-lowering medication Mevacor (lovastatin); the third had no medication but was high in plant sterols, soy protein foods, and foods rich in viscous fibers. The second and third diets were the winners in lowering cholesterol. For nine people, the plant-only diet was the most effective.

Lifestyle Tip

Add 2 teaspoons (8 g) of psyllium husks to water every morning. Stir well and drink. Besides helping lower cholesterol, it will keep you regular. Make sure to chase the glass of psyllium with a full glass of water.

Psyllium Smoothie

¼ cup (38 g) strawberries
¼ cup (38 g) blueberries
½ banana
1 cup (235 ml) water
3 ice cubes (optional)
1½ teaspoons (10 g) honey (optional)
1 teaspoon (6 g) psyllium husks

PREPARATION AND USE:

Place the fruits in a blender. Add the water, ice cubes (if desired), honey, and psyllium and blend until smooth. Enjoy!

YIELD: 1 SERVING

❷ **How it works:** *Fiber-rich psyllium seed husks, when mixed with water, form a gel that binds cholesterol in the intestine, thereby reducing its absorption into the blood. It also increases the elimination of cholesterol from the body. These fruits provide fiber and antioxidants.*

Artichokes and Garlic Dip

1 cup (235 ml) olive oil
1 garlic clove, crushed
Salt and freshly ground black pepper
2 artichokes
¼ cup (60 ml) water

PREPARATION AND USE:

Pour the olive oil into a small bowl. Mix in the garlic. Stir in salt and pepper to taste.

On a cutting board, cut the artichoke stems to 1 inch (2.5 cm) long. Snip off the sharp tips of the petals. Slice each one in half lengthwise. Scoop out the prickly "choke" inside. Fill a microwave-safe dish with the water. Lay out the four artichoke halves, cut side down, and cover with waxed paper or a lid. Microwave on HIGH until tender, about 10 minutes. Let stand for 1 to 2 minutes to cool. Pull off the leaves and dip the fleshy part into the olive oil mixture.

YIELD: 2 SERVINGS

❓ **How it works:** *Artichokes are shown to reduce LDL cholesterol. Some studies indicate that garlic reduces LDL cholesterol. It protects LDL from oxidation, discourages blood clots from forming within the arteries, modestly lowers blood pressure, helps maintain the elasticity of arteries, and slows the development of atherosclerosis.*

❗ **Warning:** *Stop taking garlic supplements two weeks before surgery. If you're taking blood-thinning medication such as warfarin (Coumadin), talk to your doctor first before adding garlic supplements or raw garlic to your diet. Garlic could potentially increase the action of the medication.*

Lifestyle Tip

Go for a walk. Exercise is one of the best ways of increasing HDL, the "good" cholesterol.

Beneficial Barley Soup

3 cups (710 ml) water
½ cup (92 g) uncooked barley
1 tablespoon (15 ml) olive oil
1 onion, finely chopped
1 teaspoon (3 g) diced garlic
½ cup (35 g) sliced mushrooms
2 tablespoons (32 g) miso paste
Pinch of freshly ground black pepper
1 cup (248 g) cubed tofu (optional)

PREPARATION AND USE:

In a large pot, combine the water and barley. Bring to a boil, lower the heat, and simmer on low heat for 30 minutes.

In a separate pan, combine the olive oil, onion, garlic, and mushrooms and sauté over medium heat until tender, about 5 minutes. Add the miso paste and pepper to the sauté pan. Then add the tofu, if using, and continue cooking the mixture for an additional 2 minutes.

Pour the sautéed mixture into the barley pot. Stir well. Ladle the mixture among four plates.

YIELD: 4 SERVINGS

❓ **How it works:** *Barley is made of the viscous, or soluble, fiber, which helps keep cholesterol from absorbing into the blood. Studies show that replacing animal protein with soy foods can lower LDL cholesterol and blood pressure, among other benefits.*

Cinnamon-Hibiscus Tea

1 teaspoon (3 g) dried hibiscus
1 teaspoon (3 g) dried rose hips
1 teaspoon (5 g) cinnamon chips, from a
    crushed cinnamon stick
1 cup (235 ml) boiled water

PREPARATION AND USE:
Combine all the dried ingredients. Pour into the boiled water and let steep for 15 minutes. Strain and drink.

YIELD: 1 SERVING

❓ **How it works:** *Preliminary research suggests that cinnamon helps reduce blood levels of cholesterol and glucose (sugar). Hibiscus contains antioxidants and helps to reduce blood pressure.*

Fact or Myth?

IF RED GRAPES ARE GOOD FOR YOUR CHOLESTEROL, RED WINE IS EVEN BETTER.

Well, yes and no. Drinking a moderate amount of wine raises HDL cholesterol levels. Red wine (made from red grapes) also contains potent antioxidants. However, red grape juice also raises HDL and provides antioxidants.) Note that a moderate amount of wine means one 5-ounce (150 ml) glass a day for women and two for men because more could do more harm than good. The skin of red grapes has other added value: antioxidants.

Hummus Dip with Celery Sticks

1 can (14 ounces, or 400 g) chickpeas, drained
    and rinsed
⅔ cup (153 g) plain low-fat yogurt
1 garlic clove, chopped
Pinch of paprika, plus more if desired
Pinch of ground cumin
Juice of ½ lemon
Olives, sliced cucumbers, and tomatoes,
    for garnish
Celery sticks

PREPARATION AND USE:
Place the chickpeas, yogurt, and garlic in a blender and blend until smooth. Add the paprika, cumin, and lemon juice and blend once more until smooth.

Pour the hummus into a serving dish and garnish with the olives, cucumbers, and tomatoes.

Add additional paprika, if desired. Serve with celery sticks.

YIELD: 4 TO 6 SERVINGS

❓ **How it works:** *Chickpeas are a rich source of soluble fiber, keeping cholesterol from absorbing into the blood. They also provide omega-3 fats, potassium, and manganese.*

Recipe Variation: Add red bell pepper sticks as a garnish, or substitute for the celery.

Wholly Guacamole

3 avocados, peeled, pitted, and mashed
Juice of 1 lime
1 teaspoon (6 g) salt
½ cup (80 g) diced onion
3 tablespoons (3 g) chopped fresh cilantro
2 small tomatoes, diced
1 teaspoon (3 g) minced garlic
Pinch of cayenne
½ teaspoon hot sauce (optional)

PREPARATION AND USE:

In a medium-size bowl, mash the avocados with the lime juice and salt. Mix in the onion, cilantro, tomatoes, and garlic. Stir in the cayenne and hot sauce, if using. Serve immediately.

YIELD: 6 SERVINGS

❓ **How it works:** *Studies show that avocado, an excellent source of soluble fiber, has 15 grams of heart-healthy unsaturated fat, helps reduce LDL, and may increase HDL cholesterol. Lab studies show that cayenne lowers cholesterol and protects it from oxidation.*

Recipe Variation: Use ½ cup (130 g) of salsa instead of the cilantro, tomatoes, and garlic.

Nuts for an Almond Snack

8 ounces (225 g) whole, raw almonds
½ teaspoon sea salt
1 teaspoon (5 ml) olive oil
Pinch of cayenne pepper (optional)

PREPARATION AND USE:

Preheat the oven to 350°F (180°C, or gas mark 4).

Spread the almonds across a glass baking dish. Add the salt and olive oil and stir to combine. Roast for 10 to12 minutes. Remove the pan from the oven and add the cayenne, if using, for extra zing. Let cool for an hour.

YIELD: ABOUT A DOZEN HANDFULS

❓ **How it works:** *Almonds, walnuts, and other nuts are rich in soluble fiber, keeping cholesterol from absorbing into the blood. They also contain heart-healthy fats. Cayenne has been seen to lower cholesterol, too, and protects it from oxidation.*

Lifestyle Tip

Substitute olive oil for butter. Olive oil is high in monounsaturated fat, which helps increase HDL cholesterol and lowers your risk of heart disease. Butter, on the other hand, is high in saturated fat. As in red meat, the saturated fat in butter and other full-fat dairy products increases both HDL and in LDL cholesterol. While HDL is considered protective, LDL contributes to arterial disease.

Fact or Myth?

WHITE BREAD CAN BE BAD FOR YOUR HEALTH.

Yes. Its refined carbohydrates quickly raise blood sugar, which can increase blood triglycerides, or fats, and elevate blood pressure. Like high cholesterol, high triglyceride levels are a risk factor for cardiovascular disease.

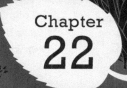

Colds

Few people make it through the winter without the familiar symptoms—sniffles, sneezes, and scratchy throat. The average adult catches two to four colds a year. Kids get at least twice that many colds. A chief reason is that the more than two hundred viruses that cause colds can survive on surfaces for hours. You push that grocery cart, borrow a pen, put away your kid's toys and then touch your finger to your nose or eyes, and—presto, you've inoculated yourself. Or someone sneezes or coughs a cloud of airborne viruses in your direction. Unless your immune system is in tip-top shape, symptoms follow in two to three days.

Fortunately, you have plenty of healing allies. The strategies outlined in Part I of this book will bolster your immune defenses. And once you get sick, those pillars will support your recovery. Eat well. Unless you don't feel up to it, you can continue to exercise, which provides natural decongesting relief. Sleep is a great healer, though a stuffy nose can interfere.

To reduce the risk of picking up other people's cold viruses or spreading yours to others, wash your hands often.

Although over-the-counter cold medications can decrease congestion, they don't cure the infection and may, in fact, prolong it. They can also create undesirable side effects. For instance, antihistamines dry and thicken secretions in your nose and elsewhere and make you feel even drowsier. To avoid a sinus infection, the goal is actually to thin respiratory mucus so it's easier to clear.

The good news is your kitchen holds a number of feel-better remedies. First, turn on the tap and drink a tall glass of cool water. Drink at least seven more glasses of warm liquids over the course of the day. Warm liquids are soothing, help increase blood circulation to the throat (and blood brings with it infection-fighting white blood cells), and speed clearance of respiratory mucus.

Next, put a kettle of water on to boil. Once it does, you have several options for recipes. You may want to try them all.

History

Long, long ago, humans were on to the fact that "colds" came in the colder part of the year, from fall to midspring. No matter the latitude or longitude, from the Sahara to Greenland, the respiratory distress came with the colder weather. Hence the name.

But so far, experiments have failed to show that getting chilled or being exposed to cold has anything to do with susceptibility to infection. (Prolonged cold exposure is, however, stressful, which can ultimately impair immune function.)

In the eighteenth century, Benjamin Franklin, while looking into the causes of the common cold, came closer to the truth. He concluded that "people often catch cold from one another when shut up together in small close rooms, coaches . . . when sitting near and conversing so as to breathe in each other's transpiration."

The cause of the common cold was identified in the 1950s (though the well-known symptoms have been with us since antiquity and described in the oldest medical text, the *Ebers papyrus* written before the sixteenth century BCE). In 1946 in Salisbury, England, the Medical Research Council set up a group called the Common Cold Unit. Through its work, the rhinovirus was isolated in 1956 and subsequently found to be a large family of some one hundred strains—and the primary cause of the so-called common cold. Other families of viruses that cause the common cold include coronaviruses, adenoviruses, parainfluenza viruses, and more.

Given the large number of viruses that cause the common cold and the frequency with which they mutate, a cold vaccine is not very likely anytime soon. Hence humankind is still stuck with coming up with ways to cope—but happily there are quite a few!

The ease with which colds are spread remains a bit of a mystery. A prominent theory since 1984 is that people spread the virus on their hands (after wiping their nose). Starting around 2002, researchers linked low blood levels of vitamin D —a vitamin made when skin is exposed to sunlight, which occurs least during the short days of winter—with increased rates of the common cold and other respiratory infections. Since then, studies indicate that adequate vitamin D intake may decrease the risk of such infections.

Traditional herbal remedies such as peppermint (somewhat decongesting), ginger (decongesting and good for coughs), yarrow (anti-inflammatory), elderflower (antiviral and makes you sweat), sage (drying), and echinacea (immune enhancing) also help.

And don't forget the chicken soup.

Fact or Myth?

YELLOW NASAL DISCHARGE MEANS YOU'VE DEVELOPED SINUSITIS.

Actually, nasal mucus normally starts out clear and thin and becomes yellower as your immune system kicks in. The yellow comes from shed white blood cells and cells lining your nose and other debris. Furthermore, most people with colds do have, as evidenced by CT scans, sinus inflammation. Some people may subsequently develop bacterial sinusitis. (See Chapter 54, on sinusitis, for more information.)

Throat Tonic

1 quart (946 ml) water

1 teaspoon (3 g) grated fresh ginger,
   or ½ teaspoon dried

¼ cup (60 ml) fresh lemon juice

2 teaspoons (14 g) honey

PREPARATION AND USE:

Boil the water and then turn off the heat. Add the ginger. Cover and steep 20 minutes and then strain. Add the lemon juice and honey. Sip the quart of tonic over the course of the day. Reheat as necessary or drink at room temperature.

YIELD: 1 QUART (946 ML) TONIC

❷ **How it works:** *The hot water is a hydrator that keeps your throat moist and also thins mucus and helps expel it. As you sip, simply breathing in the steam of the warm liquid helps with decongestion. Ginger is antimicrobial, anti-inflammatory, analgesic, immune-enhancing, and an expectorant.*

Fact or Myth?

BEING OUT IN THE COLD WILL CAUSE YOU TO CATCH COLD.

Studies show that's not true. However, being chilled stresses your body, and people who are under stress are more at risk for the common cold.

Lifestyle Tip

Eat soup. You've probably heard that chicken soup is a time-honored remedy against the common cold. Scientists have actually tried to verify why it may be helpful. It turns out that hot chicken soup hastens clearance of nasal mucus and is anti-inflammatory (and the immune system's inflammatory response creates many of the cold's symptoms). Plus the parsley, mushrooms, onions, garlic, and Italian seasonings (thyme, oregano, rosemary) so often in soup have relevant medical properties. We prefer a modified version that uses additional immune-enhancing herbs, specifically shiitake mushroom and astragalus root. Preliminary research indicates that astragalus may reduce the risk of catching colds. For details, see the Immune Soup recipe (page 325).

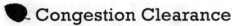

Congestion Clearance

1 quart (946 ml) water
2 to 3 drops eucalyptus essential oil

PREPARATION AND USE:

Boil the water and pour into a bowl. Add the eucalyptus essential oil. Cover your head with a clean towel. Lean over the bowl. Inhale through your nose to clear nasal congestion. (To clear lung congestion, inhale through your mouth.) Repeat three to five times a day as needed. Each time, you will need to reheat the water and add fresh plant essential oil. (Plant essential oils are volatile, meaning they vaporize quickly.)

YIELD: 1 STEAMING SESSION

❓ **How it works:** *Inhaling steam from the boiling water helps decongest nasal passages. (Breathe in slowly, as steam can burn your nose.) Oil of eucalyptus is an expectorant and antitussive (cough calming). It aids breathing by opening up bronchial tubes, easing congestion, and promoting sputum. It is also antimicrobial.*

Note: If you have asthma, try using only steam first. If steam doesn't make you cough, add 1 drop of eucalyptus oil, working up to 3 drops as tolerated. In some people with asthma, inhaling the vapors from plant essential oils may trigger coughing.

Lifestyle Tip

Take care with over-the-counter cold medications. One, they don't cure the common cold. Studies are few and most major medical groups don't recommend them as being effective.

Two, most combination products contain acetaminophen. If you combine a combination cold medication with additional acetaminophen, you might take too much of this drug, which is toxic to the liver.

Three, most products contain an antihistamine, which dries nasal secretions, as well as your mouth and other mucus-covered membranes in the body. They can also make you sleepy. (Paradoxically, kids may become agitated and have nightmares.) The dried secretions are harder to expel, which may raise the risk for developing a sinus infection.

Four, another common ingredient in cold medications is a decongestant, which does shrink mucous membranes, but also can cause nervousness and increased heart rate.

Cold Crusher

Linda's former student Gina Penka, a childbirth educator, swears by this remedy. This recipe is best prepared at least one week in advance.

1 head garlic, cloves peeled and crushed
1 medium-size horseradish root, peeled
   and coarsely chopped
1 finger-size slice of ginger, peeled and
   coarsely chopped
Apple cider vinegar

PREPARATION AND USE:

Place the crushed garlic cloves, horseradish root, and ginger in a clean, pint-size (475 ml) jar. Cover with apple cider vinegar until the fluid level clears the chopped ingredients by 1 inch (2.5 cm). Close the lid snugly. Shake.

Store in a covered cabinet. After two weeks, the chemicals in the plants will have largely moved into the vinegar. You now have two options. One is to strain and rebottle the vinegar extract and store it in the refrigerator. The second (Gina's preferred method) is to leave the herbs in the jar and eat them with the vinegar extraction.

Sip 1 to 2 tablespoons (15 to 30 ml) of this mixture at the first sign of cold symptoms. You can dilute the vinegar with herb tea or warm water. If you're feeling brave, chew a piece of garlic clove. Repeat each day for the first three days of the cold.

YIELD: ABOUT 16 SERVINGS

❓ How it works: *There is evidence that garlic stimulates the immune system and may defend against catching a cold. It may also help fight viruses. In one study, participants who took garlic supplements for twelve weeks during the winter experienced a significant reduction in colds and a reduction in the symptoms of those colds that did occur. Ginger is antibacterial, anti-inflammatory, immune-enhancing, and calms coughing. Onions, which are botanical cousins of garlic, are also immune-enhancing, anti-inflammatory, and antimicrobial. The spiciness of horseradish stimulates thin nasal secretions, which helps clear away viruses.*

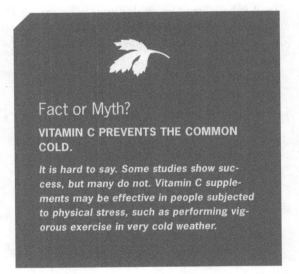

Fact or Myth?

VITAMIN C PREVENTS THE COMMON COLD.

It is hard to say. Some studies show success, but many do not. Vitamin C supplements may be effective in people subjected to physical stress, such as performing vigorous exercise in very cold weather.

Gypsy Cold-Combat Tea

3 cups (710 ml) water
1 tablespoon (2 g) dried peppermint leaves
1 tablespoon (2 g) dried yarrow flowers
1 tablespoon (2 g) dried elderflowers or
    elderberries
Honey (optional)

PREPARATION AND USE:

Boil the water. Turn off the heat. Add the herbs, cover, and steep for 20 minutes. Rewarm over low heat. Strain, sweeten with honey as desired, and sip. Drink a serving three to six times a day.

YIELD: 3 SERVINGS

❷ How it works: *This traditional European tea has been used for hundreds of years to counter symptoms of influenza. These herbs make you sweat (which helps reduce fever). Peppermint reduces respiratory congestion, pain, and headache. The steam can also help clear nasal passages.*

When Simple Doesn't Work

Zinc lozenges can reduce the duration of cold symptoms. That's because zinc inhibits the replication of cold viruses. Dosages in studies range from 4.5 to 24 milligrams of zinc (gluconate or acetate) every 1 to 2 hours while symptomatic. Side effects include a bad taste in the mouth and nausea. Avoid intranasal zinc, which has been linked to loss of the ability to smell.

The Indian herb andrographis (Andrographis paniculata) can shorten cold symptom severity and duration. Several studies have shown success with Kan Jang, a product from the Swedish Herbal Institute, that combines andrographis and eleuthero (Eleutherococcus senticosis, also called Siberian ginseng). A study in children showed this product outperformed echinacea.

Three studies have shown that, in elderly people at risk for respiratory infections, an extract of American ginseng (Panax quinquefolius) helped prevent colds.

Follow the package instructions for dosing guidelines.

Echinacea Tincture

Tinctures made with plant extracts, water, and ethanol (alcohol) are surprisingly simple to make. Vodka has the right blend of water and ethanol.

1 cup (26 g) ground echinacea root *(Echinacea purpurea)*

1½ cups (355 ml) vodka

PREPARATION AND USE:

Most echinacea root sold in natural food stores, herb stores, and online comes in small chunks. Grind it in a food mill or clean coffee grinder. Pour the ground root into a pint-size (475 ml) jar. Cover with vodka. Stir with a chopstick or other small stirring device. Add more vodka, to the point at which a good inch (2.5 cm) of liquid stands above the level of the herb. Cover tightly and shake vigorously.

Store in a cabinet, shaking daily, for at least two weeks. (If you can wait four to six weeks, great. Otherwise, you're ready to strain.)

Wash and dry your hands. Place a strainer over a bowl or large glass measuring cup. Lay a square of cheesecloth or muslin over the strainer. Pour the tincture through the cheesecloth, using a spoon to scrape out all the root. Wrap the cheesecloth around the wet root and wring as much liquid as you can from the plant. Compost the spent herb.

Pour the tincture into a clean, dry pint-size jar. Cap and store in the cupboard. It will keep for years.

At the first sign of cold symptoms, take ½ teaspoon of the tincture mixed with water or tea every 2 hours while awake. After two days, reduce the dosage to ½ teaspoon three times a day for the duration of the cold.

YIELD: ABOUT 48 DOSES

❓ How it works: *Echinacea enhances immune function and has antiviral effects against respiratory viruses. The majority of studies on echinacea show that the herb modestly reduces cold severity and duration. The reduction is only about 10 to 30 percent.*

The key to success is that a good product (the fresh juice of E. purpurea *preserved in alcohol or root extracts from* E. purpurea *and* E. angustifolia*) must be taken frequently. Ground, encapsulated herb doesn't work. Infrequent dosing doesn't work, either. One study did show success when people drank five to six cups (1.2 to 1.4 L) per day of an echinacea tea.*

❗ Warning: *Echinacea is in the same plant family as ragweed. Some people are allergic to it. If you develop any symptoms of allergy, discontinue use.*

Lifestyle Tip

If you're going to use a decongestant, nasal sprays produce fewer side effects than do oral products. They do make it easier to breathe. However, with overuse or continued use (more than a few days), the shrinkage of the mucous membranes is followed by rebound swelling. This rebound stuffiness causes people to reach for the spray bottle, perpetuating a vicious cycle that can be surprisingly hard to break.

Kid-Friendly Herbal Glycerite

Many parents prefer not to give alcohol-based extracts to children. Vegetable glycerine makes a suitable substitute. I adapted this recipe from Sunny Mavor, my coauthor for Kids, Herbs, & Health. *~ LBW*

2 tablespoons (3 g) dried echinacea root (*E. purpurea* or *E. angustifolia*)
2 tablespoons (3 g) dried echinacea leaves and flowers (*E. purpurea*)
2 tablespoons (3 g) dried lemongrass leaves
2 tablespoons (3 g) dried lemon balm leaves
1 tablespoon (2 g) dried sage leaves
1½ cups (355 ml) vegetable glycerine
1 cup (235 ml) distilled water

PREPARATION AND USE:

Using a clean coffee grinder or food mill, grind the herbs into a coarse powder. Mix the water and glycerine in a quart-size (946 ml) jar. Add the herbs and shake until the herbs are moist. Seal the lid tightly. Place in the cupboard, shaking daily, for two weeks. Strain through several layers of cheesecloth to remove herb particles. Store in a clean jar or you can use dropper bottles.

This formula is appropriate for children over twelve months of age. For kids who weigh up to 24 pounds (11 kg), start with 10 drops and work up to 15 drops three to four times a day. For kids 24 to 48 pounds (11 to 22 kg), start with 20 drops and work up to 30 drops, three to four times daily. For kids 48 to 100 pounds (22 to 45 kg), use 50 drops three to four times daily. Older, heavier kids can take adult doses (30 drops of glycerite, or about ½ teaspoon).

YIELD: 2¼ CUPS (535 ML)

❓ How it works: *Lemongrass is antioxidant and antimicrobial. Lemon balm is antioxidant and antiviral. Sage has a gentle drying effect. As mentioned previously, well-prepared echinacea products taken at recommended doses modestly decrease cold symptom severity and duration in adults. A few studies have also included children. Some have showed improvement in symptoms. A 2003 study failed to show an echinacea syrup significantly improved cold symptoms, though children did develop more skin rashes using echinacea (7.1 percent) than did those using a placebo (2.7 percent). However, a follow-up study by the same research group found that echinacea, taken over the course of the winter, decreased the risk of recurrent colds by 28 percent relative to a placebo syrup. A 2011 study showed an echinacea-based product reduced inflammation and improved quality of life in kids who had recurrent middle ear infection and throat infections.*

❗ Warning: *If ragweed allergies run in your family, try a single dose and wait several hours. If your child develops a rash, discontinue use. Other signs of allergy include runny nose and sneezing (already present with a cold) and stomach upset.*

Lifestyle Tip

If you or your child is prone to colds, consider consuming fermented foods, such as yogurt, or supplementing with probiotics. Probiotics, live microorganisms with health benefits, have been shown to prevent upper respiratory tract infections, such as colds.

Vapor Relief

Linda learned this technique from Denver herbalist Shelley Torgove and finds it instantly relieves nasal stuffiness.

1 drop ravensara essential oil

PREPARATION AND USE:
Tilt the essential oil bottle until a single drop falls onto a facial tissue. Twist the tissue so that the spot of essential oil is at the center and so you can insert that bit of twisted tissue into your nostril. So what if you look a little weird. Breathe deeply ten times and remove. Repeat with a fresh tissue on the other side. Notice the difference.

YIELD: SINGLE USE, BUT IT CAN BE REPEATED UP TO FOUR TIMES DAILY WHILE SYMPTOMATIC WITH A COLD.

❓ How it works: *Ravensara* (Cinnamomum camphora) *comes from Madagascar. The tree is the source of camphor, though a different, safer chemotype (a plant with distinct chemical constituents) is used to make the essential oil. It smells much like eucalyptus, but is gentler. Studies show it's antiseptic, anti-inflammatory, and antioxidant.*

Note: If you can't easily find ravensara essential oil, you can use eucalyptus or peppermint essential oil, which are antimicrobial, anti-inflammatory, and decongesting.

When to See the Doctor

- *Respiratory symptoms persist longer than two weeks. The common cold should resolve within seven to ten days.*
- *You develop a high fever. The common cold causes mild fever, at best.*
- *You develop pain and greenish-brown discharge from one or both nostrils.*

Chapter 23

Cold Sores

Cold sores, also called fever blisters, are lesions that occur on the lips and mouth. They start out as a group of tiny blisters. The underlying skin and mucous membrane are red and tender. The blisters often break open, releasing a clear liquid. After that, the lesion scabs over and heals within a few days to two weeks.

Herpes simplex virus (HSV) causes them. There are two types of HSV: 1 and 2. Often, HSV-1 produces cold sores, and HSV-2 causes genital herpes. Oral sex can lead to HSV-2 inoculating the mouth. Both types are highly contagious.

HSV belongs to the same viral family as the chicken pox virus. These sneaky viruses never leave us. The immune system contains but doesn't eliminate them. Instead, the viruses travel up the sensory nerves to collections of nerve cell bodies outside the spinal cord, remaining dormant until they sense you're stressed. Chronic stress increases the stress hormone cortisol, which suppresses immune function. A study of medical residents found that the stress and fatigue of working the night shift increased levels of cortisol and virus in the saliva.

The frequency of recurrence varies widely. Although 70 percent of adults carry antibodies against HSV-1, which indicates exposure, some people never get a cold sore. The initial exposure can cause no symptoms or it can result in significant illness with fever, swollen lymph glands in the neck, and painful sores in the mouth and on the lips.

Aside from stress and fatigue, other triggers that reactivate HSV include menstruation, exposure to sunlight, the common cold, flu, and fever. The first symptoms of a recurrence are often pain, tingling, burning, or itching at the site.

History

It is hard to imagine an epidemic of cold sores, but that is exactly what happened in Rome in the first century CE. To stop the spread, the emperor Tiberius banned kissing! In sixteenth-century London, even Shakespeare felt compelled to comment on the blisters "o'er ladies' lips" in his tragedy *Romeo and Juliet*. The term *Herpes simplex* was applied to cold sores in an eighteenth-century medical text by English physician Richard Boulton.

Not until the mid-twentieth century was herpes confirmed to be a virus. By the 1960s, herpes antiviral therapy began in earnest with the introduction of medications called DNA (deoxyribonucleic acid) inhibitors, which interfered with the replication of viral cells. Experimental testing of acyclovir led to its licensing by the Food and Drug Administration in 1998. Sold under the trade name Zovirax, it soon became the drug of choice for treating HSV-1.

Long before antiviral therapy was an alternative, such herbs as lemon balm *(Melissa officinalis)* were prescribed for cold sores by the Arab philosopher and physician known as Avicenna (980–1037). Sometimes combined with St. John's wort *(Hypericum perforatum)* and echinacea *(E. purpurea)*, lemon balm is still recommended today by herbal practitioners for treating cold sores. A clinical trial found that lemon balm extract, applied topically several times daily, shortens the duration and severity of the virus.

Lifestyle Tip

At the first hint of a cold sore, try dipping a cotton swab in apple cider vinegar and swiping the sore. The acid attacks the virus and helps dry up the sore. Apply clean swabs throughout the day. Throw out each swab and wash your hands to keep the virus from spreading.

 Lemon Balm Pops

2 cups (475 ml) water
¼ cup (6 g) dried lemon balm leaves,
   or ½ cup (48 g) fresh
2 tablespoons (40 g) honey

PREPARATION AND USE:

In a small pan, bring the water to a boil. Turn off the heat and add the lemon balm. Cover and steep for 20 minutes. Strain and add the honey. Let cool to room temperature.

Pour the mixture into Popsicle molds, an ice cube tray, or small (3-ounce, or 90 ml) paper cups. Freeze. Suck on the pops every couple of hours, rubbing the soothing cold on your lips. Do not hold ice to the lesion for more than a few minutes, as doing so could damage tissue; gently rubbing with ice is fine.

YIELD: 8 POPS

❷ **How it works:** *Lemon balm (Melissa officinalis) has antiviral activity against HSV and also prevents its attachment to cells. Two studies found that a cream containing 1 percent lemon balm extract applied four times a day reduced symptoms, preventing the spread of the infection, and hastened healing. Honey is a traditional and research-backed wound healer.*

Lemon Balm Tea

3 cups (710 ml) water
3 tablespoons (5 g) dried lemon balm leaves
Honey

PREPARATION AND USE:

Bring the water to a boil in a pan. Turn off the heat and add the lemon balm. Cover and steep for 15 to 20 minutes. Strain. Allow the mixture to cool to room temperature. Sip throughout the day.

YIELD: 3 SERVINGS (DOUBLE THE RECIPE IF YOU WISH TO DRINK IT MORE OFTEN.)

❓ How it works: *Lemon balm is antiviral against HSV. Also, it's important to keep drinking fluids. Don't let the pain of cold sores interfere with staying hydrated. Drink water, tea, and broth. Avoid sodas, which will irritate the lesions. Lab studies also show that several other mint family herbs (peppermint, thyme, rosemary, and sage) have anti-HSV activity. All are probably more effective as preventive strategies, stopping the viruses from multiplying before they penetrate the cells but not afterward.*

Recipe Variation: Substitute 1 tablespoon (3 g) of dried thyme, (2 g) peppermint, or (3.5 g) rosemary for one of the 3 tablespoons (5 g) of lemon balm.

Honey Lips

1 tablespoon (20 g) honey

PREPARATION AND USE:

Wash your hands. Spoon the honey into a small, clean jar or empty lip balm tin. Using a clean fingertip or gauze, apply the honey to the cold sore five or six times a day. Each time, leave on for 15 minutes and then wash off.

YIELD: MULTIPLE APPLICATIONS

❓ How it works: *Honey has antiviral and wound-healing activity. One study compared topical applications of honey versus the prescription drug acyclovir (applied topically) in sixteen adults with lip and genital herpes. The honey was superior to the drug in reducing pain and crusting and hastening healing time.*

Salt Swab

1 teaspoon (6 g) sea salt
1 cup (235 ml) warm water
A dab of unscented moisturizer

PREPARATION AND USE:

Dissolve the salt in the warm water. Dip a cotton swab into the saltwater. Gently hold the swab against the cold sore for about 5 minutes. Throw away the swab immediately. With another cotton ball, put a dab of unscented moisturizer on the sore as a lubricant. Wash your hands.

YIELD: 1 APPLICATION

❓ How it works: *Salt is a natural cleanser and healer. Sea salt contains trace minerals that soothe and heal skin that has developed a rash or become inflamed.*

Bergamot or Bust

1 teaspoon (5 ml) unscented face or body cream
1 drop bergamot essential oil

PREPARATION AND USE:

Place the face cream in a very small jar or clean, empty lip balm tin. Drop the oil into the teaspoon of lotion. Blend with a chopstick. With a clean finger or cotton swab apply a small dab to the sore. Wash your hands immediately.

YIELD: 1 TEASPOON WILL LAST FOR SEVERAL APPLICATIONS. DISCARD AT THE END OF THE WEEK.

❷ **How it works:** *Bergamot is an antimicrobial. It cannot actually kill the herpes virus but can discourage bacterial infection of the lesion.*

❶ **Warning:** *Bergamot increases photosensitivity. The sun is a common herpes trigger, so if you use bergamot, stay out of direct sunlight.*

Recipe Variation: If you don't have unscented cream or lotion, try virgin coconut oil. Better still, make the C-Salve *(calendula salve)* (page 229). Add bergamot to 1 teaspoon of this salve.

Earl Grey Tea Topical

½ cup (120 ml) water
1 Earl Grey or green tea bag

PREPARATION AND USE:

Bring the water to a boil. Add the tea bag and leave in the water only until it is soaked through. Pull it out. Allow it to cool until it is just warm and comfortable to the touch. Squeeze out the excess water, while keeping the tea bag moist. Hold the warm, moist bag against the cold sore for 15 minutes. Repeat with a fresh bag as needed.

YIELD: 1 APPLICATION

❷ **How it works:** *Earl Grey tea contains bergamot oil, which is an antimicrobial. The main ingredient is black tea, which has astringent (skin tightening) and antimicrobial effects. A component in green tea (which is processed differently than black tea) called epigallocatechin-3-gallate (EGCG) interferes with the ability of HSV to replicate.*

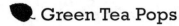 Green Tea Pops

1 quart (946 ml) water
4 green tea bags
1 tablespoon (20 g) honey

PREPARATION AND USE:

Bring the water to a boil. Add the tea bags, turn off the heat, and steep for 5 to 10 minutes. When the tea has cooled, pour it into a Popsicle mold, tray, or 3-ounce (45 ml) paper cups and freeze. Suck the pops or rub them against the cold sore. (If you used paper cups, peel back the rim until the frozen tea is exposed. That way, your fingers don't get cold as you rub the ice against the cold sore.)

YIELD: ABOUT 3 DOZEN 3-OUNCE (85 G) POPS

❷ **How it works:** *Compounds in green tea have activity against HSV, as well as against some bacteria.*

Lifestyle Tip

Some cold sore sufferers find a dab of Vicks VapoRub a soothing antidote. Apply it with a cotton ball and wash your hands afterward. While the camphor actually reduces pain and swelling by irritating the skin, it can be harmful if applied to broken skin. The menthol (from peppermint essential oil) acts as a topical analgesic. The eucalyptol (from eucalyptus essential oil) in the VapoRub contains antibacterial and antifungal chemicals. While Vicks carries these healing properties, it also keeps the cold sore from drying and cracking as it heals.

 Zinc It

1 teaspoon (5 g) zinc oxide cream
3 drops lemon balm essential oil

PREPARATION AND USE:

Put the zinc into a very small, clean jar or clean, empty lip balm tin. Drop in the oil and stir with a chopstick to blend. With a clean finger or cotton swab, dab the zinc mixture onto the cold sore. Throw away the swab and wash your hands. Repeat throughout the day, using a fresh swab each time.

YIELD: A LITTLE ZINC GOES A LONG WAY. A MERE TEASPOON (5 G) MAY GET YOU THROUGH YOUR CURRENT OUTBREAK. ONCE YOU HEAL, DISCARD THE REMAINDER AND MAKE A FRESH BATCH NEXT TIME AROUND.

❷ **How it works:** *Lemon balm essential oil is sometimes sold as "melissa." The two are one and the same. Pure lemon balm essential oil is expensive. If you can't find or can't afford it, you can substitute essential oils of tea tree, eucalyptus, or peppermint. Test-tube studies show all have activity against HSV. Discontinue use of any of these essential oils if you notice increased inflammation.*

When Simple Doesn't Work

A number of over-the-counter and prescription products can offer some relief.

As mentioned earlier, studies have shown that a standardized lemon balm cream improved symptoms and healing time for cold sores. You can find commercially prepared products at natural food stores.

- L-lysine is an amino acid. (Amino acids are the building blocks of proteins.) Several studies show that taking oral lysine supplements reduces the severity and healing time for cold sores. One study also showed that a topical formula containing lysine, zinc oxide, and other ingredients eased symptoms and sped healing. Some experts believe that increasing dietary lysine and reducing the intake of the amino acid arginine (found in higher amounts in pork, poultry, meat, oatmeal, wheat germ, eggs, peanuts, chocolate, and gelatin) helps prevent cold sores. Although studies have yet to test that theory, HSV requires arginine to make copies of itself.

- Propolis is a resinous bee product with antiviral activity against HSV. Two studies found that an ointment containing 3 percent propolis applied five times a day speeds healing.

- Vitamin C supplements (600 milligrams a day or more) and topical application of liquid vitamin C may also speed healing of cold sores.

- Abreva (docosanol) is the only over-the-counter cream for cold sores that is approved by the US Food and Drug Administration. Other over-the-counter ointments and creams can provide some relief.

If you have frequent cold sores, talk to your doctor about a prescription medication to help block recurrences. Prescription antiviral creams include penciclovir (Denavir) and acyclovir (Zorivax and generic). Oral antivirals include acyclovir (Zovirax), famciclovir (Famvir), and valacyclovir (Valtrex). All can shorten the course of cold sore attacks. Side effects for oral medications include headache, nausea, and diarrhea. Some people are allergic to the latter two medications.

Soothing Cover-Up

This recipe is an alternative to the previous mixture, for those times you'd rather not appear in public with zinc oxide smeared on your lips.

1 tablespoon (14 g) *Aloe vera* gel
3 drops lemon balm essential oil

PREPARATION AND USE:
Put the aloe gel in a small, clean jar. Stir in the drops of lemon balm oil and blend. With a clean cotton swab each time, apply a dab of the mixture several times a day. Wash your hands after touching the sore.

YIELD: THREE TO FIVE DAYS' WORTH OF MULTIPLE APPLICATIONS. AFTER FIVE DAYS, MAKE A NEW BATCH.

 How it works: *Preliminary evidence suggests that applying* Aloe vera *gel three times a day can hasten healing rates. Studies show that aloe contains chemicals that both kill bacteria and boost circulation in the tiny blood vessels at the surface of the skin.*

Baking Soda Paste

¼ teaspoon baking soda
⅛ teaspoon water

PREPARATION AND USE:
Wash and dry your hands. Cup the baking soda in one hand. Drop in the water, mixing with your finger until you have a paste. Using a clean fingertip, apply the paste over the cold sore. Let it dry for about 15 minutes. Gently wash away the baking soda. Wash your hands. Apply several times a day, making a fresh batch each time.

YIELD: 1 APPLICATION

 How it works: *Baking soda helps dry the lesion.*

Vitamin E Blast

1 vitamin E capsule

PREPARATION AND USE:
Clean and dry the lesion. Pop the capsule and saturate a cotton swab with the vitamin E oil. Hold the saturated swab on the lesion for 15 minutes. Use once for small sores, which may respond within 15 minutes to 8 hours. For large or multiple sores, repeat three times a day for three days, using a fresh swab for each application.

YIELD: 1 APPLICATION

How it works: *In two studies (both which lacked a placebo group), researchers found that applying vitamin E oil directly to a cold sore relieved pain and sped up the healing process.*

Chapter 24

Colic

Colic is defined as excessive crying in an otherwise healthy infant. "Excessive" means crying that lasts more than three hours a day for more than three days a week. During the first six months, this harmless but distressing condition afflicts about 20 percent of newborns.

Crying is typically more intense in the evening. Difficulty falling and staying asleep is common. Scientific studies suggest colicky babies aren't in pain (even though *colic* derives from the Greek word for "pain"). Nevertheless, they often look uncomfortable, their faces a furious red, legs drawn up to their belly.

The cause is unknown, though experts suspect immaturity of the nervous system or gastrointestinal system may be to blame. Compared to their more placid peers, colicky babies typically become overstimulated more easily and have more difficulty unwinding. As with most conditions of mysterious origins, a cure for colic remains elusive. Fortunately, it doesn't last forever.

History

How to soothe a colicky baby has been a concern at least since the ancient Greeks gave colic a name. Second-century physician Galen prescribed opium for fussy babies. Mothers and wet nurses smeared their nipples with opium lotions in the Middle Ages. And many a grandmother has recommended a pinkie finger dunked in bourbon to mollify a crying child.

In the twentieth century, doctors continued the tradition of sedating colicky babies with drugs: paregoric, phenobarbitol, and bentyl were a few of the "knockout drops" of choice until the practice was abandoned in the 1960s. Dr. Benjamin Spock, in his decades-long best seller *Baby and Child Care*, advised a "cry-it-out" approach—letting colicky babies cry themselves to sleep—though some psychologists and pediatricians today consider this harmful.

Introduced in the mid-1800s in England, gripe water (an over-the-counter supplement of water, sugar, baking soda, alcohol, and herbs that include chamomile, fennel, dill, and ginger) is still recommended by some pediatricians today though its effectiveness has not been confirmed. Some pediatricians oppose its use because it contains sugar and alcohol. Some of the herbs included have undergone more than the test of time. A 1993 study showed that a tea made from chamomile, vervain, licorice, fennel, and lemon balm decreased colicky crying relative to a placebo. A 2005 study showed that small amounts of simpler tea formula of chamomile, fennel, and lemon balm cut crying time by nearly two-thirds.

Hold That Baby

Your baby may not cease crying when you pick him or her up. Remind yourself that you're obeying your instincts and teaching your infant that you're reliable and trustworthy.

Your baby
You

PREPARATION AND USE:

Pick up your infant. Experiment with the position. (Some babies get more relief from being held head up; others feel better with their belly draped over someone's thighs.) The gentle pressure of your legs (or shoulders) against the baby's belly may feel good. The belly-over-the-thighs position can help expel intestinal gas. Gently rubbing the baby's back is soothing and can also help speed the process. Experiment with gentle rhythmic movement: rocking, swinging, car rides, or stroller rides. Some babies soothe to movement; others quiet to stillness. (Never roughly shake the baby, as this could rupture veins inside the baby's skull, causing a fatal injury.)

YIELD: 1 (PERHAPS INTERMINABLE) SESSION

❓ How it works: *Finding a comfortable position can help shift pressure inside the baby that may cause pain and discomfort. Slight pressure against the baby's belly can help expel gas. Soothing movement helps lull a baby to sleep.*

Swaddle Up

Swaddling is a time-honored means of soothing a baby.

Baby
A clean baby blanket

PREPARATION AND USE:

Lie the baby backside down on a blanket's diagonal. Starting with the triangle below his or her feet, carefully wrap each triangular end over the infant's legs, arms, and belly to securely enclose his or her tiny body in the blanket cocoon.

YIELD: 1 APPLICATION

❓ How it works: *Newborns startle when their arms and legs are flapping about. Swaddling helps a baby feel secure.*

Lifestyle Tip

If you are breastfeeding a colicky infant and have a family history of allergies, talk to your doctor about trying a hypoallergenic diet. Allergies may play a role in colicky crying because breast-fed babies are exposed to potential allergens in the mother's diet. In bottle-fed infants, hypoallergenic formulas can have a beneficial effect. Switching to a soy-based formula may not help, as many infants who are allergic to cow's milk are also allergic to soy.

In addition to colicky crying, other signs of allergies can include eczema, spitting up, diarrhea, stools that test positive for blood, and poor growth. Recent studies have shown that delaying the introduction of potentially allergenic foods may actually increase the odds the child will develop food allergies. For that reason, we recommend you talk to your pediatrician before making dietary changes.

Lullaby

My grandmother and mother sang an Irish lullaby called "Tura Lura." It has been a wonderful soother for the colicky babies in my life. ~ BBG

Your favorite song or "Tura Lura" (lyrics follow)

PREPARATION AND USE:

Lifting the baby against your shoulder or settling the baby on his or her tummy, gently rub the infant's back. Sing softly, using the same lyrics over and over. The rhythmic melody will gradually lull the baby to sleep.

YIELD: 1 SINGING SESSION; YOU WILL LIKELY NEED TO REPEAT THE LYRICS SEVERAL TIMES BEFORE YOUR BABY'S LIDS LOWER.

❓ How it works: *Singing and other soft, rhythmic music is a soother for colicky criers.*

Lifestyle Tip

If you buy a commercially prepared product, such as gripe water, make sure it does not contain alcohol and comes in a sterile package. Another possible problem with gripe water, a European remedy formulated with such herbs as fennel and ginger: It may also contain sweeteners, such as sucrose, that can contribute to dental cavities.

Tura Lura

Many versions of this folk song have been created over the years; you can find some on YouTube. Here are the words imprinted on my memory:

Over in Killarney, many years ago

My mother sang this song to me in tones so sweet and low

Just a simple little ditty, in her good old Irish way

I'd give the world if I could hear that song of hers today-ay

Tooh-rah looh-rah looh-rah

Tooh-rah looh-rah li

Tooh-rah looh-rah loo-rah

Hush, now don't you cry!

Tooh-rah loo-rah loo-rah

Tooh-rah looh-rah li

Tooh-rah looh-rah looh-rah

That's an Irish lullaby.

Chicken 'n Rice for Mom

2 cups (475 ml) vegetable broth, divided
2 scallions, diced
1 celery stalk, diced
1 carrot, diced
¼ cup (18 g) sliced mushrooms
½ cup (120 ml) water
¼ cup (48 g) uncooked brown rice
1 small chicken breast, cut into chunks
Pinch of salt-free seasoning

PREPARATION AND USE:

In a large pan, bring 1 cup (235 ml) of the broth to a simmer over medium heat. Add the scallions, celery, carrot, and mushrooms and cook for about 5 minutes.

Add the remaining broth, along with the water, rice, and chicken. Cover and cook for about 30 minutes until the rice is tender. Season to taste with salt-free seasoning.

YIELD: 2 SERVINGS

❓ How it works: *Studies have linked mothers' consumption of legumes (beans and peas) with colicky crying in their infants. If you eat a meal with lean meat and veggies that don't cause gas, your baby may likewise have less intestinal gas. Chicken and rice, as well as cooked carrots, scallions, and celery are on the low-flatulence list. Some nursing mothers find it helpful to avoid foods that give them gas—typically cauliflower, broccoli, Brussels sprouts, cucumbers, peppers, garlic, onions, beans, and other legumes—as well as spicy foods, caffeine, and alcohol. Brown rice is a whole-grain carbohydrate that helps a new mom keep up her energy. (And producing breast milk requires extra calories.)*

Kale and Avocado Salad

2 cups (134 g) washed kale
4 button mushrooms, sliced
4 cherry tomatoes
1 tablespoon (15 ml) olive oil
1 tablespoon (15 ml) balsamic vinegar
½ teaspoon fresh lemon juice
½ avocado, pitted, peeled, and sliced

PREPARATION AND USE:

Place the kale in a large bowl. Toss in the mushrooms and cherry tomatoes.

In a small bowl, whisk together the oil, vinegar, and lemon juice. Drizzle over the salad and toss. Divide between two plates and top each with sliced avocado.

YIELD: 2 SIDE SALADS OR 1 LARGE LUNCH SALAD

❓ How it works: *None of these ingredients are likely to produce intestinal gas. Plus they're rich in nutrients nursing moms can use: kale (protein, fiber, magnesium, and vitamins C, A, and E), mushrooms (protein, fiber, zinc, and selenium), tomatoes (carotenoids, potassium, B vitamins, and vitamins A, C, and K), and avocado (fiber, potassium, folate, and vitamins C and K).*

Lifestyle Tip

When bottle feeding, be sure that any air in the bottle is at the bottom of the bottle, not near the nipple. You want to reduce the chance that air can be swallowed as the baby feeds.

The Good Burp

A good burp doesn't always happen immediately. Be patient and persistent. You can also take a break, then return to it.

Your baby

You

A bottle or breast

A clean towel

PREPARATION AND USE:

During feedings, position your infant in the crook of your arm or against a pillow so that the baby's head is higher than his or her belly.

After the feeding, burp the baby by sitting him or her up on your lap, facing out or to the side, and patting his or her back gently but firmly; alternatively, position the baby against your shoulder and pat his or her back; finally, you can lay the infant tummy down across your lap and pat his or her back. Position the clean towel on your shoulder or lap to catch any spittle.

YIELD: 1 SESSION, WHICH MAY BE SHORT OR LONG, WITH BREAKS

❷ How it works: *During feeding, positioning the baby with head raised aids digestion and lowers gas buildup. A burp afterward helps expel any gas bubbles that have lodged in the tummy or digestive tract.*

Note: Don't burp your baby when he or she is eating fast and furiously. Pulling the infant away may cause him or her to cry and swallow more air. Wait until the baby takes a break.

Lifestyle Tip

When preparing formula, make sure it's neither too hot nor too cold. A tepid temperature will keep the baby from swallowing air during feedings.

Infant Tummy Massage

2 tablespoons (30 ml) carrier oil (apricot oil is nice)

3 to 4 drops essential oil of lavender, German chamomile, mandarin, or lemon balm

PREPARATION AND USE:

Blend the drops of essential oil of choice into the carrier oil. Lay your baby on your lap, facing you.

Dip your fingertips into the oil. Using light pressure, move your fingertips in circles around the abdomen in the direction that the large bowel empties. Start in the lower right corner of your child's belly (lower left from your perspective). Move up, under the ribs, then down the left side. Watch your baby's response. If he or she doesn't enjoy the massage, stop.

YIELD: 1 MASSAGE SESSION

❷ How it works: *Massage is calming and may also relieve colic. Your peaceful intention and the smooth movements of your hand can soothe you, too. (Your agitation only adds to your baby's distress.) Moving your fingers along the direction of the large intestine may help expel gas. Lavender, chamomile, and lemon balm are calming, antispasmodic, and expel intestinal gas. Mandarin, a member of the citrus family, calms and aids indigestion.*

Note: Don't try belly massage right after eating.

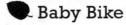 Baby Bike

You can combine this with the previous recipe for a full baby massage.

Your baby
You

PREPARATION AND USE:

On your lap, place your baby on his or her back, facing you.

Move your child's legs in a circular motion as if he or she were riding a bicycle.

YIELD: 1 SESSION

❓ How it works: *The repetitive circular motion helps expel gas from the digestive system.*

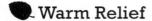 Warm Relief

A hot water bottle
Warm water
A clean towel or baby blanket

PREPARATION AND USE:

Fill the water bottle with warm, not hot, water. Test the bottle on your own skin for a few minutes to make sure it's warm but not hot. Place the water bottle over your lap and cover it with the towel or blanket. Place your baby belly down. Gently rub his or her back.

YIELD: 1 SESSION

❓ How it works: *Warmth and massage helps some colicky babies. As mentioned earlier, studies support infant massage. We don't know of studies specifically addressing the effectiveness of hot water bottles. However, many pediatricians recommend them and mention of them occurs in the pediatric literature.*

Lifestyle Tip

Treat yourself. Hire a babysitter. If you're lucky, you have family nearby who can spell you. Get out of the house. Exercise, get a massage, meet a friend, or go on a date with your partner. Caring for a colicky infant is one of the most stressful things for a new parent. Parents often feel frustrated, worried, angry, and guilty. Babies sense their parents' emotional state, which may add to the problem. If you return from an outing happy and relaxed, your infant will likely sense that. However, no research has, to our knowledge, proven that parental equanimity will dispel colic. At the very least, you'll be better able to handle the crying if you're refreshed. And, as my late Uncle Ken used to quip, "If momma ain't happy, ain't nobody happy."

🌰 Soothing Bath

In my experience, warm baths can help. When my son was an infant, he quieted if I got in the bath with him and nursed. (Caution: The baby may poop in the tub.) ~ LBW

Warm water

3 to 4 drops essential oil of lavender, German chamomile, mandarin, or lemon balm (Use only 1 to 2 drops if using a small infant tub.)

PREPARATION AND USE:

Fill an infant tub with water, checking that the temperature is pleasantly warm but not hot. Drop in the essential oil and frisk the water with your hand to disperse.

Slowly lower your infant into the water, being sure to support his or her head. Gently scoop water over the baby's chest and belly. Do not leave your infant unattended. After the bath, pat your baby's skin dry with a towel and dress.

YIELD: 1 SESSION

❓ **How it works:** *Warm water is soothing and helps calm some colicky babies. The essential oils have relaxing effects. Lavender in particular can have a muscle-relaxing or sedative effect.*

🌰 Herbal Bath Relief

1 quart (946 ml) water
¼ cup (6 g) dried catnip leaves
¼ cup (6 g) dried chamomile flowers
¼ cup (6 g) dried lemon balm leaves

PREPARATION AND USE:

In a large pot, boil the water. Turn off the heat, add the herbs, and cover. Steep for 20 minutes. Strain this infusion into warm bathwater. Check the temperature before lowering the baby into the water.

YIELD: 1 HERBAL BATH

❓ **How it works:** *All three herbs are calming and relieve intestinal gas and cramping.*

When Simple Doesn't Work

See your doctor. He or she may recommend simethicone (Mylicon or Phazyme), a medication that helps break up bubbles in the intestinal tract. You might ask your doctor about giving your baby supplements of the probiotic Lactobacillus reuteri. In a study published in the journal, Pediatrics, in 2007, the L. reuteri supplement outperformed simethicone.

🫘 Tummy Tea for Nursing Mothers

Many chemicals in these time-tested herbs for colic cross into the breast milk and deliver the needed effect to the baby.

3 cups (710 ml) water
1 teaspoon (0.5 g) dried chamomile flowers
1 teaspoon (2 g) fennel seeds
1 teaspoon (0.5 g) dried lemon balm

PREPARATION AND USE:
Boil the water in a small saucepan. Turn off the heat and add the herbs. Steep for 15 to 20 minutes. Start sipping an hour or two before your baby usually starts crying to be fed.

YIELD: 3 SERVINGS

❓ How it works: *Two studies have shown decreased crying when colicky infants drank small amounts of a tea made with herbs that relieve intestinal spasms and gas such as chamomile, vervain, licorice, fennel, and lemon balm. Fennel, vervain, chamomile, and lemon balm relax the intestines; the latter three herbs relax the nervous system. Licorice is anti-inflammatory and soothes mucous membrane linings.*

However, the general rule is, until the age of six months, infants should consume either breast milk or infant formula. They need the nutrients. Supplementing breast milk with anything risks decreasing a woman's milk supply. And, there's the risk of contamination.

Because many chemicals in herbs cross into the breast milk, a safer bet is for the mother to drink the tea.

❗ Warning: *Some people are allergic to chamomile. Also, never give honey to infants under twelve months of age because of the risk of botulism.*

Recipe Variation: Experiment with other time-honored herbs for colic, such as catnip, spearmint, dill seeds, caraway seeds, and aniseeds (not star anise).

When to Call the Doctor

Infantile colic is a benign condition that resolves with time. However, it can stress a new family. Plus, infants can and do become ill. Your pediatrician or family doctor's job is to provide support when you need it. You should call whenever you have questions or simply need reassurance. In addition, call if:

- *You suspect your infant is ill.*

- *Your baby refuses to nurse or bottle feed. (If your baby continues to wet five to six diapers a day, he or she is probably getting enough fluids.)*

- *Your infant isn't gaining weight normally. (During the first six months of life, babies gain an average of 5 to 7 ounces [142 to 198 g] a week.)*

- *You feel physically or emotionally exhausted by your baby's crying.*

- *You're concerned that you or someone else might shake or otherwise hurt the baby.*

Chapter 25

Constipation

What is the most common digestive complaint in the United States? Constipation. We probably don't need to explain the symptoms, but forgive us for stating the obvious. Stools become hard, dry, and sometimes painful to pass. Although frequency usually declines, irregularity is not the defining characteristic. Not everyone has a daily bowel movement.

Constipation is more common in seniors and affects women three times more often more than it does men. If constipation persists more than three months, it's considered chronic. The causes of constipation include the following:

- insufficient fiber and fluids (by far the most common cause)

- irritable bowel syndrome

- overuse of laxatives

- hypothyroidism

- nerve damage

- rare congenital conditions

- dietary supplements (iron and calcium)

- medications, such as:
  - bismuth (e.g., Pepto-Bismol)
  - opioid pain relievers (e.g., Vicodin and Oxycontin)

- nonsteroidal anti-inflammatory medications (e.g., ibuprofen and naproxen)
- antacids containing calcium and aluminum
- antihistamines
- calcium-channel blockers (used to lower blood pressure)

With advancing age, intestinal motility slows, allowing more time for water to be absorbed into the circulation, which leads to harder stools. Constipation and alternating constipation and diarrhea occur in irritable bowel syndrome, a condition of altered motility of the large intestine. Constipation is a common sign of hypothyroidism. Less often, the large intestine becomes obstructed. Damage to local nerves is another cause. Rare congenital conditions can also come with the absence of bowel movements.

In addition to making you uncomfortable, constipation has other negative consequences. Passage of hard stools may tear the anus, resulting in a vicious cycle where reluctance to re-experience the pain worsens constipation. Children going through toilet training are particularly vulnerable to that scenario.

Repeatedly straining to defecate can lead to hemorrhoids, varicose veins in the legs, and *diverticulosis* (a condition wherein small pouches protrude from the wall of the large intestine). In women, constipation contributes to pelvic floor prolapse (the descent of pelvic organs). In short, it's important to correct the condition.

History

With the advent of the Industrial Revolution some three hundred years ago, the Western diet and lifestyle began to change. One of the most fundamental changes included a decrease in fiber intake, along with the widespread use of refined vegetables oils, cereal grains, and sugars. With the modern age came the junk food industry and physical inactivity. The Western diet is high in refined carbohydrates and low in fiber-rich whole grains, vegetables, and fruits. The average American consumes only 15 milligrams of dietary fiber per day although the recommended intake is 25 to 35 milligrams.

In 1998, the US Food and Drug Administration approved psyllium as a supplementary source of dietary fiber. A traditional herbal remedy used as a gentle laxative for centuries in many cultures, psyllium seed husks continue to be a reliable source of soluble fiber. Taken with plenty of fluid, it is marketed under such brand names as Fiberall, Konsyl, Metamucil, Modane Bulk, and Serutan.

Lifestyle Tip

Leave yourself ample time in the morning for a relaxing breakfast. The first meal of the day often triggers a bowel movement. Being rushed can interfere with that reflexive action, mainly because the stress response slows bowel motility.

RECIPES TO TREAT CONSTIPATION

Psyllium Seed Husk Elixir

½ cup (120 ml) 100 percent apple juice
1½ cups (355 ml) water, divided
1 to 2 teaspoons (6 to 12 g) psyllium husks

PREPARATION AND USE:
Mix the apple juice and ½ cup (60 ml) of the water in a glass. Stir in the psyllium and drink the remaining water. Take two to three times a day.

YIELD: 1 SERVING

❓ How it works: *Apple juice has a laxative effect. Both black and blond psyllium husks act as bulk-forming laxatives, which means their fiber holds water in the intestine, making the stool softer and easier to pass. Studies show that psyllium can be more effective than over-the-counter stool softeners, such as Colace (docusate sodium).*

Note: Be sure to chase a glass of a psyllium beverage with an additional tall glass of water. Fiber doesn't help unless you consume water with it. In fact, insufficient water used with such products as Metamucil (whose active ingredient is psyllium husks) can make constipation worse.

A "Regular" Smoothie

This is easy—and effective! The flaxseeds and psyllium are a strong regulating combo. Instead of using an ice cube, try freezing the fruit in advance for a full, smooth texture.

½ banana
1½ teaspoons (11 g) flaxseed meal
1 teaspoon (6 g) psyllium husks
¾ cup (109 g) strawberries or (190 g) raspberries
½ cup (120 ml) almond milk

PREPARATION AND USE:

Place all the ingredients in a blender and blend well. Grind in an ice cube for a frothy finish.

YIELD: 1 SERVING

❓ **How it works:** *The fiber in psyllium and fruit help soften the stool. Flaxseed meal adds omega-3 fatty acids, which provide antioxidant and anti-inflammatory action. Flaxseeds also ought to act as a bulk-forming laxative, but research confirmation is lacking.*

Lifestyle Tip

Exercise. Regular physical activity helps stimulate the intestines. Sedentary people are more often troubled by constipation. A Scandinavian study of chronically constipated middle-aged people found that daily physical activity (30 minutes of brisk walking followed by 11 minutes of home exercises) hastened "transit time" through the large intestine and reduced symptoms of constipation.

Brocco-licious

Broccoli is rich in fiber and magnesium, both of which help regularity. Simmer it to keep its bright green appeal.

¼ cup (16 g) hulled pumpkin seeds or (28 g) slivered almonds
1 pound (455 g) fresh broccoli
1 tablespoon (15 ml) olive oil
½ to 1 teaspoon (0.5 to 1.1 g) red pepper flakes
¼ teaspoon sea salt
⅛ teaspoon freshly ground black pepper
½ cup (120 ml) water

PREPARATION AND USE:

Lightly oil a skillet using canola or olive oil cooking spray. Place over high heat, add the pumpkin seeds, and brown lightly, about a minute or two. Immediately transfer the seeds to a bowl.

Remove the larger, tougher stems of the broccoli, break the florets into bite-size pieces, and slice the remaining stems.

Add the olive oil to the pan and lower the heat to medium. Add the broccoli, red pepper flakes to taste, salt, and black pepper. Pour the water on top. Cook for 3 to 5 minutes until barely tender and still bright green. Remove immediately from the heat. Drain any remaining water. Sprinkle the pumpkin seeds on top and serve.

YIELD: 4 TO 6 SERVINGS

❓ **How it works:** *Magnesium salts (magnesium citrate, sulfate, and hydroxide) taken as supplements draw water into the intestine and stimulate motility, thereby creating a laxative effect. Magnesium is well absorbed from such vegetables as broccoli; from seeds (including pumpkin seeds) and nuts—especially almonds; and from legumes, whole grains, squash, and leafy greens. All these foods also provide fiber.*

Bean Soup Delight

A cold winter day, navy bean soup simmering on the stove, and a regulated system: all equal delight.

1 tablespoon (15 ml) canola oil

1 slice bacon (turkey or vegetarian), chopped into small bits

1 cup (160 g) chopped onion

½ cup (50 g) chopped celery

2 cans (15 ounces, or 428 g) navy beans, drained and rinsed

1 cup (235 ml) low-sodium vegetable or chicken stock

¼ teaspoon sea salt

¼ cup (85 g) honey

PREPARATION AND USE:

Place the oil and bacon bits in a large pot over medium heat and sauté for about 2 minutes. Drop in the onion and celery and sauté until the onion becomes transparent, 3 to 5 minutes. Add the beans and stir well. Pour in the stock and bring to a boil. Stir in the sea salt and honey. Lower the heat and simmer for about 15 minutes, until the beans are tender. Serve.

YIELD: 4 SERVINGS

❓ How it works: *Navy beans provide twice as much fiber as most vegetables—a whopping 9.5 grams in just ½ cup (91 g). They play a strong part in reversing constipation.*

Lifestyle Tip

Stress alters gut motility, usually in both the small and large intestines, promoting constipation. Try some of the remedies in Chapter 57 to restore your sense of peace. (For some people, however, nervousness speeds up the large intestine, triggering a bowel movement.)

Johnny Apple Treat

John Chapman, my distant cousin, was the infamous Johnny Appleseed—no joke! He spread the word that apples had medicinal qualities. They are delicious, while effective, especially for constipation. ~ BBG

1 apple

¼ cup (35 g) raisins

¼ cup (30 g) chopped walnuts

1 tablespoon (15 g) fresh lemon juice

Ground cinnamon

PREPARATION AND USE:

Coarsely grate the apple into a small bowl. Mix in the walnuts and raisins. Add the lemon juice and toss. Sprinkle with cinnamon to taste and enjoy.

YIELD: 2 SERVINGS

❓ How it works: *Fresh apples are high in fiber, which adds bulk to the stool. They contain both soluble and insoluble fiber, also called roughage.*

Super Greens with Olive Oil–Lemon Dressing

Enjoy this refreshing mix of greens—the lemon dressing adds to the zesty yet smooth flavor.

For the salad:

1 cup (20 g) arugula
1 cup (47 g) romaine lettuce
½ cup (25 g) sprouts
1 cup (40 g) torn fresh basil leaves, loosely packed
2 scallions, diced
1 avocado, peeled, pitted, and cut into chunks

For the dressing:

2 teaspoons (6 g) minced garlic
1 teaspoon (6 g) sea salt
2 tablespoons (30 ml) olive oil
2 tablespoons (30 ml) fresh lemon juice
¼ cup (30 g) dried cranberries
Freshly ground black pepper, to taste

PREPARATION AND USE:

To make the salad: Wash and drain the arugula, romaine, sprouts, and basil leaves. Toss together in a large bowl. Mix in the scallions and avocado chunks.

To make the dressing: In a small bowl, mash together the garlic and sea salt to form a paste. In another bowl, whisk together the lemon juice and olive oil and pour into a clean jar. Add the garlic paste to the jar. Close tightly and shake rapidly until combined.

Pour the dressing over the salad and sprinkle with the cranberries. Add pepper and toss.

YIELD: 4 SERVINGS

❓ **How it works:** *Olive oil has a mild laxative effect. The greens in this salad provide fiber.*

Note: Vary this recipe to use your favorite greens or just use one super green at a time! (The leftover dressing makes an excellent marinade.)

Lifestyle Tip

Eat sauerkraut—or any other fermented food. Cabbage contains fiber. Also, fermented foods are good sources of probiotics, microbes that peacefully colonize our body surfaces, providing many benefits. A study of pregnant women (for whom constipation is a common affliction) showed that a probiotics supplement containing a blend of *Lactobacilli* and *Bifidobaccilli* species significantly reduced constipation symptoms. Preliminary research also suggests that specific probiotic supplements relieve childhood constipation.

Cantaloupe with Honey-Yogurt Dressing

1 cup (230 g) plain yogurt
1 tablespoon (20 g) honey
½ teaspoon ground cinnamon
1 cantaloupe, seeded and cut into bite-size
  chunks

PREPARATION AND USE:

In a small bowl, blend together the yogurt, honey,
and cinnamon. Portion the cantaloupe among
6 small bowls. Drizzle the honey-yogurt dressing
over each serving.

YIELD: 6 SERVINGS

❓ How it works: *Yogurt contains probiotics,
living bacteria with health benefits, which promote intestinal health. Several studies have
shown that fermented dairy products (fermented
milk, in most cases) improve childhood constipation. Probiotic mixtures have been shown to
relieve constipation in pregnant women, too.
Cantaloupe contains fiber and magnesium.*

Lifestyle Tip

**Enjoy a movie night. Popcorn is a great
low-calorie way to get more fiber in your
diet, especially if low fiber is the cause of
your constipation. But skip the salt and
butter—they'll undo the benefits. Season
popcorn with a little olive oil, curry, garlic,
or a pinch of cayenne for a movie treat.**

Lifestyle Tip

**Enjoy kiwifruit, which is high in fiber—
packing about 3 grams in a single fruit.
Studies show that eating this delicious fruit
promotes motility along the entire digestive
tract. Scientists suspect that plant components other than fiber may contribute to
this effect.**

Bran Breakfast Starter

*This fiber-rich wake-up call will be the ultimate
start to your day.*

1 cup (235 ml) almond milk, plus more as
  needed
1 cup (112 g) wheat bran
1 medium-size apple or pear, cored and cut
  into chunks
1 to 2 teaspoons (7 to 14 g) honey
Ground cinnamon

PREPARATION AND USE:

Bring the almond milk to a boil in a medium-size
saucepan. Stir in the bran until well coated. Add
the fruit and honey. Lower the heat to medium and
cook for 5 to 7 minutes until the mixture thickens.
Sprinkle with cinnamon to taste and serve, adding extra almond milk as needed to create your
desired consistency.

YIELD: 2 SERVINGS

❓ How it works: *Bran is an insoluble fiber.
Because it's not absorbed in the gut, it remains,
holding water with it. Studies indicate that the
larger the size of the bran particle, the better it
works. Among fruits, unpeeled apples and pears
are leaders in the fiber arena.*

When Simple Doesn't Work

Laxatives take up a lot of drugstore shelf space. Some are relatively benign; others are better avoided altogether. Choose wisely.

- *Fiber supplements (bran and psyllium) are safe. Just be sure you take them with plenty of water.*

- *Stool softeners such as docusate (Colace and Surfak) are also safe bets. The same is generally true for lubricant laxatives, such as mineral oil, though long-term use may decrease absorption of fat-soluble vitamins (A, D, E, and K).*

- *Osmotic agents work by drawing water into the large intestine. These include magnesium salts (milk of magnesia), polyethylene glycol (MiraLax), sorbitol, and lactulose. They're generally safe. Ditto glycerin (glycerol) suppositories. Overuse of osmotic agents, however, can lead to loss of minerals. Milk of magnesia contains magnesium hydroxide, which holds water in the intestines and hastens intestinal motility. Side effects include diarrhea.*

- *Reserve stimulant laxatives for times when less harsh methods fail. These increase contractions in the large bowel. They can cause cramping and diarrhea, which depletes the body of water and electrolytes (especially potassium). Although you many have heard that frequent use can lead to dependence and damage to the large intestines, scientific study does not support such associations.*

- *Avoid stimulant laxatives if you're pregnant or nursing. If increasing fiber, water, and physical activity fail to correct constipation, some doctors recommend bulk-forming laxatives, stool softeners, lubricant laxatives (mineral oil), and sometimes osmotic laxatives. Ask your doctor before trying any over-the-counter medication or dietary supplement.*

- *Some herbal laxatives stimulate the bowel. Used at recommended doses for short periods of time (a week or less), they're generally safe for healthy, non-pregnant adults. Examples include senna (sold over the counter as Sennakot and other brands), cascara sagrada, and buckthorn. Aloe juice that contains latex from just under the leaf's skin acts as a stimulant laxative, too. However, ingesting high amounts of aloe latex (1 gram per day for several days) has been linked to kidney damage, kidney failure, and death. Also, the latex contains anthroquinones, which may cause cancer.*

- *A traditional remedy is a tablespoon (15 ml) of castor oil. If you only use this remedy occasionally, it's generally safe. Otherwise, it carries the same risk as other stimulant laxatives.*

- *Do not try enemas at home unless directed to do so by your doctor. They do cause a bowel movement, but carry the risk of bowel perforation and derangements of electrolytes.*

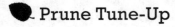 Prune Tune-Up

With its current sobriquet "dried plum," the prune is no longer the fruit of the elderly, but lends itself to enjoyment at every age, in recipes from plain to exotic.

8 pitted prunes
8 walnut halves
¼ cup (58 g) plain yogurt
1 teaspoon (7 g) honey

PREPARATION AND USE:

Slice each prune in half and insert a walnut half. Stuff the walnut completely into the prune. In a small bowl, mix the yogurt and honey together. Dip the stuffed prunes into the mixture. Enjoy throughout the day, serving the prunes as a healthy snack or dessert.

YIELD: 2 SERVINGS OF 4 PRUNES EACH

 How it works: *Whole prunes, as well as other dried fruits, such as apricots and raisins, are rich in both magnesium and fiber.*

Colon Massage

This yoga pose is an inversion of the pose called apasana, which translates roughly to "wind-removing pose."

You
A quiet place
A rug or clean floor

PREPARATION AND USE:

Lie on your back. Extend your right leg and bring your left knee toward your abdomen. Wrap your arms around your shin, just below the knee. Breathing slowly and deeply, pull your bent knee down toward your chest and move your leg a bit from side to side. Repeat on the other side. Now, bend both knees and draw them to your chest. After a few breaths, extend your legs and relax.

YIELD: 1 APPLICATION

 How it works: *Some yoga postures are thought to improve digestion by compressing and massaging the colon. (See the belly-based, depressurizing pose on page 340.)*

When to Call the Doctor

- *You've noticed a significant, unexplained change in bowel habits.*

- *Constipation is associated with significant discomfort, painful hemorrhoids, or anal fissures.*

- *You feel that bowel movements don't completely evacuate your rectum.*

- *You have chronic problems with constipation.*

- *You're pregnant. Call before you resort to over-the-counter laxatives.*

- *You're concerned about your child's bowel movements.*

Chapter 26

Coughs and Bronchitis

Coughing is the symptom that most often sends people to their doctors. Anything that irritates the airways—infection, tobacco smoke, other air pollutants, allergens, an inhaled foreign object—causes coughing. It's one of the body's defenses against illness. In fact, elderly or otherwise debilitated people are more at risk for pneumonia because they can't summon a forceful, airway-clearing cough.

The most common cause of cough is acute bronchitis. Ninety percent of the time, the infectious agent is a virus. Typically, symptoms start in the upper airways with a sore throat and runny nose. Some viruses are more likely to extend below the trachea (windpipe) into the bronchi (large airways that deliver oxygen to the lung's tiny air sacs). The mucous membranes lining the bronchi swell and generate more mucus. Cilia, tiny hairlike projections from the cell that normally move the mucus carpet upward toward the mouth, become paralyzed. The cough normally lasts three weeks, longer after a bout of influenza. Expectoration of yellowish phlegm is normal and indicates your immune system is doing its work.

Other causes of coughs: Allergic rhinitis (hay fever) and sinusitis can lead to postnasal drip, which tends to produce a nighttime cough. Gastroesophageal reflux disease (GERD, or heartburn) can cause coughing and sometimes a burning sensation. Colds can aggravate asthma, which can produce coughing, and more easily lead to bronchitis. People with cystic fibrosis are very vulnerable to lung infections.

Chronic bronchitis (cough lasting longer than three months) is common in smokers and those who live with them. Tobacco smoke compromises immune defenses, inflames the bronchial linings, increases mucus, and paralyzes the cilia. People with chronic bronchitis are more at risk of acute infection.

History

Indigenous peoples used many wild plant combinations to relieve coughs. In North America, pine bark was steeped in water to make cough syrup and pine needles chopped and soaked for tea; honey and maple syrup were mixed with teas. For millennia, Australia's Aborigines used the head-clearing vapors and mucus-removing oils of eucalyptus (E. globulus) leaves to relieve the coughs resulting from congestion, bronchitis, and sinusitis. The ancient Greeks turned to licorice and licorice teas as a remedy for coughs. Today these and many other plants used traditionally, such as peppermint, thyme, and slippery elm, are ingredients in over-the-counter cough lozenges and medicines.

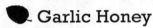 Garlic Honey

4 garlic heads
1½ cups (480 g) honey

PREPARATION AND USE:

Peel the cloves and gently squash each one with the flat of the knife. (Doing so activates an enzyme that converts an inactive chemical in garlic to one of the key ingredients.) Drop the cloves into a clean pint-size (475 ml) mason jar. Add enough honey to completely cover the garlic. Stir with a chopstick. Cap the jar. Let it sit for four to six weeks in a cool, dry place. (If you already have a cough, you can dip into the honey pot in two days.) You can eat the garlic cloves along with the honey.

YIELD: ABOUT 50 DOSES

❓ **How it works:** *Honey is antibacterial and moistening. Studies show that honey reduces nighttime cough in children more effectively than a placebo, antihistamines, and the cough suppressant dextromethorphan. Garlic is antimicrobial and an expectorant. Some of its chemicals are excreted across the lungs. Although that may give you garlic breath, the good news is some of garlic's beneficial chemicals are coming into contact with your lungs.*

❧ Old Thyme-y Honey

1 cup (43 g) dried thyme leaves or (38 g) fresh
1½ to 2 cups (480 to 640 g) honey

PREPARATION AND USE:

You have two choices for prep:

1. Pour the thyme into a clean pint-size (475 ml) mason jar. Cover completely with honey. Stir to blend (a chopstick works well for stirring). Let sit for two weeks in a sunny window. At this point, you can either call the recipe done or strain the honey, discard the herbs, and rebottle. We don't mind the thyme leaves and hate to waste the delicious honey clinging to the leaves. Store in the cupboard.

2. Put the thyme in the top of a double boiler. Add enough honey to completely cover it. Add water to the bottom pan and bring to a boil. Lower the heat to a simmer. Keeping an eye on the honey, and stirring frequently, simmer for 2 hours. You can either bottle it with the thyme leaves or strain out the thyme leaves and bottle the herb-infused honey. Take honey by the teaspoon to relieve coughing.

YIELD: ABOUT 24 DOSES (LESS IF THE THYME IS REMOVED, MORE IF IT ISN'T)

❓ **How it works:** *Thyme helps open tight airways, combats infection, calms coughs, and helps expel mucus.*

Peppermint Honey

¼ cup (80 g) honey
3 to 5 drops peppermint essential oil

PREPARATION AND USE:

Put the honey and peppermint essential oil in a small, clean jar and blend with a chopstick. Cap and store in a cupboard. Take 1 teaspoonful up to four times a day.

YIELD: 12 DOSES

? **How it works:** *Peppermint reduces chest tightness and coughing and helps clear mucus.*

! **Warning:** *This recipe is for teens and adults only. Most of the time, essential oils are used externally only. However, peppermint is safe in small amounts.*

Fact or Myth?

FOR ANY AGE, OVER-THE-COUNTER REMEDIES ARE THE QUICKEST, STRONGEST COUGH RELIEVERS.

Myth. Research indicates they're not effective in kids under six years old and carry significant risks. In fact, they are downright dangerous for kids under the age of two. In adults, expectorants don't improve outcomes. Cough suppressants, however, can make sense for teens and adults when coughing interferes with sleep. (You can't cough and sleep at the same time. Each coughing episode wakes you.)

Lifestyle Tip

Drink a lot of fluids. Staying well hydrated thins respiratory mucus, making it easier to expel.

Italian Steam

2 cups (475 ml) water
½ cup (about 24 g) Italian seasonings: fresh thyme, oregano, and/or rosemary leaves

PREPARATION AND USE:

Boil the water in a saucepan. Turn off the heat. Add a handful of the herbs and stir. Cover for 10 minutes. Remove from the heat and set on a hot pad. Remove the lid. Lean over the steaming water and cover your head with a clean towel. Breathe the vapors through your mouth for about 1 minute. Rewarm and repeat several times a day as needed. If you store the covered saucepan overnight in the refrigerator, you may reuse the next day.

Optional: After you steam, strain the liquid into a warm bath. After discarding the herbs, soak.

YIELD: ONE TO TWO DAYS' WORTH OF STEAMING

? **How it works:** *These Italian seasonings are all members of the peppermint family. As such, they relax smooth muscle (thus relaxing the airways) and discourage infection.*

Note: If you have eucalyptus trees in your area, you can substitute those leaves, crushed, for the Italian herbs.

Eucalyptus Steam

2 cups (475 ml) water
2 to 3 drops eucalyptus essential oil

PREPARATION AND USE:

Boil the water in a saucepan. Turn off the heat. Transfer the pan to a hot pad. Add 2 to 3 drops of eucalyptus oil. Bend over the pan and cover your head with a clean towel. Inhale the steam through your mouth for about 1 minute. Repeat four or five times a day. Because the essential oil vaporizes quickly, you'll need to reheat the water and add fresh eucalyptus essential oil each time.

YIELD: 1 STEAM SESSION

❓ How it works: *Essential oil of eucalyptus works against a range of bacteria and viruses. It also favorably alters immune function and helps clear excess respiratory mucus. By breathing in through your mouth, you allow the essential oil steam to come in direct contact with your throat.*

Note: Inhaling vapors from the smell of essential oils may trigger asthmatic coughing. If you have asthma, try plain steam first. If the steam doesn't trigger your asthma or worsen your coughing, add 1 drop of essential oil. If you tolerate that, work your way up to three. People with asthma usually have no problem using chest rubs that include essential oils, such as eucalyptus.

Cough-Cutting Peppermint Tea

2 cups (475 ml) water
1 teaspoon (1 g) dried thyme
3 teaspoons (5 g) dried peppermint leaves
Honey (optional)

PREPARATION AND USE:

Bring the water to a boil in a small pan. Add the herbs. Remove the pan from the heat. Cover and steep for 15 minutes. Strain and add honey, if desired. Drink the tea and inhale the steam through your mouth. Try to drink several cups a day.

YIELD: 1 SERVING

❓ How it works: *Peppermint and thyme both help calm coughs and combat infection. Peppermint can also ease throat discomfort associated with coughing.*

Note: Buy a box of peppermint tea bags and keep them handy for your this remedy.

Lemon Up

1 lemon
Less than ⅛ teaspoon freshly ground black pepper

PREPARATION AND USE:

Slice the lemon in half. Sprinkle the black pepper over one half. Suck in the liquid and swallow. Brush your teeth afterward to remove the acidity from your teeth.

YIELD: 1 SERVING

❓ How it works: *Lemon packs flavonoids and vitamin C for fighting infection. Pepper increases circulation, which helps the healing process.*

Mustard Plaster

Ask someone to assist you with the application of this remedy.

1 tablespoon (9 g) dry mustard
1 tablespoon (8 g) all-purpose flour
1 tablespoon (15 ml) warm water, plus more as needed
1 tablespoon (15 ml) olive oil

PREPARATION AND USE:

Mix the mustard and flour in a small bowl. Blend in the water. Add more water as needed to make a spreadable paste. Cover your chest with the olive oil (it will protect the skin from mustard's somewhat irritating effects). Place a clean cloth on your chest (use a bandana, thin dishcloth, or muslin—something you don't mind turning yellow).

Spread the mustard plaster over the cloth. Cover the plaster with a plastic bag.

On top, place a warm, moist hand towel (your assistant can heat it in the microwave on high for 30 to 60 seconds). After 5 minutes, remove the mustard plaster and wash your skin. Do not leave on longer, as blistering can occur.

YIELD: 1 APPLICATION

❓ How it works: *Mustard contains irritating chemicals that stimulate blood flow. The idea is that increasing blood supply promotes delivery of infection-fighting white blood cells. While the infection isn't in the skin, this plaster can create a deeper sense of warmth. This traditional remedy has not, as far as we know, been subjected to scientific study. However, many people swear by this remedy.*

Note: If you have sensitive skin or allergies, try a small test patch first. Cases of contact dermatitis (allergic skin reactions) have been reported. Do not apply to inflamed skin or open wounds.

When Simple Doesn't Work

Several studies support the use of an extract of pelargonium (Pelargonium sidoides, a South African geranium) as a bronchitis treatment. The Zulu have long used this plant. In one study, people taking it returned to work two days sooner than did those taking a placebo. You can find this product in natural food stores sold under the brand name Umcka.

Eucalyptus Chest Rub

¼ cup (55 g) petroleum jelly or unscented hand lotion

2 to 3 drops eucalyptus essential oil (half that much for pregnant women and children)

PREPARATION AND USE:

In a small bowl, blend the petroleum jelly or lotion with the eucalyptus drops. Rub on your chest. (Wash your hands before putting your fingers near your eyes or other sensitive tissues.) We recommend wrapping up in a warm sweater or blanket and sipping hot herbal tea, which will further increase circulation to your chest, thereby promoting healing.

YIELD: 1 APPLICATION

❓ How it works: *The antiviral and antibacterial essential oil of eucalyptus is absorbed across your skin to help fight congestion. It also favorably alters immune function and helps clear excess respiratory mucus.*

Fact or Myth?

YOU SHOULD ASK YOUR DOCTOR FOR AN ANTIBIOTIC IF YOUR COUGH HAS ADVANCED INTO BRONCHITIS.

Myth. Even though viruses cause the vast majority of acute bronchitis, doctors prescribe antibiotics for two-thirds of patients diagnosed with this condition. However, antibiotics kill bacteria, not viruses.

Included in the death toll are the bacteria that normally colonize your respiratory passages and intestines, peacefully protecting you from infection. That means antibiotics can weaken your defenses and give you diarrhea. Another greater risk for society is the development of antibiotic-resistant "superbugs." The American College of Chest Physicians does not recommend antibiotics to treat run-of-the-mill acute bronchitis. If your doctor whips out the prescription pad, ask why you need antibiotics.

Vicks Foot Rub

This remedy is almost as good as a foot massage.

Vicks VapoRub

PREPARATION AND USE:
Straight from the jar, put dabs of Vicks on the sole of each foot. Massage into your soles for about a minute. Cover your feet with clean socks to keep the Vicks contained and help it soak in.

YIELD: 1 APPLICATION

❓ **How it works:** *The cough-calming plant essential oils in Vicks (camphor, eucalyptol, menthol, and thymol) are absorbed across the skin. Try both chest and foot rubs to determine which is most effective for you. In other recipes, we use the plant sources of these essential oils: eucalyptus, peppermint, and thyme. Camphor comes from the camphor tree (Cinnamomum camphora).*

When to Call the Doctor

- *The sputum you expectorate has become dark green or rust-colored.*

- *You make a whooping sound at the end of a paroxysm of coughing.*

- *You have developed fever, increased respiratory and heart rates, and pain over an area of your lung.*

- *You're having difficulty breathing. (Call 911.)*

- *You have had a cough for more than a month.*

- *You have AIDS and have developed a cough.*

- *You have cystic fibrosis and have any kind of airway infection.*

- *You have asthma and an infection has significantly worsened symptoms.*

- *You have chronic bronchitis and have developed cough and fever.*

- *You have serious heart disease, such as heart failure, and have developed a cough.*

Fact or Myth?

KEEP KIDS' WHOOPING COUGH (PERTUSSIS) VACCINES UP TO DATE.

Fact. There have been recent outbreaks of whooping cough in older children and teens. These seem to be related to the vaccine losing its effectiveness. If you have a child, check with his or her pediatrician about whether a booster shot is needed.

Chapter 27

Cuts and Scrapes

From the time we take our first steps, we experience exhilaration and the associated risks—cuts, scrapes, bumps, and bruises. We humans are thin-skinned but resilient creatures. We heal and move on to new adventures.

Basic first aid takes care of small cuts (lacerations) and scrapes (abrasions). A little blood is fine. In fact, it helps clean the wound. If the wound is superficial, pour running water over it. Wash with mild soap and rinse again. Make sure you've removed foreign matter, which may infect the wound and, in the case of bits of asphalt, create a sort of tattoo.

If the area is likely to come in contact with dirt (or may stain your clothes with blood), cover with sterile gauze and tape down the edges. Change the bandage daily or if it gets wet.

If the wound is bleeding, your first step is stanch the flow by applying steady, firm pressure with your hand atop a piece of clean cloth or gauze. Hold for 5 minutes. You're helping the blood clot. If you can, hold the bleeding area above the heart. Resist the temptation to keep lifting the gauze to inspect the wound. Each time you do, you're disrupting the clotting process.

If blood soaks through, pile more gauze on top (without removing the first piece) and keep pressing. Once the bleeding stops, if blood has stuck to the gauze, leave it alone.

The same principle applies to bloody noses. Capture the fleshy part of your nose between thumb and index finger and hold firmly for 5 minutes. (A lot of people think the solution is variously to hold a tissue under the nose, squeeze the bony bridge of the nose, apply ice to the nape of neck, or lie flat. Meanwhile, blood is staining your best clothes . . . .)

History

Along with hand washing, antiseptics, and pre-treated surgical gauze, honey stands out across many centuries as one of the most useful means of treating cuts, scrapes, and wounds. The *Ebers Papyrus*, dating to around 1500 BCE, mentions the use of honey as a topical treatment for wounds. The ancient Egyptians touted honey as an integral part of healing a wound (along with washing and dressing it). Recent tests of honey found in Egyptian tombs determined it to be antibacterial.

In the days before antibiotics, infection was perhaps the greatest threat to health—and the smallest cuts or wounds could turn deadly. Today, despite the presence of antibiotic creams and gels in every home and first-aid kit, honey is making a comeback. Its antibacterial properties are being used in honey-impregnated dressings and applied to the hardest-to-heal wounds. In particular, manuka honey, made by bees that feed upon the manuka bush (*Leptospermum scoparium*), native to New Zealand and Australia, has impressive antibacterial activity relative to honey from many other sources and has been shown to be effective in treating wounds infected with methicillin-resistant *Staphylococcus aureus* (MRSA). Recent research shows that combining this honey with an antibiotic amplifies the MRSA-killing power of both agents.

Fact or Myth?

YOU SHOULD USE ANTIBACTERIAL SOAP TO WASH CUTS AND SCRAPES.

It's not necessary. Mild soap and running water (and your immune system) handily clear away microbes. Some antibacterial soaps contain triclosan, which is bad for us and the environment. It contributes to antibiotic resistance and disrupts hormone regulation. Lab research shows that it has estrogen-like activity and accelerates replication of human breast cancer cells.

Fresh Aloe Vera Gel

I keep a potted Aloe vera *plant in my kitchen, so it's handy for minor cuts, scrapes, and burns.* ~ LBW

1 *Aloe vera* plant

PREPARATION AND USE:
Wash the cut with soap and water. Slice a fleshy leaf from the aloe plant. Using clean fingernails (or a clean knife), open the leaf lengthwise. Rub the gel on the wound.

YIELD: 1 APPLICATION

❓ **How it works:** *Used since ancient times as a wound healer, the gel of this plant is antibacterial, anti-inflammatory, and soothing. Research shows that it speeds the healing of wounds.*

Note: Although some studies do show aloe gel reduced pain and hastened healing from surgical wounds, one study found that aloe actually delayed closure of the wound. Discuss with your doctor if you're having surgery.

Lifestyle Tip

If you have a puncture wound, do *not* apply herbs that speed wound healing. The problem with puncture wounds is that they don't bleed much and microbes can be deposited more deeply (than with superficial cuts and scrapes). In theory, speeding the closure of the skin can trap in microbes.

Honey-Aloe Salve

1 tablespoon (15 g) fresh *Aloe vera* gel or commercially prepared aloe gel (It should be at least 99 percent *Aloe vera.*)
1 tablespoon (20 g) honey

PREPARATION AND USE:

Wash the cut. Blend the aloe gel and honey. Apply the mix to the wound. Store the remainder in a jar in the refrigerator.

YIELD: MULTIPLE APPLICATIONS

❓ **How it works:** *Ancient Roman naturalist Pliny the Elder wrote about the virtues of aloe gel combined with honey for injuries. Aloe and honey both are antibacterial, anti-inflammatory, and enhance wound healing.*

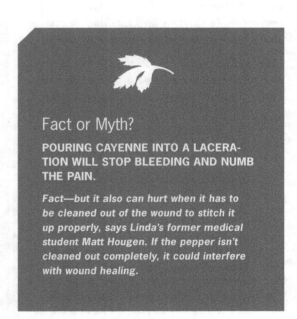

Fact or Myth?

POURING CAYENNE INTO A LACERATION WILL STOP BLEEDING AND NUMB THE PAIN.

Fact—but it also can hurt when it has to be cleaned out of the wound to stitch it up properly, says Linda's former medical student Matt Hougen. If the pepper isn't cleaned out completely, it could interfere with wound healing.

Homemade First-Aid Salve

I learned to make this salve from herbalist Sunny Mavor. It helps heal minor cuts and scrapes as well as chapped lips and hands. Because it does take some time to make, prepare in advance. It stores well, up to six months. ~ LBW

¼ cup (6 g) dried comfrey leaves
¼ cup (6 g) dried calendula flowers
¼ cup (6 g) dried St. John's wort flowers
¼ cup (6 g) dried echinacea leaves and flowers
Extra-virgin olive oil (or almond, apricot, avocado, or grapeseed oil)
Beeswax

PREPARATION AND USE:

Place the herbs in a clean pint-size (475 ml) jar. Cover the herbs with oil, stir, and add more oil until you have a good 1 inch (2.5 cm) of oil above the line of the herbs. Cap tightly. Place in a sunny window for two to four weeks. If the herbs sop up more oil, add extra oil to maintain the 1-inch (2.5 cm) margin on top.

At the end of the steeping period, the oil will have turned a greenish hue. You may also see some red color from the St. John's wort flowers. (Alternatively, you can heat the herbs and oil in a double boiler over low heat for 1 hour, stirring frequently.)

Before straining the mixture, wash and dry your hands. Rest a medium-size strainer atop a bowl. Cut a piece of cheesecloth large enough to drape over the edges. Place it on the strainer. Slowly pour the herbal oil into the strainer. Scoop out the plant parts. With your clean, dry hands, wring any remaining oil from the herbs. Discard or compost the spent herbs.

Measure the herbal oil. Let's say you ended up with 7 ounces (about 200 ml). To thicken the oil to a soft salve consistency, you need one part beeswax—1 ounce (28 g) in this case—to seven parts oil. For a firmer consistency, like that of lip balm, use one part beeswax to four parts oil.

Put water in the bottom part of a double boiler. Heat to boiling, and then lower the heat to a simmer. Pour the oil into the top of double boiler and add the beeswax. Stir until the beeswax melts, and immediately transfer it to the clean jar and cap tightly. (The salve will soon start to set.) Apply as needed. Store in the refrigerator for up to six months.

YIELD: ABOUT SIX MONTHS' WORTH OF APPLICATIONS

❓ **How it works:** *Comfrey contains allantoin, which helps "knit" wounds back together. Because it also contains chemicals that can harm the liver when taken in larger doses, you should only use this herb externally on wounds no larger than 2 inches (5 cm) in diameter. Experiments also demonstrate calendula's anti-inflammatory, antibacterial, and wound-healing properties. The same is true for echinacea, more popularly known as an immune-enhancing herb. Likewise, St. John's wort fights bacteria, reduces inflammation, and speeds healing, though that knowledge has been eclipsed by the herb's antidepressant effect.*

❗ **Warning:** *Calendula and echinacea are in the aster family, along with ragweed. If you're allergic to ragweed, you may also be allergic to these plants. If you develop skin irritation, stop using the salve. If you have a puncture wound, do not apply this salve because you want to keep the wound open to allow for proper drainage. If you have a minor burn, refrain from using this salve until the burned area cools—which can take a few hours.*

Note: Unless you grow these plants in your yard, you'll need to acquire them from an herb store or an online retailer. If the herbs aren't already chopped, break them into small pieces with a food processor or coffee mill. (Clean the coffee mill first with a cloth dampened with vodka.)

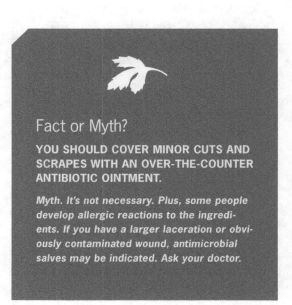

Fact or Myth?

YOU SHOULD COVER MINOR CUTS AND SCRAPES WITH AN OVER-THE-COUNTER ANTIBIOTIC OINTMENT.

Myth. It's not necessary. Plus, some people develop allergic reactions to the ingredients. If you have a larger laceration or obviously contaminated wound, antimicrobial salves may be indicated. Ask your doctor.

Thyme to Heal

1 cup (235 ml) water
1 teaspoon (1 g) crushed dried thyme leaves

PREPARATION AND USE:
Bring the water to a boil in a small pot. Turn off the heat. Add the thyme leaves and let steep until the tea cools to a temperature that is comfortable to the touch. Strain and apply to the wound with gauze or a clean cloth.

YIELD: 1 APPLICATION

❓ How it works: *The oils in this herb have a powerful antimicrobial effect; use the wash to enhance the effects of the mild soap and water you use to clean a cut.*

Tea-Tree Tincture

¾ teaspoon tea tree essential oil
½ cup (120 ml) warm water

PREPARATION AND USE:
Disperse the tea tree oil in the water by stirring. Rinse a cut or other abrasion with the liquid.

YIELD: 1 APPLICATION

❓ How it works: *Tea tree (Melaleuca alternifolia) is a shrubby tree native to Australia. The essential oil from this plant is antimicrobial and anti-inflammatory. It also promotes wound healing. Use this recipe after you have cleaned the cut with mild soap and water.*

Fact or Myth?

IF A WOUND IS BLEEDING BRISKLY, APPLY A TOURNIQUET ABOVE IT.

Myth. You may risk damaging tissue below the tourniquet. For small wounds, most people wouldn't consider using a tourniquet. Direct pressure on the wound is enough to stop the bleeding. Tourniquets are reserved for severe injuries to the limbs.

Scar Squelchers

Apply this simple recipe to the wound after the skin has begun to heal to help minimize inflammation and scarring.

Vitamin E capsule

PREPARATION AND USE:
Break open the capsule and rub the liquid onto the healing skin of the wound.

YIELD: 1 APPLICATION

❓ **How it works:** *Vitamin E has moisturizing properties that help hydrate and soften the skin and lower inflammation. Some research indicates topical applications improve healing from surgical wounds.*

Note: Alternatively, use a dab of petroleum jelly on the healing wound to keep a scab and the new skin moist. Petroleum jelly is an occlusive, which holds moisture into the skin to prevent the scab from cracking open with movement.

Lifestyle Tip

Cleansing wounds with soap and clean, cool water is sufficient for minor scrapes and cuts. Using stronger solutions, such as hydrogen peroxide, rubbing alcohol, or iodine, can actually irritate a cut, harm tissue, and slow down healing.

Backyard Bandage

Try growing comfrey in your garden for use as an immediate treatment.

1 comfrey leaf

PREPARATION AND USE:
Wash the wound thoroughly. Cut the comfrey leaf from the plant. (Mature leaves are quite large. If it's early in the growing season, you might need two leaves to cover the wound.) Rough up the leaf with your fingers and place against the wound. Wrap a clean, damp cloth around the leaves and the wound. If you can, leave in place for an hour before removing.

YIELD: 1 APPLICATION

❓ **How it works:** *Comfrey leaves and roots contain allantoin, which helps the generation of new skin cells. Research shows that abrasions healed faster with topical comfrey relative to a dummy ointment. Use comfrey only on wounds up to 2 inches (5 cm) in diameter. That precaution is due to the small risk of absorption of chemicals in comfrey that, in large quantities, can harm the liver.*

When Simple Doesn't Work

If you've stopped the bleeding and cleansed and covered the wound, watch it carefully as it heals. If the site develops any signs of infection, as noted in "When to Call the Doctor," see a doctor immediately.

Butterfly Bandage

Use for clean, straight cuts that may need to have edges pulled together to begin healing. See a doctor right away if the cut is deep, bleeding won't stop, and it appears you need stitches.

1 strip 1-inch (2.5 cm) wide strip adhesive tape (short enough to effectively draw the wound together)
Small strip of gauze

PREPARATION AND USE:

Fold the strip of tape in half, adhesive side out. At the folded top, cut a diagonal notch on each side; when you open the tape, there should be a triangle on each side, with the points directly across from each other and a small tape surface between the points.

Cut a small piece of gauze. Center the gauze on the sticky side of the tape, between the triangle points. This nonstick surface will be over the wound and must stay clean. Stick one end of the tape on one side of the cut. Pull the other end across the cut so that the edges of the cut come together. For a long cut, use two or more adhesive bandages as needed.

YIELD: 1 BANDAGE

❓ **How it works:** *Bringing together the edges of a cut promotes healing.*

When to Call the Doctor or Seek Medical Assistance

If the wound is serious, call 911.

Proceed to the emergency room if:

- *You can't remove foreign material from the wound.*
- *The laceration is on the face or neck or crosses a joint.*
- *Five minutes of steady pressure fails to stop the bleeding.*
- *The laceration is more than 1 inch (2.5 cm) long, is deep, jagged, or gapes open.*
- *You have any doubt that you need sutures (stitches).*
- *A human or animal bite broke the skin.*
- *You or your child is the victim of domestic violence.*

See your doctor if:

- *Your tetanus shot is out of date.*
- *Signs of infection develop: purulent discharge (some light yellow material is normal and indicates white blood cells are doing their job healing the wound), red streaks moving away from the wound, increased local tenderness and heat, or fever.*
- *You have diabetes (in which case you're at higher risk for poor wound healing).*
- *You have any concerns about the way the wound is healing.*

Chapter 28

Dandruff

You win some, you lose some. This principle holds true not only for economics but for human biology. For example, just as new cells perpetually form at the base of the skin and scalp, old cells slough off the surface. These cells comprise much of the dust in your house.

For some reason, we have a social stigma against visible accumulations of dead skin cells caught in our hair or dusting the shoulders of our clothes. In truth, it's all relative. Some people simply have more exuberant cell turnover, which makes the process more noticeable. In fact, dandruff affects half of us.

Dandruff can also cause itching and redness of the scalp. Heat can worsen the condition. Men have it more often than women. For many people, the scalp becomes less flaky with age.

Seborrheic dermatitis causes more severe dandruff. The affected skin and scalp becomes inflamed, very flaky, and greasy looking. Cradle cap in infants is one form of seborrheic dermatitis. Other disorders—psoriasis, eczema, fungal skin infection, and head lice—can cause scalp flakiness. A particular fungus (*Malassezia*) has now been associated with dandruff, seborrheic dermatitis, and cradle cap. It seems to thrive on excretions from the scalp's oil glands.

History

Nineteenth-century French researcher Louis-Charles Malassez identified the *Malassezia* fungus as the culprit that caused dandruff. Over the next half-century, scientists identified many forms of the fungus associated with dandruff and seborrheic dermatitis. A complicated picture emerged in which individual sensitivity and diet also play a role in determining who gets dandruff.

Throughout history, various folk and herbal remedies have enjoyed some success, such as those involving vinegar, rosemary, goldenseal, yogurt, and tea tree oil. In the last few decades, antidandruff shampoos have become popular. But the common denominator in these treatments is the same: antifungal and/or antibacterial activity. More recently, tea tree oil has been confirmed in at least two studies to be effective and well tolerated in fighting dandruff. (See "How it works" under the Tea Tree Oil Shampoo recipe on page 201.)

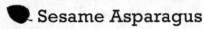 ## Sesame Asparagus

1 bunch asparagus, thick ends removed
1 tablespoon (15 ml) sesame oil
Freshly ground black pepper
1 teaspoon (3 g) sesame seeds

PREPARATION AND USE:

Preheat the oven to 450°F (230°C, or gas mark 8).

On a baking sheet, toss the asparagus spears with the sesame oil. Sprinkle with pepper to taste. Roast the asparagus for 5 minutes and then turn the spears and sprinkle with the sesame seeds. Roast for 5 minutes more until the asparagus is tender and just browned. Serve immediately.

YIELD: 2 SERVINGS

❓ **How it works:** *Low body levels of zinc and certain B vitamins can trigger dandruff. Asparagus and sesame seeds contain both zinc and vitamin B. Leafy green vegetables are excellent delivery systems for these important nutrients, as well as nuts and seeds, including pine nuts, pecans, and pumpkin seeds.*

Tea Tree Scalp Treatment

2 to 3 drops tea tree essential oil
¼ cup (60 ml) flaxseed oil

PREPARATION AND USE:

Drop the tea tree essential oil into the flaxseed oil and blend. Apply the mixture liberally to your scalp before bedtime. Wrap your head in a clean towel or cover your pillow with the towel to protect it. In the morning, shampoo and rinse your scalp thoroughly.

YIELD: 1 APPLICATION

❓ **How it works:** *Tea tree oil has antifungal properties. Flaxseed oil contains omega-3 fatty acids, which reduce inflammation that can accompany dandruff. If you have the type of dandruff caused by dry skin, the oil may help.*

Lifestyle Tip

If your dandruff appeared after you tried a new shampoo, switch to another, milder product—perhaps a fragrance-free, hypoallergenic shampoo. The same goes for other hair products. They can either irritate the scalp or lead to a buildup of oil. Hair dyes and permanents can be very irritating.

When Simple Doesn't Work

Try a medicated, antidandruff shampoo, available over the counter. The active ingredients vary from product to product. Most contain either selenium sulfide (slows the loss of old skin cells), coal tar (also slows skin turnover), zinc pyrithione (inhibits fungi and bacteria), octopirox (inhibits fungi), ketoconazole (a broad-spectrum antifungal), or salicylic acid (promotes removal of flakes). It may take some experimenting with various brands. Read the packages (noting that some products have undesirable effects on hair.) Follow the directions. Be sure to rinse thoroughly.

Rosemary Scalp Wash

1 cup (235 ml) apple cider vinegar
2 tablespoons (3 g) fresh rosemary leaves

PREPARATION AND USE:
Place the vinegar in a small pan and heat until nearly boiling. Remove from the heat, stir in the rosemary, cover the pan, and steep for 10 minutes. Strain the mixture and discard the herbs. Pour into a clean empty jar or bottle to store.

After every shampoo, mix ¼ cup (60 ml) of the solution with 2 cups (475 ml) of water. Use it to rinse your scalp thoroughly.

YIELD: 4 APPLICATIONS

❓ **How it works:** *Vinegar contains acetic acid, which is antifungal. Rosemary is an excellent antibacterial and antifungal agent.*

Fact or Myth?

DRY SKIN CAUSES DANDRUFF.

That depends. In seborrheic dermatitis, the skin and scalp are oily and the oils can favor the growth of a fungus called Malassezia. Frequent shampooing can improve dandruff but could worsen dry scalp. However, dry skin and scalp account for the fact that some people have flakier scalps in winter.

Tea Tree Oil Shampoo

¼ cup (60 ml) liquid castile soap
¼ cup (60 ml) water
½ teaspoon olive or flaxseed oil
10 to 20 drops tea tree essential oil

PREPARATION AND USE:
Place all the ingredients in a sizeable, clean squeeze bottle with a secure top. Cap and shake to combine. Part your hair in small sections. Dab the shampoo onto one small area at a time. Massage the shampoo into your scalp. Rinse.

YIELD: 4 TO 6 APPLICATIONS

❓ **How it works:** *Tea tree oil is active against some species of* Malassezia, *the fungus associated with dandruff and seborrheic dermatitis. One study found that a shampoo containing 5 percent tea tree oil significantly improved dandruff relative to a placebo. Although this study did not reveal any side effects, some people are allergic to the essential oil of this plant. If this shampoo irritates your scalp, stop using it.*

Note: You can also use this mild mixture as a general skin wash.

Lifestyle Tip

Go outdoors without a hat for about 15 minutes or so. Sun exposure helps manage some of the skin conditions that can cause scalp flakiness.

🌿 Honey Hair Mask

½ cup (170 g) honey
¼ cup (60 ml) olive oil

PREPARATION AND USE:

In a small, microwave-safe bowl, mix the honey and olive oil. Heat the mixture in the microwave on high for about 10 seconds, and then allow it to cool. Gradually work the mixture onto your scalp until it is covered. You can also coat your hair with this mask to make it shine. Cover your scalp with a shower cap or warm, damp towel for about 30 minutes. Remove the wrap and rinse well.

YIELD: 1 APPLICATION

❓ **How it works:** *Honey inhibits* Malassezia *fungi, which means it may be helpful in treating dandruff and seborrheic dermatitis, although studies have yet to investigate that possibility.*

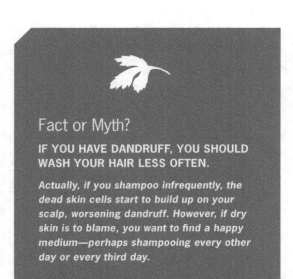

Fact or Myth?

IF YOU HAVE DANDRUFF, YOU SHOULD WASH YOUR HAIR LESS OFTEN.

Actually, if you shampoo infrequently, the dead skin cells start to build up on your scalp, worsening dandruff. However, if dry skin is to blame, you want to find a happy medium—perhaps shampooing every other day or every third day.

Lifestyle Tip

Avoid stress and fatigue, which can worsen seborrheic dermatitis. Get a minimum of 8 hours of sleep. When feelings of stress envelop you, close your eyes, breathe in deeply for four long counts, hold your breath for seven long counts, and release your breath for eight long counts. Repeat this four times and find yourself filled with a sense of well-being. See Chapters 35 and 56, on fatigue and stress, for more ideas for counteracting both.

🌿 Brush Up Relief

A good brush

PREPARATION AND USE:

Starting at your scalp, brush from scalp through hair with firm strokes. Repeat until you've covered the entire scalp and corresponding strands.

YIELD: DAILY APPLICATION

❓ **How it works:** *This brushing action carries oil from your scalp, where it causes dandruff, along your hair strands. While it fights dandruff, the repetitive brushing also brings out the shine in your hair.*

Yogurt Boost

1 cup (230 g) plain yogurt
1 tablespoon (15 ml) fresh lemon juice

PREPARATION AND USE:

In a small bowl, mix the yogurt and lemon juice.

Thoroughly massage the yogurt mixture into your scalp. Cover your scalp with a shower cap or warm towel for about 30 minutes. Remove the wrap and shampoo.

YIELD: 1 APPLICATION

❓ **How it works:** *If a case of dandruff is caused by a fungal infection, yogurt can help fight it. It contains friendly bacteria that discourage fungal infections such as Malassezia. The citric acid in lemon juice is also antifungal.*

When to See the Doctor

Make an appointment if your scalp has recently begun to flake, particularly if you also have itching and reddened patches of skin. It doesn't hurt to get a diagnosis to find out whether you have a condition such as psoriasis, eczema, fungal infection, or seborrheic dermatitis. Even if it's run-of-the-mill dandruff, your doctor might have ideas for treatment.

Cradle Cap Relief

Pure castile liquid soap
Mineral oil (optional)

PREPARATION AND USE:

Gently massage your infant's scalp with your fingers to help circulation and loosen scaly patches. Shampoo with the castile soap, rinsing the head thoroughly. Do this daily until the scaly patches disappear; then shampoo twice weekly.

If your child has a head of hair, brush it with a clean, soft brush after each shampoo and several times during the day.

For stubborn scales: To help loosen especially stubborn scales, put mineral oil on your fingertips and massage it into your baby's scalp. Wrap a warm, wet cloth around your child's head for about an hour. (Alternate two cloths, changing one cloth for a warm cloth each time it starts to cool; you must keep the wrap warm to maintain the baby's body heat.)

YIELD: DAILY APPLICATION UNTIL THE SCALES DISAPPEAR

❓ **How it works:** *Gentle massage increases circulation for smooth skin and also helps remove the dead, scaly skin of cradle cap. The mineral oil and warm cloth helps soften especially stubborn scales. The key ingredient in castile soap is skin-softening olive oil combined with the alkaline sodium hydroxide. It has no harsh artificial additives to irritate the baby's tender scalp.*

Note: Contact your doctor if the scales continue; you may need a prescription cream.

Chapter

29

Depression

No one is happy all the time. Sadness represents an appropriate response to misfortune. For the psychologically hardy, low moods soon lift. Significant loss, however, produces grief, which can endure for months (for some people, depression can complicate normal grief). Barring tragedy, most people experience episodes of low mood against a backdrop of psychological well-being.

Depression isn't part of the normal emotional fabric. It burdens people with persistent unhappiness and an inability to derive pleasure from activities, even those that once brought joy. As opposed to "the blues," it impairs a person's ability to function.

This debilitating illness is all too common. According to the World Health Organization, depression affects 121 million people around the globe and places second behind heart disease as a leading cause of disability. About 16.3 million Americans over the age of eighteen experience some type of depression. Major depression strikes 20 percent of women and 13 percent of men.

This illness does more than engender sadness. Depressed people often feel irritable, angry, worthless, and ashamed. Thinking becomes irrationally negative. ("Nothing's any good. I'm a burden. I'll never get better.") Physical symptoms include increased pain, changes in appetite, and sleep disturbances.

In addition to major depression, other depressive illnesses include seasonal affective disorder (depression during the short days of winter), premenstrual dysphoria (depression around the time of menses), dysthymia (low-level depression that endures for at least two years), and bipolar disorder (formerly called manic depression and marked by alternating episodes of depression and mania).

Major depression is a serious illness. Not only does it diminish quality of life, but it raises the risk for chronic conditions such as heart disease and stroke. Like any other disease, it warrants professional treatment.

The following recipes and tips are designed to buoy normal bouts of low mood and prevent depression. *Please do not use these remedies as a substitute for professional treatment.* If you think you are clinically depressed, get help.

History

Treating depression and other forms of mental illness have long been the focus of psychology and psychiatry. As early as the fourth century BCE, Greek physician Hippocrates speculated on the nature of mental disorders. In the early twentieth century, Austrian physician Sigmund Freud developed psychoanalysis and psychotherapy to investigate and treat emotional distress and conflict. Into the twenty-first century, great strides were made in understanding and treating psychological problems and psychiatric illnesses.

Mental *health*, in contrast, has gotten little attention through the centuries (though twentieth-century humanistic psychologists—such as Carl Rogers, Abraham Maslow, and Erich Fromm—developed theories and practices relating to human fulfillment). Then in 1998, psychologist Martin Seligman launched a new movement called positive psychology. In his 2003 book, *Authentic Happiness*, Seligman urged psychologists to focus on improving human happiness and normal life.

Shifting the scientific spotlight toward what goes *right* in human affairs, this new branch of psychology aims to enhance human strengths and virtues, such as joy, gratitude, responsibility, creativity, and achievement. What helps us to feel productive and optimistic? How do we generate positive emotions, such as altruism, hope, resilience, and mindfulness? Just what is involved in the "pursuit of happiness"? As interest in positive psychology grows, such questions loom larger. Recently, a course in positive psychology was Harvard University's most popular class.

Scatter Joy

One morning, while riding my bike to work, feeling a bit grumpy, I tried smiling and saying, "Good morning," to every creature I passed—pigeons and ducks included. I felt positively joyous once I arrived. ~ LBW

You
Another human

PREPARATION AND USE:

Smile at someone. It could be an acquaintance, friend, family member, or animal. If you feel so bold, say hello to a stranger (unless you're concerned about your safety).

YIELD: MULTIPLE APPLICATIONS

❷ **How it works:** *Smiling and spreading laughter and goodwill can reduce pain, decrease stress hormones, enhance immune function, buoy mood, and heighten alertness and creativity. Apparently your body doesn't know the difference between spontaneous mirth and simulated laughter. Either way, health benefits occur.*

Lifestyle Tip

Get regular physical activity. A number of studies confirm that exercise reduces symptoms of depression. Find something you enjoy so much you look forward to doing it each day. You don't need to join a gym. Any physical activity counts—dance, garden, clean house, jog, walk, practice yoga, bowl, or throw a Frisbee.

Light-It-Up Laughter

As the Irish proverb goes, "A good laugh and a long sleep are the two best cures for anything."

You
A friend or other optional accessories
    (e.g., a funny video, such as BBC's talking
    animal videos available on YouTube, or
    a comedy show)
A group

PREPARATION AND USE:
Start by letting out a giggle, guffaw, or chortle. Don't worry about seeming false or forced. It doesn't matter that nothing has struck your funny bone. Keep going. Soon, you might genuinely laugh—because you feel silly or downright mirthful. Laughter is contagious. Repeat the experiment in a group. If you like the experience, you might investigate whether your community offers "laughter yoga" classes.

YIELD: 1 SESSION

? **How it works:** *Humor is good medicine. If you're feeling down in the dumps, it's harder to laugh. Take cheer from the fact that emerging evidence hints that doing so can lift mood. A good laugh relaxes your body and stimulates endorphins, promoting a feeling of well-being that helps us look at stressful or unhappy situations in a new light. One National Institutes of Health study showed that it stimulates the brain to counteract depressive symptoms. "Laughter therapy" decreases chronic pain and symptoms of depression and improves quality of life and resilience in cancer survivors.*

Crack a Joke

One of my nieces learns a new joke or two in advance of social events. It's a great icebreaker.
~ LBW

You
A joke book or an Internet site with jokes
A listener

PREPARATION AND USE:
Memorize one joke. Tell it to someone. (Don't worry about your delivery. In fact, a poorly delivered joke is, in itself, comical.)

YIELD: 1 SESSION

? **How it works:** *As with laughter, joke-telling promotes a smile, if not a chuckle or all-out laughter. Besides enhancing physical well-being, laughter is a social connector. If you tell a joke that highlights the other person's own experience, it promotes appreciation and gives the teller a sense of "belonging and social cohesion," noted psychiatrist Joseph Richman, professor emeritus at Albert Einstein Medical Center in New York, in* Psychology Today.

Note: It doesn't much matter whether the other person erupts in sidesplitting laughter. People tend to laugh longer and harder at their own jokes than at those other people tell.

Gratitude Journal

Keep a gratitude journal every day of the year to record all the joy in your life—what a mood boost!

A notebook
A pen

PREPARATION AND USE:
At the end of each day, record at least three things that made you feel grateful. (Small things count. In fact, the ability to appreciate small signs of beauty and joy may be particularly helpful. Maybe someone opened a door for you. Maybe you stopped to watch a breathtaking sunset. Maybe you received a compliment at work. Maybe you were able to help another person.)

YIELD: 1 DAILY SESSION

❓ **How it works:** *Repeated studies have shown that expressing gratitude increases positive emotions and decreases symptoms of depression. In 2003, Robert Emmons and Michael McCullough published a paper called* **Counting Blessings versus Burdens: An Experimental Investigation of Gratitude and Subjective Well-Being in Daily Life.** *In brief, the researchers randomly assigned 201 college undergraduates to keep journals describing five things for which they felt grateful, five things that annoyed or bothered them, or five events that had some kind of impact. Relative to the other two groups, gratitude journalers had significantly sunnier outlooks on life. They also exercised more and experienced better moods and fewer symptoms of ill health. A similar study design showed benefits in adolescents.*

Talk to Yourself

We all do something called self-talk, in which we often dwell on the negative. But no one's perfect and misfortune befalls us all. Happier people spin their self-talk in a positive direction.

You
A past event that didn't go ideally

PREPARATION AND USE:
Conjure up a recent event that made you feel down on yourself. Write down what happened and what you thought. Was your assessment fair and kind? Why not? Now write down what went right. Write down all the positive things you could have brought to the situation. Write down how you can handle it better in the future.

YIELD: 1 SESSION

❓ **How it works:** *We become so used to our inner voice that we may stop paying attention to the tone and content of our monologues. Spend an hour paying attention. Are you hard on yourself? Critical of others? Unduly negative? Do you generalize ("I'm so stupid") or make mountains out of molehills? How would you do something better next time? Did anything go right? Focus on that. Bring more of it into your life. More and more, catch yourself grousing and try to rephrase that script.*

Cook Up Some Optimism

This easy practice becomes infectious; you'll see how the power of positive thinking in the most dire situations can help build a foundation for future challenges.

Your imagination
A piece of paper
A pen

PREPARATION AND USE:

Think of an upcoming event you're not looking forward to. Perhaps you're even dreading it. Draw a line down the middle of the page. On the left, write down all the negative, pessimistic things you're thinking. (For instance: Maybe you're going to get a root canal. You're thinking it's going to hurt, you'll have to miss work, you'll be behind schedule, you'll drool, and the dentist will keep asking you questions with his fingers in your mouth.)

On the right, list the positive. (For instance: Your dentist will use anesthesia to dull the pain. You'll likely have less pain in the long run. Your tooth will look better. Maybe you could listen to an audio book, podcast, or music while it's being done. At the very end of the list you can write that you'll have the procedure behind you.)

YIELD: 1 SESSION PER DREADED EVENT

❓ How it works: *Envisioning all aspects of a situation helps us balance the ups and downs and to see it in a neutral, if not positive, light. You may be surprised how many positive points you see in any situation. Thinking positively can gradually infiltrate all your planning and your life.*

Recipe Variation: Try positive mental rehearsal. Envision an upcoming event turning out well: Maybe it's a big presentation at work; maybe it's a meeting with a friend or sibling you've had a disagreement with. See it in every detail. Use all your senses to lay your mental foundation for a positive event.

Skip

My daughter and I periodically do this to lighten our spirits. It never fails to elicit laughter. ~ LBW

You
A sidewalk or path

PREPARATION AND USE:

Skip. We're not kidding. If you can't skip, try waltzing. If you're wheelchair-bound, turn a tight 360. If you're in bed, wave your arms.

YIELD: ENDLESS APPLICATIONS

Recipe Variations: Play hopscotch. Chalk a flower on the sidewalk. Blow bubbles.

❓ **How it works:** *We aren't sure. Maybe it takes you back to your childhood. It certainly shakes things up.*

Lifestyle Tip

Wake up and smell the coffee (or tea). This dynamic duo does more than kick-start your day. Moderate consumption of coffee (two to three cups a day) is associated with a lower risk of depression. Don't get carried away. Caffeine excess can cause anxiety, which often coexists with depression. If you're a teetotaler, you might like to know that regular consumption of green tea (three or four cups a day) has been linked to a lower risk of depression.

Sunny Mediterranean Salad

1 cup (100 g) halved and pitted black olives
1 cup (100 g) halved and pitted green olives
1 cup (150 g) halved cherry tomatoes
1 cup (135 g) cubed cucumber
¼ cup (38 g) crumbled feta cheese
½ cup (60 g) crushed walnuts
½ teaspoon minced fresh garlic
Freshly ground black pepper
1 tablespoon (15 ml) extra-virgin olive oil
¼ cup (10 g) chopped fresh basil leaves
   (optional)

PREPARATION AND USE:

Mix together the olives, tomatoes, cucumber, and feta in a large bowl. Toss in the walnuts, garlic, and pepper to taste. Drizzle the olive oil over the salad and give it one final toss. Top with the basil leaves, if using.

YIELD: 4 SIDE SALADS

❓ **How it works:** *One study found that women who ate a "traditional" diet (i.e., high in vegetables, fruit, meat, fish, and whole grains and low in sugar and processed foods) had lower odds of depression and anxiety. The inverse relationship was true for women who followed a "Western" diet (i.e., high in processed or fried foods, refined carbohydrates, sugary foods, and beer). People who follow a Mediterranean diet—a traditional diet that emphasizes vegetables, fruits, nuts, whole grains, fish, and olive oil—enjoy some protection against depression. Lastly, basil is traditionally considered an uplifting and tasty herb.*

🐟 Good-Fat Fish

4 salmon, tuna, or herring fillets (3 ounces, or 85 g)
4 tablespoons (60 ml) olive oil, divided
Freshly ground black pepper
Juice of 1 lemon
2 tablespoons (22 g) Dijon mustard
Tabasco sauce
1 teaspoon (7 g) honey
¼ cup (16 g) chopped fresh dill
Lemon wedges, for garnish

PREPARATION AND USE:

Brush the salmon with 1 to 2 tablespoons (15 to 30 ml) of the olive oil and season with the pepper. Broil for 3 to 4 minutes on each side, so that the skin is brown and firm like meat.

In a small bowl, whisk together the remaining olive oil with the lemon juice, mustard, Tabasco sauce to taste, honey, and dill. Add pepper to taste.

Drizzle the sauce over the warm fillets and serve with the lemon wedges.

YIELD: 4 SERVINGS

❓ **How it works:** *Oily fish, such as tuna, salmon, herring, and mackerel, are rich in the omega-3 fatty acids your brain needs to function properly. In susceptible people, low levels seem to increase the risk of depression.*

Lifestyle Tip

Eliminate or cut back on alcohol. It's a central nervous system depressant. Problem drinking makes people more at risk for depression. So do depressant drugs. In addition, a withdrawal symptom of amphetamines is low mood. Unfortunately, people who can't get proper treatment often self-medicate (and understandably so) with alcohol, tobacco, and illicit drugs.

Lifestyle Tip

Express your emotions. Confiding in a trusted friend, writing about thoughts and feelings, and creating expressive art are examples of outlets that can diffuse mental tension and provide perspective on inner turmoil. Rumination, on the other hand, perpetuates distress. Suppressing strong emotions, such as anger, can create a toxic stew that nourishes depression and eating disorders and lowers pain thresholds.

Cobra Pose

The cobra pose, called bhujangasana *(boo-jang-ahhs-anna) in Sanskrit, is one of a series of heart-opening yoga exercises. Although such poses are practiced to help strengthen the back, tone the abdomen, and open the chest, they are also intended to balance the body and spirit.*

You
Comfortable clothes
A pad or rug

PREPARATION AND USE:

Lie on your belly. Straighten your legs behind you. Draw your heels and toes together. Press your toenails and pubic bone against the ground.

Rest your forehead on the floor. Place your palms against the floor, fingertips spread, hands facing forward. Hug your elbows to your sides (like cricket wings).

Push down with your hands and arms so that your head, neck, and shoulders lift. All the while, keep your shoulders open, not hunched; keep your lower abdominals engaged to avoid pinching your lower back; and keep your neck in a neutral position.

Breathe slowly in and out three to five times. Lower your body. Rest. Repeat three more times.

YIELD: 1 SESSION

? **How it works:** *Emerging research shows that yoga improves mood in people without bona fide depression. In people with major depression, the addition of yoga to antidepressant medications further reduces symptoms. Also, it's a big boost just being part of a class and enjoying the socialization it brings.*

! **Warning:** *Do not try this if you have a hernia, lower back pain, or are pregnant.*

Variations: See www.yogajournal.com or YouTube for videos of easy yoga moves.

Lifestyle Tip

Serve. Compassionate acts help transcend the self. Psychological challenges tend to make us self-absorbed. Helping others is an antidote. Make a sick friend dinner. Give a family member a massage. If you're not extremely social, work at an animal shelter or help clean a public park. Volunteering makes you feel needed, builds confidence, and grows skills. A number of Internet sites can help you locate volunteer opportunities.

When Simple Doesn't Work

Several dietary supplements have antidepressant effects. However, we recommend that anyone with symptoms of depression that are severe or last more than two weeks see a doctor. The two of you can decide if dietary supplements are right for you.

The best-researched supplement for depression is St. John's wort. Studies show that for mild-to-moderate depression, standardized extracts work better than placebo treatment and are on a par with synthetic antidepressants, though with fewer side effects. Because St. John's wort can increase sun sensitivity, fair-skinned people should take precautions to avoid sunburn. Also, this herb hastens the body's breakdown of many medications, lowering levels in blood. If you're taking medication, check with your doctor before adding St. John's wort. Do not take it with prescription antidepressant drugs (serious side effects can occur). Two herbs, rhodiola and saffron, show promise in managing depression.

Studies indicate that supplements with S-adenosyl methionine (SAMe) can improve depression symptoms. Although SAMe has been shown to improve response to conventional treatment, it should not be combined with antidepressant drugs without physician monitoring. People with bipolar disorder shouldn't take St. John's wort or SAMe because of the risk of triggering mania.

Preliminary research suggests that fish oil and folic acid (a B vitamin) supplements can improve symptoms of depression.

🦀 B-eautiful Crab Cakes

16 ounces (455 g) crabmeat, flaked
1 large egg, lightly beaten
1 cup (115 g) bread crumbs
¼ cup (25 g) scallion
¼ cup (60 g) plain low-fat Greek yogurt
1 teaspoon (5 ml) fresh lemon juice
1 tablespoon (15 ml) Worcestershire sauce
½ teaspoon minced fresh garlic
Freshly ground black pepper
Olive oil

PREPARATION AND USE:

In a large bowl, mix together all the ingredients until combined. Roll and shape the mixture into eight cakes. Coat a large skillet with a small amount of olive oil and place over medium-low heat. Cook the cakes until golden brown, about 3 minutes on each side.

YIELD: 4 SERVINGS

❷ How it works: *It's easy to have a vitamin B_{12} deficiency if you don't consume animal foods: fish, meat, poultry, and eggs. Long-term vitamin B_{12} deficiency can lead to anemia, nerve damage, depression, memory loss, disorientation, and dementia. Crab is high in vitamin B_{12}. Look for stone crabs and Dungeness, which are lowest in contaminants.*

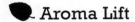

Aroma Lift

Your favorite uplifting plant essential oil

PREPARATION AND USE:

You can use essential oils in a variety of ways:

- Create blends or use them singly.
- Put a few drops in a commercial diffuser (which gently heats the oil to aerosolize the oils).
- If you don't have a diffuser, pour hot water into a bowl, add 3 drops of essential oil, and place nearby.
- You can also add 10 drops per ounce (28 ml) of unscented lotion or body oil.
- Finally, you can add 10 drops to a bath and mix well.

YIELD: 1 APPLICATION EACH

❓ How it works: *Plant essential oils bind to receptors in the nose. Nerve impulses for smell affect areas related to mood. Also, aromas are linked to memories. The small molecules in plant essential oils can also cross the skin and the respiratory linings (when you inhale the airborne chemicals) to enter the bloodstream. In a study of depressed and anxious pregnant women, a diluted blend of rose and lavender improved symptoms. Centuries of use and preliminary studies indicate that other essential oils can positively modulate mood.*

Note: Essential oil options include lemon, neroli, geranium, bergamot, clary sage, rose, lemon verbena, ylang ylang, jasmine, lavender, basil, and marjoram. (Avoid synthetic perfumes.) If you don't have any of these plant essential oils at home, go to the nearest natural food stores and sniff the sample bottles until you find a scent you enjoy. If the smell reminds you of a happy experience, that's exactly what you want.

Lifestyle Tip

Get enough sleep. Sleep deprivation can make you irritable, moody, and more vulnerable to depression. That said, depression is associated with poor sleep. It can even be one of the first signs of depression. Either way, if you can't sleep, talk to your doctor.

Mindful Massage

2 tablespoons (30 ml) unscented lotion or vegetable oil
10 to 12 drops lavender essential oil, or your favorite

PREPARATION AND USE:

In a serene setting with your favorite calming music; slowly and deliberately add the lotion to a teacup. Drop in the essential oil. Mix with a spoon or chopstick.

Dip one hand into the lotion and massage it into the opposite arm, thinking about the smooth feel of the lotion against your skin, the aroma of lavender, and the joy of the motion. When finished, pause. Appreciate your bodily sensations and the setting.

Now massage your opposite arm, then each hand, leg, and foot, focusing on the slow, soothing motion of the massage and the velvety feel of the lotion against your skin. Take an appreciative pause as you finish each body part. Finish with your face, neck, and chest. Close your eyes for a few moments, inhaling and exhaling slowly.

YIELD: 1 APPLICATION

❷ How it works: *Mindfulness, by definition, helps you focus on the present moment, which can stop you from brooding. It can also help you appreciate the beauty around you. In a study involving pregnant women, mindfulness reduced symptoms of depression and facilitated maternal-infant bonding.*

Chapter 30

Diabetes Prevention

Worldwide, diabetes is one of the most common chronic diseases. In developed countries, diabetes has reached epidemic proportions. In the United States, it's the seventh leading cause of death. The number of Americans diagnosed with diabetes tripled between 1980 and 2010, when the number topped 20 million.

In the developing world, cases of diabetes have surged, due mainly to the importation of the Western lifestyle, particularly the combination of physical inactivity and diets high in refined grains and sugar, both of which fuel weight gain and which, in turn, promotes obesity. By 2025, experts anticipate that diabetes will afflict 246 to 380 million people worldwide.

Fortunately, type-2 diabetes, which accounts for 95 percent of diabetes cases, is largely preventable. More on prevention in a minute.

The underlying problem in diabetes lies with insulin, a pancreatic hormone whose main function is to move glucose (sugar) from the bloodstream into liver, muscle, and fat cells. Without insulin, blood glucose levels climb, damaging many tissues, and the cells starve.

In type-1 diabetes, the pancreas doesn't make enough insulin. This condition often appears in childhood. In genetically susceptible individuals, some trigger (perhaps a viral infection) causes antibodies to attack the insulin-making cells of the pancreas.

In type-2 diabetes, the pancreas makes plenty of insulin, but the liver, muscles, and fat cells become insulin resistant, meaning the cells fail to respond to this hormone.

Things that promote insulin resistance include being overweight or obese, chronically stressed, sleep deprived, and physically inactive. Avoiding all of the aforementioned risks helps prevent type-2 diabetes. If you have a family history of diabetes, preventive strategies are particularly important.

A third type of diabetes, gestational diabetes, involves insulin resistance during pregnancy. About 18 percent of pregnant women develop diabetes during pregnancy (gestation). Scientists believe that certain hormones made by the placenta promote insulin resistance.

Gestational diabetes usually resolves after the birth. However, the woman is at risk for developing type-2 diabetes later on. If the pregnant woman's blood glucose isn't controlled, the fetus gains too much weight, may experience abnormally low blood glucose, and is later at risk for obesity and type-2 diabetes.

If you have diabetes, you know how important it is to control blood sugar with some combination of lifestyle modifications and medications. Consequences of chronically high blood sugar are accelerated aging of many tissues, arterial disease, heart disease and heart attack, stroke, eye disease (vision-robbing diabetic retinopathy), nerve damage, and poorly healing wounds.

The rest of this section will provide you with tips on reducing your risk for diabetes. If you already have diabetes, first discuss the use of these recipes and lifestyle tips with your doctor.

Lifestyle Tip

Mellow out. When you're stressed, the hormones cortisol, epinephrine, and glucagon rise. All three hormones raise blood glucose, thereby antagonizing insulin. For people who already have diabetes, moderate psychosocial stress can undermine glucose management. Controlling stress, on the other hand, improves glucose levels. Preliminary research supports mindfulness-based stress reduction in diabetics. (Mindfulness meditation is a practice that involves deliberately paying attention to the present moment.)

History

Diabetes was first described as "too great emptying of the urine" in an Egyptian manuscript around 1500 BCE and as "honey urine" in India around the same time. Diabetes mellitus (from the Greek) means "honeyed flow"—so named because it elevates blood sugar, leading to a heavy flow of sugary urine. As early as the fifth century, type-1 diabetes was associated with young age and type-2 diabetes with being overweight (though the distinctions weren't clearly made until 1936).

Not until the late 1800s did scientists understand that the pancreas had something to do with a diabetic's high sugar levels. It took another half-century to pin the problem on the pancreatic hormone insulin. A diagnosis of diabetes was a death sentence until 1922, when diabetics first received insulin injections. By the end of the century, biosynthetic insulin vastly improved the treatment of diabetes.

One of the great strides forward was metformin, an oral medication for type-2 diabetics, which targets the body's insulin resistance rather than increasing insulin production. Developed from goat's rue *(Galega officinalis)*, metformin is an effective glucose-lowering agent—and the future of diabetes treatment may lie with such medicinal plants. To date, more than four hundred traditional plant treatments for diabetes have been reported, although only a small number have received scientific and medical evaluation to assess their efficacy.

Roasted Veggie Explosion

1 to 2 tablespoons (15 to 30 ml) olive oil
1 large onion, quartered
2 carrots, diced
1 red or yellow bell pepper, seeded and sliced
  into strips
1 bunch asparagus, woody bottoms cut off
2 beets, peeled and quartered
4 garlic cloves, peeled
¼ cup (7 g) crushed fresh rosemary
Sea salt (optional)

PREPARATION AND USE:

Preheat the oven to 400°F (200°C, or gas mark 6).

Spray or brush a baking sheet with olive oil. Drizzle the olive oil over the vegetables in a bowl and toss to coat them. Spread the vegetables and garlic evenly across a baking sheet. Sprinkle with the rosemary and the sea salt to taste, if using.

Roast for 15 minutes and then flip the vegetables and roast for another 10 minutes. They should be browned but not overcooked.

YIELD: 6 SERVINGS

❷ **How it works:** *Fruits and vegetables contain fiber, which slows absorption of dietary sugars, and many nutrients beneficial to overall health and reducing diabetes risks. The World Health Organization recommends eating at least five portions a day to prevent diabetes. A recent study found that people who ate a greater quantity and variety of fruits and vegetables had a much lower risk of developing type-2 diabetes.*

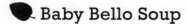 Baby Bello Soup

1 tablespoon (15 ml) olive oil
2 cups (140 g) sliced cremini mushrooms,
  divided
2 leeks, sliced and well rinsed
1 celery stalk, diced
1 small carrot, diced
¼ teaspoon minced fresh garlic
½ teaspoon grated fresh ginger
¼ teaspoon freshly ground black
  pepper
¼ cup (60 ml) chicken or vegetable stock
6 chicken bouillon cubes, or 2 tablespoons
  (12 g) bouillon grains
2 quarts (2 L) water
1 tablespoon (16 g) miso paste
Chopped fresh scallions and/or cilantro,
  for garnish (optional)

PREPARATION AND USE:

Heat the olive oil in a large pot over medium-high heat. Add 2 tablespoons (8.75 g) of the mushrooms, along with the leeks, celery, carrot, garlic, ginger, and pepper. Stir in the stock. Add the bouillon, water, and miso paste. Stir well. Raise the heat to high and bring the mixture to a boil. Cover and lower the heat to medium. Cook for 30 to 40 minutes.

Place the remaining mushrooms in another large pot. Place a strainer over that pot and pour the broth of the first pot into the second, straining out all the other contents. Steep for about 10 minutes. Enjoy the soup while it's steaming, garnished with chopped scallions or cilantro, if desired.

YIELD: 4 TO 6 SERVINGS

❷ How it works: *Mushrooms contain complex carbohydrates and fiber. Extracts of a particular button mushroom (Agaricus blazeii, which you won't find in the store but is related to portobello and button mushrooms) reduced high blood glucose. In combination with medication, this extract decreased insulin resistance in people with type-2 diabetes. No research has, to our knowledge, examined the effect of eating whole mushrooms on blood glucose.*

Lifestyle Tip

Enjoy an occasional beer or glass of wine. Moderate alcohol intake (not more than one drink a day for women, not more than two for men) correlates with a lower risk of type-2 diabetes.

🍠 Simply Psyllium Date Loaf

1⅓ cups (120 g) gluten-free oat flour
¼ cup (28 g) flaxseed meal
2 tablespoons (36 g) psyllium powder
1½ teaspoons (7 g) baking soda
5 large eggs
¼ cup (60 ml) water
¼ cup (60 ml) coconut oil, melted
1 packet (1 g) stevia
1 tablespoon (15 g) apple cider vinegar
½ cup (89 g) chopped, seeded dates
Plain nonfat Greek yogurt

PREPARATION AND USE:
Preheat the oven to 350°F (180°F, or gas mark 4).

Lightly spray a 9 x 5-inch (23 x 12.5 cm) loaf pan with canola oil. Set aside.

In a large bowl, blend the flour, flaxseed meal, psyllium, and baking soda. Stir in the eggs, water, oil, stevia, and vinegar. Fold in the chopped dates. Pour into the prepared pan and bake for about 30 minutes or until the center springs back to touch. Serve warm with a dollop of yogurt.

YIELD: 1 LOAF

❷ How it works: *Not only does psyllium husk prevent and correct constipation, but the fiber lowers cholesterol levels as well as blood glucose after a meal in people with type-1 and type-2 diabetes. It doesn't lower blood glucose in people who are not diabetics. Fiber helps you feel fuller, which can reduce calorie intake (a boon if you're trying to lose weight).*

Stevia is a South American herb whose leaves produce a sweetener that, unlike sugar or honey, does not send blood sugar skyrocketing. Lab research also indicates it has antidiabetes activities.

Flaxseed Breakfast Delight

¼ cup (28 g) flaxseed meal
¼ cup (60 ml) nonfat milk or almond milk
1 large egg
1 teaspoon (7 g) honey
¼ cup (35 g) seeded and cubed apple
1 tablespoon (7.5 g) crushed walnuts
At least 1 teaspoon (2 g) ground cinnamon (see How it works.)

PREPARATION AND USE:

Pour the flaxseed meal into a microwave-safe breakfast bowl. Stir in the milk, egg, and honey. Microwave on high for about 30 seconds. Stir the cereal, then fold in the apple and walnuts. Stir in the cinnamon. Microwave for another 30 seconds. Enjoy.

YIELD: 1 SERVING

❓ **How it works:** *Flaxseed consumption can improve some measures of disease in people with type-2 diabetes. Studies show that a compound in flaxseed called* lignan *(also called* lignin*) can improve some measures of disease in people with type-2 diabetes. Some research indicates that two species of cinnamon—Ceylon or "true" cinnamon* (Cinnamomum verum, *a.k.a.* C. zeylanicum) *or Chinese cinnamon* (Cinnamomum cassia, *or* C. aromaticum)— *lower blood glucose. Other studies have failed to find a significant effect. Because it's cheaper, Chinese cinnamon is what you'll find in most supermarkets. Look for Ceylon cinnamon in specialty stores.*

Caff It Up

1 quart (946 ml) water
4 teaspoons (8 g) Earl Grey or other black caffeinated tea
8 ice cubes
Handful of fresh, whole mint leaves
Stevia
4 lemon slices
4 orange slices

PREPARATION AND USE:

Boil the water. turn off the heat, add the tea, and brew for 3 to 5 minutes. Pour the tea through a strainer into a pitcher. Stir in the mint leaves. Add stevia to taste. Chill the brew for 1 hour. Add two ice cubes to each of four glasses. Pour the minted tea over the ice cubes. Garnish each glass with slices of lemon and orange.

YIELD: 4 SERVINGS

❓ **How it works:** *Coffee and tea drinkers enjoy some protection from diabetes. Caffeine alone is associated with a reduced risk. Take it easy. Too much caffeine can make you jittery and sleepless.*

Lifestyle Tip

Sleep well. Chronic sleep deprivation and poor quality sleep increase the risk of obesity and diabetes.

Buckwheat Blueberry Pancakes

1½ cups (180 g) buckwheat flour
1 packet (1 g) stevia
2 teaspoons (5 g) ground cinnamon
1 teaspoon (5 g) baking soda
3 tablespoons (45 ml) olive oil
2 cups (475 ml) buttermilk
1 cup (145 g) blueberries

PREPARATION AND USE:

Combine the flour, stevia, cinnamon, and baking soda in a large bowl. Drizzle in the olive oil and begin stirring. Slowly pour in the buttermilk and continue to stir, mixing only until the ingredients are just combined and still lumpy. Fold in the blueberries.

Wipe a griddle with olive oil and heat it over medium heat. Ladle the batter for the pancakes on the hot griddle. Lower the heat to medium-low, cook, and turn when the top side shows bubbles—about 2 minutes. Cook the other side for about a minute until browned.

Suitable toppings include a dollop of yogurt, a few additional fresh blueberries (or other fresh fruit), or a small amount of peanut butter. Resist the urge to smother the pancakes with syrup, honey, jam, or jelly—sugary substances that will stimulate a rapid rise in blood glucose.

YIELD: 3 TO 4 SERVINGS

Lifestyle Tip

Get a diabetes-fighting magnesium boost from a handful of roasted pumpkin seeds. About ¼ cup (35 g) of the seeds boasts 300 milligrams of magnesium; that's 95 percent of the recommended daily dose.

❷ **How it works:** *Buckwheat flour packs a magnesium punch. Whereas low magnesium levels seem to raise the risk of type-2 diabetes, eating a diet high in magnesium has been linked to reduced risk of developing type-2 diabetes. Studies show that just 100 milligrams put adults at a 15 percent lower risk of developing the disease. Aside from buckwheat, good sources of magnesium include spinach, beans lentils, almonds, peanuts, cashews, and wheat bran. Barley, yogurt, and halibut are other terrific sources.*

Cinnamon Super Oats

½ cup (40 g) whole or steel-cut oats (not instant)

1 cup (235 ml) water

1 tablespoon (9 g) golden raisins

½ apple with skin, chopped and seeded

1 to 2 teaspoons (2.5 to 5 g) ground cinnamon

2 tablespoons (14 g) flaxseed meal

1 tablespoon (18 g) psyllium powder

1 tablespoon (15 g) nonfat Greek yogurt

½ banana, chopped

PREPARATION AND USE:

Mix the oats, water, raisins, apple, and cinnamon in a medium-size, microwave-safe bowl. Microwave on high for about 3 minutes. Stir in the flaxseed meal and psyllium powder. Top with yogurt and chopped banana.

YIELD: 2 SERVINGS

Lifestyle Tip

Exercise every day. Walking counts. Physical activity improves your tissues' sensitivity to insulin. Regular exercise also adds muscle mass and burns calories, making it easier to manage blood glucose and body weight.

❓ How it works: *Studies show that oats and oat bran can lower blood glucose and improve insulin function in people who are healthy, diabetic, or at risk for diabetes. Compounds in flaxseed called lignans can reduce some disease markers, including blood glucose, in people with type-2 diabetes. Psyllium fiber helps lower blood levels of cholesterol and glucose (sugar) in people with type-2 diabetes. The apples help make the cereal naturally sweet and rich and add fiber and flavonoids. Diets rich in apples have been linked to a modest decreased risk of developing type-2 diabetes. As noted in the earlier recipe, research shows that liberal use of cinnamon may lower blood glucose.*

California Cactus Salad

2 medium-size cactus pads (nopales)

1 tablespoon (15 ml) olive oil

3 garlic cloves, minced

½ cup (120 g) canned black beans, rinsed and drained

¼ cup (25 g) chopped scallion

¼ cup (4 g) chopped fresh cilantro

1 tablespoon (15 ml) fresh lime juice

1 teaspoon (4 g) sugar

½ teaspoon ground cumin

¼ teaspoon dried chipotle powder, or about 1 tablespoon (9 g) minced chipotle pepper in adobo

2 medium-size tomatoes, seeded and diced

6 cups (330 g) shredded lettuce

2 tablespoons (19 g) crumbled queso fresco

PREPARATION AND USE:

Carefully trim off the eyes from each cactus pad with a vegetable peeler or knife and remove any spines from the green skin; rinse the fruit thoroughly. Cut the cactus pads into thin strips.

Heat the oil in a large nonstick skillet over medium-high heat. Add the cactus and garlic and sauté for 7 to 8 minutes or until the cactus is tender. Combine the cactus mixture with the remaining ingredients, except the lettuce and cheese.

Arrange one-quarter of the lettuce on each of four plates and top each with one-quarter of the cactus mixture and one-quarter of the cheese.

YIELD: 4 SERVINGS

Lifestyle Tip

Avoid refined carbohydrates, added sugars, and trans fats (which are mainly manmade). An excess of any or all of them can promote unhealthy weight gain, increasing the risk of diabetes. All increase the risk of cardiovascular disease. Refined carbohydrates and sugars raise blood sugar and triglycerides (body fat) and tax insulin. If you eat real food (fruits, vegetable, fish, meat, seeds, and nuts) rather than processed food, you will naturally remove these items from your diet.

❓ **How it works:** *Prickly pear cactus has both fiber and pectin. Some studies show that the fruit can help lower blood glucose by lowering the absorption of sugar in the stomach and intestines. Some researchers also think it lowers cholesterol levels and kills viruses. One study showed that the species* Opuntia streptacantha, *specifically its broiled—not raw—stems, helped decrease blood glucose levels in patients with type-2 diabetes.*

Note: You can find nopales at Hispanic food markets, if not at your own supermarket.

Artichokes with Pepper Dip

2 garlic cloves, divided
1 cup (230 g) plain Greek yogurt
2 tablespoons (12 g) chopped fresh mint
¼ teaspoon ground cumin
⅛ teaspoon cayenne pepper
Dash of olive oil
2 artichokes

PREPARATION AND USE:

Mince one garlic clove. In a bowl, mix the yogurt, minced garlic, mint, cumin, cayenne, and olive oil. Refrigerate for at least 1 hour.

While the dip is chilling, snip the sharp tips of the artichoke petals and trim the stem to about 1-inch (2.5 cm) long. Fill a large pot with about two fingers of water and drop in the other garlic clove. Place the artichokes in a steamer basket.

Bring the water to a boil and steam the artichokes until you can pierce the bottom of the stems with a fork and the leaves easily pull away, about 30 minutes.

Serve the artichokes warm with the cool dip.

YIELD: 2 SERVINGS

❷ How it works: *Artichoke petals and hearts are rich in fiber. Also, artichoke is related to milk thistle. Milk thistle extracts improve fast blood glucose, cholesterol levels, triglycerides, and other indicators of risk in people with type-2 diabetes. Regular consumption of cayenne and chiles may also help regulate insulin levels after a meal.*

When Simple Doesn't Work

If you have any concerns about your health, make an appointment to see your doctor as soon as possible. Simple tests can determine whether you have diabetes. A number of medications can improve insulin function. In type-1 diabetes, and in more severe type-2 diabetes, insulin injections are necessary.

Also, American ginseng (Panax quinquefolius) and Asian ginseng (Panax ginseng) extracts have been shown to reduce blood glucose. To avoid hypoglycemia (abnormally low blood sugar), diabetics taking medications need to consult with their physician before taking ginseng.

Fabulous Fenugreek Stir-Fry

This easy, crunchy side dish is a great addition to almost any meal.

1 large sweet onion, diced
2 celery stalks, diced
1 red or yellow bell pepper, seeded and diced
1 teaspoon (4.5 g) whole fenugreek seeds
1 tablespoon (15 ml) canola oil

PREPARATION AND USE:
Combine all the ingredients in a bowl, ensuring everything is coated with the oil. Transfer to a large skillet and sauté over medium heat until the onion is transparent, 8 to 10 minutes.

YIELD: 2 SERVINGS

❷ How it works: *Fenugreek* (Trigonella foenum-graecum), *a plant cultivated in India, North Africa, and the Mediterranean, contains soluble fiber and beneficial components. Preliminary studies show that the powdered, defatted seeds lower glucose, cholesterol, and triglyceride levels.*

Fenugreek seems to benefit people with both types of diabetes. In one study, type-2 diabetics who added fenugreek to their regimen were able to reduce their medications by 20 percent. Study dosages have ranged from 2.5 milligrams of encapsulated seed powder taken twice a day to 25 to 100 grams of ground seeds divided into two doses and mixed into such foods as bread.

Chapter 31

Diaper Rash

Diaper rash is so common among infants it's practically a rite of passage, along with adolescent acne and menstrual cramps. That said, the condition deserves care to prevent it from becoming severe and uncomfortable.

The appearance varies from a few red, irritated spots to redness over the entire diaper area. Inflammation can make the skin look puffy and feel warm.

What causes the rash is prolonged contact between diaper contents and an infant's sensitive skin. Wastes in urine can break down to ammonia, which is very irritating. Redness can also occur in areas where the diaper chafes the skin. Another possibility is contact allergy to chemicals in commercial diaper wipes or detergents used to wash cloth diapers. There are, however, things you can do to control it.

History

As long as there have been babies in diapers (of one kind or another), there have been parents dealing with diaper rash. In the ancient world, the Egyptians and others who knew how to make cloth for diapers didn't know how to prevent rashes in their diapered babies.

For millennia, babies were swaddled. Native Americans swaddled babies in rabbit skins (or seal skins, farther north) stuffed with soft moss or grass. The Paiute, a tribe of the Great Plains, treated rashes with softened sagebrush—grinding the dried leaves to make a kind of talcum. In Europe, swaddling—usually with linsey-woolsey (a strong, coarse fabric), wool, or cotton cloth—was changed in sections but infrequently. Diaper rash was treated with burnt flour or powdered club moss.

Japanese farmers of the seventeenth century came up with a novel solution: a wooden bassinet holding a mattress with a hole for the baby's buttocks. The baby's waste collected in lower layers of ash, rags, and straw, and the baby stayed dry while the parents worked. In warm places in the world, even today, toddlers go without pants; in China, children often wear pants with a hole cut out of the bottom.

The modern diaper came into use with the Industrial Revolution and the invention of the safety pin. As the awareness of bacteria and viruses became more common, mothers began to wash diapers in boiling water—thus killing infectious microbes and reducing diaper rash. The introduction of one-use, disposable diapers (Pampers were the first, in 1961) also helped. Today's superabsorbent diapers, coupled with barrier creams to protect babies' sensitive skins, make it easier to keep babies clean and dry—and help control diaper dermatitis.

The Big Change

Warm water

Castile or other mild, nonscented soap (Use soap only if the area is soiled.)

Commercially prepared ointment or herbal salve

PREPARATION AND USE:

Remove the wet or dirty diaper. Wash the diaper area with a cotton ball moistened in warm water. If the area is dirty, bathe with mild soap (avoid commercially prepared fragranced wipes). Gently pat dry. Apply a commercially prepared ointment or an herbal salve to the diaper area.

YIELD: 1 APPLICATION

❷ **How it works:** *Immediate cleansing, drying, and lubricating of the diaper area with mild, natural ingredients helps keep the baby's skin fresh and supple.*

❶ **Warning:** *Do not use powders, especially talcum powder. Inhaled talcum particles can cause lung disease. Cornstarch can worsen a yeast infection.*

Fresh and Fluffy

This safe, easy wash for cloth diapers is gentle enough for baby's skin.

Hypoallergenic detergent

½ cup (120 ml) vinegar

PREPARATION AND USE:

Place soiled cloth diapers in the washing machine and add hypoallergenic detergent. Run the diapers through a full cycle, adding the vinegar to the rinse cycle. Dry as usual.

YIELD: 1 LOAD OF LAUNDRY

❷ **How it works:** *A hypoallergenic detergent minimizes allergic reactions. Such reactions will manifest as a rash limited to the areas the diaper contacts the skin. Vinegar is an antibacterial.*

Lifestyle Tip

Change the diaper frequently, at least every 2 hours, until your baby begins urinating less often. Poopy diapers are hard to miss. Change these immediately, and then gently cleanse the diaper area with water or an unscented wipe.

Baby Sitz Soother

Soaking will help soothe the diaper area, especially if the skin is very raw.

2 tablespoons (28 g) baking soda

PREPARATION AND USE:
Pour warm water into a basin large enough to soak the baby's bottom. Mix in the baking soda. Soak the infant in the bath for 10 to 15 minutes. Pat your infant dry, paying attention to the diapered area. Repeat once or twice more as needed throughout the day.

YIELD: 1 APPLICATION

❓ **How it works:** *Sitting in a warm bath is therapeutic for many babies. Cleansing the area with soothing warm water and baking soda will help counter the acidity of the affected area.*

❗ **Warning:** *Be sure to stay with your baby constantly while he or she is in the tub.*

Baking Soda Sponge Bath

1 tablespoon (14 g) baking soda
1 cup (235 ml) water

PREPARATION AND USE:
Place the baking soda and water in a sterilized jar and stir or shake until the baking soda is dissolved. Soak a clean washcloth with the solution.

Thoroughly, yet gently, cleanse the affected area. Pat the area dry with a second clean washcloth. Use the solution throughout the day with a clean washcloth each time to avoid contamination.

YIELD: 1 TO 3 APPLICATIONS

❓ **How it works:** *Baking soda cleanses soiled areas and helps to neutralize the acidity of the urine.*

Air Time

Your baby
A clean towel

PREPARATION AND USE:

Remove the diaper from your baby. Clean and dry baby's bottom, but don't apply ointment. Lay the baby on a clean towel, leaving his or her bottom bare.

Let the air do its handiwork for several hours, if possible. Feel free to apply ointment before diapering your baby again.

YIELD: 1 SESSION

❓ How it works: *An occasional break from diapers and ointment gives your baby's skin a chance to breathe. Air contact dispels the moisture and the friction of wet skin against the diaper that precipitates a rash.*

Lifestyle Tip

When applying the diaper, avoid having tape the adhering to the skin because this can irritate the skin.

Skin-Healing Calendula Oil

You'll find dried calendula in herb stores, some natural food stores, and through online retailers. Calendula is an easy-to-grow annual. Plant it in pots or your garden. (Make sure you're plant-ing Calendula officinalis, *not garden marigold,* Tagetes erecta, *or* T. patula*).*

1 cup (25.5 g) dried calendula flowers
1½ cups (355 ml) oil (e.g., almond, apricot, or olive), plus more as needed

PREPARATION AND USE:

If the flower heads are whole, grind in a clean coffee grinder or food processor. Pour the flowers into a clean jar (pint-size [475 ml] should work well). Pour in the oil until you've covered the flowers. Stir with a wooden spoon or chopstick.

Add another ½ to 1 inch (1.3 to 2.5 cm) of oil atop the herb and tightly screw on the lid. Place the jar inside a paper sack or box (to protect from ultraviolet rays). Set near a window or other warm area. Shake daily for one to two weeks. The oil will now be tinged a deep yellow.

Line a strainer with cheesecloth or muslin. Strain. With clean, dry hands, wring as much oil as you can from the cloth-wrapped herbs. Feel free to massage the oil on your hands into your skin. It feels and smells wonderful!

Pour the oil into a clean, dry bottle and cap tightly. Store in the refrigerator. Apply to clean skin as needed. Discard or compost the herbal matter.

YIELD: MULTIPLE APPLICATIONS

❓ How it works: *Calendula has anti-inflammatory, antibacterial, antifungal, and wound-healing properties. One study showed that calendula cream improved diaper rash better than an aloe-based cream did. The oil protects the skin. However, even though calendula is antifungal, do not apply it if your baby develops a fungal infection. You don't want to apply oils, salves, and ointments that could trap in moisture, which promotes fungal growth.*

❗ Warning: *Calendula is in the same plant family as ragweed, which means some people are also allergic to it. If you have a family history of allergies, apply calendula to a small patch of your baby's skin (an area that isn't already affected by diaper rash). It can take up to forty-eight hours for a skin rash to appear.*

Note: If you can't wait two weeks, you can make this oil much sooner by substituting the recipe on page 230 that uses coconut oil.

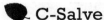

C-Salve

1 cup (235 ml) calendula oil (page 228)
¼ cup (55 g) grated beeswax

PREPARATION AND USE:

Make the oil as instructed in the previous recipe. Pour the oil into a saucepan over low heat. Add the beeswax. Stir continuously until the beeswax melts, taking care not to burn the oil. Spoon a little of the mixture onto a clean plate and pop it in the freezer for a minute or two. If you like the consistency, you're ready to jar. If you want a firmer consistency, add more beeswax and melt. If you desire a less solid consistency, add more calendula oil.

While the mixture is still warm, pour it into a clean glass jar or tin. Screw on the cap. The salve will soon solidify. Store in a cool place. Apply the salve as needed.

YIELD: MULTIPLE APPLICATIONS

❓ How it works: *Beeswax adds a soothing, protective factor. It also turns the oil into a consistency that's less messy to apply. Do not apply if your baby has developed a fungal infection.*

When Simple Doesn't Work

Not everyone has time to whip up an herbal salve. You can find a number of over-the-counter creams and ointments at the drugstore: calendula cream, zinc oxide cream, A + D (lanolin, petrolatum, mineral oil, cod liver oil, and beeswax), and Boudreaux's Butt Paste (which contains zinc oxide, a proprietary blend of Peruvian balsam, mineral oil, petrolatum, and paraffin).

For more severe cases, your baby's doctor may recommend a mild over-the-counter hydrocortisone cream. Ask the doctor which strength to purchase. Strong steroid creams are not appropriate for infants. Also, make sure an infection isn't present that requires instead an antifungal or antibacterial cream.

 Calendula Butter

If you can't wait to make an herbal oil as in the calendula recipe on page 228, here's a faster method.

½ cup (120 g) virgin coconut oil
½ cup (120 g) shea butter
1 cup (25.5 g) dried calendula flowers

PREPARATION AND USE:
Fill the bottom of a double boiler with about 2 inches (5 cm) of water. Place the coconut oil and shea butter in the top of the double boiler. Heat the water below until the oils melt. Lower the heat to low. Add the calendula flowers and stir. Add more coconut oil if necessary so that the flowers are saturated and swimming in oil. Wait at least 1 hour (4 hours, if you have time), stirring frequently. You don't want to burn the oil. Remove the pot from the heat and carefully dry any water that has condensed on the bottom of the pan. (You want to avoid getting water in the oil.)

Line a strainer with the muslin or cheesecloth and place over a bowl. Strain the warm oil. Fold the cloth around the herbs and with clean, dry hands, wring out as much oil as possible. Pour the liquid into a clean, dry jar and cap tightly. Discard or compost the herbal matter. Store in the refrigerator or cool cabinet. The oils will become solid again. Apply as needed.

YIELD: MULTIPLE APPLICATIONS

❷ How it works: *Like calendula, coconut oil is anti-inflammatory. It also absorbs easily and protects the skin. Do not apply if your baby has developed a fungal infection.*

Note: If you can't easily find shea butter, you can use only coconut oil. The end product will be less solid, but still excellent.

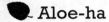 **Aloe-ha**

If you don't have an ointment on hand, aloe can bring soothing relief.

1 *Aloe vera* plant

PREPARATION AND USE:

Break off a leaf from the aloe plant. Cut a small wedge in the leaf to access the gel. Squeeze the gel into a bowl. Cleanse the baby's bottom with warm water or a mixture of baking soda and water (see "Baking Soda Sponge Bath" on page 227). Allow it to dry thoroughly. Spread a thin layer of aloe gel across the diaper area. Apply a diaper.

YIELD: 1 APPLICATION

❓ **How it works:** *Topical* Aloe vera *gel is anti-inflammatory, pain-relieving, antibacterial, and discourages the growth of yeast. One study found that an aloe cream helped heal diaper rash, though calendula cream was found to be even more effective.*

Note: Alternatively, you can buy aloe creams and gels over the counter at a pharmacy or health food store.

Lifestyle Tip

Fit is everything! Attach diapers comfortably to allow air to circulate and avoid rubbing and irritation between skin and diaper. Make sure they fit well around the leg. If leaks are happening often, try going down a size.

When to Call the Doctor

- *Two days of home treatment haven't improved the rash.*

- *The rash is getting worse. Signs can include blisters, pus, or other discharge from the skin, and extension of the rash beyond the diaper area.*

- *Your infant seems ill—has a fever, is excessively irritable, lethargic (won't easily awaken), refuses to eat. Call right away. If your pediatrician's office is closed, proceed to the emergency room.*

- *If the rash is concentrated in a ring around the anus, your baby may be allergic to something in his or her diet. Try discontinuing any recent new foods. It might also be something you're eating, if you are still breast-feeding your baby. Ask your doctor's advice.*

- *The combination of warmth, wetness, and vulnerable skin promotes yeast infections. Yeast infections are particularly common—even more so when a breast-feeding mother or her infant takes antibiotics. It often starts in the skin folds and spreads. Topical antifungal creams usually clear the problem. Get a diagnosis first. Bacteria can also infect the diaper area.*

Diarrhea

A long list of maladies can cause diarrhea. Infections are a common cause of acute diarrhea. Accompanying symptoms often include nausea, vomiting, mild fever, cramping, and general malaise. Microbes infecting the gastrointestinal tract include viruses (rotavirus and Norwalk virus), bacteria (*E. coli, Salmonella, Shigella, Campylobacter,* and *Vibrio cholerae),* and protozoa (giardia and amoebas). Toxins produced by bacteria also make us sick.

Food allergies and intolerances (e.g., lactose intolerance) can cause gas, crampy pain, diarrhea, and vomiting. Allergic foods also cause hives and swelling of respiratory linings.

Food poisoning and consumption of poisonous foods (e.g., poisonous mushrooms) usually also cause vomiting. Antibiotics disrupt the normal microbial ecosystem to cause diarrhea. Overconsumption of fruit and fruit juice loosens stools. Fear and extreme anxiety can trigger a precipitous emptying of the bowels.

Some chronic conditions are associated with recurrent diarrhea. In irritable bowel syndrome (also called spastic colon), a condition of altered bowel motility, diarrhea may alternate with constipation. Inflammatory bowel diseases, which include Crohn's disease and ulcerative colitis, result in recurrent diarrhea

(which may contain blood or pus), fatigue, fever, abdominal pain, and trouble maintaining weight. In celiac disease, consumption of gluten (a protein in certain grains) leads to an immune system attack on the intestinal lining. Hyperthyroidism speeds bowel activity, which means there isn't enough time for water to be absorbed into the blood.

Chronic conditions require careful medical management. If allergies or intolerance upset your stomach, avoid those foods. Allergy testing, careful food diaries, and elimination diets (removing all potential culprits for several days, then slowly reintroducing them one at a time) can help pinpoint the offending foods.

Food poisoning and *infectious gastroenteritis* (inflammation of the stomach and intestines) usually resolve within twenty-four to seventy-two hours. During that time, it's important to rest and replace fluid losses with clear liquids—but not simply water. You also need salt and sugar. Steer clear of apple juice and prune juice, which loosen stools. Because you may temporarily lose the ability to digest dairy, skip that food group until several days after you recover. The foods you eat should be bland, relatively low in fiber, and easy to digest. This chapter offers some recipes you can try.

History

We Americans often take for granted clean water and food. (The adoption of most clean water technologies in the United States dates from the early twentieth century.) Before improvements in hygiene and sanitation, many people died at an early age from gastroenteritis and other infections. Many parts of the world still lack proper sewage, clean drinking water, and food refrigeration—and in those places people still die from diarrheal diseases. In 2010, an estimated 780 million still lacked safe drinking water and 7.6 million children died before age five. Infections caused 4.9 million (64 percent) of those deaths, including 801,000 deaths from diarrhea.

Fact or Myth?

MOST PEOPLE WASH THEIR HANDS AFTER USING THE BATHROOM.

Not so much. An observational study in a college campus washroom revealed that 61 percent of the women and 37 percent of the men washed their hands with soap and water. A 2007 Korean survey found that, although 94 percent of respondents swore they washed their hands after using public restrooms, only 63 percent of those observed actually did. Again, women more often washed their hands. Hand washing after using the toilet and before eating is one of your best strategies for avoiding diarrhea from transmission of disease-causing microbes. In fact, consistent hand washing can reduce the number of episodes of diarrhea by about 30 percent.

RECIPES TO PREVENT AND TREAT DIARRHEA

BRATT Diet

In pediatric practice, the diet recommended after twenty-four hours of clear liquids is the BRATT diet: bananas, cooked rice, applesauce, tea, and toast. Round it out with saltine crackers and soup.

Bananas
Rice
Applesauce
Tea
Toast

PREPARATION AND USE:

Alternate these foods throughout the day. Although we generally prefer whole grains, we recommend low-fiber white rice and white bread when coping with diarrhea. Be sure to eat applesauce, not raw apples, which loosen stools.

YIELD: AS MANY APPLICATIONS AS NEEDED

❓ **How it works:** *These low-fiber, bland foods high in carbohydrates are easy for an inflamed intestinal tract to digest. Once the diarrhea is under control after twenty-four hours of clear liquids, the BRATT diet helps the body make its way back to accepting a balanced diet including fats, proteins, and fibers. Once you can tolerate bland foods for twenty-four hours, feel free to return to fiber-rich foods.*

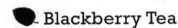 Rehydration Drink

For the first day, stick to clear liquids. This is a variant of the recipe on page 394, adapted from the Rehydration Project. This nonprofit international group works to curb the high death rate of children in developing countries from infections.

¼ cup (60 ml) fresh orange juice
2 cups (475 ml) room-temperature water
¼ teaspoon baking soda
2 teaspoons (14 g) honey

PREPARATION AND USE:

Combine the orange juice and water in a small pitcher. Stir in the baking soda until dissolved. Stir in the honey until dissolved.

YIELD: 2 SERVINGS

❓ How it works: *The biggest risk associated with diarrhea is dehydration. Children and the elderly are most vulnerable. This drink replaces depleted water, salt, potassium, and sugar. The baking soda also helps correct losses of alkaline fluid.*

Blackberry Tea

If you have access to blackberry (or raspberry) leaves or roots, this time-honored recipe can help slow the flow.

3 cups (710 ml) water
2 tablespoons (3 g) chopped dried
    blackberry leaves, or 4 tablespoons
    (24 g) fresh honey

PREPARATION AND USE:

Boil the water. Add the leaves. Turn off the heat, cover, and steep for 15 to 20 minutes. (If you also add blackberry roots, turn the heat to low and simmer for 20 minutes.) Strain. Sweeten with honey, to taste.

YIELD: 3 SERVINGS

❓ How it works: *Blackberry tea is an astringent, which gently contracts and helps dry tissues in the intestinal tract.*

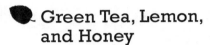 Green Tea, Lemon, and Honey

1 cup (235 ml) water
2 teaspoons (4 g) loose green tea
1 teaspoon (7 g) honey
1 teaspoon (5 ml) fresh lemon juice

PREPARATION AND USE:

In a saucepan, boil the water and add the tea. Turn off the heat, cover, and steep for 1 to 3 minutes. In a cup, mix the honey and lemon juice. Strain out the tea leaves and pour the tea into the honey mixture.

YIELD: 1 SERVING

❓ How it works: *Green tea is astringent and it inhibits major food-borne bacteria, such as* E. coli, Salmonella typhimurium, *and* Staphylococcus aureus. *Lemon is astringent, too, and contains vitamin C and bioflavonoids, which support the immune system. The essential oils in citrus fruits also discourage bacteria such as* E. coli *and* Salmonella. *Honey is anti-inflammatory, soothing, immune system–enhancing, and antibacterial.*

Lifestyle Tip

Practice good kitchen hygiene. Improper food preparation can cause bacterial infection. Use different knives and cutting boards for raw meats and fruits and vegetables. And refrigerate foods as noted on the labels.

Barley Water

Like the recipe for rice water (page 390), this will help with rehydration.

¼ cup (46 g) uncooked barley
3 cups (710 ml) water
Salt or honey (optional)

PREPARATION AND USE:
In a saucepan, combine the barley and water. Bring to a boil. Lower the heat to low. Cook the barley gently for 1 hour. Strain out the barley, filling a bowl with the water. Allow th barley water to cool. Add a pinch of salt or 1 teaspoon (7 g) of honey, as desired, before drinking.

YIELD: 1 SERVING

 How it works: *Barley and rice water restore fluids and reverse electrolyte imbalance.*

Moderating Miso

Try this simple, brothy variation of the miso recipe on page 299. The addition of garlic makes this a super-bacterial foe.

¼ cup (64 g) miso paste
2 cups (475 ml) water
1 scallion, chopped
2 garlic cloves, minced

PREPARATION AND USE:
Spoon the miso paste into a bowl. Boil the water in a saucepan and lower the heat to low. Pour ¼ cup (60 ml) of boiled water into the bowl with the miso, and stir until the mixture is smooth. Add the miso mixture to the remaining water in the saucepan. Stir until fully blended. Add the scallion. Stir in the garlic just before serving (by not cooking the garlic, you maintain it's key ingredients).

YIELD: 2 SERVINGS

How it works: *Miso, which is made from fermented soybeans, contains probiotics. In research showing that probiotics shorten the course of diarrhea, volunteers received supplemental bacteria. Scientists have not yet studied miso as a remedy for diarrhea. But it will help correct loss of salty and alkaline fluid. Raw garlic inhibits a number of bacteria, viruses, protozoa, and worms.*

Quickie Chickie Soup

1 cup (235 ml) water
1 chicken bouillon cube, crushed
½ cup (80 g) uncooked egg noodles
1 tablespoon (14 g) minced, precooked chicken breast
Freshly ground black pepper
Dried sage or thyme
1 garlic clove, minced

PREPARATION AND USE:
Bring the water to a boil and reduce the heat to low. Sprinkle the crushed bouillon cube into the water. Stir until the bouillon is fully dissolved. Stir in the egg noodles and chicken pieces. Add pepper and sage or thyme to taste. Stir in the garlic just before serving.

YIELD: 1 TO 2 SERVINGS

How it works: *While the broth is both nutritious and easy on the digestive system, the sodium from the bouillon helps restore electrolytes to the depleted system. The small amount of chicken helps your system begin acclimating to small amounts of protein.*

The Big Apple—Sauced

½ cup (120 ml) water
2 unpeeled apples, cored and cut into chunks
¼ teaspoon ground cinnamon
1 tablespoon (20 g) honey

PREPARATION AND USE:

Pour the water into a saucepan. Add the apples, cinnamon, and honey and stir together. Cook the mixture over medium heat for about 15 minutes or until the apples are soft. Let the apple mixture cool and mash with a fork.

YIELD: 3 TO 4 SERVINGS

❷ How it works: *Apples, particularly the peels, contain pectin. If you've ever made jam, you known that pectin draws water to make a gel. In that way, it reduces watery diarrhea. Because raw apples are harder to digest, it's better to consume cooked apples. If you don't feel up to cooking, use store-bought applesauce. Cinnamon contains the antibacterial agent cinnamaldehyde. Honey is anti-inflammatory, soothing, and inhibits some bacterial species.*

Skinny Oats

½ cup (40 g) rolled oats
1 cup (235 ml) water
½ teaspoon ground cinnamon
1 teaspoon (14 g) honey (optional)

PREPARATION AND USE:

Mix together the oats, water, and cinnamon in a microwave-safe dish. Heat on high for 3 minutes. (Alternatively, combine the oats and cinnamon in a dish or measuring cup. Boil the water in a small pan, and then stir in the oats and cinnamon. Lower the heat to medium-low and cook, stirring occasionally, for 5 to 8 minutes until the oats reach your desired consistency.)

Add the honey, if desired. Let cool and eat.

YIELD: 1 TO 2 SERVINGS

❷ How it works: *Oats are soothing to irritated linings and contain a complex carbohydrate that enhances immune function. Honey has anti-inflammatory and antibacterial properties. Cinnamon is antibacterial.*

Lifestyle Tip

Make toast. Toast a slice of white bread or an English muffin, and then spread with raspberry, blueberry, or blackberry jam. All these fruits have astringent properties.

Fact or Myth?

WHEN TRAVELING IN DEVELOPING COUNTRIES, DRINK AND USE ONLY BOTTLED WATER, BUT IT'S OKAY TO BRUSH YOUR TEETH WITH TAP WATER.

Myth. Even a little impure water goes a long way toward attacking your system with bacteria. Stick to bottled water for brushing.

When Simple Doesn't Work

You may want to go to the pharmacy to buy an antidiarrhea medication. But note: Diarrhea represents a nonspecific defense against infectious agents and toxins. Normally, you don't want to stop it. Don't use an over-the-counter antidiarrhea remedy, such as Lomotil, without discussing it first with your doctor. Pepto-Bismol is okay to take (unless the sick person is under the age of eighteen, due to the small risk of a serious condition called Reye's syndrome). The active ingredient in this over-the-counter medication is bismuth subsalicylate. It seems to soothe irritated tissues and may kill some bacteria.

Probiotic supplements containing particular bacterial strains (Lactobacillus rhamnosus, Lactobacillus GG, L. ruteri, L. casei, and L. rhamnosus) have been shown to shorten the duration of diarrhea in children. A combination of Bifidobacterium bifidum with either L. acidophilus, L. bulgaricus, or Streptococcus thermophilus has been shown to shorten the course of diarrhea in children and decrease the risk of traveler's diarrhea. Probiotic supplements also reduce the odds of developing antibiotic-induced diarrhea.

Also, goldenseal and Oregon grape roots contain berberine, which has been shown to treat diarrhea caused by giardia and such bacteria as E. coli.

 # Carob Shake

2 small or 1 large banana, chopped
½ cup (65 g) raspberries (optional)
½ cup (115 g) plain yogurt (Read the label to buy a yogurt with probiotic organisms.)
1 tablespoon (6.5 g) carob powder
1 tablespoon (20 g) honey

PREPARATION AND USE:

Combine the bananas and raspberries, if using, in a blender and blend until smooth. Add the yogurt, carob powder, and honey and fully blend. Serve.

YIELD: 1 SERVING

❓ How it works: *Carob (locust bean) contains locust bean gum, a polysaccharide that binds water. Tannins in carob have an astringent effect. Bananas are a bland, soothing food. They provide needed sugars and potassium. The probiotics, or good bacteria, in some yogurts can help relieve infectious diarrhea—the kind encountered by travelers—by fighting the bad bacteria in the intestines. Whereas many dairy products are difficult to digest during a bout of infectious diarrhea, yogurt can often be tolerated.*

Lifestyle Tip

Add a squeeze of lime to water. A 2011 study found that straight lime juice inhibited all tested strains of E. coli. So did lime juice plus garlic and ginger. Because straight lime juice is hard to swallow, we recommend instead squeezing a tablespoon (15 ml) of juice into an 8-ounce (235 ml) glass of water.

Soothing Carrot-Ginger Soup

2 cups (475 ml) water

1 cup (130 g) scrubbed, chopped carrot

2 tablespoons (28 g) unsalted butter

1 teaspoon (7 g) honey (optional)

½ tablespoon fresh lemon juice

¼ teaspoon ground ginger

1 vegetable bouillon cube

PREPARATION AND USE:

Bring the water to a boil in a saucepan. Add the carrot and cook about 7 minutes until tender. Meanwhile, melt the butter in a skillet over low heat and stir in the honey, if using. Mix together the lemon juice and ginger in the skillet. Strain the carrots, reserving the liquid, and stir into the skillet mixture. Pour the carrot cooking liquid back into saucepan and add the bouillon cube. Add the skillet mixture to the saucepan and cover. Simmer for about 5 minutes.

YIELD: 2 SERVINGS

❓ **How it works:** *Carrot soup and carrot juice are traditional remedies for diarrhea. Carrots are rich in a number of vitamins, many of which support immune health, and also minerals, including potassium, which diarrhea depletes. They also supply sugars. Cooked carrots are easier to digest than raw. Ginger is antibacterial and eases upset stomachs.*

When to Call the Doctor

The following are signs that you have something other than run-of-the mill infectious diarrhea, which usually resolves within seventy-two hours.

- *Diarrhea lasts more than three days. (For babies younger than six months of age, call if diarrhea lasts more than a day.)*

- *Signs of significant dehydration occur: urinating less than every 8 hours, light-headedness, weakness, poor skin turgor (you pick up a pinch of skin and it stays up, rather than popping back down), sunken eyes, and dry mouth, skin, lips, and eyes (no tears with crying).*

- *Severe abdominal pain and/or a fever over 101°F (38.3°C) accompanies diarrhea.*

- *Blood or pus appears in stool.*

- *Prolonged or recurrent diarrhea follows recent foreign travel or a camping trip.*

- *Diarrhea seems to be associated, along with other symptoms, with a new medication.*

Chapter 33

Dry Skin

For people living in arid climates, dry skin and chapped lips may be constant challenges. People with eczema and psoriasis also have dry, easily irritated skin. Age-related changes in the skin make it drier. Xerosis is the medical term for excessive dryness.

Oily substances (lipids) made by the sebaceous glands and cells within the epidermis (outer skin layer) prevent dryness. As anyone who has weathered adolescence knows, hormones make the skin oily. Specifically, androgens ("male" hormones made by both sexes) increase oil production. Heredity, humidity, age, ultraviolet light exposure, and other factors affect the relative oiliness of skin.

With age, sebaceous (oil) glands secrete less sebum. There's also a decrease in lipids made by cells within the epidermis. Decrease in skin oil makes hair less lustrous.

Essential fatty acid deficiency can also dry skin and eyes.

Dry skin feels rough and looks scaly. You may also notice white flakes and patches of reddened skin. Itching is common. Don't give in to the urge to scratch, as doing so causes inflammation, breaks down the epidermis (top layer of skin), and introduces microbes into deeper layers.

The concern is more than aesthetic. Our largest organ, the skin forms a barrier against the outside world. It helps keep water from escaping and inhibits disease-causing microorganisms, ultraviolet light, and noxious chemicals from penetrating deeper. The skin's oils play an essential role in that barrier function. Some lipids discourage colonization with fungi and bacteria. Furthermore, dry skin more easily cracks, which not only hurts but also creates breeches in the barrier. Skin more easily becomes inflamed and infected.

History

Perhaps we should take our cues from Cleopatra and the ancients. Her skin care secrets included milk and honey baths and aloe (Aloe vera) rubs. Egyptians used plant oils as moisturizers for the whole body. Romans made skins creams of beeswax, olive oil, and rose water. The ancient Greeks used honey as a moisturizing rub. Grecian women also used a paste of fresh berries and milk as a facial mask. Through the ages, staying out of the sun was common advice for maintaining a moist, dewy skin—right up to our grandmothers' time and well into the twentieth century. Our mothers and grandmothers also recommended cold creams, made largely of beeswax, distilled water, and mineral oil, for removing dirt and softening dry skin.

In the late nineteenth century, advertising entered the skin care picture—with Pears' soap. Posters of ivory-skinned stage actress Lillie Langtry, the first woman to endorse a commercial product, touted the soap's purity. With Pears' soap also came biochemistry.

By the twentieth century, when Madison Avenue began to market skin-care products, moisturizers, lotions, and creams had turned into a chemical soup of alcohols, preservatives, synthetic fragrances, and petroleum-based compounds, some of them carcinogenic and likely to trigger allergies.

In this century, however, interest in safer alternatives is leading us back to reconsider the beauty secrets of the ancients—and choose products free of parabens, phthalates, polyethylene glycols (PEGs), sodium lauryl sulfate, and more. (For ingredients in thousands of skin-care products, consult the Environmental Working Group's cosmetic database at www.ewg.org/skindeep/.)

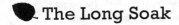

RECIPES TO PREVENT AND TREAT DRY SKIN

The Long Soak

Mild soap
Moisturizer

PREPARATION AND USE:

Take a quick shower to clean your skin, using a mild soap. Draw a warm bath. Step in and relax. If you're a reader, bring a magazine or paperback book with you. Once your toes and fingertips begin to pucker, you're done. Pat dry and immediately apply a moisturizer. Repeat the treatment a couple of times a week.

YIELD: 1 APPLICATION

❓ How it works: *Cleansing in the shower before you soak allows your skin to take in fresh, clean water from the bathtub. Covering your damp skin with a moisturizing lotion will seal in that water, keeping your skin soft and supple.*

Lifestyle Tip

Load up on vitamin C by eating plenty of fruits and vegetables. Collagen, the chief protein in skin, requires vitamin C for its production. Vitamin C also keeps capillary walls strong, to prevent easy bruising.

Coconut Oil Rub

Extra-virgin coconut oil

PREPARATION AND USE:
Take a shower or bath. Gently pat your skin dry to remove most but not all of the water. Massage in coconut oil.

YIELD: 1 APPLICATION

❓ How it works: *Pure coconut oil is an emollient, which leaves the skin soft and supple. It penetrates the skin quickly with its rich blend of saturated fatty acids, which help replace fats lost from the skin. We recommend virgin coconut oil, which is made from fresh coconut meat without the use of chemicals and high heat, thus creating a higher-quality oil.*

All-Natural Makeup Remover

Coconut oil (also try olive or almond oil)

PREPARATION AND USE:
Dab two to four cotton balls with enough oil for each eye and the general face. Gently swab eyes, cheeks, and lips to remove makeup. Gently wipe off the excess with a warm, damp washcloth. Rinse your face with water and pat it dry, leaving the skin damp.

YIELD: 1 APPLICATION

❓ How it works: *Rather than drying out your face by washing it with soap, the coconut oil will cleanse and lubricate skin. It's especially beneficial for the eye area, where rubbing can damage sensitive skin and wrinkles are more pronounced when the skin is dry.*

❀ Avocado Rub

¼ avocado, peeled and pitted

PREPARATION AND USE:
In a small bowl, mash the avocado (feel free to use the rest of the avocado in the next recipe). Rub into dry skin. Allow 5 minutes for the avocado to absorb into the skin. Use the damp cloth to remove residual green fruit.

YIELD: 1 APPLICATION

❓ How it works: *Avocado is packed with healthy fats—monounsaturated fatty acids and linoleic acid—that counter dry skin.*

Skin-Salvation Salad

6 ounces (168 g) salmon
2 tablespoons (30 ml) olive oil, divided
3 cups (90 g) torn, well-rinsed spinach
1 avocado, peeled, pitted, and cut into chunks
¼ cup (25 g) pitted and sliced black olives
¼ cup (30 g) crushed walnuts
Freshly ground black pepper
2 tablespoons (30 ml) balsamic vinegar
1 tablespoon (15 ml) fresh lemon juice

PREPARATION AND USE:

Preheat the oven to broil. Brush the salmon with 1 tablespoon (15 ml) of the olive oil and place in a baking pan. Broil the salmon for 15 minutes.

Meanwhile, toss together the spinach, avocado, olives, and walnuts in a large bowl. Remove the salmon from the oven when the fish flakes with a fork and allow it to cool for several minutes. Cut the salmon into chunks and toss into the salad. Sprinkle the salad with pepper to taste.

In a small bowl, whisk together remaining tablespoon (15 ml) of the olive oil and the vinegar and lemon juice to make a dressing. Drizzle the dressing over the salad and give the salad a final toss.

YIELD: 3 TO 4 SERVINGS

Lifestyle Tip

Eat plenty of orange and yellow veggies, such as carrots, squash, and papaya. Vitamin A deficiency, although uncommon, can cause severe dry skin, as well as other signs and symptoms. The body can convert alpha-carotene, beta-carotene, and beta-cryptoxanthin to vitamin A.

How it works: *Cold-water fish, such as salmon or tuna, are high in omega-3 fatty acids. One of the symptoms of omega-3 fatty acid deficiency is dry skin and eyes. Avocado is rich in the good fats monounsaturated fatty acids and linoleic acid. One study found these fats helpful for psoriasis, although there is no research on dry skin in particular. Olives and olive oil are rich in fatty acids as are walnuts, which are packed with omega-3 fatty acids.*

Lifestyle Tip

Make more use of an avocado mask than the much-celebrated clay masks. Clay absorbs the skin's oils, while avocado returns needed oils to the skin.

Cocoa Butter Beauty Balm

Tropical peoples have long used coconut oil as a moisturizer.

Cocoa butter (see note)

PREPARATION AND USE:
Smooth the cocoa butter onto the dry area. Use lotion instead of cream if you have a large skin area to cover.

YIELD: 1 APPLICATION

❓ How it works: *Cocoa butter has high saturated fat content and several oils, including oleic acid, which counter dryness. It also has antiseptic effects. One study found it was as effective as mineral oil in improving skin hydration and surface oils in people with very dry skin.*

Note: Pure cocoa butter is available as lotion or cream at a pharmacy or health food store.

 ## Luscious Lanolin

Made by the oil glands of sheep, lanolin is a fatty substance harvested from sheep's wool and used for effective emollients and ointments.

Lanolin cream or lotion (see note)

PREPARATION AND USE:
Smooth over the dry area.

YIELD: 1 APPLICATION

❓ How it works: *Lanolin is an occlusive agent, forming a barrier against water loss. It also helps soften skin. Some people are sensitive to it. An alternative, petroleum jelly (petrolatum) has a similar action. However, some people prefer not to use it because, as the name suggests, it's a by-product of the petroleum industry. It does, however, hold in moisture.*

❗ Warning: *Don't apply if you have a skin fungal infection, as sealing in moisture will promote fungal growth. Also stay away from lanolin if you're allergic. If you're not sure, apply a nickel-size spot of lanolin to skin. An allergic rash can develop anytime from a couple of hours to a couple of days after application.*

Note: You can buy lanolin at a health food store or pharmacy or online.

 ## Glistening Glycerol

Glycerol is a useful humectant, a substance that fends off moisture loss.

¼ cup (60 ml) water, boiled and cooled
½ teaspoon vegetable glycerin
½ teaspoon almond oil (You can also use avocado oil for especially dry skin.)

PREPARATION AND USE:
In a small bowl, whisk together the water and glycerin. Add the almond oil and whisk to combine. Pour the mixture into a sterile container and cap tightly. Wash your face gently before applying. Smooth the moisturizer over clean skin with clean fingertips. Store the product in a cool, dry place.

YIELD: ABOUT TWO WEEKS' WORTH OF TWICE-DAILY APPLICATIONS

❓ How it works: *Glycerin helps hold moisture in the skin, but works best when paired with oil or other moisturizing vehicles because glycerin draws water to it and by itself can make the skin feel dry. However, the addition of water and almond or avocado oil provide a counterbalance by moisturizing.*

Jojoba on Hand

Because jojoba (pronounced ho-HO-ba) oil is so stable, you can keep a huge bottle on hand for ages without it going bad. I order liter-size bottles.
~ LBW

1 scoop of your daily facial moisturizer
3 drops jojoba oil

PREPARATION AND USE:

Put your usual scoop of moisturizer into your palm and add the jojoba oil. Mix together with your fingertips. Smooth over your face and neck in gentle, circular motions.

YIELD: 1 APPLICATION

❓ **How it works:** *Jojoba "oil" is actually liquid wax derived from the seeds of the jojoba plant. This emollient is not greasy, penetrates the skin easily, and does not clog pores as oil-based lotions and creams can do. It's also antiviral.*

Note: Alternatively, you can apply jojoba oil directly to your skin by dropping a few drops onto your fingertips, and then applying gently to the skin below eyes, your face, and neck.

Lifestyle Tip

Use mild soaps. Highly touted antibacterial and deodorant soaps have been found to be no more effective than mild soaps and can actually irritate and dry out skin. Plus some of them (particularly those containing the agent triclosan) are bad for the environment and contribute to antibiotic resistance.

Vera Smooth Skin

1 *Aloe vera* plant

PREPARATION AND USE:

Remove an aloe leaf and clip the end. Squeeze out the gel. Smooth over the skin beneath your eyes in a gentle, circular motion. Continue this action over the rest of your face and neck.

YIELD: 1 APPLICATION

❓ **How it works:** *Aloe gel has been shown to increase skin hydration and reduce water loss from the skin.*

Note: Alternatively, for the rest of your body, buy aloe gel at a pharmacy or whole foods store. (The few leaves on your plant may not produce enough gel to cover your body!)

Rosemary Gladstar's Luscious Moisturizer

You'll need a good blender to mix the oils and water to mix in this recipe, which I adapted from Rosemary Gladstar's Family Herbal. Rosemary, one my favorite herbalists, looks much younger than her chronological age. ~ LBW

⅔ cup (160 ml) distilled water
⅓ cup (80 ml) *Aloe vera* gel
¾ cup (175 ml) almond oil (or try apricot
    or grapeseed)
½ teaspoon lanolin
⅓ cup (80 ml) virgin coconut oil
1 tablespoon (14 g) grated beeswax
1 tablespoon (14 g) shea butter

PREPARATION AND USE:

In a mixing bowl, blend the distilled water and aloe gel. Fill half the bottom of a double boiler with water. Add the almond oil, lanolin, coconut oil, beeswax, and shea butter to the top pan.

Over low heat, warm the ingredients until they liquefy and stir to blend. Pour the oil mixture into a blender and let cool until the mix becomes semisolid, but not solid, 60 to 90 minutes.

Turn on the blender at high speed. Slowly drizzle in the aloe mixture. Blend the ingredients until you have a thick white mixture. Pour into a clean jar and cap tightly. Store the mixture in the refrigerator or other cool location. Apply as needed.

YIELD: A LITTLE MORE THAN 2 CUPS (ABOUT 16 OUNCES [475 ML]). THE NUMBER OF APPLICATIONS DEPENDS ON HOW GENER-OUSLY YOU APPLY IT.

❷ **How it works:** *This mixture of water and these oils creates a moisturizer, which adds or seals in water.*

You've Got Grape Skin

6 red grapes
Water
Your moisturizer

PREPARATION AND USE:

Wash the grapes and cut them in half. Boil the water. Remove from pot from the stove and lower your head over it. Corral the vapors by draping a towel over your head. Let your face steam for 5 minutes. Gently rub the open halves of the grapes across your forehead and over your cheeks, chin, and neck. Rinse your face with cool water. Pat dry with a cool, damp washcloth. Apply your usual moisturizer.

YIELD: 1 APPLICATION

❷ **How it works:** *Alpha-hydroxy acids (AHAs) include citric acids (in citrus fruit), glycolic acid (in cane sugar), lactic acid (in yogurt), malic acid (apples), and tartaric acid (grapes). These exfoliate, act as humectants, and increase skin pliability. Studies show that lotions containing AHAs improve dry skin.*

Note: Instead of grapes, use ½ cup (115 g) of mashed papaya and paste it over your face after the steam treatment. Let it sit for 5 minutes and rinse. If your skin is sensitive, carefully apply to a small area first to check for breakout. Papaya might cause an allergic reaction in some people. Test a patch on the inside of your wrist before ap-plying it to larger areas of skin.

Sea Salt Scrub

1 cup (236 g) sea salt
½ cup (120 ml) apricot, olive, almond,
   or grapeseed oil
Your moisturizer

PREPARATION AND USE:
Fully blend the salt and oil in a clean, dry jar.
Set aside.

Shower so that your skin is damp. While still in the shower, turn off the water, scoop out several fingerfuls (about 2 tablespoons [28 g]) of the mixture and scrub your arms and legs, avoiding any wounds or scratches. Rinse thoroughly. Pat yourself dry. Apply your regular moisturizer. Store the bottle of salt scrub in a cool area.

YIELD: ABOUT A WEEK'S WORTH OF APPLICATIONS TO ARMS AND LEGS.

❓ How it works: *Exfoliants remove dead skin cells to reduce the scaliness of dry skin.*

❗ Warning: *The oil may make the floor of the shower slippery while using this. Step carefully and rinse the floor thoroughly when finished.*

Note: Alternatively, mix white or brown sugar with the oil, instead of salt.

When to Call the Doctor

- *You develop a rash. (If any of these home remedies or a new commercially prepared skin-care product make you break out, stop using it. See your doctor if the rash persists.)*

- *Home treatment does not improve dryness and itching.*

- *You develop signs of skin infection: redness, swelling, and discharge.*

When Simple Doesn't Work

If you've tried these recipes and your skin is still dry to scaly, speak to your doctor or dermatologist about recommended over-the-counter and prescription creams and lotions to counteract dryness.

Chapter 34

Earaches

The ear has three main parts: the outer (the ear lobe and ear canal), middle (the small space just behind the eardrum), and inner ear (the fluid-filled structures that translate mechanical vibrations into nerve impulses).

Problems in the inner ear cause disturbances in hearing and balance, but not pain. Dental problems (including teething in kids) can cause pain that seems to come from the ear.

Trauma and infection of the outer ear hurt. Bacterial and fungal infections in the ear canal—as can happen to swimmers—cause itching, redness, a feeling of fullness in the ear canal, diminished hearing, and increasing pain. Antibiotic eardrops fight bacterial infection; antifungal drops kill fungi; and steroid eardrops can decrease inflammation.

Middle ear pain is caused by a pressure differential between the middle ear and throat. Earaches during childhood usually stem from middle ear infection. By the age of five, 80 percent of children have had at least one episode.

What happens: The Eustachian tube connects the middle ear, which is normally an air-filled space, with the throat. Something—cigarette smoke, bacteria, viruses, or allergens—inflames the Eustachian tube. Inflammation obstructs the tube, which traps microbes that entered from the throat. The

microbes multiply. Accumulating fluid (from infection and inflammation) creates pressure against the eardrum, which hurts.

Infants and small children are more vulnerable because their Eustachian tubes are shorter, more horizontal, and floppier, making collapse and obstruction of the tube easier.

Signs and symptoms of a middle ear infection include irritability, fever, batting or pulling at the ear, difficulty sleeping, decreased hearing, loss of balance, decreased appetite, and discharge from the ear. Blood-tinged pus exiting the ear is a sign that the eardrum has ruptured. Often the pain immediately subsides. The eardrum usually heals itself. Nevertheless, you should see the doctor. Unless recommended by your doctor, do not instill eardrops into the ear canal if you suspect a ruptured eardrum. Doing so could further contaminate or irritate the now-exposed middle ear. If the doctor prescribes an antibiotic or steroid eardrop, by all means use it.

Doctors diagnose outer and middle ear infections by examining the ear with a lighted instrument called an otoscope. They may also withdraw fluid from the middle ear with a small needle and send it off for culture. To prevent children's middle ear infections, it helps to stay up to date on immunizations, particularly the

Haemophilus influenza type b (Hib), seasonal influenza virus, and pneumococcal conjugate vaccines.

In addition, stay away from tobacco smoke. It impairs the immune system and inflames the respiratory linings. Inflammation and swelling in the Eustachian tube can obstruct it, which increases the risk of middle ear infection.

History

The cries of children suffering from earaches have plagued parents for millennia. The ancient Chinese, Egyptians, and Greeks used garlic (*Allium sativum*) oil to remedy earaches. Native Americans concocted mullein (*Verbascum thapsus*) teas and drops made from the leaves of the chaparral (*Larrea tridentata*). Eclectic physicians (nineteenth- and early twentieth-century doctors who relied heavily on American medicinal plants) commonly prescribed eardrops made with mullein or St. John's wort (*Hypericum perforatum*). More recently, the European Scientific Cooperative on Phytotherapy recommended dried mullein flowers made into a tea.

In the United States, pediatricians have routinely treated children's middle ear infections with antibiotics—despite the fact that 80 to 90 percent of middle ear infections resolve within a week without antibiotic treatment. In European countries, such as the Netherlands, doctors do not prescribe antibiotics in mild cases and instead recommend anesthetic eardrops (plus or minus oral analgesics) for pain relief.

In 2004, in response to antibiotic resistant bacteria, the American Academy of Pediatrics (AAP) recommended doctors refrain from prescribing antibiotics for children with signs of mild infection, and instead reserve these medications for more severe cases. However, a 2010 study found that the AAP guidelines didn't change the rate at which doctors wrote such prescriptions.

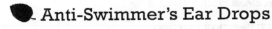

Anti-Swimmer's Ear Drops

1 teaspoon (5 ml) white vinegar
1 teaspoon (5 ml) rubbing alcohol

PREPARATION AND USE:

Pour the ingredients into a sterile bottle with a dropper (or a small squeeze bottle; just use a sterile bowl and clean teaspoon). Cap and shake vigorously to combine (or stir them together in a bowl first and then add to bottle). Squeeze 2 to 3 drops into each ear before and after swimming or bathing (or pour 1 teaspoon [5 ml] into each ear). Tip the head to one side, so the solution reaches the ear canal, and then tip the head back, so that the mixture drains out.

YIELD: 1 APPLICATION FOR EACH EAR

❓ How it works: *Mildly acidic solutions help restore normal pH and an environment less hospitable to bacteria and fungi.*

Lifestyle Tip

If you have an infant, know that breast-feeding provides immune protection against a number of infections, including middle ear infections.

If you do bottle-feed, elevate your baby's head. Never put a baby to bed with a bottle. Doing so increases the odds that fluid will travel from the Eustachian tube into the middle ear. It also increases the risk for dental cavities.

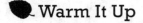 Warm It Up

A hot water bottle or warm washcloth
A clean cloth

PREPARATION AND USE:
Lie on your side, the painful ear up. (Or ask your child to do the same.) Check that the hot water bottle or washcloth is warm but not too hot. If using a hot water bottle, cover the outer ear with a clean cloth first. Apply the warmth until the bottle or cloth cools. Reheat and apply again if needed.

YIELD: 1 APPLICATION

❓ **How it works:** *Warmth relieves ear pain. Cold can also do the trick. Determine which works best in your case. This treatment relieves symptoms and may increase circulation to the area. However, it does not directly combat the infection, and you should see the doctor for antibiotics or other treatment if necessary.*

Note: If your child finds cold more soothing, use a bag of frozen peas, first covering the ear with a cloth.

Lifestyle Tip

Antihistamines and decongestants relieve middle ear congestion. Myth. Studies show that neither over-the-counter medication has any significant benefit. Both carry the risk of side effects, especially in children.

Rice Ear Warmer

1 cup (195 g) uncooked rice (any variety)

PREPARATION AND USE:
Pour the rice into a clean athletic sock and knot the top. Microwave the rice-filled sock on HIGH for 30 seconds. Check the warmth level: the rice-filled sock should be warm but not too hot. Lie down with the painful ear up. Apply the warm sock to the ear. If it is too warm, apply it on top of a clean, soft cloth.

YIELD: 1 APPLICATION

❓ **How it works:** *Heat helps relieve the pain of earache.*

Fact or Myth?

DON'T GET NEAR PEOPLE WHO HAVE A MIDDLE EAR INFECTION: YOU COULD CATCH IT.

Myth. They aren't contagious. Still, you don't want to share the dirty cotton swabs of a person who has an infection. Staying clean and dry is the rule for avoiding swimmer's ear.

Olive Oil Ear Drops

Warm olive oil dropped into the ear canal can relieve middle ear pain and also help soften earwax.

1 tablespoon (15 ml) olive oil

PREPARATION AND USE:

Put the olive oil in a small, sterile bottle with a dropper and cap it securely.

Fill a saucepan halfway with water. Heat the water on the stove top until warm but not boiling. Turn off the burner. Hold the capped bottle in the hot water for 5 minutes or less—just until the oil is warm. Test the temperature on your inner wrist.

Position the person with ear pain on his or her side, painful ear up.

Drop in 2 to 3 drops of warm oil (you are loosely plugging the ear canal with oil) and have the person stay in position for 10 to 15 minutes. If your child has the earache, read to him or her (or sing or tell stories) to keep him or her still. Repeat up to four times a day. When the child sits up, blot the oil the runs out of the ear with a clean cloth, cotton pad, or facial tissue.

YIELD: 1 APPLICATION

❓ How it works: *Warmth relieves ear pain, and warm olive oil is a time-honored remedy. However, one study did compare olive oil (that had not been warmed) to prescription anesthetic drops and found that the latter was more effective. You can always try the home remedy first. If that doesn't bring relief, call your doctor.*

❗ Warning: *Do not instill olive oil in the presence of blood-tinged purulent discharge from the ear canal (a sign of a ruptured eardrum). Also refrain from using oil if you plan on seeing the doctor within the next few hours, as the oil will interfere with a proper ear exam.*

Fact or Myth?

IF YOU HAVE SWIMMER'S EAR, WEARING EARPLUGS WILL BLOCK OUT THE WATER AND ALLOW YOU TO CONTINUE SWIMMING UNTIL THE INFECTION CLEARS.

Myth. Refrain from using earplugs until an infection is fully cleared. Then clean them with an alcohol swab before using the earplugs again. Also, if you're prone to swimmer's ear, watch for warnings at the pool or swimming area that indicate high bacterial counts. Keep your head out of the water on those days.

Herbal Eardrops

This formula eased ear pain when my children were young. ~ LBW

1 tablespoon (2 g) dried St. John's wort flowering tops

2 tablespoons (3 g) dried calendula flowers

1 tablespoon (2 g) dried mullein

½ cup (120 ml) extra-virgin olive oil

2 garlic cloves, minced

1 vitamin E capsule

PREPARATION AND USE:

Place the herbs in a clean coffee mill or food processor and process until powdered.

Heat water in the bottom of the double boiler. Once it boils, lower the heat to low.

Pour the oil into the top pan. Add the garlic. Stir in the herbs and cover the pot. Heat over as low a heat as possible for 30 to 60 minutes, stirring frequently. Do not allow the oil to burn or water to get into the oil. Remove the pot from the heat.

Let cool. Strain through muslin or a double layer of cheesecloth. Squeeze as much oil as you can out of the herbal matter. Discard or compost the herbs.

Bottle the oil. To help preserve the oil, puncture the vitamin E capsule into the bottle. Refrigerate the mixture for up to one year. Drop 2 to 3 drops of warm herbal oil into the affected ear as described in the previous recipe.

YIELD: ⅓ TO ½ CUP (80 TO 120 ML), FOR MULTIPLE APPLICATIONS

❓ How it works: *Three studies have shown that herbal eardrops reduce pain from middle ear infections in children as well as or better than anesthetic eardrops. Otikon, the herbal oil used in the studies, contains garlic, mullein, calendula, and St. John's wort in olive oil. Garlic* (Allium sativum) *is antimicrobial against viruses, bacteria, and fungi. Mullein* (Verbascum thapsus), *St. John's wort* (Hypericum perforatum), *and calendula* (Calendula officinalis) *have activity against some viruses and bacteria, counter inflammation, and ease pain. Calendula also fights some fungi, though these can infect the outer, but not the middle ear.*

Fact or Myth?

DIDN'T YOUR GRANDMOTHER TELL YOU NOT TO PUT ANYTHING SMALLER THAN YOUR ELBOW INTO YOUR EAR?

Well, it's a fact. Don't put cotton swabs, hairpins, or anything else in your ear canal to dig out wax or scratch an itch. You risk packing the wax deeper and injuring the ear canal and eardrum. If you're prone to swimmer's ear, use a cotton ball or towel to dry your outer ear after showering, bathing, and swimming.

High and Dry

Fight swimmer's ear by taking action immediately after swimming or bathing.

A clean, soft cloth
Your ears

PREPARATION AND USE:

After swimming, immediately dry your outer ears gently and thoroughly with the cloth. Tip your head to one side, letting the water drain from one ear. Dab away that moisture. Repeat the action with the other ear.

YIELD: 1 APPLICATION IN EACH EAR

❓ How it works: *Bacteria and fungi thrive in warm, moist conditions. Plus, public swimming pools, lakes, and oceans contain bacteria. Removing water from the ear eliminates a potential breeding ground.*

Note: Alternatively, you can use a blow-dryer, but do so with care: I turn it to low and hold it at least a foot (30 cm) away from your ear. Excessive heat and noise can cause damage.

When Simple Doesn't Work

Middle ear pain can be relieved by anesthetic eardrops, such as Auralgan and Aurodex. In the United States, most pharmacies require a doctor's prescription. Oral pain relievers, such as acetaminophen (Tylenol) and ibuprofen (Motrin and Advil), can also relieve discomfort. Do not give children or teens aspirin. Do not exceed recommended dosages. Note that applying warmth to the ear and using the other remedies here may relieve discomfort, but do not directly combat the infection.

Go Pro (Biotics) Summer Pops

2 cups (400 g) honey vanilla Greek yogurt
  (or your favorite)
1 tablespoon (15 g) fresh orange juice
1 cup (170 g) sliced fresh strawberries
1 cup (145 g) fresh blueberries

PREPARATION AND USE:

In a blender, combine the yogurt and juice. Gradually add the strawberries and blueberries and pulse until fully blended.

Spoon the yogurt mixture into a Popsicle mold with 8 impressions or into 8 paper cups. Insert sticks (for the paper cups, you can use plastic spoons or snip sturdy plastic straws in half to create holders). Freeze for 2 to 4 hours until firm. To remove, dip the cups or mold briefly into warm, not hot, water, pull out, and enjoy! Remove them all at once and wrap in individual resealable plastic bags to eat at your leisure.

YIELD: 8 SERVINGS

❓ How it works: *Live-culture yogurt and kefir contain bacteria similar to those normally present in your intestinal tract. The friendly bacteria and fungi that colonize your bodily surfaces promote immune system function and defend against disease-causing microbes. The five studies investigating the ability of oral probiotics (usually taken as supplements) to prevent recurrent middle ear infections in infants and children have yielded mixed results. However, studies have shown that probiotics help prevent respiratory infections. The significance is that colds and influenza set the stage for middle ear infection.*

Note: Because their intestines aren't mature enough to digest dairy products, children under the age of twelve months should not consume milk. However, if your infant is six months old or older, is not allergic to milk, and doesn't have an allergic condition such as eczema, yogurt is fine. The bacterial cultures in yogurt digest much of the lactose (milk sugar) and casein (milk protein).

When to See the Doctor

You or your child:
- *has a mild to moderate earache for more than two to three days*
- *has severe ear pain*
- *has significant symptoms of swimmer's ear or middle ear infection*

You:
- *notice discharge leaking from the ear canal*
- *have a sick infant under six months of age*
- *have a toddler under two years of age who has ear pain and fever*
- *have any concerns or questions about your child's health*

Your infant or child:
- *is extremely irritable and inconsolable*
- *has become listless or lethargic*

Chapter 35

Eye Health

Sight is one of our most cherished senses. We navigate, read, appreciate art, admire sunsets and flowers, and connect with loved ones by gazing into these "windows of the soul."

Some eye-related conditions are relatively mild, short-lived, easily treatable, and can occur at any age. Other eye conditions are chronic. More than 14 million Americans over age twelve have a visual impairment. Excluding conditions such as nearsightedness and farsightedness (which are caused by the shape of the eye, not disease) leaves more than 3 million with the age-related diseases macular degeneration, cataracts, glaucoma, and retinopathy.

A recent survey found that the prevalence of these diseases rose more than 20 percent between 2002 and 2008—an upsurge driven in large part by an increase in diabetes. Because these conditions become more common with advancing age, the graying of the baby boomer generation only adds to the problem.

Some of the age changes in the eye happen nearly universally and, therefore, aren't considered diseases. For instance, loss of elasticity in the eye's lens makes it difficult to focus on nearby objects. We compensate with reading glasses. Other age changes reduce night vision.

Most of the other eye diseases become more common with age because they require years of wear and tear to develop. Some of them have a strong genetic component. But genetic vulnerability only rarely dictates destiny. Reducing risky lifestyle habits and improving diet can improve the odds of clear vision.

History

The ancient Egyptians fought disorders of the eye with a variety of agents: ointments made from copper, sulfur, even beef liver, along with urine eyewashes! Rubbing an eye with an onion was prescribed for dry eyes. Like the Babylonians, the Egyptians believed that eye problems came from demons. A person with a squint or cataract might cause a demon in another's eye—perhaps the origin of the "evil eye." The Romans, also superstitious about diseases of the eye, used amulets to ward off eye troubles: necklaces made of cherry seeds tied on a string or green lizards caught under a full moon in September and draped around the neck.

For millennia, herbalists promoted eye health with a number of herbs, including ginkgo (Ginkgo biloba) and bilberry (Vaccinium myrtillus). Today we know the powerful antioxidant properties of these herbs improve circulation and protect against cell damage and the degenerative eye problems that come with aging. Ginkgo extracts improve circulation and help maintain the health of the retina (retinal cells trigger impulses that go from the optic nerve to the brain to form images). A concentrated ginkgo leaf extract seems to improve vision in patients with glaucoma.

Bilberry, along with its antioxidant properties, contains anthocyanins, plant chemicals that strengthen blood vessels and put the blues, purples, and reds into many other berries, including the bilberry's botanical cousins, the blueberry and cranberry. Human studies from the 1980s reinforced the promise of bilberries in managing cataracts, glaucoma, and diabetic retinopathy. Later studies confirm that bilberry extracts protect against these major eye disorders and macular degeneration as well. Leaf and berry extracts also have an antidiabetic effect—a relevant action, given the high risk of eye diseases among diabetics.

Lifestyle Tip

Get B: B vitamins also protect the eye. Several studies support the use of pyridoxine (vitamin B_6), vitamin B_{12}, and folic acid. Likewise, thiamine (vitamin B_1), niacin (vitamin B_2), and riboflavin (vitamin B_2) protect against cataracts. Supplementing with single B vitamins can unbalance others. Ask your doctor whether he or she recommends a B-complex supplement or a multivitamin and mineral blend formulated for eye health.

 ## Go Walk

A good pair of shoes
You

PREPARATION AND USE:
Walk for 30 minutes every day. Supplement walking with bike riding, jumping jacks, or pushups.

YIELD: 1 SESSION

❓ How it works: *Regular physical activity helps you stave off cardiovascular disease, diabetes, and being overweight—three risk factors for chronic eye diseases.*

 ## Veggie-Rich Couscous

1¼ cups (219 g) uncooked couscous
½ teaspoon freshly ground black pepper
3 tablespoons (45 ml) olive oil, divided
1 yellow squash, chopped
1 yellow bell pepper, chopped
3 broccoli florets, sliced lengthwise
1 cup (235 ml) vegetable stock
2 tablespoons (8 g) chopped fresh dill

PREPARATION AND USE:
Combine couscous and peppers in a bowl. Stir in half of the olive oil to coat. Add the remaining oil to a skillet over high heat with the vegetables. Sauté them for 2 to 3 minutes until barely braised.

Heat the vegetable stock to boiling in a small pan. Add the braised vegetables to the couscous and combine. Pour the boiling stock over the couscous mixture and stir. Cover the bowl with aluminum foil and steam for 5 minutes. Fluff with a fork, fold in the chopped dill, and serve.

YIELD: 4 SERVINGS

How it works: *Vegetables are staples of the Mediterranean diet, which is a great example of a plant-based diet. Meals focus on fruits, vegetables, whole grains (such as couscous), nuts, olives, olive oil, and fish. Studies show that this dietary pattern, rich in vegetables, protects against cataracts and glaucoma in diabetics, a population at high risk for eye disease. Another study showed that eating at least three servings a day of antioxidant-rich vegetables reduced cataract risk.*

Bright and Beautiful

Go for vegetables high in carotenoids, the plant pigments responsible for yellow, orange, and red hues.

4 medium-size yellow summer squashes, sliced lengthwise
1 red bell pepper, sliced lengthwise and seeded
1 tablespoon (15 ml) olive oil
1 red onion, sliced into rings
Freshly ground black pepper

PREPARATION AND USE:

Preheat the oven to 425°F (220°C, or gas mark 7).

Lightly spray a baking sheet with the olive oil or canola cooking spray. Put the squash and bell pepper slices on the sheet. Drizzle the olive oil over the top and toss. Line up the pieces so they are not overlapping. Sprinkle the sliced onion over the top. Grind the black pepper over the vegetables. Roast for 30 minutes, turning over the veggies halfway through. Serve hot.

YIELD: 6 SERVINGS

How it works: *Among other virtues, these colorful vegetables are full of antioxidants. Furthermore, yellow, orange, and red-colored plants contain fat-soluble plant pigments called carotenoids that are, among other benefits, strong antioxidants. Two carotenoids, lutein and zeaxanthin, accumulate in the macula. Their yellow color allows them to filter out damaging blue and ultraviolet light. Higher dietary intake seems to protect against macular degeneration and cataracts. In fact, getting these nutrients from food is just as good, and possibly better, than popping them in supplement form.*

🌿 Hail to Kale!

1 bunch of kale (about a pound [455 g]),
  washed, stems and ribs removed
4 teaspoons [20 ml] olive oil, divided
½ cup (120 ml) water
2 garlic cloves, minced
2 teaspoons (10 ml) vinegar
Cayenne pepper
¼ cup (28 g) crushed pecans

PREPARATION AND USE:

Chop the kale into small pieces. In a large skillet,
heat 1 tablespoon (15 ml) of the olive oil over medium heat. Add the kale and toss it in the oil for
about a minute. Add the water, cover, and steam
over low heat for about 10 minutes.

When done, push the kale to one side. To the
open area of the skillet, add the final teaspoon
(5 ml) of oil and the garlic, cooking the garlic for
about 40 seconds. Remove the skillet from the
heat and stir the garlic and kale together. Mix in
the vinegar. Sprinkle the kale with cayenne pepper to taste and toss in the pecans. Serve warm.

YIELD: 4 SERVINGS

❓ How it works: *Green leafy vegetables are
important dietary sources of lutein. Kale tops the
list of foods rich in lutein and zeaxanthin. Other
good sources include other green leafy vegetables (spinach, Swiss chard, collards, mustard,
beet and turnip greens, and romaine lettuce),
winter squash, okra, broccoli, Brussels sprouts,
green peas, pumpkin, carrots, and tangerines.*

🌿 Blueberry-Bilberry Waffle Toss

*Research shows that bilberry extracts defend
against cataracts and glaucoma and improve diabetic and hypertensive retinopathy.*

¼ cup (38 g) blueberries
¼ cup (30 g) dried bilberries (If bilberries
  are not available, double the blueberries
  to total ½ cup [75 g].)
¼ cup (39 g) sliced, pitted cherries or
  strawberries
¼ teaspoon ground nutmeg
¼ teaspoon ground cinnamon
4 whole-grain toaster-style waffles
1 cup (230 g) low-fat Greek yogurt

PREPARATION AND USE:

Combine the fruit in a bowl, sprinkle with the
spices, and toss. Place a nonstick skillet over
medium-high heat. Pour in the fruit and toss continuously for about a minute to soften.

Toast the waffles. Top each waffle with a dollop of yogurt. Cover the yogurt with the fruit (the
fruit will be especially sweet because the quick
cooking brings out their flavor).

YIELD: 2 TO 4 SERVINGS

❓ How it works: *Many blue-, purple-, and
ruby-colored berries owe their color to a type
of flavonoid called anthocyanins, a potent
antioxidant and blood-vessel strengthener.
Top sources include bilberries, blackberries,
blueberries, huckleberries, pomegranates,
black currants, cherries, elderberries, cranberries, and eggplants. The blueberry is related to
the bilberry, which is native to Europe. Whereas
blueberries' inner flesh is white, bilberries' is
blue, making them higher in anthocyanins.*

Anthocyanins protect the retina (light-sensitive layer at the back of the eye) and help regenerate a pigment in the eye responsible for seeing under low illumination. Although initial studies suggested the bilberries improved night vision, more recent trials didn't pan out. Volunteers in these studies were young and had normal night vision. We don't yet know whether bilberry might help elders with deteriorating night vision. Bilberries, however, have shown promise in improving retinopathy (disease of the retina) caused by diabetes and high blood pressure.

Note: Unless you live in Europe, you probably won't find fresh bilberries. You can order them dried from herbal retailers. The blueberry is an accessible runner-up for eye health.

Lifestyle Tip

Wear sunglasses when outside during the day. Ultraviolet light—and yes, UV penetrates clouds—damages several structures in the eye. The reflective power of snow, pale sand, and water magnifies the effects. Sunglasses should block 99 to 100 percent of UVA and UVB (two bands of ultraviolet light). When you're recreating outdoors, wear wrap-around sunglasses or goggles. A broad-brimmed hat heightens eye protection. If you wear corrective lenses, request the UV-protective coating and get a pair of prescription sunglasses.

Lifestyle Tip

Manage blood glucose. High blood sugar contributes to cataracts and damages small arteries, including the delicate blood vessels in the retina, leading to diabetic retinopathy. If you have diabetes, work closely with your health practitioner to maintain your glucose levels within the normal range. See Chapter 30, on diabetes prevention.

Black Currant Smoothie

You'll find black currants year-round in the frozen food section of your grocery store, but can buy this sweet and delicate berry in stores in mid- to late summer.

1 cup (145 g) fresh or frozen black currants
1 banana, chopped
1 cup (235 ml) pure pomegranate juice
3 tablespoons (38 g) plain nonfat Greek yogurt

PREPARATION AND USE:
Put all the ingredients in a blender. Blend until smooth.

YIELD: 1 SERVING

? How it works: *One study found that an extract of black currant (Ribes nigrum), an anthocyanin-rich berry like the bilberry, sped vision adaptation to the dark and also reduced eye fatigue. Other anthocyanin-rich berries include blueberry, cranberry, raspberry, elderberry, and strawberry. The pomegranate juice adds an extra jolt of anthocyanins and other antioxidants.*

Note: If black currants are out of season, try bilberries, blueberries, or strawberries.

Eye-Enhancing Oysters on the Half Shell

¼ cup (60 ml) white wine vinegar

2 teaspoons (6 g) diced shallot

2 teaspoons (10 ml) fresh lime juice

¼ packet (0.25 g) stevia

1 teaspoon (2 g) freshly ground black pepper

1 tablespoon (4 g) finely chopped fresh dill

1 dozen oysters, shucked

PREPARATION AND USE:

In a small bowl, fully blend the vinegar, shallot, lime juice, stevia, and pepper. Cover the mixture and refrigerate for an hour. Mix in the fresh dill just before serving.

Arrange the oysters on a plate of ice to serve. Drizzle the mixture over each oyster. Remove each oyster with a small fork or oyster fork and enjoy.

YIELD: 2 SERVINGS

❓ How it works: *Oysters are rich in zinc, an anti-inflammatory mineral that contributes to antioxidant enzymes in the body and seems also to support eye health. Other zinc-containing foods include crab, veal liver, roast beef, mutton, toasted wheat germ, pumpkin seeds, dark chocolate, and peanuts.*

❗ Warning: *Never eat an oyster if it emits a sulfurlike smell.*

Hot-E-Cakes

1 cup (130 g) whole wheat flour

¼ cup (28 g) toasted wheat germ

½ teaspoon ground cinnamon

1 whole egg

½ cup (120 ml) almond milk

¼ teaspoon almond extract

Water, as needed

Honey or agave nectar

½ cup (75 g) fresh blueberries

1 teaspoon (5 ml) canola oil

½ cup (115 g) vanilla yogurt

1 batch of fruit from Blueberry-Bilberry Waffle Toss (page 258) (optional)

PREPARATION AND USE:

In a medium-size bowl, mix the flour, wheat germ, and cinnamon.

In a separate bowl, whisk together the egg, almond milk, and almond extract. Stir the wet mixture into the dry until fully combined. Add water as needed for your desired consistency. Add a small amount of honey or agave to taste. Fold in the blueberries.

Place a large skillet over high heat. Disperse half the canola oil over the skillet. Pour enough batter for two pancakes onto the skillet (you'll be making a total of eight), adding the rest of the oil as needed to line the skillet. Flip the pancakes when bubbles begin to appear on top—don't overcook. They are ready when golden brown.

Top with dabs of yogurt and the fruit mixture from the Blueberry-Bilberry Waffle Toss—or your favorite juice-sweetened berry jam or jelly.

YIELD: 4 SERVINGS OF 2 PANCAKES EACH

❷ **How it works:** *Toasted wheat germ contains vitamin E and zinc, two nutrients included in research-backed supplements for eye health. Other good dietary sources of vitamin E and zinc include sunflower seeds, almonds, hazelnuts, and peanuts.*

Recipe Variation: If you desire, add crushed almonds or hazelnuts, also high in vitamin E.

Lifestyle Tip

Avoid tobacco smoke. Smoking is the leading cause of preventable death. It generates free radicals, damages the eye, and escalates the risk of arterial disease, which indirectly harms the eye.

Lifestyle Tip

Eye drops to reduce redness only work for a short time. Later, the blood vessels on the eye's surface enlarge again. Use with caution, as these drops can irritate the eye and do nothing to clear up conjunctivitis.

Lifestyle Tip

Enjoy a daily glass or two of green tea. Extracts in green tea protect against diabetes and heart disease (two risk factors for eye diseases) and defend against damage to the lens (where cataracts form) and retina.

Strawberry-Kiwi Parfait

2 cups (400 g) vanilla nonfat Greek yogurt
½ cup (85 g) sliced strawberries
½ cup (89 g) peeled and diced kiwifruit
½ cup (55 g) crushed pecans

PREPARATION AND USE:

Divide the ingredients in half and layer them into two tall glasses the following way: a layer of yogurt followed by a layer of kiwi, crushed pecans, yogurt, strawberries, crushed pecans, and a layer of yogurt. Add the remaining kiwi and strawberries on top. Enjoy!

YIELD: 2 SERVINGS

❷ **How it works:** *Kiwis and strawberries are packed with vitamin C, another important antioxidant for eye health. Sources include all fresh plants, particularly red peppers, oranges, grapefruit, kiwifruits, green peppers, broccoli, strawberries, and tomatoes. Many of those plants are also rich in carotenes.*

🐟 Tuna Once

Unless you're a strict vegetarian, put fish on the menu two times a week. This recipe makes four portions, but you can reserve two for use in Tuna Twice, Curried, on this page.

4 tuna steaks (4 ounces, or 115 g)
2 tablespoons (28 ml) olive oil
2 teaspoons (7 g) minced fresh garlic
1 tablespoon (15 ml) soy sauce
1 tablespoon (4 g) crushed fresh oregano
1 tablespoon (15 ml) fresh lemon juice
Pinch of freshly ground black pepper

PREPARATION AND USE:

Rinse the tuna steaks and place in a shallow baking dish. Pierce the steaks with a fork so the marinade will penetrate them.

In a small bowl, whisk together the olive oil, garlic, soy sauce, oregano, and lemon juice. Baste the steaks with the marinade, cover, and refrigerate for a hour.

Preheat the broiler. Transfer the steaks to a broiler pan. Broil the steaks for 4 minutes on each side until opaque.

YIELD: 4 SERVINGS (OR 2 SERVINGS, KEEPING THE OTHER TWO FOR THE FOLLOWING RECIPE)

❓ **How it works:** *Oily fish are rich in the omega-3 fatty acids eicosapentaenoic acid (EPA) and docosahexaenoic acid (DHA). The retina requires these fatty acids to function properly. Studies show that people who consume more fish have a 38 percent reduction in macular degeneration. The omega-3 fatty acids also ameliorate dry eye syndrome, which becomes more common with age.*

🐟 Tuna Twice, Curried

Use the other two steaks in the previous recipe to top lunchtime salads or in this yummy curried tuna salad mix on whole wheat crackers with a side of sliced red peppers.

2 tuna steaks, cooked (4 ounces, or 115 g)
2 tablespoons (30 g) plain low-fat Greek yogurt
2 tablespoons (22 g) brown mustard
1 teaspoon (5 g) prepared horseradish
3 tablespoons (45 ml) pickle juice
2 tablespoons (18 g) chopped pickle
1 tablespoon (10 g) minced onion
Curry powder

PREPARATION AND USE:

Cut the tuna into small chunks and place in a bowl. Mash in the yogurt, mustard, horseradish, and pickle juice. Fold in the pickle and onion. Sprinkle in curry powder to taste. Serve.

YIELD: 2 SERVINGS

❓ **How it works:** *Tuna's omega-3 fatty acids promote eye health as noted above. Turmeric, the key spice in curry, contains curcumin, which creates the yellow color and packs a powerful anti-inflammatory and antioxidant punch. Curcumin shows promise in combating glaucoma and macular degeneration. The antioxidant-rich red peppers add eye-health benefits.*

Lifestyle Tip

If you develop a sty, refrain from pressing on it. You may worsen the inflammation and spread the infection.

Eye Flush

If you have something in your eye, do not rub it—doing so could scratch the surface of your cornea. If gentle flushing does not work, call your doctor.

Lukewarm water (best if distilled or boiled)

PREPARATION AND USE:
Fill a small, sterile cup with lukewarm water. (If you have a particle in your eye, you probably won't take the time to boil the water first or shop for distilled water. You just want to get rid of the thing.)

Hold your head back and let the water run into your eye to help dislodge the particle. Look in the mirror to track the journey of the particle. Do not touch it until it swims to the corner of your eye and can be removed without touching the eye itself. You can also pull your upper eyelash and then lower eyelashes away from your eye as you flush. This maneuver may help clear material trapped under the eyelid.

YIELD: 1 APPLICATION

❓ **How it works:** *Clean, preferably distilled, lukewarm water is the safest way to help dislodge a particle from your very sensitive eye.*

Note: If a chemical splashes in your eye, simply turn on the tap and stick your eye into the flow. You can also get in the shower to flush your eye. If you get an acid or alkali or other toxic chemical in your eye, flush first and then proceed to the emergency room.

Lifestyle Tip

If you have blepharitis, conjunctivitis, a sty, or any other eye inflammation, take a break from wearing contact lenses. If your lenses are the disposable type, start with a new set once the inflammation clears. If your lenses irritate your eyes, see your eye doctor.

 ## Allergic Conjunctivitis (Pinkeye) Wash

This remedy makes sense if your eyes are pink because of allergies, a swim in the pool, or a viral infection. If you have bacterial pinkeye, see the doctor.

1 cup (235 ml) water
½ teaspoon noniodized salt (e.g., pickling or canning salt)

PREPARATION AND USE:
If you're using tap water, boil it. If you have distilled water, the microbes and impurities have already been removed. Pour the water in a sterile bowl. Add the salt, stir, and let cool to room temperature. Pour the mixture into an eyecup. Lower your face until your eye is in the cup. Blink several times. Clean the eyecup in hot soapy water before repeating with the other eye. Apply three to six times throughout the day. Keep the solution covered between uses. Discard any leftover solution at the end of the day.

YIELD: ONE DAY'S WORTH OF APPLICATIONS

❓ **How it works:** *Your tears are salty. You're making a solution that is similar to tears to wash away allergens such as pollen, chemicals (e.g., soap, or chlorine), pollutants, and viruses.*

Green Tea Eye Wash

1 cup (235 ml) water
1 teaspoon green tea leaves
½ teaspoon noniodized salt (e.g., pickling or
   canning salt)

PREPARATION AND USE:
Boil the water. Turn off the heat and add the green tea leaves.

Simmer covered for 5 minutes. Strain through clean muslin or cheesecloth into a cup. Mix in the salt. Let cool to room temperature.

Pour into the eyecup, as directed in the previous recipe. Soak each eye for about 60 seconds, blinking the eyelids. Sterilize the eyecup between washing each eye and after each use. Repeat three to six times a day. Keep the solution covered between uses. Discard the solution at the end of the day.

YIELD: ONE DAY'S WORTH OF APPLICATIONS

❓ How it works: *Green tea is astringent, which helps contract swollen tissue. It's also antibacterial and antiviral against some of the microbes causing pinkeye. However, please don't use this formula as a substitute for proper medical treatment.*

Lifestyle Tip

Protect the health of your heart and arteries. High levels of triglycerides (blood fats), cholesterol, and blood pressure increase the risk of conditions such as cataracts, hypertensive retinopathy, and macular degeneration. See Chapter 40, on heart health.

Sty in the Eye

The main treatment of sties is a warm compress.

Very warm water

PREPARATION AND USE:
Soak a clean washcloth in the water. Apply to the eye for about 15 minutes, warming the water and washcloth again as it begins to cool. Put the washcloth into the laundry hamper when finished. Repeat three to six times during the day, using a clean washcloth each time.

YIELD: ONE DAY'S WORTH OF APPLICATIONS

❓ How it works: *The warm, almost hot, compress, promotes blood flow (and the delivery of white blood cells) to the sty and speeds healing. A sty usually heals on its own within a week. In the meantime, keep the area clean and stay away from wearing eye makeup or contact lenses.*

❗ Warning: *See your doctor if the infection is not healing or appears to spread.*

Tea Compress

You can use this remedy in lieu of the warm compress recipe above. It also helps reduce bags under the eyes.

¼ cup (60 ml) water
1 green or black tea bag

PREPARATION AND USE:
Boil the water. Pour into a cup. Drop in the tea bag. Let steep for 1 minute. Check the temperature. When it's warm but not cool, apply it to a sty or to puffy areas under your eye. Use a fresh bag for each eye as needed.

YIELD: 1 APPLICATION

❓ How it works: *Green tea is astringent, which helps contract swollen tissue. It's also antibacterial and antiviral.*

When Simple Doesn't Work

A large trial called the Age-Related Eye Disease Study found that six years of supplementation with vitamin C (500 milligrams), vitamin E (400 IU), beta-carotene (15 milligrams), and zinc (80 milligrams) significantly slowed the progression of macular degeneration. Studies that have lasted a shorter duration did not produce such benefits. Higher intake of antioxidants, zinc, and omega-3 fatty acids (such as those found in fish) may decrease the risk of developing macular degeneration in those at high genetic risk.

The Age-Related Eye Disease Study 2, published in 2013, investigated whether adding lutein and zeaxanthin and/or omega-3 fatty acids (the type found in fish) further reduced the risk of progression to advanced macular degeneration. Unfortunately, the results did not show additional benefit.

The research is less clear for whether antioxidant supplementation prevents or slows the progression of cataracts. Some researchers note that, to prevent cataracts, antioxidants need to be started before the age of fifty.

For people at risk for eye diseases, fish oil supplements, which contain the omega-3 fatty acids DHA and EPA, may have merit. DHA helps maintain the retina's function with age. Fish oil also reduces symptoms of dry eye, which is especially common in women.

Mirtogenol (a product combining standardized bilberry extract with pycnogenol, a patented extract of French maritime pine bark) improved blood flow and reduced pressure within the eye, suggesting application in glaucoma. Pycnogenol alone may also slow progression of retinopathy caused by diabetes or arterial disease.

Ginkgo (Ginkgo biloba) extracts improve blood flow to the retina (the light-sensitive tissue at the back of the eye). Preliminary research indicates that a concentrated ginkgo leaf extract improves vision in people with glaucoma.

When to Call the Doctor

If you develop pinkeye, you may need to see the doctor. If your eyes are pink because you've been swimming or standing near the fire, you'll be fine if you simply give your eyes a break from the irritant. If you have allergies, prescription medications can help. Viral conjunctivitis is usually accompanied by symptoms of a viral respiratory infection. Bacterial conjunctivitis merits a trip to the doctor for antibiotic eye drops.

Also, keep up with annual eye exams, more often if your doctor recommends it. Most of these conditions come on so slowly that people may not develop noticeable symptoms until the disease has become severe. Early detection and prompt treatment can prevent significant visual loss.

The following signs and symptoms indicate you need to see your doctor soon:

- *signs of bacterial conjunctivitis (redness, discharge, awakening with crusty eyelids, increased sensitivity to light, and a foreign-body sensation)*

- *decreased ability to read and do other up-close work*

- *halos around lights*

- *increased glare from sunlight and artificial light*

- *loss of acuity in the center of your visual field (central vision) or at the edges (peripheral vision)*

- *chronic eye dryness or irritation*

- *redness of the whites of your eyes, especially if you have eye discharge*

Signs that you should seek emergency treatment:

- *sudden, unexplained loss of vision or double vision*

- *flashing lights or floating objects in your vision*

- *severe pain in or around your eye*

- *redness, swelling, and tenderness of the tissue around the eye*

- *trauma to your eye*

- *a toxic chemical in the eye (If you get chlorine, an acid, or another toxic chemical splashes into your eye, flush for 5 minutes first and then proceed to the doctor.)*

- *a foreign body stuck in your eye (If you have small particles in your eye, you may be able to remedy the problem by rinsing your eye with clean water. If an object is protruding from the surface of your eye, don't try to remove it. Tape a paper cup over the eye and have someone take you to the emergency room.)*

Chapter 36

Fatigue

Far too many Americans drag through their days feeling weary and downright exhausted. In a survey of American workers, 38 percent reported feeling fatigued within a two-week period.

In a 2005 survey of 4,500 male and female twins, about 37 percent of the people reported extreme fatigue at some point in their lives. In addition, nearly 23 percent had experienced prolonged fatigue (longer than one month), and almost 16 percent had chronic fatigue (lasting more than six months). The women were two to three times more likely to feel run down as men. Specifically, 75 percent of the women reported fatigue, versus 25 percent of the men. The women also developed "fatiguing illness" at younger ages. We'll leave it up to our readers to speculate on why women are more vulnerable, though differences in genetics, hormones, and social demands (working and caring for family) could certainly be factors.

The most common reasons for feeling worn out are sleeping too little and being overscheduled—two familiar and coexisting problems in America. Another related issue is chronic stress overload, which leads to burnout (emotional detachment, apathy, and low energy). Ill-advised yet common solutions to coping with stress by eating junk food, smoking, or drinking heavily only compound the problem.

Fatigue can be physical, mental, and emotional. Repetitive activities in any one dimension can tire you out. If you exercised harder or longer than usual, you'll feel physically depleted. If you've been problem-solving for hours, your head will feel fuzzy. Staring endlessly at a computer screen fatigues the eyes. If you've been upset or have been comforting someone else, you may feel emotionally spent. The solution to overdoing it is to give yourself breaks.

Fatigue is a normal reaction to taxing yourself. If you feel better after you relax and get a good night's sleep, you're okay. Nevertheless, you should take care not to wear yourself out very often.

A number of medical conditions can also cause persistent physical fatigue unrelieved by rest, including the following:

- Anemia makes you tired because your red blood cells aren't carrying enough oxygen.

- Acute infections are often accompanied by fatigue, as well as other telling symptoms (e.g., body aches, sore throat, cough, vomiting, and diarrhea).

- Chronic infectious illnesses such as AIDS, viral hepatitis, mononucleosis, and Lyme disease are also exhausting.

- Sleep disorders such as obstructive sleep apnea, restless legs syndrome, and narcolepsy lead to daytime sleepiness.

- Psychological disorders, particularly depression, interfere with sleep and cause daytime fatigue.

- Other chronic diseases associated with fatigue include diabetes, heart failure, hypothyroidism, chronic obstructive lung disease, cancer, adrenal insufficiency, and celiac disease (or other conditions that impair intestinal function).

- Surgery, even a minor procedure, can set a body back.

- Pregnancy, while not a disease, shifts hormones and puts unique demands on the body.

- Medications such as antihistamines, some antidepressants, chemotherapy, and some blood pressure medications cause sedation or fatigue. (If you take a medication that has sapped your energy, discuss the matter with your doctor. Please don't abruptly stop a prescription medication on your own.)

History

Twenty-first-century fatigue comes with a litany of woes: low energy, lassitude, lethargy, trouble concentrating, and even mild depression. But fatigue is nothing new. First-century Greek physician Dioscorides wrote about it in his medical text *De Materia Media*, documenting the medicinal benefits of an herb he called *rodia riza* to treat fatigue. (It was later renamed *Rhodiola rosea*.) Chinese emperors sent expeditions to Siberia to bring back the precious "golden root" for preparations that strengthened vitality and promoted long life. Centuries later, Viking warriors are thought to have taken rhodiola to boost endurance on their long-distance sea journeys and campaigns. Rhodiola's root has been used to fight fatigue and boost energy in traditional medicine in Russia and the Scandinavian countries for centuries.

Rhodiola is categorized as an adaptogen, a substance that safely helps us cope with stress. Russian and Scandinavian scientists have researched rhodiola for half a century. More recently, American and Canadian scientists have conducted studies. Some research shows that rhodiola decreases stress-induced fatigue and enhances mental performance in fatigue. (See "When Simple Doesn't Work" on page 277 for other fatigue-fighting adaptogenic herbs.)

RECIPES TO PREVENT AND TREAT FATIGUE

Breakfast Boost Omelet

Handful of well-rinsed baby spinach or kale
3 large or 4 small shiitake mushrooms
2 teaspoons (10 ml) olive oil
2 large eggs
1 tablespoon (15 ml) milk
Pinch of dried or fresh thyme
Pinch of freshly ground black pepper

PREPARATION AND USE:

Wash and pat dry the leafy greens. Tear into bite-size pieces, removing any thick stems. Wash, dry, and slice the mushrooms.

Heat the oil in an omelet pan over medium heat. Sauté the mushrooms until they soften and brown.

Scramble the eggs and milk in a bowl. Stir in the thyme and pepper. Pour over the mushrooms. When the center begins to gel, turn with a spatula to cook the other side, 2 to 3 minutes.

Place the greens on one side of the omelet and fold the omelet in half. Remove from the pan and serve.

YIELD: 1 SERVING

How it works: *You literally need to break your overnight fast in the morning. If you find yourself crashing before lunch, a nutritious breakfast might be the solution. The olive oil and the protein in the eggs supply long-lasting energy. (Cereal and baked goods, particularly if made from refined grains, give you a quick boost followed by a quick decline in blood glucose.) Leafy greens contain a host of vitamins, including calcium, magnesium, and B vitamins—all of which are needed in energy processes. Shiitakes contain fiber, minerals (potassium, magnesium, selenium), the B vitamin folate, and, when grown under ultraviolet light, vitamin D. They also taste delicious and promote immune health. Some studies indicate that additional magnesium improves symptoms of chronic fatigue syndrome. However, these studies used intramuscular injections of the mineral.*

Lifestyle Tip

Shun junk food. Foods high in sugar, refined carbohydrates, and trans fats are high in calories but low in nutrition. These foods actually create stress on a cellular level, which can simply add to feelings of fatigue. Be aware that, when we feel exhausted and overwhelmed, most of us reach for comfort foods. Now you know better. Retrain yourself to instead meditate, exercise, or try one of the healthy snacks in this chapter.

Sweet Pot-assium Energy Push

2 quarts (2 L) water
4 large sweet potatoes
2 tablespoons (30 g) plain Greek yogurt
1 teaspoon (5 ml) olive oil
Freshly ground black pepper
1 tablespoon (20 g) honey or agave nectar (optional)

PREPARATION AND USE:

Heat the water in a large pot over medium heat.

Peel the potatoes and cut them into chunks. Add the chunks to the hot water and simmer until tender, about 20 minutes. Reduce the heat to low. Drain the potatoes, place back in the pan, and return the pan to the low heat.

Mix the yogurt and olive oil until completely blended.

Mash the potatoes, adding the yogurt mixture and mashing until smooth. Add pepper to taste. If desired, mix in honey to taste.

Serve warm.

YIELD: 4 SERVINGS

How it works: *If your system is low in major nutrients, such as potassium, you'll feel the fatigue. Give your system an energy boost with potassium-rich veggies and fruits. Sweet potatoes, avocados, baked potatoes with their skin, edamame, and papayas deliver up to a whopping 1,000 milligrams per serving out of the recommended daily intake of 4,700 milligrams.*

Pick-Me-Up Snack

If your energy sags between meals, try this healthy snack.

1 apple, cored and sliced
1 tablespoon (16 g) peanut butter
1 large carrot, sliced lengthwise
1 hard-boiled large egg
Freshly ground black pepper

PREPARATION AND USE:
Put dabs of peanut butter on the apple and carrot slices. Shell the egg and sprinkle with pepper. Enjoy and face your next few hours with energy.

YIELD: 1 SERVING

❓ **How it works:** *Fatigue can result from eating too little and eating the wrong things. For instance, sweets cause a brisk but transient spike in blood sugar, but provide few nutrients. Instead, choose whole-food snacks, such as hard-boiled eggs, nuts, peanuts, carrots, and apples, which provide calories and the vitamins and minerals needed for energy production. Fresh fruits and vegetables are high in vitamin C and other antioxidants which counter the free radicals that lead to oxidative stress, which has been linked to fatigue. Antioxidants counter that effect. In a 2012 study, an intravenous infusion of vitamin C (not something to try at home) reduced fatigue in office workers.*

 ## Water on Hand

If you are thirsty, you're already dehydrated—a cause for fatigue. Drink up.

Fresh purified water
Lemon slices, crushed fresh mint, or cucumber slices

PREPARATION AND USE:
Pour water into a glass or, if you're on the go, a bottle. Add zing to the taste by adding one of the suggested options.

YIELD: 1 SERVING

❓ **How it works:** *One symptom of dehydration is fatigue. Staying hydrated helps. And if you add lemon slices or lemon juice to your water, you're adding vitamin C and flavonoids that are also antioxidant. Drink at least eight 8-ounce (235 ml) glasses of water a day and more when you're active. Drink when you're thirsty. (The elderly may need help getting the amount they need because they don't have acute thirst sensation.) Go for two glasses in the morning, two glasses an hour before physical activity, sipping during the activity, and another two glasses afterward. Drink your other glasses in the late morning and early evening. Avoid drinking water 2 hours before bedtime, so you'll sleep the night through. You'll know you're getting enough water if you're urinating four to seven times a day. If you urinate less and your urine looks dark, you're probably dehydrated.*

20-Minute Fix

You

A pair of athletic shoes

PREPARATION AND USE:

Ride your bike, take a brisk walk, do jumping jacks, or perform another activity. Sustain your activity for 20 minutes. Feel the energy fill your body. Repeat at least three to five times a week.

YIELD: 1 SESSION

❓ How it works: *Research suggests that frequent moderate exercise can boost energy and spirits. One study showed that riding a stationary bike for just 20 minutes three times a week at an easy pace significantly raised energy levels. If you have a medical condition, such as diabetes or heart disease, ask your doctor's advice about a reasonable exercise program.*

 ## Bed Check

You

Your bed

A clock

PREPARATION AND USE:

Go to bed 15 minutes earlier than usual. Try it for a week. If you feel better, try for a half hour earlier. Finally, try an hour earlier until you reach a full 8-hour sleep.

YIELD: 1 SESSION

❓ How it works: *Getting at least eight hours of sleep leaves you refreshed and helps you face challenges with a clear mind. During a magazine interview, pioneer sleep researcher, author, and Stanford professor William Dement, MD, once told author Linda White that most Americans link their fatigue and ill health to insufficient sleep. For more information, read Chapter 46, on insomnia.*

Iron Out Fatigue: Easy, Yummy Clams

Iron helps battle anemia, a major cause of fatigue. Women who menstruate heavily are at particular risk. A simple blood test can establish whether you need extra iron.

3 dozen clams (these can be little- or medium-neck)

3 tablespoons (42 g) unsalted butter

2 garlic cloves, minced

1 small onion, diced

½ cup (120 ml) white wine

¼ cup (15 g) chopped fresh parsley

Freshly ground black pepper

Lemon wedges, for garnish

Loaf of crusty whole wheat bread, sliced

PREPARATION AND USE:

Thoroughly wash the clams, throwing away any that have an odor.

Over medium heat, melt the butter in a large pan. Add the garlic and onion and braise for about 3 minutes; do not allow them to burn. Pour in the wine and stir well. Increase the heat to medium-high and cook until the wine boils. Add the clams. Cover the pan and steam the clams, stirring occasionally, for 8 to 10 minutes, until they open. Throw away any clams that are still closed: they are likely bad. Toss in the fresh parsley, sprinkle the clams and broth with pepper, and stir the clams once more.

Transfer the clams to a large serving bowl. Pour the clam broth over them and serve the clams steaming hot, garnished with lemon wedges. Serve with the bread: it's perfect for sopping up the clam broth.

YIELD: 4 APPETIZER SERVINGS

How it works: *Although beef liver and chicken liver top the list for iron-rich sources, shellfish is a major contender. Clams, oysters, and mussels have the same amount—about 3.5 milligrams per serving, (about eight clams). Spinach and dark leafy greens, beans, and tofu are among the best vegetable-based iron sources.*

Date Night

A night with friends can put spark back into your life. Do something that makes you glad.

You
A significant other or a good friend

PREPARATION AND USE:
Go for a meal (or let someone wait on you). Take in a movie or other cultural event. Go dancing. Play Frisbee by moonlight. Swap massages.

YIELD: 1 SESSION PER WEEK

 How it works: *A night out with friends is fun and life-affirming and makes you feel vital. Socially connected people general enjoy better health. Playtime is also critical—and a healthy habit we tend to neglect in our workaholic society. The only caveat is that if you stay out too late or drink too much alcohol, you will likely feel weary rather than energized the next day.*

Lifestyle Tip

Stop smoking and stay away from others' smoke. In addition to many other toxic substances, tobacco smoke contains carbon monoxide, which reduces the oxygen-carrying capacity of your blood.

 # 50-Minute Breather

This is a great alternative to the water cooler break.

You
A timer

PREPARATION AND USE:
Set the timer for 50 minutes. When it goes off, do something physical for 10 minutes. Stand and stretch. Walk around the block. (If a co-worker will go with you, you add social stimulation.) Climb the stairs in your building.

Turn on your favorite tunes and dance.

YIELD: 1 SESSION

 How it works: *Most people can't concentrate for longer than an hour. Some experts say we can't even stay focused for that long. Short breaks refresh and ultimately improve productivity.*

Fact or Myth?

IT'S NORMAL TO FEEL TIRED AS YOU GROW OLDER.

Myth. A loss in some hormones associated with youthful vigor accompanies normal aging. Also, sleep becomes lighter, which means you awaken more easily and spend less time in deep stages of sleep. However, healthy elders continue feeling energetic. Naps are a healthy option for anyone feeling an afternoon dip in alertness.

Fact or Myth?

EXERCISING WILL JUST MAKE YOU MORE TIRED.

Myth. Exercise is the key to energy. Make time for physical activity each day. It refreshes mentally, emotionally, and, when done in moderation, physically. More extreme exercise, however, does cause temporary fatigue. You'll also sleep better at night. (Just avoid vigorous exercise before bed, as doing so can keep you awake.) If you have a serious disease, get medical clearance first. If you have chronic fatigue syndrome, work with your health practitioners to make sure you don't overexert yourself and thereby trigger a relapse. However, research does show that properly paced exercise improves these chronic conditions.

 # Mini Work Break

If you can't take a 10-minute break, short exercises can "reset" your brain.

You
Your office or cubicle
A chair

PREPARATION AND USE:

Energize One: Wall Tap: Stand up and touch one wall, and then walk to the other and touch it.

Energize Two: Arm Wrap: Stand up and wrap your left arm over your right, crossing your palms, too. Raise your elbows to shoulder height and press your palms away from your face. Hold for 10 to 20 seconds. Repeat on the other side.

Energize Three: Leg Wrap: Sitting at your desk, lift your feet and cross your right leg over the left. Repeat on the other side.

Energize Four: Infinity Trace: Extend your right arm in front of you. Hold out your thumb and trace the infinity sign (a sideways figure eight). Follow the motion with your eyes, without moving your head. Repeat with your left arm.

YIELD: 1 SESSION

❓ How it works: *Standing up and touching walls is a simple way to take a short, physical break and reset the brain. According to experts who study how to teach in ways that better match the way the brain learns, activities that cross the sides of your body—as in the arm and leg wraps and the infinity trace—stimulate and refresh the brain. Wrapping your arms and legs also stretches some muscles and temporarily constricts circulation. When you release, you feel a pleasant flush of fresh blood.*

Savasana

The translation of savasana *from Sanskrit is "corpse pose," which sounds morbid but is meant to suggest that we arise from this "little death" feeling restored.*

You

A quiet, comfortable place

A blanket

An eye pillow or clean cloth

Soft music (optional)

A bolster (optional)

PREPARATION AND USE:

Lie on your back. Cover your eyes to block out the light. Cover your body with the blanket if you need it to stay warm and comfortable. Play soft, music, if you wish. If you have low back pain, slide a bolster under your knees. Pull your shoulder blades underneath you to open your chest. Rest your arms comfortably away from your sides, palms up. Separate your feet hip-width apart and let your feet turn out. Let the floor or mattress take all your weight. Feel yourself melting into it. Breathe easily. Let go. Let go again. Try to remain in this pose for at least 5 minutes.

YIELD: 1 SESSION

? How it works: *This yoga pose is a great antidote for people who have trouble relaxing and doing absolutely nothing. A 2012 study found that, compared to nonpractitioners, people who regularly practiced yoga—and there's more to it than this final restorative pose—were more likely to have improved well-being, better sleep, and less fatigue. They also tended to eat a plant-based diet and avoid tobacco smoke. Another 2012 study concluded that mindfulness meditation (paying relaxed attention to the present moment) improved the long-term mental fatigue that so often follows a stroke or traumatic brain injury. You don't have to have injured your brain to reap the benefits.*

Note: Alternatively, lie with one hand over your heart and the other over your belly. Feel your heartbeat and the rise and fall of your belly and chest as you breathe.

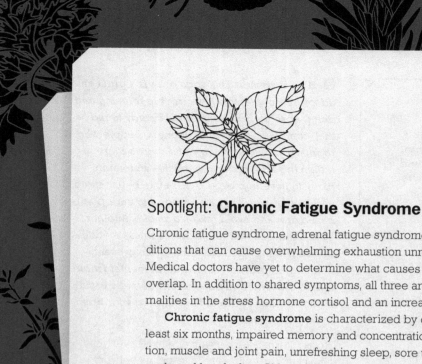

Spotlight: **Chronic Fatigue Syndrome**

Chronic fatigue syndrome, adrenal fatigue syndrome, and fibromyalgia are three conditions that can cause overwhelming exhaustion unrelieved by ample sleep and rest. Medical doctors have yet to determine what causes them. These three syndromes overlap. In addition to shared symptoms, all three are usually accompanied by abnormalities in the stress hormone cortisol and an increase in inflammatory chemicals.

Chronic fatigue syndrome is characterized by deep-seated fatigue lasting at least six months, impaired memory and concentration, exhaustion after physical exertion, muscle and joint pain, unrefreshing sleep, sore throat, tender lymph nodes in the neck, and headaches. Although the cause is unknown, some infectious agents have been linked to the disease.

The hallmark of **fibromyalgia** is chronic pain in muscles and ligaments, especially in the neck, shoulders, back, and hips. Fatigue, difficulty concentrating, poor quality sleep, and depression are also common.

Adrenal fatigue syndrome has only recently been recognized. Most of the time, the problem with chronic stress is an excess of the adrenal hormones epinephrine (adrenaline) and cortisol. In adrenal fatigue, cortisol is abnormally low. A prominent theory is that excessive stress (including a taxing illness) can cause the syndrome. People feel tired, achy, and lightheaded. Weight loss and low blood pressure may occur.

No magic bullet cures any of these syndromes. Recovery can be slow and requires a lot of patience, which presents a challenge to the hard-driving types who may be most vulnerable.

Legs Up the Wall Pose

If you stand or sit for hours on end, the legs-up-the-wall pose is refreshing.

You
A wall in your house or office

PREPARATION AND USE:

Lie with your legs up against the wall. Relax in that pose for 15 minutes.

YIELD: 1 SESSION

❷ **How it works:** *Lying in this position helps return any blood pooling in your legs to your heart. That improved circulation of blood and the period of relaxation has a restorative effect.*

Life Assessment

A journal
A pen

PREPARATION AND USE:

Keep a daily log of the social changes in your life. Track new challenges and look for patterns that may be stressful.

YIELD: 1 SESSION

❷ **How it works:** *By identifying your schedule and challenges in your social sphere, you can better determine how to face and change them to your benefit. Potential stressors include falling in love, falling out of love, losing a loved one, caring for a sick family member, or having difficulty getting along with friends, family, or co-workers. Getting a new job or losing your job consumes energy. Might you be a workaholic? Have you simply scheduled your life so tightly (even with great things) that you have no time to relax?*

When Simple Doesn't Work

Through the ages, herbalists have recommended herbs that help restore vigor in the face of debility. In Ayurvedic (traditional Indian) medicine and traditional Chinese medicine, practitioners recommended herbs such as ashwaghanda (Withania somnifera), ginseng (Panax ginseng), and schisandra (Schisandra chinensis). Native Americans used a different species of ginseng (Panax quinquefolius). Rhodiola (Rhodiola rosea) and eleuthero (Eleutherococcus senticosus, also called Siberian ginseng) became popular in Russia.

Research shows that rhodiola decreases fatigue during stress and improves mental performance in fatigue. Eleuthero and schisandra have been shown to enhance endurance and mental performance in fatigued people. In one study, a concentrated extract of eleuthero wasn't generally effective in people with chronic fatigue syndrome, though it did help people with less severe symptoms. Although these herbs are generally safe, they are not intended to be used as crutches. If you are chronically exhausted, get a proper medical evaluation first.

Essential Oil Lift

Peppermint essential oil

PREPARATION AND USE:

Place 5 to 10 drops of the oil on a cotton ball. Place the cotton in a clean jar and cap it. Whenever you need a boost, open the jar and sniff.

YIELD: MULTIPLE SNIFFS

❓ How it works: *A study showed that an inhaled mixture of peppermint, basil, helichrysum, and rose water reduced perceptions of mental exhaustion and burnout. Other essential oil candidates for countering fatigue include jasmine, basil, eucalyptus, lemon, rosemary, cardamom, cinnamon, cedarwood, cypress, and patchouli.*

When to See the Doctor

- *Despite your efforts to follow a healthy lifestyle, you feel tired much of the time.*

- *You habitually awaken feeling unrefreshed.*

- *Your bed partner notices that you snore most nights. If you've also been observed to intermittently hold your breath at night, make an appointment as soon as possible.*

- *You feel chronically fatigued and have numerous points that are tender to the touch.*

- *You have other symptoms such as unexplained weight loss, recurrent diarrhea, frequent infections, or any other signs of illness.*

- *You feel sad, irritable, hopeless, and have lost interest in activities that previously gave you pleasure.*

Chapter 37

Hay Fever and Seasonal Allergies

For many people, spring is the sneezin' season. Other symptoms of hay fever (allergic rhinitis in the medical world) include nasal congestion and itchy and watery nose and eyes. If you only have these symptoms a couple of months, consider yourself lucky. Some people have a year-round condition called perennial rhinitis. Triggers include pollen, molds, dust mites, animal dander, and other airborne offenders.

Allergic and perennial rhinitis tends to run in families, along with asthma and atopic dermatitis (eczema). In recent decades, the prevalence of all three conditions has risen. A warmer climate with longer growing seasons is expected to increase the pollen load for hay fever sufferers.

The underlying problem is immune system hypersensitivity. The immune system detects a speck of ragweed pollen and reacts as though an army of streptococci had invaded. In response, white blood cells produce a type of antibody called immunoglobulin E (IgE), which binds to mast cells, immune system cells involved in allergic reactions. Once IgE binds to mast cells, the latter release histamine and other inflammatory chemicals that cause those well-known symptoms.

Conventional treatment calls for avoiding known allergens and taking medication, such as antihistamines, to reduce symptoms. Side effects include excessive drying of the mouth, nose, and throat. The older antihistamines, such as diphenhydramine (Benadryl) and chlorpheniramine, also cause drowsiness. Newer antihistamines, such as loratadine (Claritin) and fexofenadine (Allegra), are less sedating. Intranasal steroid sprays and other medications can manage symptoms in people with persistent symptoms. Finally, immunotherapy ("allergy shots") may be used to desensitize people to allergens (the substance that causes an allergic reaction).

History

Humans have suffered from hay fever for millennia. But it was not until 1819 that British physician John Bostock first described this allergy, noting it was a periodical condition causing itchy eyes, sneezing, and congestion. In 1869, a researcher performed a skin test—applying pollen to a small break in his skin—and introduced the idea that sensitivity to pollen causes hay fever. A century later in 1965, Armenian physician and pharmacologist Roger Altounyan, while researching medicinal plants traditionally used to treat asthma, derived a drug called cromolyn from khella *(Ammi visnaga)*. Cromolyn stabilizes mast cells, thereby preventing them from spilling their inflammatory chemicals. Doctors still prescribe cromolyn nasal sprays and eye drops to manage allergic rhinitis.

Fact or Myth?

WHEN YOUR NOSE IS CLOGGED, YOU HAVE TO BLOW REALLY HARD TO GET OUT ALL THE MUCUS.

Myth. Blowing too hard can make mucus back up into your sinuses, causing even more pressure, discomfort, and infection. Press your finger against one nostril and blow gently from the open one. Then repeat on the other. Try using steam to help thin mucus and make it easier to expel by blowing gently. Afterward, wash your hands!

RECIPES TO PREVENT AND TREAT HAY FEVER

 ## Blushing Apple Smoothie

½ cup (78 g) pitted fresh cherries
½ English cucumber, peeled
1 apple, cored and peeled
½ cup (65 g) fresh raspberries
1 tablespoon (10 g) chia seeds
½ cup (120 ml) water
6 ice cubes

PREPARATION AND USE:
Place all the ingredients in a blender and blend until smooth.

YIELD: 3 SERVINGS

❓ How it works: *Bioflavonoids, which are found in many fruits, vegetables, nuts, and seeds, are antioxidant, antihistamine, and inhibit histamine release. The fruits in this smoothie are rich in vitamin C, which blocks histamine release from mast cells. People with higher levels of vitamin C have lower levels of histamine. This vitamin also acts as an antioxidant and enhances immune function. Some but not all studies suggest vitamin C supplements can improve asthma and allergy.*

Probiotic Salad

2 cups (340 g) sliced strawberries
1 cup (150 g) sliced red seedless grapes
1 apple, cored and sliced
1 celery stalk, sliced
¼ cup (35 g) raisins
½ cup (115 g) plain Greek yogurt
¼ cup (25 g) crushed almonds
Pinch of ground cinnamon

PREPARATION AND USE:

In a large bowl, mix the fresh fruits, raisins, and celery together. Fold in the yogurt. Chill for 30 minutes. Toss with the almonds and serve with a pinch of cinnamon.

YIELD: 2 SERVINGS

❷ How it works: *People with a genetic predisposition to asthma, allergic rhinitis, and eczema have a different microbial ecosystem in their intestines than allergy-free people do. Yogurt contains live, health-promoting microbes (probiotics) that benefit immune health. Supplemental probiotics have been shown to reduce certain allergic symptoms in children.*

Chia Breakfast Pudding

2 cups (475 ml) almond milk
5 tablespoons (59 g) chia seeds
1 banana, sliced
2 teaspoons (14 g) honey
Ground cinnamon

PREPARATION AND USE:

In a saucepan, heat the milk to just before boiling; do not boil. Stir in the chia seeds. Remove from the heat and let stand for about 10 minutes, stirring a few times, until the mixture begins to gel. Reheat the mixture until it is your desired warmth. Divide between two dishes and top each with ½ banana, 1 teaspoon (7 g) of honey, and a sprinkle of cinnamon.

YIELD: 2 SERVINGS

❷ How it works: *Chia seeds (also hemp seeds and flaxseeds) contain omega-3 fatty acids, which are anti-inflammatory. In addition to consuming more of these healthful fats, we recommend you reduce intake of foods that contain fats that increase inflammation, such as meat and processed foods. A study in pregnant Japanese women showed that eating more meat correlated with more symptoms such as watery eyes and nose. On the other hand, greater consumption of fish (a good source of omega-3 fats) correlated with less allergic rhinitis.*

In-the-Bag Onion Soup

Leave the onion skins in a muslin bag in the soup until you serve it, so the antihistamine agent quercetin will have its strongest effect.

2 teaspoons (10 ml) olive oil

2 cups (320 g) thinly sliced sweet white or yellow onion, skins reserved

2 cups (320 g) thinly sliced red onion, skins reserved

2 teaspoons (6 g) minced fresh garlic

¼ teaspoon freshly ground black pepper

¼ teaspoon sugar, or ½ packet (1 g) stevia

2 tablespoons (30 ml) dry white wine

1 quart (946 ml) low-sodium vegetable stock

½ teaspoon chopped fresh thyme, or ¼ teaspoon dried

PREPARATION AND USE:

In a large saucepan, heat the olive oil over medium heat. Add the onion and sauté, stirring for 5 minutes. Add the garlic, pepper, and sugar and stir. Lower the heat. Continue to cook for another 20 minutes, adding small amounts of stock to keep moist. Meanwhile, place the reserved onion skins in a muslin bag.

Stir the wine into the pot and, after 1 minute, add the bag with the skins, remaining stock, and thyme. Lower the heat to low and simmer for 1 hour. Leave the onion skins in the broth until just before serving and then remove the muslin bag.

YIELD: 4 SERVINGS

Fact or Myth?

A HUMIDIFIER WILL HELP SOOTHE YOUR ALLERGIES.

Yes and no. While moisture can soothe dry sinus passages, dust and mold can gather in the humidifier and actually do more harm than good. Clean and change the filter often and use distilled water. The high minerals in tap water encourage bacteria growth, which may cause further irritation.

❷ **How it works:** *The skin and outer ring of onions contain the substance quercetin, which has an antihistamine effect. In a study of people with year-round allergic nasal symptoms, quercetin significantly inhibited histamine release. Furthermore, substances in onion called thiosulfinates seem to have anti-inflammatory activity and can inhibit bronchoconstriction (airway narrowing as occurs in asthma). Other foods with quercetin are grapefruit, red wine, apples, garlic, cayenne pepper, cabbage, and tea.*

Wakame Seaweed Salad

Juice of 2 honey tangerines or 1 Valencia orange
About ½ cup (10 g) dried wakame
2 tablespoons (30 ml) toasted sesame oil
A splash of hot sauce
2 tablespoons (16 g) sesame seeds

PREPARATION AND USE:

Place the tangerine juice into a bowl. Add enough seaweed to cover the juice. Let sit for about 20 minutes while the juice is absorbed. (Add more seaweed if the juice is not all absorbed.) Stir in the oil and hot sauce. Mix in the sesame seeds.

YIELD: 1 SERVING

❓ How it works: *A Japanese dietary analysis of pregnant women found that seaweed stood out as protective against allergic rhinitis. Wakame, which is a type of seaweed, is rich in omega-3 fatty acids, vitamins, and minerals. It's also high in sodium; so take care if you're on a salt-restrictive diet.*

Broiled Red Peppers

This is a specialty from the kitchen of Barbara Grogan's dear friend Sophia Eorio, who makes peppers, olive oil, and garlic a healthy part of her family's diet; her daughter Lisa whips up several batches ahead of time, and then makes divine roasted pepper sandwiches for drop-in lunch guests.

2 teaspoons (10 ml) olive oil
4 red bell peppers, cut in half, stemmed, and seeded
6 garlic cloves, sliced thinly

PREPARATION AND USE:

Preheat the oven to 450°F (230°C, or gas mark 8) and then turn it to broil. Spread a baking sheet with the olive oil. Cover with a layer of garlic and top with a layer of peppers. Place the baking sheet on the top rack of the oven. Broil for 15 to 20 minutes until the pepper skins blacken.

Transfer the peppers and garlic to a platter and let cool, about 15 minutes.

Place the peppers and garlic in a resealable plastic bag and store in the refrigerator. Remove the skins from the peppers (optional) and serve the roasted pepper and garlic in salads, sandwiches, soups, pastas, and more.

YIELD: 4 SERVINGS

❓ How it works: *Studies link higher intake of beta-carotene with fewer allergies. Foods rich in beta-carotene include red peppers, romaine and other green and red-leaf lettuces, kale, carrots, spinach, dandelion greens (buy or pick in an area where pesticides haven't been used and where they have not been grown near the street), collards, cabbage, beet, mustard, and turnip greens, pumpkin, sweet potatoes, and winter squashes, such as butternut squash.*

Note: Make sure to broil, not roast, the peppers. Roasting overcooks them.

Lifestyle Tip

Try these tips to reduce your exposure to allergens:

- **Always use air purifiers with HEPA (high-efficiency particular air) filters.**

- **Vacuum at least once a week with a vacuum cleaner equipped with an HEPA filter.**

- **Favor bare floors (i.e., easier to clean) over rugs and carpets.**

- **If you're allergic to pollen, close your windows. Consider exercising indoors until the season passes. Leave your shoes at the door.**

- **If you're allergic to a pet you own and love, wash him or her once a week. In between, wipe down his or her fur with a damp cloth.**

- **To reduce dust mite exposure, cover pillows and mattresses with impermeable covers. Wash bedding weekly in hot water.**

- **Exterminate cockroaches.**

- **Call in a specialist to remove household mold.**

 ## Honey-Sage Tea

Popular lore has it that local honey (made by bees visiting local plants) can reduce hay fever symptoms. New studies are confirming the benefits of honey.

2 cups (475 ml) water
2 teaspoons dried, crushed sage leaves
2 tablespoons (40 g) honey

PREPARATION AND USE:

In a small saucepan, bring the water to a boil. Add the sage. Turn off the heat. Cover and steep for 15 minutes. Stir in the honey. Sip and enjoy.

YIELD: 1 LARGE OR 2 SMALL SERVINGS

❷ How it works: *For nasal secretions, sage (Salvia officinalis) has a drying and anti-inflammatory effect. A Finnish study was able to confirm that, for people allergic to birch pollen, consuming steadily greater amounts of birch pollen honey between November and March (before hay fever season) had significantly fewer symptoms come spring. Do not give honey to infants under twelve months of age because of the small risk of botulism.*

Antiallergy Artichokes

For the artichokes:

6 artichokes, tops sliced off, tips and stems
   trimmed

1 tablespoon (18 g) salt

Juice of 1 lemon

For the dressing:

3 tablespoons (45 ml) olive oil

1 tablespoon (10 g) minced fresh garlic

2 tablespoons (28 ml) fresh lemon juice

¼ teaspoon freshly ground black pepper

½ teaspoon salt

PREPARATION AND USE:

To make the artichokes: In a large pot, bring
2 cups (475 ml) of water to a boil (the water
depth should equal about 2 inches [5 cm]).

Add the artichokes, salt, and lemon juice.
Cover and lower the heat. Steam about 30 minutes, until the artichoke bottoms can be pierced.
Drain and let cool. Slice in half and remove and
discard the fuzzy center of each artichoke.

To make the dressing: Combine all the dressing ingredients in a bowl.

Brush the artichokes with the dressing. Lay
face up in the broiler or face down on an outdoor or indoor noncharcoal grill and cook over
medium heat, turning once, for a few minutes.
Remove when browned lightly and serve.

Enjoy by peeling off each petal and tearing off
the flesh at the bottom with your teeth. And finally,
slice into the delicious heart of the artichoke. If
you like, make an extra batch of the dressing
for dipping.

YIELD: 6 SERVINGS

❓ How it works: *The artichoke plant is related
to milk thistle, whose seeds have antihistamine
properties. A concentrated extract of milk thistle
seeds was shown to be as effective as the antihistamine medication Zyrtec. Artichoke contains
polyphenols (including flavonoids) that act as
antioxidants and may boost immunity.*

When Simple Doesn't Work

*Several studies in children and adults sup-
port the use of a special extract of a plant
called butterbur (Petasites hybridus). It
appears to be as effective as Zyrtec and
Allegra. If you buy this supplement, make
sure the product promises it's free of compounds called pyrrolizidine alkaloids. In a
study of sixty-nine patients with hay fever,
58 percent rated freeze-dried, encapsulated nettles (Urtica dioica) effective, and
48 percent said the herb was as good as or
better than previously used medicines.*

🍃 Saltwater Nasal Rinse

This recipe is recommended by the American Academy of Allergy, Asthma & Immunology. You'll need a sterile syringe—either a soft rubber ear bulb syringe or an infant nasal syringe, or neti pot (nasal irrigation pot sold in natural food stores).

1 tablespoon (18 g) iodide-free salt
1 teaspoon (5 g) baking soda
1 cup (235 ml) lukewarm distilled or boiled
  water

PREPARATION AND USE:

In a clean bowl, mix the salt and baking soda. Add 1 teaspoon (6 g) of the mixture to the sterile water. (Store the remaining dry mixture in an airtight container.) Draw the saline solution into the syringe bulb or pour into the neti pot.

Tilt your head downward over the sink and rotate to the left. Gently squeeze (or pour) about ½ cup (120 ml) of the solution into your right nostril. Breathe normally through your mouth. After a brief lag, the solution should come out through your left nostril.

Rotate your head to the right and repeat the process on the left side. Gently blow your nose to remove excess water and prevent the solution from going into your ear. After using the rinse, fully clean the syringe. Repeat two to three times a day during hay fever season.

YIELD: 1 APPLICATION (BOTH NOSTRILS)

❓ How it works: *The saltwater literally washes away allergens of hay fever. Furthermore, solutions that are saltier than your own body fluids (including mucus) help draw out extra moisture. A recent study in children with hay fever found that this so-called hypertonic saline rinse twice daily was more effective than a less salty rinse (closer to the salt concentration in bodily fluids),*

When to Call the Doctor

- *Hay fever is making you miserable.*

- *You suspect you have a sinus infection. Hay fever can block the drainage ducts from the sinuses. Clues of sinus infection include worsening congestion, a feeling of fullness or pain over the cheekbone or forehead, fever, and a green or brown nasal discharge (versus the clear discharge from hay fever).*

- *You suspect you or your child has developed a middle ear infection. The inflammation associated with hay fever can block a tube that runs between the middle ear and throat. Children are particularly at risk.*

which was more effective than no nasal wash at all. The American Academy of Allergy, Asthma & Immunology even posts this recipe on its website (www.aaaai.org/conditions-and-treatments/treatments/saline-sinus-rinse-recipe.aspx).

Note:

- Make sure to use pickling or canning salt containing no iodide, anticaking agents, or preservatives, which can irritate the nasal lining.

- Make a weaker solution if you experience burning or stinging.

Chapter 38

Headaches: Migraine, Tension, and Sinus

Headaches can be a miserable—and for some people, daily—experience. They come in different varieties, with tension headaches being the most common. Tight muscles in the neck, shoulders, and/or face create a viselike constriction. These headaches may evolve over the course of a taxing day.

In a condition called bruxism, people clench or grind their teeth, resulting in pain in the jaw and temples. Some people clench mainly at night and do so unwittingly. The main clue is morning face pain that subsides over the course of the day. Chewing gum or eating hard candy can aggravate the condition.

Migraines cause repeated episodes of intense, throbbing pain. The pain is usually localized to one side, centering on the temple, around the eye, or at the back of the head. About 20 percent of migraines are preceded by auras, which are marked by sensory distortion. Sensations are usually visual (blind spots in the vision, jagged lines, or flashing lights) but can also affect hearing, taste, and smell.

Cluster headaches, also called suicide headaches, center around one eye. Several headaches may occur in a single day. Or the cluster of headaches can stretch over a couple of months.

Medical treatment for headache includes nonsteroidal anti-inflammatory medicines, such as aspirin, acetaminophen, ibuprofen, and naproxen. People with migraines may take prescription medications such as the "triptans." Doctors typically prescribe medications taken daily to prevent frequent migraines.

People with what are called "frequent daily headaches" may get them due to a rebound effect from pain relievers. In other words, the medications create a vicious cycle.

History

Headache sufferers, despite their pain, might take heart that they are not subject to various nostrums of the ancient world. For headache relief, the Egyptians used a strip of linen to bind a clay crocodile to the head of those experiencing headaches. Tenth-century physician Ali ibn Isa recommended binding a dead mole to the head instead.

But things did improve. Medieval European herbalists, like ancient Greek physicians before them, used feverfew (*Tanacetum parthenium*) to manage fever, as you might expect, but also for migraine headaches. In 1978, a British health magazine described the case of a woman who found that eating three feverfew leaves (which are quite bitter) daily for ten months stopped her migraines. (Unfortunately, in some people, chewing the leaves can produce mouth ulcers, tongue inflammation, and swelling of the lips.) Most of the research that followed indicated that feverfew extracts can both help prevent and reduce the frequency and severity of migraines. These extracts are usually well tolerated or produce only mild side effects such as stomach upset.

RECIPES TO PREVENT AND TREAT HEADACHES

Ginger-Feverfew Elixir

2 cups (235 ml) water
1 teaspoon (3 g) finely grated fresh ginger, packed
1 teaspoon (2 g) chopped fresh feverfew leaves, or ½ teaspoon dried
Honey or agave nectar

PREPARATION AND USE:

Bring the water to a boil. Add the ginger and simmer, uncovered, for 10 minutes. Remove from the heat and add the feverfew leaves. Cover and steep for 15 to 20 minutes. Strain out the ginger and feverfew. Stir in honey to taste, and serve hot.

YIELD: 2 SERVINGS

❓ **How it works:** *Ginger reduces pain and inflammation. Its antinausea effect may help counteract nausea associated with migraines. Research indicates that feverfew extracts help prevent migraines, possibly due to anti-inflammatory effects and the prevention of the*

arterial constriction in the brain that contributes to these headaches. Fresh leaf extracts seem to work better than dried. Two studies have shown that special extracts combining ginger and feverfew can help to stop an evolving migraine.

Note: Feverfew is bitter; honey or agave will help the medicine go down.

Honey-Cinnamon Coffee

We used nondairy milk in this recipe because, for some people, allergies to cow's milk protein can trigger migraines. ~ LBW

1 cup (235 ml) freshly brewed coffee
¼ cup (60 ml) almond or other nondairy milk
¼ teaspoon vanilla extract
2 tablespoons (40 g) honey
¼ teaspoon ground cinnamon

PREPARATION AND USE:

In a saucepan, combine the coffee, nondairy milk, and vanilla. Warm until hot, but do not boil. Stir in the honey until dissolved. Stir in the cinnamon.

YIELD: ABOUT 2 SERVINGS

❓ **How it works:** *Caffeine has a paradoxical effect on migraines. For people who consume it infrequently, it can help break a migraine. Scientists aren't sure exactly how it works, but point to mild analgesic action and effects upon blood vessel diameter and certain brain chemicals. Caffeine also increases the absorption of pain-relieving medications, which is why it's often combined with acetaminophen or aspirin for headache treatment. However, regular consumption of higher doses of caffeine (more than 300 milligrams, or about 3 cups [710 ml] of coffee a day) can contribute to the development of migraines. Withdrawal from caffeine can also make the head throb.*

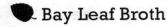

Bay Leaf Broth

1½ quarts (1.4 L) water
1 onion, diced
1 garlic clove, minced
⅛ teaspoon dried thyme
⅛ teaspoon dried rosemary
1 bay leaf
1 celery stalk, halved
⅛ teaspoon sea salt
Freshly ground black pepper

PREPARATION AND USE:

Stir together the water, onion, garlic, thyme, and rosemary in a pot. Add the bay leaf and celery. Bring to a boil. Lower the heat to low, cover, and simmer for 1 hour. (The longer you simmer the bay leaf, the more it infuses the broth with its healing properties.) Remove the bay leaf and celery. Season with salt and pepper to taste. Pour the steaming broth into mugs and enjoy.

YIELD: 6 SERVINGS

❷ **How it works:** *Herbal experts, such as James Duke, Ph.D., recommend bay leaves for preventing migraines. The leaves contain some of the same chemicals as feverfew. Studies show that they block bodily chemicals that dilate arteries. (In migraines, exaggerated dilation of arteries painfully stretches nerves.) To date, no studies have investigated its use in preventing migraines.*

Lifestyle Tip

Stay hydrated. Drink water or any other beverage without dairy or caffeine, which, in some people, can aggravate migraines. Dehydration can lead to headache.

Essential Oil Anti-Pain Massage

1 tablespoon (15 ml) carrier oil (try almond, apricot, or olive)
3 to 5 drops peppermint essential oil

PREPARATION AND USE:

Place the oils in a clean, small jar. Cover tightly with a lid. Shake until combined. Massage into sore areas: neck, shoulders, jaw, or temples. Take care not to touch your eyes. When finished, lie down in a quiet place with your eyes shut.

YIELD: 1 APPLICATION

❷ **How it works:** *Two studies show that peppermint essential oil, applied topically, helps relieve tension headaches. It seems to inhibit pain nerve receptors. In addition, massage is effective in relieving tightness in the tender neck, shoulder, and head muscles by increasing blood flow.*

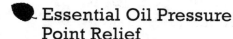 Essential Oil Pressure Point Relief

1 drop peppermint essential oil
1 drop lavender essential oil

PREPARATION AND USE:

Put a drop each of peppermint and lavender essential oil in one palm. Spread onto your fingers. Press your fingers into the muscles paralleling the spine between the base of your skull and your neck (about two finger widths on either side of your spine).

YIELD: 1 APPLICATION

❓ How it works: *As in the previous remedy, peppermint essential oil relieves headaches by inhibiting nerve receptors. Inhalation of lavender essential oil has also been shown to reduce migraine headache pain as well as nausea and sensitivity to light. Studies also show that this acupressure point and others can relieve pain in people with chronic headaches.*

🌶 Hot Headache Relief

I use a commercial capsaicin ointment; this recipe naturally delivers capsaicin, the constituent of chile peppers that both creates heat and reduces pain. ~ LBW

2 teaspoons (10 ml) unscented hand cream
¼ teaspoon cayenne pepper

PREPARATION AND USE:

In a small, clean bowl, blend the hand cream and cayenne. Massage into your neck and shoulders.

YIELD: 1 APPLICATION

❓ How it works: *Cayenne contains capsaicin, which interferes with the ability of nerves that transmit information about pain from the periphery to the brain. (Pain, though very real, is all in your head. If the brain doesn't get the news—well, what pain?) You can find over-the-counter ointments standardized for capsaicin in drugstores. Research suggests that special capsaicin preparations applied inside the nose (which we don't recommend you do with cayenne pepper or commercial ointments) can help block cluster headaches—severe, one-sided headaches that come in waves.*

❗ Warning: *Do not touch your eyes when mixing or using this remedy. Also, this mixture could stain clothes. Expect to feel heat at the site of the application. Start with small amounts until you see how you respond.*

🌰 Put It on Ice

When a headache attacks, keep a cool head!

½ cup (115 g) crushed ice
3 drops lavender essential oil

PREPARATION AND USE:
Place the ice in a resealable plastic bag and seal. (A good substitute is a bag of frozen peas or corn.) Wrap the bag of ice in a damp washcloth and secure with a safety pin. Dot the essential oil onto the cloth and spread across the cloth with your fingertips. Apply the wrapped bag to the painful area, with the cloth against your skin.

YIELD: 1 APPLICATION

❓ How it works: *Cold reduces inflammation. For some people, cold feels better than heat. Do what works for you. In one study, 71 percent of patients who used a frozen gel pack during a headache found it an effective pain reliever and about half reported that it immediately decreased pain. Another study found that cold applications reduced the frequency of exercise-induced headaches in children. You can also alternate cold packs with hot packs. In theory, this technique narrows (cold), then dilates (warm) blood vessels, creating a flushing effect. For throbbing headaches, end with cold.*

🌰 Some Like It Hot

1 Homemade Neck Cozy (page 425)

PREPARATION AND USE:
Microwave the neck cozy on high for 60 to 90 seconds. Wrap around your neck and relax. You can also lie down and drape the neck cozy over your forehead and temples.

YIELD: 1 APPLICATION

❓ How it works: *Heat relaxes tight muscles and encourages blood flow to areas to which it's applied—neck, shoulders, and head. As noted previously, you can alternate hot and cold packs. If you have tight muscles from a tension headache of teeth clenching, you might want to end the cycle with heat to keep those muscles relaxed.*

Lifestyle Tip

Take a nap. Lie down in a quiet place and get some shut-eye. Sleep can be the best medicine for a headache. Sleep deprivation increases pain sensitivity. People with migraines report more insomnia than do people without these headaches. Researchers hypothesize that increased sleep might help manage the condition. A 2007 study revealed that chronic migraine sufferers who received information to help them get more sleep experienced a significant reduction in headache frequency and intensity.

When Simple Doesn't Work

Studies are mixed on the use of feverfew to ease headaches, though the majority are positive. A recent ten-week study found that acupuncture, which alone can reduce headaches, combined with feverfew was more effective than either used alone. Three studies have shown success following use of a special, concentrated extract of butterbur (Petasites hybridus) to prevent migraines. Commercial products containing butterbur remove plant substances called pyrrolizidine alkaloids, which can harm the liver. Take as directed.

Other supplements with some support for preventing migraines include riboflavin (a B vitamin), coenzyme Q10, magnesium, and alpha lipoic acid. A few studies support chiropractic manipulation for relief of chronic headaches. Biofeedback is also a treatment for migraine and tension headaches—electrodes attached to the skin give information that helps a person manage headaches by influencing blood flow to the brain.

 # Six-Point Neck Stretch

When you feel a migraine coming on, do this multiple stretch slowly in a dark, quiet place—you'll find yourself relaxing away your headache.

You, in comfortable clothes
A dark, quiet place

PREPARATION AND USE:

Sit or stand with your torso erect. Bend your neck, as though trying to touch your chin to your chest (don't force it). Clasp your hands at the base of your neck, elbows pointing down. Let the weight of your arms gently pull your head forward (no force is necessary to feel a stretch). Hold for ten slow inhalations and exhalations. Imagine the muscles letting go.

Point your nose in the direction of your right shoulder (you're looking down with your head angling to the right). Place your left palm on the back of your head, fingers pointing toward your right ear. Pull your head gently to the left and down. Hold for slow inhalations and exhalations. Gently release. Repeat to the left.

Now, tilt your head sideways, right ear heading toward right shoulder. Wrap your right arm over your head, palm against your left ear. Hold. Repeat on the other side.

Finally, lie face up on a firm, comfortable surface. Press your head back into the surface (as though into a headrest). If you can't lie down, lace your fingers behind your head. Press your head into your hands, while resisting with your hands. Release. Take a moment to lie still and enjoy some relief from muscle tension.

YIELD: 1 SESSION

❷ **How it works:** *Tension can be a migraine trigger. Loosening your neck and shoulder muscles when your head begins to throb may help arrest a migraine. Keeping muscles relaxed daily may help cut down on migraine frequency.*

Journal Away Your Headache

If your headaches are frequent, it's worthwhile to keep a journal to help identify triggers.

A journal
A pen

PREPARATION AND USE:

Each day for a week, write down your activities and what you eat. How long you keep the journal depends upon the frequency of your headaches: If you get more than one headache per week, journaling for one week will suffice. If headaches are monthly, write each day during that period of time.

In your journal, see if you can link daily events to headaches. Keep in mind there can be a lag of up to twenty-four hours between a food trigger and a migraine. Also, rather than pinpointing a single cause, you may find that a convergence of several factors may culminate in a headache. Possible triggers are as follows:

- Skipped meals

- Food allergies—Common food allergens are found in dairy, wheat, peanuts, tree nuts, and shellfish. Often people have other symptoms of allergies (intestinal distress, rash, nasal congestion, and even severe respiratory distress).

- Foods high in tyramine, a natural breakdown product of the amino acid tyrosine that arises when some foods are aged, smoked, or fermented—Examples include aged cheese, cured meats, smoked fish, red wine, sauerkraut, pickles, kimchi, soy sauce, and miso soup.

- Food ingredients and food additives such as excessive caffeine, chocolate, aspartame (artificial sweetener), monosodium glutamate (MSG), and nitrates and nitrites (in cured meats, such as bacon, ham, and hot dogs)

- Stress overload

- Tension in neck, shoulders, and face muscles—Note what activities caused the muscle tension (e.g., working on a computer, reading, sleeping on a certain pillow, feeling or emotionally upset)

- Disrupted or insufficient sleep

- Jet travel

- Hormonal changes—Note the time of your menstrual cycle

- Exposure to tobacco smoke or other air pollutants

- New medications

- Use of pain medications (overuse of which can cause rebound headaches)

YIELD: 1 DAILY SESSION

❓ **How it works:** *Looking at your daily activities, the foods you eat, and the stressful situations you endure will help you identify and avoid migraine triggers.*

🍂 Press Away the Pain

You

A quiet place

PREPARATION AND USE:

Open your left palm and extend your fingers. Place the thumb and index finger of your right hand on either side of the web between thumb and index finger on your left hand. Press on the meaty portion near the second metacarpal (the bone leading to your index finger). Press with firm pressure and massage in a circular motion for 2 full minutes. Repeat on the other side.

Here's another acupressure exercise. Sit and bend your head forward. Rest your fingers on the sides of your head above your ears. Press the tips of your thumbs into the bony protuberances of your occiput (the back of your head above the junction with your spine). Massage firmly in a circular motion. At the start, these points are tender, though discomfort dissipates with steady, firm pressure.

YIELD: 1 SESSION

❓ **How it works:** *Acupressure can help reduce pain and nausea of headaches. Massaging these points regularly may also reduce the frequency of recurrent headaches. According to the ancient Chinese practice of acupressure, the fleshy web part of the hand is an acupoint that lies on a pathway connected to your head. Pressure on that point relieves head pain. Studies comparing the effectiveness of muscle-relaxing drugs with a month of acupressure treatments showed acupressure gave more effective headache relief.*

❗ **Warning:** *Do not stimulate the point in the flesh between your thumb and index finger if you are pregnant, particularly in your last trimester. Doing so may trigger uterine contractions.*

When to Call the Doctor

Seek immediate medical care for the following signs:

- *severe pain, especially if it's unlike anything you've ever experienced*

- *severe headache accompanied by stiff neck and fever*

- *persistent or recurrent headache that seems to becoming worse or more frequent*

- *headache accompanied by other symptoms, such as pain or weakness anywhere in your body or loss of vision, that's not a symptom you have gotten before with a migraine*

- *severe or persistent headache after a head injury (other warning signs include nausea, vomiting, memory loss, and trouble concentrating)*

- *You have a history of high blood pressure or of severe headaches.*

Schedule an appointment for the near future if:

- *You suspect you have never been evaluated for frequent or incapacitating headaches.*

- *You have sinus pain and other signs suggestive of a sinus infection. (See Chapter 55, on sinusitis.)*

Chapter 39

Heart Health

Here's the bad news: Heart disease is the number one killer in America. Now for the good news: Heart disease is largely preventable—and small steps can make a big difference to your heart health. For example, even one hour of physical activity a week in an otherwise sedentary lifestyle is a good start.

The most common heart problem is coronary artery disease (also called coronary heart disease). The coronary arteries encircle the heart, supplying it with oxygen and nutrients and carrying away wastes. Like other arteries in the body, the coronary arteries can become diseased. The usual culprit is atherosclerosis, a condition in which fatty material is deposited within the arterial walls (see page 314). Atherosclerosis impairs circulation to the heart and other tissues in the body and increases blood pressure. The heart now has to pump blood through narrowed, rigid arteries. It's hard work. Like any other overused muscle, the heart hypertrophies, or thickens. Eventually, it starts to give out, leading to congestive heart failure.

The sooner you take steps to protect your heart the better. Here are some ways to have a healthier heart:

- Steer clear of tobacco smoke. Most smokers die not from lung disease but from diseases of the arteries and heart. Smoking increases heart disease risk for a factor of two to four. It decreases the oxygen available to the heart, elevates blood pressure, damages the arteries (including the heart's coronary arteries), and increases blood clotting. If you smoke, talk to your doctor about getting off nicotine.

- Get moving. Sedentary behavior increases heart disease risk. On the other hand, physical activity has multiple cardiovascular benefits. If the weather's inclement, exercise indoors. Try to be physically active at least 30 minutes each day. If you don't have a full half hour, shoot for three 10-minute intervals. You needn't exercise intensely. One study in older women showed that walking and vigorous exercise similarly reduced the risk of cardiovascular events (e.g., angina, heart attack, heart failure, and sudden cardiac death).

- Eat foods that support heart health. Make "strive for five"—five servings of fruit and vegetables daily—your mantra. Consume fish twice a week. If you eat meat, choose lean cuts.

Avoid fried foods and processed foods (most of which are high in sugar and unhealthy fats).

- Cut down on sweets, such as candy, bakery goods, sodas, juices, and other sweetened beverages. Excess sugar drives up blood triglyceride levels, a risk factor for cardiovascular disease.

- Keep to a healthy weight. Being overweight and obesity are key risk factors. If you've tried to lose weight without success, ask your doctor for advice.

- Tame stress. Repeated and prolonged stress increases inflammatory chemicals in the body, elevates blood pressure, and makes platelets stickier—all factors that promote heart attack. In vulnerable people, extreme stress can trigger heart attack, irregular heart rhythm, and sudden cardiac death. (See the recipes "Feel the Gratitude" [page 301] and "Heart-Soothing Pulse Check" [page 303] for easing stress.)

- Get enough sleep. Sleep deprivation raises the risk for heart disease and heart attacks. (See Chapter 46, on insomnia, for tips on sleeping better.)

- Spend time with friends. Social health promotes cardiovascular health.

- Keep regular appointments with your doctor to make sure your blood pressure and cholesterol within normal limits (see Chapters 21 and 42, on cholesterol and high blood pressure).

- Control your blood sugar if you have diabetes. People with diabetes are at much higher risk of developing heart and arterial disease.

- Meet with a therapist if you think you might be depressed, anxious, or are having trouble controlling anger. Heart disease raises the risk for depression and vice versa. Personalities marked by frequent anger and hostility have a risk of heart disease and a heart rhythm disturbance called atrial fibrillation.

History

The technological age has made life less strenuous physically—and people more prone to heart disease. Heart disease was not even described in the medical literature until 1912, and the first heart surgery was not performed until 1938. The arrival of automation meant not only less physical activity but also changes in diet that clogged arteries and led to heart attacks. Food became processed and mass-produced. Rather than eating whole foods, from plants and animals, we dined on foods rich in unhealthy fats, refined grains, and added sugars. This so-called Western diet made us fatter and clogged our arteries. Heart disease became the number one killer.

Lifestyle Tip

When you're feeling stressed, go for a brisk walk, talk to a friend, rethink the situation, or otherwise unburden your heart. Undue stress is hard on the heart. Physical activity, social support, and adjusting your attitude all defuse stress.

Go Fish! Quick Salmon Salad Spread

Use smaller crackers and add capers for a party-perfect recipe—what guest wouldn't want to have a heart-healthy good time?

1 can salmon, drained (6 ounces, or 168 g)

2 tablespoons (20 g) minced red onion

1 tablespoon (15 ml) fresh lemon juice

1½ teaspoons (7.5 ml) olive oil

⅛ teaspoon freshly ground black pepper

2 tablespoons (30 g) low-fat cream cheese

4 large, whole-grain crackers

4 slices tomato

1 large romaine lettuce leaf, cut in half

PREPARATION AND USE:

In a medium-size bowl, combine the salmon, onion, lemon juice, oil, and pepper. Spread the cream cheese on each cracker. Spread the salmon mixture over the cream cheese. Top with tomato and lettuce.

YIELD: 2 SERVINGS

❓ How it works: *Cold-water fish, such as salmon, mackerel, sardines, and herring, contain heart healthy omega-3 fatty acids called DHA (docosahaenoic acid) and EPA (eicosapentae-noic acid). These so-called fish oils decrease inflammation and triglycerides, raise HDL (good) cholesterol, discourage blood from clotting within the arteries, inhibit progression of atherosclerosis, stabilize heart rhythm to reduce the risk of sudden cardiac death, and possibly lower blood pressure. Regular consumption of fish—about two servings a week—correlates with a lower the risk of heart disease. Avoid fried fish, which has the opposite effect.*

Recipe Variation: Substitute two slices of rye or pumpernickel bread halved for the crackers.

 Mediterranean Food-cation

People with exceptional longevity reside in regions called "Blue Zones." One is Sardinia. And one of their secrets to a long, heart-healthy life seems to be diet—both the foods, such as fresh fruit and vegetables, and the leisurely pace of preparing and enjoying them. Eggplant is at its best from August through October, yielding yummy tastes and textures. Don't cut off the skin! It's packed with antioxidants.

1 medium-size eggplant, sliced into 6½-inch (16.5 cm) thick rounds

2 teaspoons (10 ml) olive oil

½ teaspoon salt-free herbal seasoning, divided

2 tablespoons (30 g) store-bought or home-made pesto

¼ teaspoon freshly ground black pepper

PREPARATION AND USE:

Preheat a pan over medium-high heat until hot. Brush both sides of the eggplant slices with the oil. Sprinkle with half of the salt-free seasoning. Cook the eggplant slices for 5 minutes on one side or until browned. Turn and cook for about 3 more minutes or until tender. (You may also roast them in the oven.) Transfer to a plate. Spread each slice with 1 teaspoon (5 g) of pesto and sprinkle with the remaining salt-free seasoning and the pepper.

YIELD: 2 SERVINGS

❓ How it works: *The Mediterranean diet emphasizes vegetables, fruits, legumes, whole grains, and olive oil and minimizes animal foods (which contain cholesterol and saturated fats). Eggplant, a commonly consumed vegetable in this traditional diet, is particularly helpful because it contains viscous fibers that lower cholesterol.*

Several studies have linked the Mediterranean diet with better heart health. A 2013 Spanish study published in the New England Journal of Medicine *assigned people at high risk for cardiovascular disease to a Mediterranean diet with supplemental extra-virgin olive oil, a Mediterranean diet with extra nuts, and a control diet designed to reduce fat intake. At the end of the five-year trial, both Mediterranean diets significantly reduced heart attacks, strokes, and other cardiovascular calamities relative to the reduced-fat diet.*

Fact or Myth?

MEN MORE OFTEN DIE OF HEART DISEASE.

Myth. Heart disease is the number one killer of women and men alike. Women tend to develop symptoms of heart disease later in life—after menopause. But they are more likely to die from a heart attack than men are. A big reason is that atypical warning signs (see "When to Call the Doctor") can masquerade as heartburn or incipient influenza, leading to a delay in treatment.

Resveratrol-Rich Mulled Wine

I use this festive drink throughout the holidays. As guests walk in the door, the scent is as soothing and welcoming as the taste. ~ BHS

1 bottle (1.5 L) red wine
1 tablespoon (7 g) ground cinnamon
1½ teaspoons (3 g) ground cloves
1½ teaspoons (3 g) ground ginger
1½ teaspoons (3 g) ground nutmeg
Grated zest of 1 lemon
Grated zest of 1 orange (Slice and reserve the orange.)
Honey
Extra ground cinnamon, for sprinkling

PREPARATION AND USE:
Place a large pot over low heat. Pour in the wine. Combine the spices and citrus zest in a tea satchel or tie into a piece of cheesecloth and place in the pan. Heat for 30 minutes. Stir in honey to taste. Pour the wine through a strainer into a decanter. Pour into mugs and top with a sprinkling of cinnamon and a slice from the zested orange.

YIELD: ABOUT 8 MUGS

❓ How it works: *Red grapes, purple grape juice, and red wine contain resveratrol and other flavonoids that protect the heart and blood vessels. Some studies have linked moderate alcohol consumption with cardiovascular benefits. However, high amounts of alcohol damage the heart. If you prefer not to drink alcohol at all, you can instead consume resveratrol and other flavonoids in red grapes, berries, and peanuts.*

❗ Warning: *Women should drink no more than one 5-ounce (150 ml) glass of wine; and for men, the limit is two 5-ounce (150 ml) glasses. Always ask your doctor about the limit for you.*

Nut-ritious Salad

I add a mixture of almonds, pecans, and Brazil nuts to this for an extra boost of heart-healthy omega-3s. ~ BHS

1 cup (55 g) torn lettuce or salad mix
1 tangerine, seeded and separated into
   sections
¼ cup (30 g) crushed walnuts
2 tablespoons (14 g) flaxseed meal
¼ cup (60 ml) olive oil
¼ cup (60 ml) balsamic vinegar

PREPARATION AND USE:

In a bowl, combine the lettuce, tangerine sections, and walnuts. Sprinkle in the flaxseeds. Toss. Shake together oil and vinegar and sprinkle over the top. If not using all the dressing, store the rest in the refrigerator.

YIELD: 1 MAIN COURSE SERVING OR 2 SIDE SALAD SERVINGS

❓ How it works: *Walnuts are rich in omega-3 fatty acids and polyphenols (compounds with potent antioxidant and anti-inflammatory effects). Studies have linked consumption of walnuts with a reduced risk of cardiovascular disease. These nuts seem to lower blood cholesterol, reduce inflammation, and improve arterial function. They also have omega-3 fatty acids, as do flaxseeds (and flaxseed oil). The body converts the fatty acids in plants to EPA and DHA.*

10-Minute Miso Soup

This quick meal is short on prep time and long on benefits—it's antiaging, antioxidant, immune-boosting, and full of vitamins. And it's versatile. Slice and dice leftover veggies (onions, carrots, corn, peas, and tomatoes) from the fridge for added nutrition and flavor. It's a warm comfort at the end of a good day's work.

1 quart (946 ml) water
1½ teaspoons (3 g) instant dashi (Japanese
   vegetable stock)
½ cup (124 g) cubed tofu
½ cup (35 g) sliced mushrooms
1 tablespoon (14 g) dried wakame, soaked
   in water
½ cup (125 g) miso paste
2 tablespoons (12 g) chopped scallion

PREPARATION AND USE:

Place a medium-size pot over high heat. Add the water and bring to a boil. Add the dashi and stir to dissolve. Lower the heat to medium-low. Add the tofu and mushrooms. Drain the wakame and add to the pot. Simmer for 2 minutes.

Spoon the miso paste into a bowl. Ladle about ½ cup (120 ml) of hot broth into the bowl and stir until the miso has dissolved and the mixture is smooth.

Turn off the heat (the remaining broth should not be boiling hot or the miso will become mealy). Add the miso mixture to the pot and stir well. Divide the soup among four bowls, top with chopped scallion, and serve immediately.

YIELD: 4 SERVINGS

❓ How it works: *Miso and tofu are both made from soybeans. Both soy products contain chemicals called isoflavones. Research has linked a higher consumption of isoflavones from dietary soy with a reduced risk of heart attack and stroke.*

❗ Warning: *Miso soup may not be the best choice for your meal plan if you monitor your sodium intake, as a 1-cup (235 ml) serving of miso soup contains 382 to 630 milligrams of sodium. The American Heart Association recommends that you limit your daily sodium to 1,500 milligrams or less. Consuming too much sodium regularly may elevate high blood pressure.*

Fact or Myth?

THE FRENCH HAVE MORE HEART DISEASE THAN AMERICANS.

Myth—For years, medical experts puzzled over the "French paradox." Despite consuming a diet high in cholesterol and saturated fat—butter, cheese, rich sauces, meat—French people have lower rates of coronary artery disease (and obesity). The hypothesized secret? Moderate amounts of red wine. That, and French people savor smaller portions than Americans. Don't take this theory as free license to imbibe. High amounts of alcohol can increase blood triglycerides and blood pressure and damage the heart.

🍃 Do the Chai-Chai

In Ayurvedic medicine, chai spices are considered sattvic: they calm, vitalize, and increase mental clarity, all key to stress reduction and heart health.

1 cup (235 ml) water
1 tea bag Darjeeling or other preferred tea
½ teaspoon ground cinnamon
½ teaspoon ground ginger
3 cardamom seeds
3 whole cloves
3 peppercorns
1 teaspoon (7 g) honey, or 1 packet (1 g) stevia
¼ cup (60 ml) nonfat milk

PREPARATION AND USE:

Put the water in a small saucepan. Add the tea bag, spices, and sweetener. Bring to a boil and simmer for 2 minutes. Add the milk. Strain the tea into a teapot.

YIELD: 1 SERVING

❓ How it works: *Studies have linked regular consumption of green and black tea with a lower risk of cardiovascular disease. Consumption of tea, whether it's green or black, benefits the heart and arteries. Cardamom, ginger, and cloves decrease platelet stickiness. (Platelets are blood cell fragments that form clots. When blood clots develop within the coronary arteries or brain arteries, heart attack or stroke develops.) Pepper contains piperine, which lab studies show lowers blood pressure. In one study involving the addition of dietary cinnamon in people with diabetes, cinnamon decreased blood levels of glucose (sugar) and cholesterol, both of which are risk factors for heart disease. In a subsequent study, only glucose significantly declined.*

● Feel the Gratitude

I first learned about HeartMath from a student working in a cardiac rehabilitation center. A central idea of HeartMath is that slow, deep breathing and positive feelings, such as gratitude, reduce stress and improve heart health. Research backs up those tenets. ~ LBW

A quiet room
Your imagination

PREPARATION AND USE:

Find a comfortable seated position. Let your eyelids fall. Think of something you feel grateful for or happy about. Notice how you are feeling. Imagine those positive feelings pulsing out from your heart so others can feel them.

YIELD: 1 SESSION

❷ How it works: *Healthy hearts exhibit significant heart rate variability, meaning the pulse normally varies subtly with respiration—slower with inhalation and faster with exhalation. Loss of heart rate variability, as can happen with chronic stress, is a risk factor for heart disease. Meditation, laughter, and slow, deep breathing improve heart rate variability. Studies show that positive emotions such as gratitude also improve heart rate variability.*

Note: The heart generates electromagnetic energy in pulses, which is what an electrocardiogram (ECG) measures. Some people believe you and others can feel them.

When Simple Doesn't Work

At your annual physical, talk to your doctor about your heart-healthy routine. If you follow a healthy lifestyle through good diet, exercise, and personal relationships (see Part 1 of this book), yet feel fatigued or have reduced ability to exert yourself, your doctor may prescribe a series of tests such as stress test, echocardiogram (echo), or electrocardiograpm (EKG).

Lifestyle Tip

Drink a cup (235 ml) of pomegranate juice or sprinkle the fleshy arils on salads and whole-grain cereals. Research indicates that drinking the juice and eating the fruit protects against cardiovascular disease. In people who already have coronary artery disease, drinking a cup a day for three months improved stress-induced reductions in blood flow to the heart.

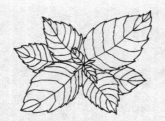

Spotlight: **Green Tea**

Green tea—which comes from the *Camellia sinensis* shrub, just as black and oolong teas do—is currently receiving much attention as an antidote to cardiovascular disease. The difference between green, black, and oolong teas lies in the processing.

Black and oolong tea are allowed to oxidize, which changes the chemical composition. A soon as the leaves are picked, green tea is steamed to prevent the leaves from oxidizing. This allows green tea to retain greater amounts of naturally occurring chemicals called catechins, a special type of flavonoid with multiple health benefits. For example, green tea catechins are antioxidant, which means they counter the tissue-damaging free radicals that contribute to aging and most chronic illnesses.

The number one chronic illness in America is heart disease. Green tea reduces several cardiovascular risk factors. Some studies suggest it improves cholesterol profiles, lowers blood sugar levels, and helps maintain healthy body weight. Furthermore, studies link regular green tea consumption with a lower risk of heart attack and stroke. Preliminary research suggests a reduction in diabetes as well. Regular consumption of green tea offers a number of additional benefits:

- lowers the risk of bladder, esophageal, ovarian, pancreatic, and possibly breast and prostate cancer
- protects the nervous system
- sharpens concentration and alertness
- helps prevent or delay the onset of Parkinson's disease
- may inhibit a toxic protein called beta-amyloid thought to underlie Alzheimer's
- reduces dental plaque and gingivitis
- increases bone mineral density
- promotes the growth of healthy bacteria in the intestines
- heals genital warts (a special green tea extract ointment applied topically)
- helps heal sunburn and protect against skin cancer

As with most things, more is not better. Three to five 8-ounce (235 ml) cups of tea a day is sufficient. Higher amounts may cause stomach upset and jitteriness (the latter because of the caffeine content). Also concentrated green tea extracts (such as those used in weight-loss products) have been linked to liver injury.

Heart-Soothing Pulse Check

When I'm feeling stressed or having trouble relaxing into sleep, I find that becoming aware of my heartbeat grounds me. I close my eyes and picture my heart beating slowly, steadily, and strongly. ~ LBW

You

PREPARATION AND USE:

Sit in a chair. Find your pulse: Good locations are on the thumb side of your inner wrist and in the neck just below the angle of the jaw. Count the number of heartbeats inside of 15 seconds. Multiply the number by four to calculate the beats per minute.

Close your eyes. Straighten your spine so that the back of your head, shoulders, and sacrum line up. Rest your palms on your thighs.

Inhale slowly for a count of four, pause, and then exhale slowly for a count of six. Notice how your collarbones and ribs rise and your abdomen moves outward with deep inhalation, then fall with exhalation. Repeat ten times. Check your pulse again.

YIELD: 1 SESSION

❷ **How it works:** *This complete relaxation slows your heart rate and helps lower blood pressure, which lowers strain on the heart. Long-term stress elevates blood pressure, which strains the heart and also sets the stage for atherosclerosis. Eventually, the normal heart-rate variability is lost.*

Note: Unless you were already very relaxed, this activity probably slowed your heart rate.

When to Call the Doctor

If you or someone else develops any symptoms suggestive of an impending heart attack, do not take a chance. Immediately dial 911. Remember: Minutes matter. While awaiting the ambulance, chew a 325-milligram tablet of aspirin, and then wash it down with water. Doing so helps discourage blood clots from forming within the coronary arteries.

Warning signs of a heart attack include:

- *discomfort in the center of the chest that lasts more than a few minutes or that goes away and comes back—It can be uncomfortable pressure, squeezing, fullness, or pain.*

- *unexplained shortness of breath, even if it appears without chest discomfort*

- *discomfort or pain in one or both arms, the neck, jaw, back, or stomach*

- *other signs: cold sweats, nausea, or lightheadedness.*

Chapter 40

Heartburn and Gastritis

Fourteen to 20 percent of American adults have at least occasional heartburn. The medical name, gastroesophageal reflux disease (GERD), describes the basic problem—a backwash of acidic stomach contents into the esophagus. Normally, a band of muscle at the end of the esophagus (the lower esophageal sphincter) prevents this reverse movement. Thanks to that sphincter, most people can eat and stand on their head without heartburn.

The causes of GERD include laxity of the lower esophageal sphincter, slow emptying of the stomach, obesity, and hiatal hernia (a condition whereby the upper stomach slides above the diaphragm, a dome of muscle that normally separates the lungs from the stomach and intestines). Pregnant women may develop heartburn due to the pressure exerted by the developing fetus.

The typical symptoms of GERD, usually worse after meals, are burning pain behind the breastbone and occasional nausea. Reflux that occurs during the night can fracture sleep (even when people aren't aware of the burning). If acidic material ascends high enough, it can cause coughing, sore throat, hoarseness, dental erosion, and worsened asthma.

After a doctor diagnoses GERD, he or she will usually recommend lifestyle modifications. Two important strategies are eating smaller meals and staying upright for a few hours after eating. People can also elevate the head of the bed 4 to 6 inches (10 to 15 cm) by slipping blocks or large books under the mattress. Although sleeping on a second pillow keeps the head elevated, in back sleepers, that position can compress the abdomen, causing reflux.

Because excess abdominal fat creates pressure against the stomach, causing reflux, doctors recommend their overweight patients slim down. Studies show that weight loss can resolve GERD. In addition, stay away from tobacco smoke, which worsens GERD.

History

Presidents (Clinton and Bush 2), famous football players (including John Elway), and singer Celine Dion, among others, have reportedly suffered from heartburn. Although the fast-food, stressed-out American culture may aggravate the condition, even the ancients suffered from it.

Around 200 CE, Roman physician Galen coined the term *heartburn*, noting that the condition often mimicked diseases of the heart. Remedies have included teas made from chamomile grown in monastery gardens of the Middle Ages and the tissue-coating licorice root extracts and slippery elm bark teas used by Native Americans and early settlers. Modern herbalists still recommend these herbs.

In 1958, physicians identified acid as the agent that caused the burning sensation associated with acid reflux. Since the 1990s, proton pump inhibitors, such as Prilosec and Nexium, which reduce gastric acid production, have also been used to treat GERD. While these drugs are useful, potential side effects include deficiencies in magnesium and vitamin B_{12} kidney inflammation, stomach cancer, bone fractures, intestinal infections, and pneumonia.

Fact or Myth?

PEOPLE WITH GERD SHOULD AVOID PEPPERMINT AND SPEARMINT.

Myth. Although it's true that mint relaxes the lower esophageal sphincter, it also relaxes the pyloric sphincter, the band of muscle between the stomach and small intestine. In that way, mint increases the emptying of stomach contents into the small intestine. Furthermore, mint has not been shown to worsen GERD symptoms.

RECIPES TO PREVENT AND TREAT HEARTBURN

Lemon Zesty Squash

Zesting requires care: This part of the lemon—the outermost skin—has a zingy citrus flavor without being bitter. Breaking into the white pith just below will bring out the bitterness.

2 large organic lemons, washed and dried
1 tablespoon (15 ml) olive oil
1½ teaspoons (8 ml) fresh lemon juice
⅛ teaspoon freshly ground black pepper
2 cups (240 g) chopped zucchini
¼ cup (10 g) chopped fresh basil
1½ tablespoons (6 g) crushed fresh oregano

PREPARATION AND USE:

With a lemon grater or zester, zest (remove the outermost skin) the lemons; set aside.

In a small bowl, whisk together the olive oil, lemon juice, and pepper. Set aside.

Steam the zucchini for about 10 minutes until tender but still firm. Drain and transfer to a serving bowl while still warm. Drizzle the oil mixture over it. Add lemon zest, basil, and oregano and toss. Serve warm.

YIELD: 4 SERVINGS

❓ **How it works:** *Citrus peels contain D-limonene, a naturally occurring chemical that provides the characteristic flavor and fragrance. Taking limonene as a supplement has been shown to reduce heartburn. Exactly how it works isn't known. Limonene may protect the esophagus from stomach acids and increase normal motility of the esophagus.*

When Simple Doesn't Work

Melatonin, better known as a hormone that regulates sleep, also affects the gut. Some of the effects protect the esophagus, stimulate the lower esophageal sphincter to contract, and diminish stomach acidity. Animal studies show melatonin protects the esophagus from the harmful effects of stomach acid. However, human studies of using melatonin for this purpose are preliminary. As mentioned earlier, one study found that a product containing melatonin and other natural supplements more effectively relieved GERD symptoms than did the drug omeprazole (Prilosec). Discuss melatonin supplementation with your doctor first, especially if you're taking medications.

Mild symptoms of GERD may be relieved by over-the-counter antacids. The Food and Drug Administration has approved some H2 blockers (a type of acid-decreasing medication) for over-the-counter use for up to two weeks. For more severe conditions, doctors typically prescribe a different type of acid-blocking medication called proton pump inhibitors.

In addition to relieving symptoms, the goal is to prevent the damaging effects of re-fluxed stomach acids, such as sore throat, damage to tooth enamel, and esophageal inflammation (which, over the long term, can scar and even cause cancer in the esophagus).

 # E-ssential Breakfast

This delicious mix contains vitamin E and plant chemicals to stave off stomach acid.

1 tablespoon (15 ml) canola oil
1 medium-size sweet onion, diced
1 block (14 ounces, or 390 g) firm tofu, cut into small cubes
1 cup (100 g) pitted and sliced black olives
⅛ teaspoon turmeric
⅛ teaspoon freshly ground black pepper
1 tablespoon (3 g) chopped fresh basil
2 tablespoons (18 g) sunflower seeds

PREPARATION AND USE:

Heat the oil in a skillet over medium heat. Braise the onion until tender and translucent. Stir in the tofu and olives and continue to cook, stirring and sprinkling with the turmeric and pepper, 5 to 7 minutes. Remove from the heat and toss in the basil and sunflower seeds. Serve.

YIELD: 4 SERVINGS

❓ **How it works:** *Turmeric contains the anti-inflammatory and antioxidant compound curcumin. In lab experiments, curcumin reduces esophageal inflammation. The outer rings and peel of onion contain the flavonoid quercetin. Quercetin combined with the vitamin E—found in canola oil, sunflower seeds, and olives—has been shown in experiments to reduce stomach acid and esophageal inflammation.*

Oatmeal and Slippery Elm Porridge

The inner bark of the slippery elm has been used as a traditional treatment for gastrointestinal flare-ups.

1 cup (235 ml) water
½ cup (40 g) rolled oats
¼ cup (about 13 g) slippery elm bark powder
¼ teaspoon ground cinnamon
Honey, stevia, or agave nectar

PREPARATION AND USE:
Boil the water in a saucepan. Add the oats, slippery elm bark powder, and cinnamon. Stir until the oatmeal is cooked, adding more water as needed. Sweeten to taste.

YIELD: 1 TO 2 SERVINGS

❷ **How it works:** *Slippery elm and oatmeal are anti-inflammatory and soothing to irritated mucous membranes—in this case, those lining the lower esophagus. In addition to containing mucilaginous substances, slippery elm can stimulate gastrointestinal mucus secretion. (Mucus coats and protects all mucous membranes.) You can find powdered slippery elm in natural food stores.*

Chamomile, Peppermint, and Licorice Tea

1½ cups (355 ml) water

1 teaspoon (1 g) dried chamomile flowers or the contents of a chamomile tea bag

1 teaspoon (1 g) dried peppermint leaves

¼ teaspoon licorice root, or ¼ teaspoon aniseeds or fennel seeds

PREPARATION AND USE:

Boil the water in a saucepan. Turn off the heat. Add the herbs. Cover and steep 20 minutes. Strain and sip.

YIELD: 1 TO 2 SERVINGS

❓ How it works: *Chamomile, peppermint, and licorice relieve symptoms of indigestion. Chamomile and licorice are anti-inflammatory. Peppermint speeds emptying of the stomach and reduces pain. Do not use licorice daily for more than two weeks. Long-term use can cause water retention, lower potassium, and elevate blood pressure. Occasional use is fine. If you have high blood pressure or take a diuretic, use anise or fennel instead.*

When to Call the Doctor

- *You have yet to be evaluated for heartburn and have symptoms more than twice a week.*

- *You develop signs of extension of reflux to your throat and mouth (sore throat, sinusitis, or loss of tooth enamel).*

- *Acid reflux causes you to awaken repeatedly during the night.*

- *You develop severe pain in your upper abdomen.*

- *You vomit blood or material that resembles coffee grounds.*

- *You aren't sure whether your chest pain is from heartburn or a heart attack. The pain of heartburn tends to be sharp and burning; heart attack more often causes a feeling of chest tightness and pressure, as well as dizziness, sweating, and shortness of breath. However, the two can be difficult to distinguish. If you suspect a heart attack, dial 911.*

Chapter

41

Hemorrhoids

Hemorrhoids are commonplace and generally benign, which doesn't make them any less of a nuisance. They are varicose (widened) veins in the anus and rectum. Anything that increases pressure within these veins can cause them: pregnancy, straining due to constipation, chronic cough, and chronic liver disease.

Internal hemorrhoids lie within the rectum. A common sign is the presence of small amounts of bright red blood with a bowel movement. The swollen veins may sag outside the anus. External hemorrhoids appear under the skin at the anus. In addition to bleeding when passing stool, these can cause pain, especially if a clot forms within one. Anal itching occurs when hemorrhoids interfere with hygiene, though the symptom can also indicate allergies, parasites, and other conditions.

Treatment involves correcting the underlying cause, easing the discomfort of hemorrhoids with topical ointments, and, when needed, minor surgery. For tips on resolving constipation, refer to page 183.

History

Rumor has it that Napoleon Bonaparte, Karl Marx, Marilyn Monroe, and Jimmy Carter suffered from hemorrhoids. But they are by no means a modern malady. One of the oldest discomforts known to humans, hemorrhoids have been treated by many cultures, including the Babylonians who described them in 2250 BCE. The Egyptians applied poultices of dried acacia leaves. The ancient Greek physician Hippocrates used several methods, including a hot iron to burn the hemorrhoid off. A Roman remedy called for two dove or pigeon eggs, boiled and piping hot, inserted into the anus. A gentler seventh-century method was to pray to St. Fiacre, the patron saint of hemorrhoids. In the twentieth century, several approaches became common, including dietary modification; nonsurgical methods, such as rubber-band ligation (to cut off blood supply to the hemorrhoid); and in severe cases, surgical removal.

Fiber-Up Bran Muffins

1 cup (80 g) uncooked multigrain hot cereal
1 tablespoon (12 g) flaxseeds
1 cup (125 g) all-purpose flour
1 tablespoon (14 g) baking powder
½ teaspoon baking soda
½ teaspoon salt
½ teaspoon ground cinnamon
2 tablespoons (6 g) stevia powder
1 banana, mashed
½ cup (125 g) applesauce
½ cup (120 ml) almond milk
2 large eggs
¼ cup (60 ml) olive oil
1 teaspoon (5 ml) vanilla extract
½ cup (55 g) chopped pecans
Honey, for serving (optional)

PREPARATION AND USE:

Preheat the oven to 350°F (180°C, or gas mark 4).

Mix together all the dry ingredients in a large bowl. Add the banana, applesauce, almond milk, eggs, oil, and vanilla. Stir until the batter is moist and thick. Stir in the pecans. Place twelve muffin liners in a muffin tin. Spoon the batter evenly into each cup.

Bake for about 15 minutes or until the muffins are golden brown. Do not overbake. Serve warm with honey.

YIELD: 12 MUFFINS

❓ How it works: *Constipation and hard stools passing through the anus contribute to hemorrhoids. A diet rich with fiber from bran, fruit, and vegetable sources, with plenty of water, helps get you regular and allows easy, nonaggravating passage.*

🥄 Horse Chestnut Soother

1 cup (235 ml) water
1 teaspoon (4 g) dried horse chestnut seeds (see note)

PREPARATION AND USE:

Boil the water. Add the seeds and simmer for 15 minutes. Allow the tea to cool. Soak a piece of clean gauze or cloth in the mixture and apply to irritated tissue as needed.

YIELD: 1 SET OF APPLICATIONS

❓ How it works: *Horse chestnut seed extract is a traditional treatment for varicose veins and hemorrhoids. Constituents are anti-inflammatory, astringent, and a tonic to veins, which reduces swelling and bleeding. Multiple studies show special extracts taken by mouth and applied topically reduce a condition called chronic venous insufficiency.*

⚠ Warning: *Do not consume the above recipe. Without special processing, horse chestnut seeds can be toxic when taken internally.*

Note: Dried horse chestnut seeds are available online or at natural food stores.

Lifestyle Tip

A dab of petroleum jelly on hemorrhoids can protect them from irritation. It's an ingredient in many commercially prepared hemorrhoid treatments.

Lemon Relief

1 cup (235 ml) warm water
3 tablespoons (45 ml) fresh lemon juice

PREPARATION AND USE:

Mix the lemon juice into the warm water and drink first thing in the morning.

YIELD: 1 SERVING

 How it works: *Lemons contain flavonoids, plant pigments with health benefits. Flavonoids act as antioxidants (thus protecting the blood vessel linings from free radical damage) and promote formation of collagen (a protein found in blood vessels, skin, and many other tissues). They also have an astringent (contracting) effect on blood vessels. A glass of warm water with lemon juice first thing in the morning may also stimulate bowel activity.*

Fact or Myth?

STRAINING WHILE ON THE TOILET IS USUALLY NECESSARY WHEN RELIEVING YOURSELF.

Myth. People in a hurry often strain, which puts pressure on the veins in the lower rectum and contributes to hemorrhoids. Make a routine for yourself where you set aside time for a daily movement without rushing.

Lifestyle Tip

In the shower, cleanse your anus gently with warm water and mild soap. Afterward, gently pat the area dry or dry gently with a blow-dryer on low. Doing so will inhibit bacteria from becoming trapped in hemorrhoids and thereby decrease itching.

Very Berry Orange Fruit Salad

This fresh and easy recipe includes the bilberry, a cousin to the blueberry that is chock-full of antioxidants—and flavor.

1 cup (145 g) blueberries, divided
1 teaspoon (5 g) Dijon mustard
1 tablespoon (15 g) grapeseed or canola oil
Juice of 1 lemon wedge
¼ cup (30 g) dried bilberries
½ cup (85 g) sliced strawberries
1 orange, peeled, sectioned, and seeded
1 celery stalk, diced
½ cup (60 g) chopped walnuts
2 cups (60 g) baby spinach, rinsed and drained

PREPARATION AND USE:

Blend half of the blueberries with the mustard, oil, and lemon juice in blender for an easy dressing; set aside.

Mix together the remaining berries in a large bowl. Toss the orange sections, celery, and walnuts into the berries. Spread a spinach base on two plates. Divide the fruit salad evenly between each plate and top with the blueberry dressing.

YIELD: 2 SERVINGS

(Continued)

❓ How it works: *Fruit provides fiber to promote bowel regularity. Berries and citrus fruits are rich in flavonoids, which help maintain the health of blood vessels, increase the tone of veins, and decrease inflammation. Anthocyanidins, a subtype of flavonoid with particular vascular benefits, create the red, blue, and purple in these berries. A concentrated flavonoid product containing the citrus flavonoid hesperidin has been shown successful in reducing signs and symptoms of varicose veins and hemorrhoids. Special extracts of bilberries, a near relative of blueberry, help improve chronic venous problems.*

Note: Bilberries are native to Europe and generally not available fresh in the United States. You can buy them from online retailers and local herb shops. They're not as juicy as many other dried berries. Sample a few before first to see how you like them. Alternatively, just double the blueberries in this recipe.

🍃 Witch Hazel Soothing Wipe

1 teaspoon (5 ml) witch hazel

PREPARATION AND USE:
Moisten facial or toilet tissue with the witch hazel and gently wipe the affected area.

YIELD: 1 APPLICATION

❓ How it works: *Witch hazel is high in flavonoids and tannins. The former help maintain blood vessels, reduce inflammation, and inhibit enzymes that degrade the architecture of veins. The latter have an astringent (tightening) effect.*

Note: You can find witch hazel decoctions (water extracts) in most pharmacies.

🍃 Salty Sitz Bath

½ cup (144 g) salt

PREPARATION AND USE:
Run a warm bath and mix in the salt. Sit for 15 minutes, three times a day. Pat dry afterward.

YIELD: 1 APPLICATION

❓ How it works: *The warm, salty water relieves congestion in the pelvic circulation and reduces inflammation.*

Note: If you don't have a bathtub, you can find a sitz bath at most drugstores. This simply fits over the toilet and you sit in it to bathe the anal area.

When Simple Doesn't Work

- *Several studies show that commercial horse chestnut extract taken internally and applied externally reduces varicose veins. (In oral preparations, processing of the horse chestnut seeds' toxic chemicals are removed and the seeds' active chemicals are concentrated.) A French study showed improvement in hemorrhoids.*

- *You can buy rubber or air-filled "doughnuts" at pharmacies to sit on for comfort.*

Cold Comfort

3 ice cubes

PREPARATION AND USE:

Crush the ice cubes, put in a resealable plastic bag, and seal. Wrap the bag in a clean washcloth. Lie in a comfortable position and apply to the anal area for 15 minutes. Apply in the morning and again at night.

YIELD: 1 APPLICATION

❓ **How it works:** *Ice is among the most effective ways to reduce swelling and inflammation.*

 # Legs-up-the-Wall Pose

You
A wall

PREPARATION AND USE:

Start by lying with one side against a wall. Tuck your knees toward your chest, swivel your buttocks 90 degrees toward the wall, and extend your legs skyward. Your objective is to end up lying on your back with your legs up the wall and your buttocks close to the wall's base.

If that maneuver is awkward, lie on your back at a 90-degree angle to the wall and scoot closer until your buttocks are near the base of the wall. Straighten your legs as far as you can comfortably go.

Breathe slowly, noticing how your belly rises and falls. Stay with your legs elevated for 10 to 15 minutes.

YIELD: 1 SESSION

❓ **How it works:** *Elevating your legs reduces pressure in the veins in the lower body. This pose is also very relaxing, particularly after a busy day.*

Note: If this posture is difficult, try lying on your back with your legs bent over the seat of a chair. More simply, you can lie on your back and slide a bolster (or sofa cushion) under your legs.

Lifestyle Tip

Use moistened toilet paper or baby wipes to clean the affected area instead of dry paper, which has a tendency to irritate.

When to Call the Doctor

- *You experience bleeding with a bowel movement. Make sure something other than hemorrhoids is not causing the bleeding.*

- *You notice increased pain. You may have developed an infection or a blood clot within a hemorrhoid or other problem requiring medical extent.*

- *A hemorrhoid extends beyond the anus and cannot be gently pushed back in.*

Chapter 42

High Blood Pressure

It's dubbed the "silent killer" for good reason. This sneaky disease exhibits no signs or symptoms until significant damage is done. The first sign might be a heart attack or stroke—the leading causes of death in the United States. Some 65 million Americans have high blood pressure, or hypertension.

The rate is particularly high in African Americans. One study found that the rate of hypertension was nearly 48 percent in blacks versus 31 percent in whites. Furthermore, despite comparable treatment, blood pressure less often returned to normal in African Americans. Different ethnic groups may respond differently to blood pressure–lowering medications.

Blood pressure has two readings, measured in millimeters of mercury (abbreviated "mm Hg"). The top number reflects systolic pressure—the highest pressure, reached when the heart contracts. The bottom number reflects diastolic pressure—the lowest pressure just before the heart contracts again. Ideally, systolic pressure is lower than 120 mm Hg and diastolic pressure is lower than 80 mm Hg. Prehypertension is defined as a systolic blood pressure between 120 and 139 or diastolic blood pressure between 80 and 89 mm Hg. The threshold for hypertension starts at 140 systolic, 90 diastolic.

Hypertension damages arteries and taxes the heart. Pressure in the arteries comes from the force of the heart's contraction, the volume of blood, and the narrowness and stiffness of the arteries. With age, arteries lose elasticity. Atherosclerosis, a condition marked by fatty deposits in the arterial walls, can both cause and result from hypertension. Other consequences of hypertension can be heart disease, stroke, kidney damage, and vision-robbing eye disease.

Lifestyle changes can help lower blood pressure. They include reducing dietary salt, eating a plant-based diet, quitting smoking, exercising regularly, losing excess weight, and managing stress.

Doctors also prescribe medications: diuretics to increase loss of water in urine, beta blockers to slow the heart, and other medications aimed at dilating the arteries. If you're taking a prescription medication to lower blood pressure, do not stop—not without a discussion with your doctor. None of the following remedies is intended as a substitute for standard medical care.

History

For millennia, healers felt pulses and listened to hearts by pressing an ear to their patients' chest. The stethoscope became available in the middle of the nineteenth century. The sphygmomanometer—an instrument for measuring blood pressure—finally became available at the close of that century. Until then, doctors had no way to measure blood pressure.

Fact or Myth?

EXERCISE REDUCES BLOOD PRESSURE.

Fact. Studies show that regular qigong practice lowers blood pressure. Pronounced chee gung, this moving meditation takes practitioners through a series of rhythmic movements and breathing techniques. Participants inhale as they lift their arms and exhale as the arms fall. The National Center of Complementary and Alternative Medicine website has videos on qigong and a similar Asian practice called tai chi at http://nccam.nih.gov/video/taichiDVD.

Hibiscus Cooler

5 cups (1.2 L) water
½ cup (72 g) dried hibiscus calyces
1 cup (235 ml) pure pomegranate or cranberry juice
Juice of ½ lemon

PREPARATION AND USE:

Boil the water in a nonreactive (enamel or stainless-steel) pot. Remove from the heat. Add the dried hibiscus. Cover and steep for 15 minutes. Strain. Add the pomegranate and lemon juices. Drink warm or cold.

YIELD: 4 SERVINGS

❓ How it works: *Studies show simply drinking tart, delicious hibiscus tea lowers blood pressure in people with prehypertension and moderate hypertension. One study found that hibiscus tea (consumed before breakfast for four weeks) compared favorably to the blood-pressure-lowering medication captopril. Regular consumption of hibiscus tea also lowers LDL cholesterol and triglycerides (blood fats) and raises HDL (good) cholesterol. Both pomegranate and cranberry can lower blood pressure. All of these plants are rich in antioxidant and cardiovascular-protecting plant compounds called flavonoids.*

Note: Pomegranate juice is naturally sweet. If you use cranberry juice, which is very tart, add honey or agave nectar to taste.

The calyx in hibiscus forms a cup under the petals. You can find dried hibiscus in bulk in some natural food stores and in Mexican food stores, where they may be sold as "flores de Jamaica."

Heart-Healthy Cocoa Smoothie

Incorporating small amounts of cocoa or dark chocolate into your daily diet can protect your heart and blood vessels.

1 large banana
1 cup (235 ml) almond milk
2 to 3 (10 to 15 g) tablespoons unsweetened cocoa powder
1 tablespoon (20 g) honey or agave
1 teaspoon (2 g) flaxseeds

PREPARATION AND USE:
Combine all the ingredients in a blender or food processor and blend until smooth. Enjoy!

YIELD: 1 TO 2 SERVINGS

❓ **How it works:** *Chocolate and cocoa power come from dried beans of the cacao tree. The flavonoids in chocolate and cocoa reduce blood pressure—the darker the chocolate, the higher the flavonoids. Cocoa powder also contains fiber, which can help curb cholesterol, as do the flax seeds.*

Lifestyle Tip

Visualize! Close your eyes and imagine the dial on a blood pressure cuff slowly falling. Studies show that guided imagery (thoughts and images that evoke calm) and biofeedback (a technique that allows people to see changes in such measurements as heart rate and blood pressure with relaxation) lower blood pressure.

Go Fish! Hors d'Oeuvre

In our household, when Dad opened a can of sardines, it was a special occasion. They were delicious doled out on simple saltines. Little did we know that we were keeping our blood pressure in check. ~ BBG

1 can (8- to 12-count) oil-packed sardines
12 to 16 whole-grain crackers
Lemon wedges
Sprigs of parsley

PREPARATION AND USE:
Spread each cracker with a half sardine. Squeeze lemon juice on top. Add parsley to garnish. Enjoy!

YIELD: 4 SERVINGS

❓ **How it works:** *The omega-3 fatty acids in fish oil have been shown to reduce blood pressure in people with mild hypertension, mainly from fatty fish, such as mackerel and salmon. Sardines are at the top of the list.*

Spice it, Don't Salt it

Have fun finding new tastes that lead you away from salt, the intake of which can boost blood pressure. These delectable alternatives sprinkled on your favorite dishes will help curb your salt cravings. Experiment with different flavors. Be bold!

Try cayenne pepper, coriander, black pepper, nutmeg, parsley, cumin, cilantro, ginger, rosemary, marjoram, thyme, tarragon, garlic or onion powder, bay leaf, oregano, dry mustard, or dill.

PREPARATION AND USE:
Use your seasoning of choice in recipes or over foods in place of salt. In addition to being salt-free, many of these options, such as garlic and ginger, benefit your heart and circulation.

YIELD: 1 SERVING

How it works: *In ancient times, salt (sodium chloride) was so valuable people used it for currency. Needless to say, people use salt sparingly to season and preserve food. Because most processed foods are laden in salt, modern humans consume more than is good for them. Whereas people once consumed about 100 milligrams a day of sodium, the current sodium average intake has soared to 3,400 milligrams (8.5 grams), far exceeding the American Heart Association's recommended cap of 1,500 milligrams (less than 1 teaspoon [6 g]) a day. Extra sodium attracts extra water in the vascular system, which then raises blood volume and, therefore, blood pressure. African Americans tend to be especially sensitive to salt.*

Substituting salt with herbs and spices makes food taste great and benefits heart health. Multiple studies show that reducing salt intake lowers blood pressure. A 2010 analysis published in the Annals of Internal Medicine *estimated that if the food industry reduced average sodium intake by 9.5 percent, the United States would save $32.1 million on medical costs—not to mention lives otherwise lost to heart attack and stroke. In the meantime, read food labels for sodium content.*

Lifestyle Tip

It's best to poach, bake, broil, or sauté your fish in a little olive oil or broth. Grilling, as tasty as it is, generates carcinogens. And deep-frying oils aren't healthy to begin with—worse, high heat oxides oils.

Veggie Bake with Olive Oil and Garlic

Your customized veggie combinations deliver great taste and healthy benefits.

3 tablespoons (45 ml) olive oil, divided
Any vegetables in your fridge (about 3 cups, or 680 g), chopped
1 teaspoon (3 g) minced fresh garlic
1 can (14 ounces, or 400 g) low-sodium, chopped tomatoes, drained
1 can (14 ounces, or 400 g) chickpeas, drained and rinsed
Salt-free seasonings, such as coriander, cayenne, parsley, or tarragon
2 zucchini, sliced into thin sheets

PREPARATION AND USE:
Preheat the oven to 350°F (180°C, or gas mark 4). Place 2 tablespoons (30 ml) of the olive oil in a large skillet over medium heat and add the chopped veggies and garlic. Sauté for about 5 minutes. Add the tomatoes and chickpeas and mix to combine. Add your choice of salt-free seasonings to taste. Remove from the heat.

Spread the remaining tablespoon (15 ml) of olive oil on the bottom of an 8-inch (20 cm) square baking dish. Cover with a layer of zucchini. Spread the sautéed mixture evenly across the zucchini base. Add a layer of zucchini on the top. Sprinkle with oil. Bake for 30 minutes.

YIELD: 6 SERVINGS

How it works: *The American Heart Association recommends a diet high in vegetables, legumes, and fruit and low in salt and animal foods. Studies show that a plant-based, Mediterranean diet with liberal amounts of olive oil reduces age-related blood pressure. Other studies show that garlic can modestly reduce blood pressure.*

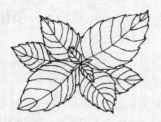

Spotlight: **Chocolate**

Chocolate and cocoa come from the fruit, cacao beans, of the *Theobroma cacao* tree. Traced to as early as 1400 BCE in Latin America, chocolate was likely first consumed as a bitter drink called *xoacatl*, brewed from cacao beans. Ancient Maya and Aztecs believed cacao it had magical powers, so sipping it was mainly for royalty, hence the name "food of the Gods." When the Spanish invaded the Americas in the 1500s, they "discovered" cacao. In 1544, Mayan nobility brought cacao with them on a visit to the Spanish court.

For centuries, people relished chocolate as a "sinful" treat. The medical profession demonized it as unhealthy. Researchers have shown that the right kind of chocolate has plenty of life-promoting properties. What's the right kind? We're talking cocoa powder or dark chocolate, labeled as having 70 or 80 percent cocoa content.

Cocoa powder is made by grinding the cacao beans and removing the cocoa butter. Look for pure cocoa powder. Chocolate is made from chocolate liquor, sugar, cocoa butter, plus or minus other ingredients. Compared to dark chocolate, milk chocolate contains fewer cocoa solids (about 30 percent) plus powdered and condensed milk.

Those cocoa solids contain flavonols—plant polyphenols that have strong anti-inflammatory and antioxidant properties. Flavonols help improve circulation, lower blood pressure, and reduce the risk of heart disease.

One study of 30,000 women in Sweden showed that eating one to two 1-ounce (28 g) servings a week of dark chocolate high in cocoa content was linked with a 32 percent lower risk of women developing heart failure. Frequently eating small servings of dark chocolate helps reduce blood pressure and lowers the risk of stroke. Here's a buying guide for chocolate:

- Look for a product high in nonfat cocoa solids. The higher the content, the greater the flavonols and their antioxidant power.

- Natural cocoa powder or unsweetened baking chocolate have the highest flavonol levels. Put it back if you see bad fats listed, such as partially hydrogenated vegetable oil or palm oil.

- Curb your chocolate consumption. A 2-ounce (55 g) serving contains about 300 calories.

Blueberry and Banana Smoothie

1 ripe banana
¾ cup (109 g) fresh or (116 g) frozen blueberries
¾ cup (175 ml) pomegranate juice or almond or nonfat soy milk
Pinch of ground cinnamon

PREPARATION AND USE:

Combine all the ingredients, except the cinnamon, in a blender and blend until smooth. Sprinkle with the cinnamon. Serve.

YIELD: 1 TO 2 SERVINGS

❓ How it works: *Bananas are a rich source of potassium. Taking potassium has been shown to reduce blood pressure. Supplementation may be particularly helpful for people who normally consume too much salt and relatively too little potassium (most Americans) and also for African Americans. Also, diuretics can rob the body of potassium. Blueberries lower blood pressure. Their color comes from potent flavonoids that protect cholesterol from oxidation and maintain the health of blood vessels. A pinch of cinnamon, high in fiber, is an anticholesterol perk.*

Depressurizing Tonic

For an extra punch, Linda substitutes hibiscus tea for the liquid in this recipe.

2 teaspoons (10 ml) apple cider vinegar
1 cup (235 ml) water or pomegranate juice

PREPARATION AND USE:

Mix the vinegar and liquid. Drink the tonic once a day.

YIELD: 1 APPLICATION

❓ How it works: *Apple cider vinegar, an apple product, contains flavonoids. Apple cider vinegar has been used as a tonic for blood pressure and other ailments for centuries. Recent animal and preliminary human studies show that the flavonoid quercetin in apples may help lower blood pressure and improve heart health.*

❗ Warning: *Check with your doctor before using. Large doses of apple cider vinegar over a long period of time can burn the mouth and throat or erode tooth enamel; it may also counteract medications for heart and kidney disease.*

Lifestyle Tip

Be mindful. Studies show that a regular meditation practice can help manage hypertension. So create your own meditation: Mindfully brush your hair or rub lotion on your legs. Or simply repeat a mantra, with your eyes closed and body in a relaxed posture. Being mindful means you're not thinking about anything else, but focusing instead on all the sensations (touch, smell, and sound) of the present moment, such as of the brush's movement through your hair.

 # Melonmania

In general, whole fruit contains fiber and phytochemicals that are just plain good for you. The potassium in melon helps control high blood pressure.

2 cups (340 g) seeded honeydew melon
   chunks
2 cups (300 g) watermelon chunks

PREPARATION AND USE:

Mix the fruit in a large bowl. Don't remove the seeds from the watermelon chunks. See why below.

YIELD: 2 TO 4 SERVINGS

❷ **How it works:** *All melons, especially honeydew, contain potassium. As noted earlier, reducing dietary intake of sodium and optimizing intake of potassium can help bring blood pressure under control. Eat your watermelon, seeds and all. The seeds of watermelon have a juice that contains L-citrulline, an amino acid the body converts to L-arginine, another amino acid, which relaxes arteries. A 2013 study in older women found that consumption of a watermelon supplement reduced arterial stiffness and blood pressure.*

Purple Potato Salad

One study showed that overweight people who ate purple potatoes twice a day for a month lowered their blood pressure.

For the salad:

3 medium-size (or 6 small) purple potatoes, scrubbed thoroughly

2 large eggs

1 celery stalk, diced

½ onion, diced

1 tablespoon (4 g) crushed fresh dill

Pinch of freshly ground black pepper and paprika or cayenne, or your choice of other salt-free seasoning

For the dressing:

1 cup (230 g) plain low-fat yogurt

3 tablespoons (45 g) deli brown or honey mustard

1 packet (1 g) stevia

PREPARATION AND USE:

Place the potatoes and eggs in separate pots of water and bring both to a boil. Boil the potatoes for about 20 minutes until tender. Bring the eggs to a boil, then remove from the heat, cover, and set aside for 10 to 12 minutes. Let cool.

Cut the potatoes, including their skin, into bite-size chunks and place in a medium-size bowl. Peel, dice, and add the egg whites (toss the cholesterol-rich yolk). Add the celery, onion, dill, and seasonings.

In a separate bowl, mix together the yogurt, mustard, and stevia. Fold into the salad and serve.

YIELD: 4 SERVINGS

❓ **How it works:** *These spuds have high levels of chlorogenic acid, shown to reduce blood pressure. And they're antioxidant-rich—one key to reducing inflammation that causes heart disease.*

When to Call the Doctor

If you monitor your blood pressure at home, make an appointment to see your doctor should pressure exceed the normal range (140/90) more than twice. If your blood pressure rises above 180/110, call your doctor immediately.

If you are on blood-pressure-lowering medication and develop undesirable side effects, call your doctor's office for an appointment. (Do not stop the medication unless medical staff instructs you to do so.) Side effects vary with the type of medication. Beta-blockers tend to cause the most problems (insomnia, cold hands and feet, tiredness, depression, slow heart rate, and erectile dysfunction). For more information, go to the American Heart Association website at www.heart.org/ HEARTORG/Conditions/HighBloodPressure/ PreventionTreatmentofHighBloodPressure/ Prevention—Treatment-of_High-Blood-Pressure_UCM_F002054_Article.jsp.

If you have hypertension, the following signs and symptoms necessitate emergency treatment:

- *sudden onset of blurry vision*

- *severe pulsating headache*

- *pain or pressure in the chest, arm, or shoulder*

- *sudden confusion, loss of consciousness, or inability to talk, move, or smile*

Chapter 43

Immune System Support

Microorganisms are everywhere—in the air, soil, and water. Humans are like small planets colonized by billions of bacteria and fungi. The bacteria carpeting our intestinal tract alone outnumber our own cells by a factor of ten. Fortunately, most of these tiny denizens benefit us by manufacturing vitamins, outcompeting disease-causing microbes, and otherwise contributing to immune function.

Nevertheless, a large number of microbes—viruses, bacteria, fungi, protozoa, and worms—can make us sick. So if they're everywhere, why aren't we sick all the time? You guessed it: the immune system. This complex association of organs, cells, and molecules protects us from anything foreign and potentially harmful: "bad" microbes, cancer cells, splinters, toxic chemicals. Ideally, it refrains from attacking harmless pollen, animal dander, and our normal cells. But allergies and autoimmune diseases do occur.

Certain people have more trouble maintaining a healthy immune system than others. Elderly people often have diminished immune defense. Chronic sleep deprivation causes imbalances in the immune system and results in increased inflammation. Chronic stress overload dampens immune system function. Certain medications (corticosteroids and chemotherapy) and procedures (radiation therapy) suppress the immune system. Surgical procedures stress the body and also raise the risk for infection. Finally, some diseases either present at birth or acquired later (AIDS, mononucleosis, leukemia, and diabetes) impair the immune system.

Fortunately, a host of simple lifestyle choices and a few nutritional supplements can ironclad your immune system. Key among them is taking care of yourself. Undue stress, sleep deprivation, a diet of processed foods high in sugar and fat, social isolation, and inactivity undermine general health and the immune system.

History

For millennia, people didn't understand the nature of infectious illnesses. The intricacies of the immune system are still being worked out. One of the earliest known references to immunity from disease occurred in 430 BCE in the ancient city-state of Athens. Greek historian Thucydides noted that those who had recovered from a plague epidemic could tend to the sick without falling ill again.

The same was true of smallpox. Seventeenth-century healers in the Middle East, Africa, India, and China introduced material from smallpox scabs into the nose or skin of healthy people. The procedure largely protected against smallpox, though the inoculation did kill a few people.

Meanwhile, Europeans observed that milkmaids exposed to cowpox (a relatively mild disease), were often immune to smallpox. In 1796, English physician Edward Jenner inoculated his gardener's eight-year-old son with material from a milkmaid's cowpoxed hands, thereby protecting the boy from smallpox. Jenner published his results, which spurred other doctors to replicate the results.

Based on the work of many others over centuries, in the midnineteenth century, chemist and microbiologist Louis Pasteur developed the theory that microorganisms cause communicable diseases. At the end of the nineteenth century, German physician and scientist Paul Ehrlich helped to explain in detail the antigen-antibody reaction—when a toxin or other foreign substance induces an immune response by producing antibodies—another huge advance in immunology. In recent years, significant advances in immunology have come from cell cloning and recombinant DNA technologies—genetically engineered DNA usually incorporating DNA from more than one species of organism—that further explain fundamental aspects of immune system function.

 Harvest Colors Veggie Roast

This sweet and succulent dish is packed with antioxidants, which help counter unhealthy free radicals.

1 sweet potato or yam, sliced into chunks
2 carrots, sliced into chunks
2 red, yellow, or orange bell peppers, seeded and sliced into chunks
1 tablespoon (15 ml) olive oil

PREPARATION AND USE:
Preheat the oven to 400°F (200°C, or gas mark 6). Combine the vegetables and spread across a baking sheet. Brush with olive oil on each side. Roast for 25 minutes, flipping half way through, and serve.

YIELD: 2 TO 4 SERVINGS

❓ **How it works:** *Plants contain a number of molecules that promote our immune function. Examples include the carotenoids and flavonoids that give fruits and vegetables their beautiful colors and act as antioxidant and anti-inflammatory agents. That's important because as the immune system goes about its business of dispatching microbes, it stirs up inflammation and oxidation. Furthermore, carotenoids directly contribute to immune function.*

Pumpkin Pleasure Soup

This easy-to-prepare autumn soup will warm you to your bones and provide nutrients that support immune system function.

3½ cups (406 g) fresh pumpkin, or
    2 cans (15 ounces, or 528 g) pure pumpkin
    purée (if pumpkin is not in season)
Enough water to just cover the fresh pumpkin,
    if used
2½ cups (570 ml) low-fat coconut milk
1 teaspoon (6 g) salt
½ teaspoon ground nutmeg
¼ teaspoon ground allspice
Freshly ground black pepper
2 tablespoons (30 g) brown sugar (optional)

PREPARATION AND USE:

Cut the pumpkin into chunks and place in a large pan. Barely cover the pumpkin with water. Bring to a boil. Lower the heat and simmer for about 20 minutes. Puree the pumpkin, using a stand or immersion blender, and keep it warm. (Alternatively, place the canned pumpkin in a large pan without water and heat.)

Stir in the coconut milk, salt, nutmeg, allspice, and pepper to taste. Serve warm.

YIELD: ABOUT 4 SERVINGS

❓ How it works: *Pumpkin is rich in carotenoids, which neutralize free radicals and support immune health. Our bodies convert some of these carotenoids to vitamin A, which is also critical for proper immune function. Many spices are antibacterial, including cinnamon, nutmeg, and allspice.*

Feel Better Fruit Salad

This naturally sweet, fresh salad is delicious year-round. Add a dab of Greek yogurt for a dessert.

½ cup (80 g) cantaloupe chunks
1 apricot, cut into chunks
½ cup (83 g) guava chunks
½ cup (70 g) papaya chunks
1 ripe persimmon, peeled, seeded, and cut
    into chunks (see note)
Ground cinnamon

PREPARATION AND USE:

Mix the fruit in a large bowl. Sprinkle with cinnamon. Chill and serve.

YIELD: 4 TO 6 SERVINGS

❓ How it works: *Antioxidant carotenoids and flavonoids create the colors in fruits and vegetables. When eaten fresh, all also provide vitamin C, which also benefits the immune system.*

Note: Choose a ripe persimmon, as they are bitter when unripe. To see how to prepare a persimmon, go to www.wikihow.com/Eat-a-Persimmon.

◗ Immune Soup

Years ago, herbalist and author Brigitte Mars told me about this recipe. Since then, I've adapted the recipe and make it at the first sign a family member has a cold. ~ LBW

2 tablespoons (30 ml) olive oil
1 large onion, chopped
2 chicken breasts (skin removed), or 1 pound (455 g) extra-firm tofu
1 quart (946 ml) vegetable or chicken stock
1 quart (946 ml) water
4 to 6 fresh shiitake mushrooms, or 8 to 10 dried
1 cup (100 g) chopped celery,
2 cups (260 g) chopped carrots or other root vegetables
4 to 5 astragalus roots
2 teaspoons (2.8 g) dried thyme
1 teaspoon (1. g) dried rosemary
1 teaspoon (1 g) dried oregano
½ teaspoon dried sage
4 garlic cloves, minced
2 tablespoons (8 g) chopped fresh parsley
Cracked pepper (optional)

PREPARATION AND USE:

In a large stockpot, heat the olive oil over medium heat. Add the onion and sauté until soft, 3 to 5 minutes. If using chicken, sauté it, too, adding ¼ cup (60 ml) of the stock or water to keep it from sticking. Once the chicken is cooked through, 7 to 10 minutes on each side, remove it from the pot, cube it, and place it in the refrigerator.

In the same pan, sauté the mushrooms over medium heat until gently browned, 3 to 5 minutes. Add the remaining stock and the remaining water. Bring to a boil. Add the remaining vegetables and astragalus roots. Lower the heat, cover, and simmer for 30 minutes. Add the tofu now (if you're using it rather than chicken) and the thyme, rosemary, oregano, and sage. Simmer for another 20 minutes or until the vegetables are tender. Return the chicken to the pot and heat over low heat another 5 minutes. (You should have enough liquid to generously cover all the vegetables. If not, add more water.)

Turn off the heat. Fish out the astragalus roots, which are too fibrous to eat. Add the garlic, parsley, and, if desired, cracked pepper to taste. Serve.

YIELD: 4 HEARTY SERVINGS

❷ **How it works:** *Shiitake mushrooms, garlic, and onions all enhance immune function. Garlic and onion are also antimicrobial. If you can't find shiitake mushrooms, all mushrooms contain complicated polysaccharides called beta-glucans, which enhance immune system function. Astragalus root also contains polysaccharides and other chemicals that support the immune system. You may find the dried roots (which look like tongue depressors) in the bulk section at your natural food store or order them online. Chinese medicine doctors use extracts of this root to enhance immune function in people being treated for cancer (radiation and chemotherapy often suppress immune function). Studies support that use. Rosemary, thyme, and oregano all carry antimicrobial action.*

Recipe Variations: Feel free to experiment with the seasonings. You can, for instance, use curry spices instead of Italian seasonings. Rather than using vegetable or chicken stock, you can blend 2 tablespoons (32 g) of white miso paste with 1 quart (946 ml) of hot water.

Medicinal Mushroom Sauté

Maitake is Japanese for "dancing mushroom." Perhaps people danced for joy upon finding this treasure (also called hen of the woods) in the wild.

1½ teaspoons (8 ml) olive oil
2 teaspoons (10 g) butter
1½ teaspoons (8 ml) balsamic vinegar
1 pound (455 g) fresh maitake mushrooms
1 garlic clove, minced

PREPARATION AND USE:
Place the oil and butter in a large skillet and melt over medium heat.

Stir in the balsamic vinegar. Add the mushrooms. Sauté for about 15 minutes or until tender.

Add the garlic at the end of the cooking time and sauté for about a minute: active ingredients in garlic do not survive prolonged cooking. Sprinkle the mushrooms over a bed of wilted spinach for a delicious salad, fold them into an omelet, or enjoy them alone, as a side dish.

YIELD: 4 TO 6 SERVINGS

❓ How it works: *Maitake mushrooms, along with shiitake, are among the top medicinal mushrooms. Shiitake has antiviral, anticancer molecules called interferons. Studies show complex polysaccharides from the maitake mushroom enhance immune function and also have anticancer effects.*

Recipe Variation: Substitute shiitake mushrooms for maitake mushrooms, which are harder to find fresh, or make a mix. If you use dried mushrooms, 3 ounces (85 g, about ⅓ cup) will substitute for a pound (455 g) of fresh. First, reconstitute by soaking in boiling-hot water for 20 minutes (save the water for soup stock).

Fact or Myth?

KEEPING YOUR VACCINATIONS UP TO DATE IS VITAL.

Fact. Vaccines prevent illness by exposing you to the microbe or fragments of it—inactivated or weakened so that you don't get sick. Your immune system "learns" that microbe. So when you're exposed to the actual microbe later on, you don't get sick. For more information about immunizations go to the Centers for Disease Control and Prevention website at www.cdc.gov/vaccines.

Lifestyle Tip

Hug a tree. Studies show that spending time in forested areas increases certain immune markers. Some of the effects may be due to relaxation and some from the aroma of essential oils from such plants as coniferous (e.g., pine), eucalyptus, and bay trees.

Holy Mackerel

Use a gas grill (charcoal has carcinogens) or broiler year-round to bring out the flaky and succulent taste.

4 Spanish mackerel fillets
2 tablespoons (30 ml) olive oil
Salt and freshly ground black pepper
¼ teaspoon paprika
8 slices lemon

PREPARATION AND USE:

Preheat the broiler. Use vegetable cooking spray to grease a baking dish.

Rub the tops of the fillets with olive oil. Place skin side down in a baking dish. Sprinkle with the salt, pepper, and paprika. Broil for about 7 minutes until the fish begins to flake. Serve with the lemon slices.

YIELD: 4 SERVINGS

❷ How it works: *Mackerel is a good source of vitamin D, which supports immune function. Mackerel, as well as sardines, salmon, oysters, and tuna, are also kings of omega-3 fatty acids, which help reduce inflammation.*

Fact or Myth?

IF MODERATE REGULAR EXERCISE IS KEY TO ENHANCING THE IMMUNE FUNCTION, HEAVY EXERCISE MUST BE EVEN BETTER.

Myth. Extreme amounts of exercise tax your immune system.

Lifestyle Tip

Eat an orange. Citrus fruits are high in vitamin C and flavonoids. Your immune system needs vitamin C, which acts as an antioxidant and also produces an antiviral, anticancer molecule called interferon. In traditional Chinese medicine, oranges are recommended for managing indigestion and coughs. In recent years, studies conflict as to whether vitamin C prevents the common cold. Still, it never hurts to eat fresh fruits and vegetables containing vitamin C and other important nutrients. Vitamin C is not very stable, so eat vitamin C-rich foods raw. Other food sources include kiwifruit, guavas, papayas, peppers, strawberries, cantaloupe, fresh thyme or parsley, tender fresh kale, fresh broccoli, red cabbage, and peppers.

Nut Pick-Me-Up

We love this recipe for parties—little do the guests suspect they are consuming nutrients that support the immune system.

½ cup (75 g) unsalted peanuts
½ cup (73 g) unsalted almonds
¼ cup unsalted (36 g) sunflower seeds
1 teaspoon (5 ml) olive oil
1 teaspoon (6 g) sea salt

PREPARATION AND USE:
Preheat the oven to 350°F (180°C, or gas mark 4). Mix the nuts with the olive oil. Spread across a baking sheet. Bake for about 10 minutes. Remove from the oven and sprinkle with the salt. Let cool for an hour before serving. Pop a handful into your mouth.

YIELD: FIVE ¼-CUP (38 G) SERVINGS

❓ How it works: *Peanuts, almonds, and sunflower seeds are rich in zinc and vitamin E. The immune system needs vitamin E as an antioxidant and to manufacture important regulatory molecules. Low zinc intake impairs immune function. If you take supplements, take care not to overdo it. The recommended intake is 11 milligrams for men and 8 milligrams for women (11 milligrams for pregnant women). Too much zinc from supplements can cause problems. But you can't go wrong with eating zinc-rich foods, including oysters, crab, wheat germ, and pumpkin and squash seeds.*

Simply (Probiotic) Sauerkraut

1 head cabbage, shredded
1 teaspoon (6 g) sea salt
Vinegar

PREPARATION AND USE:

Toss together the cabbage and salt in bowl. Knead the salted cabbage until the water is extracted and the cabbage becomes limp. Pack the mixture into a mason jar so that no air bubbles remain and it is submerged in liquid. Cover and leave at room temperature for one to three weeks until it is sour to the taste. Transfer to the refrigerator. To each serving, add a few drops of vinegar for extra flavor.

YIELD: 4 SERVINGS

? How it works: *Probiotics are live microorganisms similar to those that normally colonize mucous membranes—the slippery linings in the respiratory system, digestive system, and vagina. We ingest them in fermented foods and as supplements. Some probiotic strains strengthen the immune system and may even protect against respiratory infections. The sauerkraut you buy in stores is usually pasteurized, which kills the good (while also killing the bad) bacteria.*

Note: The key to fermenting correctly is to keep the solid cabbage well below the liquid, so pack cabbage firmly, with liquid on top, and don't expose it directly to air while it ferments.

When Simple Doesn't Work

Unfortunately, there's no magic bullet for shoring up the immune response. Management lies primarily with removing the underlying cause, whenever possible. Simple measures include making sure you're getting enough sleep and keeping your stress levels under control.

Supplements can correct deficiencies in zinc and vitamins A, C, D, and E. Ask your doctor whether he or she recommends a multivitamin and mineral supplement. A blood test can screen for vitamin D deficiency and guide supplementation.

Some of the herbs that enhance immune system function in the recipes can be taken as concentrated extracts in liquid and tablet form. In addition to shiitake (Lentinula edodes), maitake (Grifola frondosa), and astragalus (Astragalus membranaceous), other herbal immune tonics include echinacea (Echinacea purpurea, E. pallida, E. angustifolia), ginseng (Panax ginseng, P. quinquefolius), and eleuthero (Eleutherococcus senticosus). If you have a serious disease, especially if you're undergoing treatment for cancer, discuss supplements with your doctor. Some of these herbs have been studied in cancer patients and seem not to interfere with treatment. In theory, people with autoimmune disorders should not take immunostimulating herbs. They definitely shouldn't be used by people taking immunosuppressant drugs in advance of receiving an organ or tissue transplant.

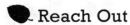 Reach Out

Make one gesture every day to build a strong social circle.

You
A friend

PREPARATION AND USE:
Take a walk and talk.

YIELD: 1 SESSION

❓ **How it works:** *Loneliness is bad for your health. Feeling socially isolated activates the stress response, generates inflammatory chemicals, and impairs some aspects of immune function. Social support, on the other hand, improves outcomes in serious immunological challenges, such as cancer and HIV infection. It may even protect against the common cold. When researchers put rhinoviruses (one of the viruses causing the common cold) in the nose of volunteers, those with more social ties were less likely to get sick and, if they did, they had fewer symptoms for a shorter period of time. Healthy sexual relationships also improve markers of nonspecific immune function.*

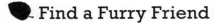 Find a Furry Friend

Cuddling with a pet has an immediate positive effect on your system.

You
A friendly domesticated animal

PREPARATION AND USE:
Pat or cuddle the pet. Feel yourself relax.

YIELD: 1 SESSION

❓ **How it works:** *To experiment, researchers asked college students to pet a stuffed dog or a live dog. Those who petted the real dog had a significant increase in infection-fighting antibody in their saliva. Those caressing the stuffed dog simply felt silly.*

🐾 Foot Massage

2 teaspoons (10 ml) lotion or oil (almond, olive, grapeseed, or apricot)
2 drops peppermint or lavender essential oils

PREPARATION AND USE:
Sit in a comfortable position. Draw one foot toward you or onto your lap. Apply a teaspoon (5 ml) of lotion or oil to your palm. Using firm pressure, massage into your feet. If you're feeling tired, blend one or two drops of peppermint essential oil into the lotion or oil. If you're getting ready for bed, use lavender oil instead.

YIELD: 1 APPLICATION

❓ **How it works:** *Several studies have shown immune benefits from foot reflexology treatments. In reflexology, the feet and hands are thought to contain regions that correspond to specific organs and other body parts. In theory, applying firm pressure to representative areas helps heal illness in the body.*

Circulation-Boosting Salt Scrub

This scrub leaves skin feeling toned and silky while enhancing blood circulation for a healthier, livelier you.

1 cup (240 g) sea salt (avoid regular table salt, which is harsh on skin)
½ cup (120 ml) olive oil
5 drops peppermint oil

PREPARATION AND USE:
Put the salt in a small bowl. Mix in the olive oil so that mixture is moist and holds together but is not overly oily. Drop in the peppermint oil, blending with each drop.

Soften your skin by soaking in a tub for 10 minutes. Drain the tub, pat yourself dry, and sit on the side of the tub. Apply a small amount of the scrub to each leg. With a warm, moist washcloth, slowly scrub each leg, not rubbing too hard and moving upward, toward your heart. Repeat with your arms and torso, always toward your heart. Rinse off in a warm shower. Finish with a burst of cold water.

YIELD: 3 TO 4 APPLICATIONS

❓ How it works: *Massaging in salt and essential oils increases blood circulation. Warm water dilates blood vessels (making you look pink). The quick burst of cold water at the end constricts blood vessels. The total effect is immediate invigoration, cleansing, and ultimate relaxation.*

Note: The oil creates a slippery surface, so step carefully.

When to Call the Doctor

- *You notice that you seem to catch more than your fair share of infectious illnesses. (Note: If you work or live with small children, you're exposed to more infectious microbes and may well have more minor illnesses, such as colds and infectious diarrhea.)*

- *You develop a serious infection or a milder but lingering infection.*

- *You have traveled to a foreign country or may have consumed unsanitary water while camping and now have persistent symptoms of infection.*

- *You develop symptoms of an overactive immune response, such as asthma (coughing and wheezing), eczema (itchy rash), or hay fever.*

- *You develop infections uncommon in healthy individuals—oral fungal infections, pneumonia caused by bacteria, fungi, or protozoa.*

- *You're at high risk of HIV infection (e.g., practice unsafe sex, have anal intercourse, have multiple partners, have had more infectious illnesses, or use intravenous drugs).*

- *You develop recurrent fever, night sweats, and weight loss.*

- *You have an immunodeficiency disease and develop a fever, cough, vomiting, diarrhea, or any other sign of infection.*

Chapter
44

Indigestion and Irritable Bowel Syndrome

Everyone has an Achilles' heel. For many Americans, the weak point is the gut. It may not take much—a change in diet, some added stress—to create gastrointestinal (GI) distress. For some people, the symptoms are felt in the upper part of the GI system; for others, the lower GI system generates discomfort.

Dyspepsia is another term for indigestion. Symptoms, which originate from the stomach and first part of the small intestine, include pain or burning high in the abdomen (below the tip of the breastbone), early satiety (feeling full after a few bites), feeling heaviness after eating, and belching. For many people, symptoms coincide with mealtimes.

Likewise, lower GI symptoms are often associated with meals. They can include gas, bloating, and cramping. In a condition called irritable bowel syndrome (IBS), additional symptoms include diarrhea and/or constipation.

Dyspepsia and irritable bowel syndrome fall into the category of "functional" rather than "organic" disorders. In the former, the problem lies with the performance of the system, but without visible signs of disease. In organic disorders, there is a visible lesion such an ulcer. Examples include peptic ulcers and inflammatory bowel diseases.

The potential causes of functional bowel conditions are multiple. They include stress overload; hypersensitivity of intestinal nerves; imbalances in the bacterial ecology of the intestines; food allergies and intolerances; medications, such as nonsteroidal anti-inflammatory drugs and antibiotics; and chronic diseases, such as hypothyroidism, diabetes, anxiety, and depression.

History

For millennia, people around the globe have consumed bitter foods and beverages to enhance the digestive process. The Romans drank wine infused with bitter herbs. In the early 1800s, German physician Johann Siegert, a surgeon general in Simón Bolívar's Venezuelan army, developed angostura bitters as a tonic and remedy for soldiers' upset stomachs and later established a distillery to produce it. The drink soon became widely popular.

To this day, Europeans traditionally precede the main course with aperitifs—alcohol infused with bitter fruits and herbs—meant to whet the appetite. Examples include Campari, Cynar, and vermouth. The bitters prime the digestive process. Research shows that stimulating bitter taste receptors does, in fact, augment appetite and digestion. Similarly, after the meal, a bitter digestif may be served to help diners digest their meal. In this case, the alcohol contains carminatives, herbs that relieve gas and bloating. Examples include ouzo (anise), sambuca (anise, licorice, and elderberries), limoncello (lemons), and Pernod (star anise, mint, and coriander). As herbalists know, you can enjoy digestive bitters and carminatives—without alcohol. That's a good thing for people who also experience heartburn, a condition aggravated by alcohol.

Lifestyle Tip

Take a warm bath. Sitting in a warm tub can spell relief when you have intestinal gas buildup. The muscles relax and allow the wind to escape.

RECESPES TO PREVENT AND TREAT INDIGESTION

 ## Light Your Fire Salad

Traditional Chinese medicine practitioners speak of "digestive fire." If you experience burning sensations with meals, don't let this description alarm you. It refers to stimulating enzymes to better digest your food.

1 cup (20 g) torn arugula
1 cup (50 g) torn endive
1 cup (40 g) torn radicchio
2 tablespoons (30 ml) balsamic vinegar
1 garlic clove, minced
Freshly ground black pepper, to taste
¼ cup (60 ml) olive oil
¼ cup (20 g) shaved Parmesan cheese

PREPARATION AND USE:
Toss together the greens in a large bowl and set aside.

Pour the vinegar into a large salad bowl. Add the garlic and few sprinkles of pepper. Drizzle the olive oil into the bowl, stirring briskly with a whisk until the mixture is light brown. Empty the bowl of greens into the salad bowl with dressing. Toss. Sprinkle with the Parmesan shavings and serve immediately.

YIELD: 4 TO 6 SERVINGS

❓ **How it works:** *Herbalists have long used digestive bitters, drunk before the meal, to jump-start digestion. A European tradition is eating a salad of bitter greens after the main meal. Bitters stimulate bile and digestive enzymes.*

Mango Summer Aperitif

This elegant yet easy aperitif stimulates your appetite and prepares your digestive system for a meal. Aperitif comes from the Latin verb aperire, "to open."

2 cups (350 g) mango chunks, frozen
¼ cup (120 ml) Muscat or Dolce dessert wine
1 bottle (750 ml) dry champagne, chilled

PREPARATION AND USE:

Partially thaw the mango chunks. Blend the mango in blender. Add the dessert wine and blend slightly. Fill champagne flutes half-full with the mango mixture. Top with chilled champagne and serve.

YIELD: 6 SERVINGS

❓ **How it works:** *Dry champagne stimulates digestion. In addition to being rich in essential nutrients, mango contains fiber, which promotes healthy intestinal microbes and regular bowel movements.*

Note: Alcohol aggravates heartburn. If you have this condition, consider substituting pomegranate juice for the alcohol.

Après-Dinner Digestif

In France, a digestif, often brandy or a liqueur, is sipped after meals to aid digestion. You can make your own, with digestion-aiding fennel.

2 tablespoons (12 g) fennel seeds
½ cup (50 g) fresh, chopped fennel stalks
    and leaves
1½ cups (355 ml) vodka
Honey

PREPARATION AND USE:

Put the fennel seeds, stalks, and leaves into a clean pint-size (475 ml) jar. Pour the vodka over the plant matter until you have a good 2 inches (5 cm) of alcohol above the top of the fennel. Cap and shake well. Place in a cupboard for one to two weeks, shaking occasionally.

When ready, place a strainer over a small mixing bowl. Lay a square of cheesecloth over the strainer, with about an inch (2.5 cm) of extra material hanging over the sides of the strainer. Carefully pour the contents of the jar through the cheesecloth.

Use a spoon to scoop out all the fennel onto the cheesecloth. With clean hands, gather the edges of the cheesecloth. Squeeze out as much of the liquid as you can into the bowl. Remove the strainer. Discard the spent fennel.

Measure the amount of liquid. To that amount, add half as much honey. (For instance, if you have 1 cup [235 ml] of fennel extract, stir ½ cup [160 ml] of honey into it.) Wash and dry the jar and pour your digestif into it. Store in the refrigerator or in the freezer for a cold, refreshing drink. After dinner, pour 1 ounce (28 ml) of the drink into a small digestif glass and sip. You may also dilute it with 1 tablespoon (15 ml) of water.

YIELD: MULTIPLE SMALL SERVINGS

❓ How it works: *Fennel is in the parsley family, along with carrots, celery, anise, caraway, and licorice. All have value for the digestive tract. Fennel is a carminative herb, meaning it helps expel gas from the stomach and intestines. It's also traditionally used to relieve nausea and vomiting, inflammation, and intestinal spasms.*

Note: An herbal extract with alcohol and water (and vodka contains a good balance of the two) is called a tincture. The addition of honey creates a liqueur that's sweet enough to enjoy in small amounts without cutting it with water. Feel free to try to the recipe without honey. If you do, we recommend diluting it with water before consuming.

🖤 After-Dinner Digestive Snack

1 tablespoon (6 g) aniseeds
1 tablespoon (6 g) fennel seeds

PREPARATION AND USE:

Put the seeds into a small, clean jar, cap, and shake to mix. After dinner, put ¼ teaspoon of the seed mixture into the palm of your hand and pop into your mouth. Savor the taste as you chew.

YIELD: 24 SERVINGS

❓ How it works: *See the explanation in the previous recipe for fennel. Also a member of the parsley family, anise has similar properties to fennel. It relieves bloating, flatulence, nausea, cramping, and poor appetite. Both seeds also freshen the breath.*

Fact or Myth?

A HEALTHY DIGESTIVE TRACT MEANS STAYING AWAY FROM PROCESSED FOODS.

Fact. Processed foods are often high in refined carbohydrates and unhealthy fats. Both increase the risk of obesity, cardiovascular disease, and diabetes. Refined carbohydrates can also worsen chronic constipation. Some people are sensitive to additives, such as artificial colorings, preservatives, gluten, and lactose.

Lifestyle Tip

If gas and bloating commonly afflict you, try eliminating foods that tend to promote intestinal gas: cruciferous plants such as cabbage, Brussels sprouts, uncooked cauliflower, and broccoli, beans, lentils, raw pears and apples, dairy products, whole grains, and carbonated beverages. Fructose and artificial sweeteners (including those that are found in candy and gum) can also cause intestinal distress.

Warming Digestive Tea

These herbs and spices are both sweet and slightly bitter to improve digestion.

1 tablespoon (2 g) dried peppermint leaves
1 teaspoon (2 g) fennel seeds
1 teaspoon (2 g) aniseeds
1 teaspoon (5 g) cinnamon chips, from a crushed cinnamon stick
½ teaspoon cardamom seeds
2 cups (475 ml) water

PREPARATION AND USE:
Combine the peppermint and spices in a clean jar.

Boil the water in a saucepan. Add the spice mixture. Cover and steep for 15 minutes. Strain and enjoy before and after meals.

YIELD: 2 SERVINGS

❓ How it works: *See previous descriptions of anise and fennel. Cardamom also relieves intestinal spasms, gas, bloating, and flatulence. Peppermint relieves pain, cramping, and gas. Studies show that encapsulated peppermint oil significantly reduces symptoms of irritable bowel syndrome and dyspepsia.*

Chamomile Tea Variation

2 cups (475 ml) water
1 teaspoon (0.5 g) dried chamomile flowers
1 teaspoon (0.5 g) dried peppermint leaves
¼ teaspoon caraway seeds

PREPARATION AND USE:
Boil the water in a saucepan. Turn off the heat. Add the herbs and seeds and cover. Steep for 15 minutes. Strain and sip.

YIELD: 1 LARGE OR 2 SMALL SERVINGS

❓ How it works: *Caraway and chamomile relieve cramping and gas and stimulate digestion. Combination herb products containing these and other herbs and spices have been shown to relieve dyspepsia and irritable bowel syndrome.*

Fact or Myth?

WHEN YOU HAVE AN IRRITATED DIGESTIVE SYSTEM, DRINK CARBONATED BEVERAGES.

Myth. They actually contain acid and can increase digestive problems. When you have an upset stomach, also avoid other acid-laden foods, such as citrus fruits and tomatoes.

A Digestive "New Leaf"

1 artichoke
Water
Pinch of salt
1 teaspoon (5 ml) fresh lemon juice
1 tablespoon (15 ml) olive oil
1 teaspoon (3 g) minced fresh garlic

PREPARATION AND USE:

Slice off the artichoke top, trim the thorny tips and stem, and place in a steamer basket. In a pot, place about 2 inches (5 cm) of water, the salt, and the lemon juice and bring to a boil. Steam the artichoke in the pot, covered, for about 30 minutes (until the bottom of the artichoke can be pierced).

In a clean bowl, stir together the olive oil and garlic. Remove the artichoke from the pot and allow it to cool. Pull off each artichoke petal and dip it into the olive oil mixture. Enjoy pulling the flesh off the base of the petal with your teeth.

When all the petals are pulled away, scoop out and discard the fuzzy center. The fleshy artichoke heart remains. Slice it and enjoy on a salad or just plain. Many think it's the best part.

YIELD: 1 SERVING OR 2, IF CUT IN HALF

❓ How it works: *Artichoke, a botanical relative of milk thistle, is the main ingredient in the Italian bitter aperitif Cynar. Milk thistle seeds are a bitter digestive tonic and also protect the liver and stimulate it to make bile. The seeds are one ingredient in a botanical formula shown to reduce symptoms of irritable bowel syndrome and dyspepsia. Although artichoke hasn't been as well researched, studies have shown that leaf extracts also significantly reduce dyspepsia and irritable bowel syndrome.*

Lifestyle Tip

Avoid fatty meals and any other foods that trigger your symptoms. Healthy oils (e.g., olive, flaxseed, safflower, and canola) are fine. But fried foods are hard to digest and add calories.

Fiber-Fresh Salad

This salad is both light and fresh—and it works as dessert as well as dinner.

1 tart green apple, skin on, cored and diced
1 mango, peeled, pitted, and cubed
¾ cup (75 g) crushed almonds
¼ cup (60 g) plain yogurt
½ teaspoon ground cinnamon
¼ teaspoon ground ginger
4 fresh mint leaves, for garnish

PREPARATION AND USE:

Place the apple and mango in a bowl. Stir in the almonds.

In a separate small bowl, stir the spices into the yogurt. Toss the fruit mixture with the spiced yogurt. Garnish with the mint.

YIELD: 4 SERVINGS

❓ How it works: *In addition to being packed with essential nutrients, apples, mangoes, and almonds are rich in fiber, which improves intestinal function and decreases constipation. Yogurt contains probiotic organisms, which have been shown to ease functional disorders such as irritable bowel syndrome.*

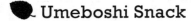 Umeboshi Snack

Umeboshi is a salty, pickled Japanese plum. The taste is tart and zingy.

1 cucumber
Umeboshi paste (see note)
1 teaspoon (3 g) sesame seeds, toasted

PREPARATION AND USE:
Wash and slice the cucumber into sturdy rounds, leaving the skin on. Add a very thin layer of *umeboshi* paste to each cucumber slice. (The taste is tangy and refreshing: a little goes a long way.) Sprinkle with sesame seeds. Serve this quick and refreshing snack between meals or as an appetizer.

YIELD: 8 APPETIZER SERVINGS

❓ **How it works:** Umeboshi *stimulates digestion, starting with increased salivation. The fiber in sunflower seeds contributes to overall bowel health. Soluble fiber inside the cucumber peel helps with digestive problems if you have constipation. Peel the cucumber if it causes you to have gas or diarrhea.*

Note: You can buy *umeboshi* paste in a local Asian food store.

Problem Foods Tracker

Food allergy and intolerance can create many of the symptoms of functional bowel conditions.

A journal
A pen

PREPARATION AND USE:
Keep a careful list of the foods you eat and your visceral reactions to these foods. True food allergies usually create more dramatic symptoms, including non-GI problems, such as hives and swelling in the respiratory tract. Food intolerances, however, can be more subtle. Examples include intolerance to lactose (in dairy products) and gluten (in many grains). Share your findings with your doctor, who can also help you identify possible culprits.

YIELD: 1 SESSION

❓ **How it works:** *Keeping daily track of what you eat and how it affects you may help you identify foods that upset your digestive function. Note that food allergies are caused by the immune system and typically create obvious reactions (diarrhea, nausea, vomiting, hives, eczema, and swelling of the lips, mouth, and throat). Food intolerance, on the other hand, comes on more gradually and creates more subtle symptoms of gastrointestinal upset. Once you identify foods you suspect don't suit you, we recommend you meet with your doctor before radically changing your diet.*

● Digestion-Calming Child's Pose

You
A rug or mat

PREPARATION AND USE:

Get down on all fours. Distribute your weight between your hands and lower legs. Spread your knees wider than your toes. With an exhalation, lay your torso between your thighs and rest your head on the ground. Let your belly relax.

Pull your hips back toward your heels. Your arms can extend straight ahead or rest alongside your outer shins. Rest. Repeat.

YIELD: 1 SESSION

❷ How it works: *This pose is called* balansana, *or child's pose. Along with such yoga postures as the cobra (see page 211), it gently stimulates abdominal muscles, intestines, and circulation to internal organs. Because your bottom is higher than your head in the child's pose, you may also experience relief from intestinal gas. Yoga also relieves stress that contributes to indigestion. Plus, it's safe for all ages and abilities. A 2011 Dutch study showed that yoga lessons significantly reduced abdominal pain in kids with functional bowel disorders, such as irritable bowel syndrome.*

When Simple Doesn't Work

Many of the gas-forming foods mentioned in this chapter are otherwise good for you. Rather than giving them up, try Beano, a product that contains alpha-galastosidase, an enzyme that digests the type of sugar found in beans and many vegetables.

If you notice that intestinal distress occurs after consuming dairy products, you might be lactose intolerant. A simple breath test, which your doctor can order, can determine whether you have it. If you are, you can either give up dairy (except fermented products, such as yogurt and kefir) or take lactase supplements.

For people with chronic digestive complaints, another condition to rule out is gluten sensitivity (also called gluten intolerance). In gluten sensitivity, the problem may arise from overexposure to dietary gluten. Celiac disease, which is more serious, is an autoimmune condition marked by destruction of the villi (fingerlike projections in the small intestine) in response to dietary gluten. Symptoms include fatigue, diarrhea, abdominal pain, bloating, and weight loss. If untreated, every organ system may ultimately become involved. Blood tests can screen for immune reaction to gliadin, a component of gluten. Treatment involves scrupulous avoidance of gluten.

Also, doctors can prescribe medications to relieve intestinal symptoms. For more information, go to National Digestive Diseases Information Clearinghouse (http://digestive.niddk.nih.gov).

Depressurizing Pose

This is not a yoga pose, but has the same relieving effect as the wind-removing yoga pose called Colon Massage (see page 184).

You
A rug or mat
A pillow

PREPARATION AND USE:
Lie on your belly on a rug. Slide a pillow under your groin, so that your hips are above your stomach.

YIELD: 1 SESSION

❓ **How it works:** *This posture can allow intestinal gas to escape.*

When to Call the Doctor

If simple home remedies fail to relieve indigestion and intestinal upset, call your doctor's office for an appointment. A number of diseases and medications can interfere with proper digestion. Your doctor can determine whether a treatable condition underlies your GI symptoms and rule out organic problems, such as ulcers and celiac disease.

Stress-Check Journal

For most people, stress and anxiety impair digestion and worsen symptoms of indigestion. Think about it from an evolutionary standpoint. If you're fleeing a tiger, digesting lunch becomes a low priority.

A journal
A pen

PREPARATION AND USE:
Over the course of a week, write down what makes you feel stressed or anxious. How does stress affect your gut? Describe what's going on during mealtimes: Are you reading the newspaper (which is rarely filled with cheerful news)? Checking e-mail? Feeling irritated with family members? Meeting with a client? Driving your car? What happens if you eat in a quiet setting and do nothing but focus on the meal?

YIELD: 1 SESSION

❓ **How it works:** *During the stress response, blood is diverted away from the intestines, bowel motility slows, and enzyme production slackens. Chronic stress also makes you more sensitive to pain coming from the gut. Identifying stressful situations takes you a step closer to avoiding or controlling them.*

Chapter 45

Influenza

Influenza, or flu, is a highly contagious viral respiratory illness. In an average year, 5 to 20 percent of Americans will develop influenza, more than 200,000 will wind up in the hospital, and more than 36,000 will die. Those most vulnerable are people older than age sixty-five and younger than age two, as well as pregnant women and people with chronic medical conditions.

The virus spreads from person to person via respiratory droplets—tiny drops of moisture released into the air when an infected person talks, coughs, and sneezes. Bystanders may inhale the viruses through their mouths or nose. Flu viruses can also survive on inanimate objects for two to eight hours. If, after handling this object, you touch your eye, nose, or lip, you have inoculated yourself.

Signs and symptoms of influenza include sore throat, stuffy nose, cough, body aches, headache, fatigue, fever, and chills. Whereas the common cold mainly causes symptoms from the neck up, influenza causes more total-body misery. Also, coughing is more pronounced. Contagion begins the day before symptoms develop and extends for a week after symptoms begin. Most symptoms resolve within three to six days. However, fatigue and cough can linger for a few weeks.

History

At least ten flu pandemics, or global epidemics, have been recorded in the last three centuries. The 1918–1919 influenza pandemic, however, was by far the most devastating, killing an estimated 50 million people worldwide and infecting perhaps ten times that number. More than 600,000 died in the United States alone.

The deadly virus hit at a vulnerable time—the end of World War I. More people lost their lives in this pandemic than had died in the war. Classified as an influenza A (H1N1) virus, this flu caused sneezing, coughing, and fever, progressing to pneumonia. It then produced a cytokine storm—an overreaction of the immune system that was often fatal.

In 2004, the Centers for Disease Control and Prevention (CDC) began testing viruses containing subsets of the eight genes of the 1918 virus. In reconstructing the virus, researchers learned which genes were making the virus so harmful. Two types of antiviral drugs, rimantadine (Flumadine) and oseltamivir (Tamiflu), have been effective against influenza viruses similar to the 1918 virus. Such research is part of ongoing preparedness for treating future pandemics.

Garlicky Honey

1 head garlic, cloves separated and peeled
2 thin slices onion
Honey

PREPARATION AND USE:

Using the flat of a knife, gently crush each clove—just enough to crack it open. Place the garlic cloves in a pint-size (475 ml) jar. Layer on the onion. Cover the garlic and onion with honey and cap the jar. Let the mixture sit in a warm place overnight. Take a spoonful of the honey to coat your throat; eating the garlic and onion will also provide relief. If you prefer not to eat the garlic and onion, you can strain the honey into a separate jar.

YIELD: MULTIPLE SERVINGS

❷ **How it works:** *Honey is soothing to inflamed respiratory passages and antibacterial (though the issue here is a viral infection). It's safer than over-the-counter cough remedies and at least as effective. Garlic is expectorant (helps clear respiratory mucus) and antimicrobial, including antiviral activity against influenza. Special extracts have been shown to decrease flu symptom severity. Onion is a close botanical relative of garlic and contains similar sulfur-containing compounds. It's antimicrobial and is used in folk medicine to clear respiratory mucus and open tight airways.*

Mom's Chicken Soup

Sometimes called Jewish penicillin, chicken soup has been used to soothe flu and colds since the twelfth century.

1 chicken (3 to 4 pounds, or 1.4 to 1.8 kg), fully washed
2 quarts (2 L) water
1 large onion, peeled and quartered
6 carrots, grated, divided
4 garlic cloves, peeled, minced, divided
1 can (28 ounces, or 80 g) crushed tomatoes
2 celery stalks, sliced thinly
1 cup (90 g) uncooked bow-tie pasta
Freshly ground black pepper
2 tablespoons (8 g) fresh dill

PREPARATION AND USE:

Place the chicken in a large pot and cover it with the water.

Add the onion, three of the chopped carrots, and two of the minced garlic cloves.

Bring the water to a boil, then turn down the heat, cover the pot, and simmer for about an hour. When the chicken is cooked through, remove it to let cool.

Pour the broth through a strainer and throw away (or compost) the vegetables. Return the broth to the original pot. Skin the chicken, tear it apart, and add the pieces to the pot. Add the tomatoes, celery, and the three remaining chopped carrots. Stir in the pasta, ground pepper, and dill. Cook until the pasta is tender enough to eat. Add the remaining two minced garlic cloves. Serve warm.

YIELD: 8 SERVINGS

❓ How it works: *For eight hundred years, chicken soup has headed the list of flu relievers. Recent scientific evidence shows mild support for the notion that chicken soup reduces congestion and other cold symptoms. Drinking warm liquids will keep you hydrated and help ease a sore throat; the steam helps to clear nasal passages. Add garlic at the end of the cooking time to take advantage of its immune-enhancing and flu-fighting ingredients, which heat destroys. Dill relaxes smooth muscle—the kind that encircles the lower airways, which may help ease chest tightness.*

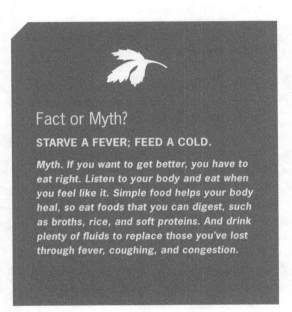

Fact or Myth?

STARVE A FEVER; FEED A COLD.

Myth. If you want to get better, you have to eat right. Listen to your body and eat when you feel like it. Simple food helps your body heal, so eat foods that you can digest, such as broths, rice, and soft proteins. And drink plenty of fluids to replace those you've lost through fever, coughing, and congestion.

🍄 Mushroom Tom Yum Soup

An alternative for Mom's time-honored chicken soup, this recipe is a version of Thailand's most beloved soup, Tom Yum. This vegetarian version is chock-full of herbs, spices, and vegetables whose soothing powers cater to flu sufferers.

2 lemongrass stalks
1 quart (946 ml) vegetable stock
2 teaspoons (10 ml) fresh lime juice, divided
2 teaspoons (5 g) grated fresh ginger
½ to 1 teaspoon (0.5 to 1 g) dried, crushed
   cayenne pepper
½ cup (35 g) sliced shiitake or maitake
   (hen of the woods) mushrooms
1 red bell pepper, seeded and chopped
¼ cup (33 g) thinly sliced carrot
½ cup (124 g) cubed extra-firm tofu (optional)
1 cup (235 ml) coconut milk
3 garlic cloves, minced
2 scallions, sliced into thin rings, for garnish
3 tablespoons (3 g) fresh cilantro leaves,
   for garnish

PREPARATION AND USE:

Cut away and discard the tough bottom ends (4 to 6 inches [10 to 15 cm]) of one or two lemongrass stalks. Chop the more tender stalks until you have 3 tablespoons (15 g).

Pour the stock into a large pot over medium-high heat. Add the lemongrass and bring to a boil. Boil for about 5 minutes. Lower the heat to a simmer and stir in 1 teaspoon (5 ml) of the lime juice, the ginger, ½ teaspoon of the cayenne, and the mushrooms. Simmer for 5 minutes more.

Stir in the bell pepper, carrot, and tofu, if using, and simmer until the vegetables are tender, 5 to 10 minutes more. Lower the heat to low and stir in the coconut milk and garlic. (Note: By adding the garlic last you will preserve its active, flu-fighting ingredients.) Heat for another 2 minutes, adding the remaining teaspoon (5 ml) of lime juice and, if you like heat, another ½ teaspoon of cayenne pepper. Serve the soup garnished with sliced scallion and cilantro leaves.

YIELD: 2 LARGE BOWLS OR 4 SMALL CUPS

❷ **How it works:** *As stated earlier, garlic is expectorant and fights infection—it should be added at the end of cooking to preserve active ingredients. Onion helps clear respiratory mucus and opens the airways. Shiitake and maitake enhance immune function. In lab studies, shiitake protects against influenza infection. Ginger settles the stomach and decreases pain and inflammation. Preliminary research indicates lemongrass decreases pain and fever. The spicy nature of ginger, cayenne, and lemongrass all have a warming effect and thin nasal mucus, making it easier to clear.*

Lifestyle Tip

Get a yearly vaccination against influenza ("flu shot"). It's one of your best strategies for avoiding the flu. Each year, researchers formulate a vaccine that protects against strains predicted to be common during flu season. The CDC recommends that people older than six months get vaccinated each year. The vaccine doesn't protect against other viruses that cause flulike symptoms. While you may still develop influenza, your symptoms will be relatively mild.

❮ Button-It-Up Omelet

Whether raw or cooked, 1 to 2 cups (70 to 140 g) of white button mushrooms a day during flu season may give a boost to the immune system to help derail flu symptoms.

1 tablespoon (15 ml) olive oil
¼ cup (40 g) diced onion
1 garlic clove, minced
1 cup (70 g) sliced mushrooms
1 cup (30 g) baby spinach leaves, rinsed and drained (optional)
4 large eggs
½ teaspoon dried thyme
½ teaspoon dried oregano
Freshly ground black pepper

PREPARATION AND USE:

Pour the oil into a medium-size skillet over medium-high heat. Add the onion, garlic, mushrooms, and, spinach, if using, and sauté for about a minute. Transfer the mixture to a bowl and set the skillet aside.

In a separate bowl, whisk the eggs until fluffy, adding the thyme, oregano, and ground pepper. If needed, re-oil the bottom of the same skillet. (You may have enough oil left over from sautéing the vegetables, especially if you use an omelet pan.) Pour the eggs into the skillet, again over medium-high heat. Allow the egg to cook until the sides begin to set. Flip it to the other side and layer the cooked vegetables on top. Once the bottom side cooks, fold in half and serve.

YIELD: 2 SERVINGS

How it works: *Like more exotic mushrooms, button mushrooms contain beta-glucans, highly branched polysaccharides that enhance immune function. In lab experiments, mushroom extracts increased activity in certain white blood cells. In a study in healthy adults, daily consumption of button mushrooms for a week led to a significant increase in antibodies in saliva. Mushrooms also contain antioxidants.*

As noted earlier, garlic is antimicrobial, with activity against influenza viruses. Cooking for more than a very short time, however, will deactivate key ingredients. Thyme and oregano are antimicrobial. Thyme also helps relax tight airways and calm coughs.

Fact or Myth?

DRINK PLENTY OF ORANGE AND GRAPEFRUIT JUICE TO CALM YOUR FLU-RELATED COUGH.

Myth. The acid in citrus can actually irritate your throat and make your cough worse. You do want to stay hydrated and take in the immune-boosting vitamin C that citrus provides—so drink up and enjoy other juices, such as carrot, spinach, pomegranate, grape, or pineapple juice. Pineapple juice, which contains an anti-inflammatory agent, can relieve sore throat. Take it easy on juice, however, which is high in sugar. (Sugar can impair some white blood cells.) All fresh plants provide vitamin C.

Lifestyle Tip

Influenza viruses are very contagious. Basic hygiene measures can prevent the flu's spread:

- Wash your hands (and your small children's hands) frequently with soap and water or use an alcohol-based hand sanitizer.

- Sneeze or cough into a tissue or your elbow.

- If you or your child falls ill, stay home. The contagious period stretches from the day before symptoms strike to five to seven days thereafter. The CDC recommends people stay home until they're without fever for twenty-four hours.

Lifestyle Tip

Listen to soothing music. This strategy may be especially helpful if you're feeling stressed. A study in college students showed that quiet music reduced stress symptoms and boosted IgA, antibodies found in the nose, ears, respiratory passages, and digestive tract. One study found that, among elders, making music lifted mood and increased certain immune cells.

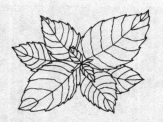

Spotlight: **Why Do We Keep Getting the Flu?**

Some viral infections—chickenpox, for instance—stimulate lifelong immunity. We're perennially vulnerable to influenza viruses because they continually undergo genetic modification, presenting our immune system with new challenges each season.

Most of the time, these genetic alterations are small and lead to the usual, relatively mild seasonal influenza. Greater genetic shifts result in more disease because our immune system lacks familiarity with the viral strain.

You've probably heard about various types of "swine flu" and "bird (avian) flu." Often, viruses only infect a certain species. Viruses with bigger genetic shifts usually occur when the virus "jumps" from one species to another. In pigs, which can become infected with viruses from humans and birds, genes can become rearranged to create a new virus that's highly virulent to humans.

Take, for example, an American tourist who visits an Asian market, complete with live ducks and pigs. One of his souvenirs is a novel, virulent influenza virus. A couple of days later, he boards his return flight, feeling a bit under the weather. Before the plane lands, he's started coughing, inoculating travelers who continue on to other destinations. A pandemic is born.

Elderberry Syrup

Most herb stores and online bulk herb retailers carry European black elderberries (Sambucus nigra). American elderberry (S. canadensis), which is similar, grows in some regions of the United States. Verify the species of local varieties before consuming. Use only ripe, black elderberries, never red elderberries, which are poisonous.

3 cups (710 ml) water

1 cup (120 g) dried elderberries

2 tablespoons (28 g) cinnamon chips, from a crushed cinnamon stick

1 tablespoon (8 g) fresh, grated ginger, or 2 teaspoons (4 g) dried

¾ cup (240 g) honey

2 teaspoons (10 ml) brandy

PREPARATION AND USE:

Bring the water to a boil in a quart-size (946 ml) saucepan. Add the elderberries, cinnamon chips, and ginger. Lower the heat and simmer, uncovered, for 40 minutes. The water level should reduce by almost half, but you should still have enough water to adequately cover the herbs.

Drape a piece of cheesecloth over a large strainer and balance it atop a glass measuring cup or a bowl. Strain the herbs. Fold the cheesecloth around the herbs and wring out the remaining liquid. If you have more than 1½ cups (355 ml) of liquid, return it to the pot and simmer until it reduces to 1½ cups (355 ml). Add the honey. (To make a syrup, the ratio of strong tea to honey should be 2:1.) Stir to blend. If the liquid is warm, the honey should dissolve easily. If not, return to heat until it does. Add a splash (about 2 teaspoons [10 ml]) of brandy to preserve. Refrigerate. The mixture is good for three months.

At the first sign of influenza (or after a recent exposure), take 1 tablespoon (15 ml) four times a day. Give children half that dose. This remedy is not appropriate for infants.

YIELD: MULTIPLE SERVINGS

❓ How it works: *European black elderberries (Sambucus nigra) have immune-enhancing and antiviral activity against influenza and other respiratory viruses. Three small studies have demonstrated that special elderberry extracts reduced symptom severity and duration in people with influenza. The first two studies used a proprietary extract sold as Sambucol. The dose was 4 tablespoons (60 ml) a day for adults, and 2 tablespoons (30 ml) a day for children. Cinnamon and ginger are warming, pleasant tasting, immune-enhancing, and antioxidant. Ginger inhibits some respiratory viruses, though it may not fight influenza viruses. It also counters inflammation, fever, pain, and cough—all of which can accompany the flu.*

⚠ Warning: *The seeds of unripe elderberries contain substances called cyanogenic glycosides, which, if ingested can be toxic. Red elderberries are poisonous.*

Recipe Variation: You can also make this syrup without the brandy and use as a delicious topping to yogurt, oatmeal, and pancakes.

Lifestyle Tip

Ramp up the humidifier. The extra moisture will help calm a dry, hacking cough.

⬤ Brake the Aches Bath

Some plant essential oils reduce pain. Examples include eucalyptus, pine, rosemary, peppermint, and ginger. You can find them at most natural food stores.

1 cup (240 g) Epsom salts
A blend of essential oils, totaling 10 to 15 drops (Use half as much for a child.)

PREPARATION AND USE:
Drop the essential oils into the Epsom salts. (If you have 5 different essential oils, you could add 2 drops of each.) Add the salts to hot, but not scalding, bathwater. Blend the salts into the water with your hand. Get into the bath and soak. If you can, sip a mug of hot Gypsy Cold-Combat Tea (see page 158) during your soak.

YIELD: 1 APPLICATION

❓ How it works: *A warm bath can help reduce aches and pains. The moisture from a bath or shower will also help loosen congestion in the respiratory tract.*

❗ Warning: *Do not use this remedy if you are pregnant.*

Note: Be sure to get out of the bath if it cools too much and you start to shiver. Becoming chilled could make you feel worse.

⬤ Beginner's Tai Chi

You
Comfortable clothes
A quiet setting in your home or outdoors

PREPARATION AND USE:
Stand straight, feet slightly apart and weight evenly distributed. Relax your knees, lower back, and shoulders. Breathe in and out slowly.

Open your fingers and extend your arms in front of you, palms facing each other. With your fingertips pointing upward, move your extended arms down, sinking your body down slowly at the same time. With your fingertips facing downward, slowly raise your arms and body. Slowly and evenly draw your hands in toward your tummy, and then pull them up and push them out in a circular motion, keeping your elbows slightly bent. As you make the circular motion, rhythmically move your entire body up and down, up and down.

Fact or Myth?

INFLUENZA CAUSES NAUSEA, VOMITING, AND DIARRHEA.

Myth: Influenza viruses have an affinity for the respiratory tract, but some strains can cause intestinal distress, along with the usual symptoms such as sore throat and cough. When people say, "stomach flu," they're referring to gastrointestinal symptoms caused by entirely different viruses, as well as by bacteria and parasites.

Make four sets of circles. Pause. Reverse the movement of your arms so they are making circles in the opposite direction as you move up and down. Make four sets of opposite circles. Bring your body to the upright position. Draw your hands in toward your chest, palms facing but not touching. Pull your palms apart, as far as shoulder width, and then bring them back, nearly together, in an open-and-close movement. Repeat four times.

YIELD: 1 SESSION

❓ How it works: *This is an opening movement in tai chi, an Eastern moving meditation practice. A 2007 study found that tai chi could help your body make the most of the seasonal flu shot. Seniors practiced tai chi or qigong (a similar practice of meditative movements linked to breath) three days a week for an hour, for three weeks. During the first week, they received a flu vaccine. Subsequent blood tests showed that, compared to elders not participating in tai chi or qigong, the study group had significantly higher antibody responses. This is great news as declining immune system function in old age typically weakens response to immunizations.*

Other studies show other types of moderate exercise also maintain immune function. However, when you are gripped by those first feverish days of flu, take a break from exercise and rest instead.

When Simple Doesn't Work

If you seem vulnerable to respiratory viral infections, a special extract of American ginseng (Panax quinquefolius) called Cold-FX has been shown to reduce the risk of developing influenza and colds and lessen symptoms of those illnesses that do occur. Concentrated extracts of Asian ginseng (Panax ginseng) also protect against influenza and improve the immune response to influenza vaccines. Extracts of eleuthero (Eleutherococcus senticosus, or Siberian ginseng) have been shown to help prevent viral respiratory infections, including the flu.

Taking vitamin D supplements during the winter months (when levels of this vitamin are at their lowest) appears to reduce flu risk. Discuss supplementation with your doctor.

Conventional medications, such as Tamiflu (oseltamivir), reduce the duration of influenza infections. Ibuprofen and acetaminophen can relieve body aches and headaches, but do not treat the infection. Do not give teens or children aspirin.

🫐 The D-Licious Fish

Three ounces (85 g) of salmon carry 794 IU of vitamin D, nearly the entire 1,000 IU a day recommended for the body to fight the respiratory upsets that accompany flu. Check the index for additional salmon recipes.

2 salmon steaks or fillets (3 ounces or 85 g)
2 teaspoons (10 ml) olive oil
Freshly ground black pepper
1 lemon, sliced

PREPARATION AND USE:
Preheat the oven to 375°F (190°C, or gas mark 5).

Place a sheet of aluminum foil on a baking sheet. Place the salmon on the foil (if using fillets, place skin side down) and baste with the olive oil. Rub in the ground pepper. Cover each steak with the lemon slices. Fold the foil into a tent over the fish. Bake for about 20 minutes until the fish just flakes with a fork. Serve.

YIELD: 2 SERVINGS

❓ **How it works:** *Salmon is a go-to food for vitamin D; it also contains anti-inflammatory fatty acids. Vitamin D also helps the immune system function optimally. Many people have suboptimal blood levels of this vitamin. Several studies have linked low levels of vitamin D with a higher risk for respiratory infection. Some studies further suggest that dietary supplementation may lower the risk of respiratory infection.*

When to Call the Doctor

- *Your child under age two may have influenza.*

- *You suspect you have influenza and are pregnant, over age sixty-five, or have a chronic illness, such as lung disease (asthma or chronic obstructive lung disease), heart disease, or diabetes.*

- *Your nasal discharge lasts more than ten days, becomes green, or is accompanied by facial or tooth pain—the signs of a bacterial sinus infection.*

- *Your fever rises above 103°F (39.5°C).*

- *You fever lasts more than three days.*

- *You develop shortness of breath or wheezing.*

- *Symptoms have not improved after three to five days of home management.*

- *You start feeling worse rather than better.*

Chapter 46

Insomnia

"To sleep, perchance to dream." Hamlet's reflection was for him, and for millions of Americans, wishful thinking. At any one time, up to a quarter of the population has insomnia, defined as an inability to fall and/or stay asleep. Nearly everyone has had at least one fretful night. Unfortunately, 10 percent of adults have chronic insomnia. For a variety of reasons, women are more often troubled with insomnia than are men.

Chronic insomnia erodes quality of life. Compared to their rested peers, people who don't get enough sleep are at risk for accidents (including car crashes and falls), infections, depression, weight problems, high blood pressure, heart disease, and diabetes. Poor concentration and thinking skills erode productivity. Tired people miss more work and decline social engagements. The personal and societal impact is enormous.

Ideally, treatment resolves the underlying problem that keeps the person awake: psychological stress, anxiety, depression, heartburn, chronic cough, night sweats associated with menopause, frequent urination in older men with enlarged prostates, sleep disorders, and more. Sometimes all that's needed is to improve what's called "sleep hygiene." That means you use your bed only for sleep and sex. In addition:

- Don't do any of the following in bed: pay bills, argue, do homework, or watch television. It's also a good idea not to do mentally stimulating things just before bed, either.

- Create soothing bedtime rituals.

- Find time for physical activity each day, but avoid vigorous exercise just before bed. Stretching is fine.

- Go to bed and arise at more or less the same time every day. Most people need about 8 hours of sleep a night. (And your brain keeps track of any accumulating debt.) Give yourself a cushion of 30 minutes for falling asleep.

- Make your bedroom a warm, dark, inviting place. Even low light can disrupt melatonin, a hormone that regulates sleep and other rhythms. Cover glowing LED lights with a cloth. Turn your alarm clock to face the wall.

- Banish self-defeating thoughts. The problem with chronic insomnia is a dread of bedtime. Welcome it. Each night is a fresh start.

If you wake up in the middle of the night, stay calm. Don't look at the clock. Get out of bed. Do something relaxing. When you're sleepy, slip between the sheets. Researchers have begun to unveil historical documents suggesting that humans have long had two sleeps separated by a period of wakefulness. If so, waking in the night is normal.

History

Sleep—and the lack of it—has been a concern for millennia. Ancient Egyptians prescribed opium for insomniacs. Of course, opium and its derivatives aren't safe. Many safer herbs have a long tradition of use as sleep aids: hops, lemon balm, skullcap, passionflower, California poppy, and valerian. Both King George III and Abraham Lincoln reportedly slept on pillows stuffed with hops, a remedy still recommended by modern herbalists. Scientific study shows that many sedative herbs act on the brain in a similar way to modern sleep medications—but without side effects. The best-researched sleep herb is valerian.

Lifestyle Tip

Drink a cup of chamomile tea. Used as a tea, the herb German chamomile has been a popular sleep remedy since ancient times. It has sleep-promoting and antianxiety effects. A preliminary study showed significant improvement in daytime functioning but only small benefits for sleep quantity and quality in a group of chronic insomniacs taking a chamomile extract. Drink tea at least an hour before bedtime to avoid being awakened by a full bladder.

 ## Lavender Foot Massage

1 ounce (28 g) carrier oil (e.g., almond, apricot, grape seed, jojoba, or olive oil)
12 drops lavender essential oil (half as much for pregnant women and children)

PREPARATION AND USE:

Pour the oil and lavender essential oil into a clean jar. Cap and shake. Wash and dry your feet. Sitting comfortably, draw a foot into your lap. Pour a palmful (about 1 tablespoon [15 ml]) of scented oil into your palm and massage into your foot. Take your time. Switch feet. If it's a chilly night, put on clean socks. Crawl into bed.

YIELD: 1 APPLICATION

❓ How it works: *Lavender is calming. The essential oil crosses the skin to enter the blood. It also enters via the lungs when you inhale the aroma. Massaging your feet literally takes you out of your busy head to help you settle down for the night. A 2013 study found inhalation of a blend of calming essential oils (lavender, Roman chamomile, and neroli) lowered anxiety and improved sleep quality in cardiac patients in the intensive care unit (a place notorious for disrupting sleep). You don't have to be sick to get the benefits. A study in healthy Japanese students showed that nighttime inhalation of lavender made them feel more refreshed come morning.*

Variation: Ask a friend or partner to rub your feet (or back) for you. Feel free to experiment with other calming essential oils, such as Roman chamomile, bergamot, rose geranium, melissa (lemon balm), neroli, jasmine, ylang ylang, and sandalwood. What's important is whether you find the aroma relaxing.

Scented Sleep Pillow

2 to 3 drops lavender essential oil

PREPARATION AND USE:
Cover your pillow with a fresh pillowcase. Rub a couple of drops of lavender essential oil into your palms. Run your palms over the pillowcase to transfer the soothing scent.

YIELD: 1 APPLICATION

❓ How it works: *Studies show that lavender essential oil has a calming effect on the nervous system. In a study of women going through menopause (a change that often disrupts sleep), smelling of lavender improved sleep quality.*

 ## Sleep-Promoting Salt Bath

2 cups (480 g) Epsom salts
10 drops lavender essential oil

PREPARATION AND USE:
Blend the salts and lavender drops in a clean bowl. Draw a warm bath. Pour in the ingredients and disperse with your fingertips. Turn off the electric lights. Light a candle. Slip into the warm, aromatic water. Relax. After you emerge and towel off, crawl into bed.

YIELD: 1 APPLICATION

❓ How it works: *Warmth helps you relax and sleep. So does lavender. Another theory is that the bath raises your body temperature slightly. Afterward, your temperature falls to normal. That downward shift simulates a decline in body temperature that normally occurs with sleep. Epsom salts are magnesium sulfate. Unpublished research suggests that soaking in an Epsom salt bath can increase blood levels of magnesium, which has a relaxant effect on tense muscles.*

Fact or Myth?

TAKE A NIGHTCAP TO BRING ON A GOOD NIGHT'S SLEEP.

Myth. Alcohol can help you fall asleep. However, as the body breaks down alcohol to a more toxic intermediary chemical (acetaldehyde), sleep becomes restless and fragmented. Moderate your alcohol intake: no more than one glass for women, two for men. If you enjoy a drink, have it with dinner and then quit.

Lifestyle Tip

For you travelers, supplements containing the hormone melatonin are helpful for jet lag and other shifts in daily rhythm. Most studies have used 2 to 8 milligrams, taken for up to three days before departure at the time corresponding to bedtime at the destination. Travelers can also take advantage of sunlight to get in sync with the new time zone. Early morning light will shift your clock earlier (earlier awakening, earlier to bed). Bright light later in the day shifts your clock later (later to bed and to rise). Because melatonin levels decline with age, supplements also seem to help elderly people with insomnia. Discuss that option with your doctor.

Lavender Bath Bomb

1 cup (221 g) baking soda
½ cup (65 g) cornstarch
½ cup (120 g) Epsom salts
½ cup (197 g) powdered citric acid (see note)
1 tablespoon (15 ml) water
2 teaspoons (10 ml) lavender essential oil
1 tablespoon (15 ml) melted coconut oil or
    vegetable oil

PREPARATION AND USE:

In a large glass bowl, combine all the dry ingredients. Whisk until smooth.

In a separate small glass bowl, mix together the liquids (they will not blend perfectly). While continuing to whisk the dry ingredients, slowly add the liquid, about 1 teaspoon (5 ml) at a time—do not add too quickly or the ingredients will react. The final consistency should be like damp (not wet) sand and should hold together in a clump. If too dry, add another teaspoon (5 ml) of oil mixed with a teaspoon (5 ml) of water. If too wet, add small amounts of cornstarch.

Press into muffin tins, filling halfway. Once dry, pop out the bombs and store in a tightly capped jar. Add one bomb to a warm bath and soothe away.

YIELD: 8 TO 12 BOMBS, DEPENDING ON THE SIZE OF YOUR MOLD

❷ How it works: *The warmth of the bath soothes and relaxes. The Epsom salts relax the muscles. The lavender is calming.*

Note: You can buy powdered citric acid in a natural food store, grocery store, or crafts store.

Worry Pad

A pad of paper
A pen

PREPARATION AND USE:

Before you go to bed, write down anything that's troubling you. After you write your list, say to yourself, "All of this can wait till the morning."

If you awaken in the night with worries, write them down, too, to help put them out of your mind.

YIELD: 1 SESSION

❷ How it works: *Thoughts of tomorrow's agenda can interfere with relaxation in the present. Writing down your troubles can help release them. Sometimes the concern is simply that you might forget to do something. If you write it down, you have a visible to-do list to address in the morning. Tell yourself that now you can let go.*

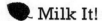 ## Milk It!

1 cup (235 ml) milk
Honey or stevia
1 cardamom seed or 1 clove, crushed

PREPARATION AND USE:

Heat the milk with the cardamom in a small pan. Bring to a boil and then lower the heat to low. Simmer for 3 minutes. Add honey or stevia to taste. Simmer for 1 minute more. Remove from the heat and cover. Set aside for 5 minutes. Strain. Drink the warm milk before going to bed.

YIELD: 1 SERVING

❓ **How it works:** *A cup of warm milk has long been revered as a sleep aid. It was once thought that milk's tryptophan (an amino acid that forms the backbone to the brain chemical serotonin and the hormone melatonin, both of which influence sleep) was the key ingredient. However, more recent studies suggest that commercially sold milk doesn't really improve sleep. Scientists hold that warm milk before bed is simply soothing—even if it's all in your head. Cardamom has been traditionally used to settle the digestive system.*

Fact or Myth?

NAPPING IS ONE GOOD WAY TO GET THE SLEEP YOU NEED.

Yes and no. Studies show that a well-timed nap can help you function better and help lower blood pressure. However, a long, late nap could throw your nighttime sleep schedule—and your important quota—off track.

Lifestyle Tip

Chill on the caffeine. It takes 5 hours for your body to eliminate half of the caffeine circulating in your blood—double that time in women who are pregnant or on oral hormonal contraceptives. If you want to sleep, avoid late afternoon and evening consumption. And be aware that many soft drinks, green and black tea, chocolate, and "energy" drinks contain caffeine. Some medications (e.g., decongestants and certain antidepressants) can aggravate sleep problems. Diuretics taken late in the day can lead to nighttime bathroom trips. Talk to your doctor about taking medications in the morning.

When Simple Doesn't Work

Herbal remedies can quiet the mind. Valerian (Valeriana officinalis) is the best researched. A 2010 analysis of eighteen published human studies concluded that the majority resulted in subjective improvements in insomnia without significant side effects. Herbalists report that a small proportion of people find that valerian stimulates rather than diminishes mental activity. One study found that a combination of valerian and hops (Humulus lupulus—an ingredient in beer) reduced insomnia. Another study showed that the combination of valerian and lemon balm (Melissa officinalis) helped children with restlessness and poor sleep. Other subtly sedative herbs include California poppy (Eschscholzia californica), skullcap (Scutellaria lateriflora), passionflower (Passiflora incarnate), and German chamomile (Matricaria recutita). You can find combination products that contain several sleep-enhancing herbs.

Count Your Blessings (Instead of Sheep)

You

Your worry pad (page 354)

PREPARATION AND USE:

After you write down any niggling worries, list three things you're feeling grateful about. They needn't be big things. If it's raining, you might feel grateful for the sound of raindrops on windowpanes and your dry, warm bed.

YIELD: 1 SESSION

❓ How it works: *Studies have shown that people with a sense of gratitude (something you can actively cultivate) sleep better. A study in people who had problems sleeping found that feelings of gratitude led to more positive expectations about sleep, which subjectively improved sleep quality. That message is important because a few nights of insomnia can generate a sense of anxiety about sleep, which worsens the situation. Focus instead on what's going right.*

🔦 Total Body Scrunch

You

Your bed

PREPARATION AND USE:

Lie on your bed. Draw your tailbone down to protect your low back. Lift your arms and legs (the Superman pose). Release.

Roll onto your back again, pull your whole body into a ball, knees to chest, arms wrapped around legs. Scrunch your face and pull it toward your knees. Release back onto the bed.

Let go. Really let go. Feel how warm and relaxed your muscles are. Feel the way the mattress and pillow support you.

If you awaken in the night, repeat this exercise out of bed, if you're sharing space with a partner.

YIELD: 1 SESSION

❷ How it works: *Complete muscle exertion helps you fully relax, bringing you closer to sleep. In the evening, light yoga or stretches can also help bring you closer to sleep. With practice, you can lie down, do a mental body scan, and quickly release any identified areas of tension.*

🔦 Sleepy-Time Quick Flex

You

Your bed (or a soft pad or rug)

PREPARATION AND USE:

Lie on your back. Sequentially tighten and release every muscle in your body:

hands	buttocks
arms	stomach
feet	neck
legs	

Scrunch your face. Open your eyes wide and stick out your tongue as far as you can. Now totally relax. Sink into the mattress and pillow. Repeat if you awaken in the middle of the night.

YIELD: 1 SESSION

❷ How it works: *Progressive muscle tightening and relaxation helps you focus on how warm and heavy the muscles feel, making you drowsy. Repeat this all the way up your body, ending at your neck and face. When you finish, you should feel quieter physically and mentally.*

Count Your Breaths

You
A quiet place

PREPARATION AND USE:

Breathe in, making the inhalation as long and as slow as you can. Count silently. It doesn't matter whether you count slowly (one-one thousand, two-one thousand) to four or to ten. Exhale as long and as slowly as you can, again counting silently. Repeat until you relax and feel sleepy.

YIELD: 1 SESSION

❓ **How it works:** *Similar to counting sheep, this exercise makes it hard to think about other things, so you begin to relax. The slow breaths calm your nervous system. Studies show that, even in people with serious medical conditions, the breath work used in yoga (plus or minus yoga poses) improves sleep quality.*

When to Call the Doctor

Insomnia is underrecognized and under-treated. Because doctors often don't inquire about sleep quality, you will likely need to bring up the fact that yours isn't good. Let your doctor know when:

- *It takes more than 30 minutes to fall asleep.*

- *You awaken during the night.*

- *You feel unrefreshed when you arise and/ or sleepy during the day—despite attempts to allow yourself enough time in bed.*

- *You have symptoms or signs of a sleep disorder (snoring and breath-holding during the night, unpleasant sensations or movements in limbs that keep you awake, etc.).*

Chapter 47

Menopause

Menopause is like climate change writ small. The woman's climate becomes more tropical, but at somewhat unpredictable moments. Like global warming, menopause can be inconvenient, such as when you're standing before a group of college students and have to stop mid-lecture to pare down to your camisole.

In menopause, the ovaries shut down for business. Estrogen and progesterone fall dramatically. Menstrual periods cease. (Yes, there is good news. That, and the hair on your arms and legs thins—seemingly by migrating to your chin.)

The average age of natural menopause is fifty-one. The long warm-up period is called perimenopause. It can last for years. Progesterone often wanes before estrogen, which can lead to more frequent, heavier periods. Some women also notice mood swings and more frequent headaches. As estrogen levels plummet, hot flashes occur. Night sweats and other menopause-related changes can interrupt sleep. Concentration may waver. Vaginal tissues become thinner and drier. Sex drive can decline—though some of that is psychological (whether you find yourself and your mate attractive). The skin, mouth, and eyes may also become drier. Some women breeze through perimenopause to menopause; others suffer.

For years, conventional treatment has focused on hormone replacement therapy (HRT)—the name for the combined use of estrogen and progesterone. Women at risk for breast cancer can't use any kind of HRT. Alternative prescription medications can help. So can lifestyle changes, such as incorporating breathable materials (e.g., a mattress pad without the rubberized backing or wearing cotton nightclothes) to combat sleep-interrupting night sweats.

History

An Egyptian medical text dated 2000 BCE advises: "If a menopausal woman has pain or makes trouble, pound her hard on the jaw." Some five hundred years ago, a more enlightened approach appeared in a Renaissance medical text recommending exercise and an herbal remedy—a "decoction of myrrh and apples." Fast-forward to the 1890s, when women had the option of taking a pharmaceutical made from pulverized cow ovaries.

In 1942, Premarin (a blend of estrogens extracted from the urine of pregnant mares) hit the scene. Later, progestins (synthetic progesterone) were added to protect against estrogen-induced uterine cancer. Marketing campaigns promised women extended youth and vitality.

Then, in 2002, a large study linked hormone replacement therapy with an increased risk of breast cancer, heart attack, and stroke. However, many of the volunteers were well past menopause and all took the same dose of Premarin and progestin—a combo called Prempro. Nevertheless, the findings left doctors and women alike at a loss for a safe solution. Recently released results from a study in younger women (forty-two to fifty-eight years old) suggest that a lower dose of Premarin or estradiol (the body's natural form of estrogen) plus a more natural form of progesterone relieves menopausal symptoms and improves depression, anxiety, and cognitive (mental) function without cardiovascular disease risk.

Meantime, in a historical 180, many women have become interested in traditional herbs, such as black cohosh, used by Native Americans. In the 1980s, German researchers began to study the effects in menopausal women of a concentrated extract called Remifemin—with significant results. Some studies have even shown black cohosh extract comparable to HRT. However, a 2006 study comparing placebo (a dummy pill), black cohosh, a multibotanical formula, soy, and HRT showed that only the hormones were actually effective.

Goddess Celebration Journal

Many women find this time of life liberating and exhilarating. You've accomplished much. Accept and celebrate your status as a Wise Woman.

A blank piece of paper
A pen

PREPARATION AND USE:
Find a quiet place. Make a list of your accomplishments.

Follow with a paragraph reflecting on your life as a twenty-year-old woman. Reflect on which woman you would rather be: the new you or the old you.

YIELD: 1 SESSION

❓ **How it works:** *Spending dedicated time to recognize and record your accomplishments reinforces your self-respect and joy and helps you look toward the future.*

Lifestyle Tip

Try a lubricant. Dealing with vaginal dryness is no fun. Try a water-soluble—not oil-based—lubricant. Some studies have shown that oil can cause irritation over time.

Practice portion control. Eating smaller meals throughout the day means taking in fewer calories and helps prevent the weight gain that often accompanies menopause and contributes to frequency of hot flashes.

Artery-Enhancing Olive Oil Dressing

Menopausal women are at greater risk for heart disease. Keep your heart tuned up with this healthy dressing.

¼ cup (60 ml) extra-virgin olive oil
¼ cup (60 ml) red wine vinegar
¾ teaspoon dried oregano
¼ teaspoon salt substitute
Pinch of freshly ground black pepper

PREPARATION AND USE:
Combine all the ingredients in a blender and blend. Pour over salads rich in leafy green vegetables.

YIELD: ⅓ CUP (80 ML) DRESSING (REFRIGERATE LEFTOVERS)

❓ How it works: *Extra-virgin olive oil, which is good for the heart and arteries, helps menopausal women guard against cardiovascular disease. Leafy greens in salads provide calcium and other nutrients to help stave off bone loss. Plus, filling up on lightly dressed salads (rather than, say, French fries) can help stave off the weight creep that often affects women past menopause.*

Leafy Greens and Tofu Sauté

Substitute any combination of your favorite greens in this recipe. Mustard greens and kale are good dietary sources of calcium and magnesium.

2 cups (72 g) Swiss chard
2 cups (60 g) baby spinach, rinsed and drained
2 cups (40 g) arugula
2 cups (134 g) kale
1 tablespoon (15 ml) vegetable oil
1 block (14 ounces, or 400 g) firm tofu, cut into 1-inch (2.5 cm) chunks
1 garlic clove, minced
1 teaspoon (5 ml) water
¼ cup (30 g) walnut halves and pieces
¼ cup (35 g) raisins or (30 g) dried cranberries

PREPARATION AND USE:
Tear the greens into small pieces.

Heat the oil in a large skillet or wok over medium heat. Add the tofu and sauté for about 5 minutes. Add the garlic and sauté for about a minute. Increase the heat to medium-high and add the greens. Stir with a wooden spoon until wilted. Reduce the heat to low and add the water. Cover and allow to steam for 3 minutes. Mix in the walnuts and raisins and serve.

YIELD: 4 SERVINGS

❓ How it works: *Tofu, made of soybeans, contains isoflavones (plant substances that act as phytoestrogens—they stimulate estrogen receptors). Research indicates that consuming soy protein (20 to 60 grams a day, which provides 34 to 76 milligrams of isoflavones) can reduce hot flashes. Also, soy foods, leafy dark greens, and walnuts are rich in bone-friendly minerals, such as calcium and magnesium. Studies indicate that consumption of more soy isoflavones slows bone loss after menopause.*

Tea for Sage Women

This earthy and pungent tea can help ground women as menopause takes flight.

2 cups (475 ml) water
1 tablespoon (2 g) crumbled dry sage leaves,
 or 2 tablespoons (5 g) chopped fresh
Honey (optional)

PREPARATION AND USE:
Boil the water. Turn off the heat and add the sage. Cover and steep for 10 minutes. Strain. Add honey, if desired, to taste.

YIELD: 1 LARGE SERVING OR 2 SMALL SERVINGS

❓ How it works: *Sage is a traditional remedy for excessive perspiration. It also contains a chemical called geraniol that acts as a phytoestrogen. A 2011 Swiss study showed that a fresh sage extract taken for eight weeks significantly reduced hot flashes and associated menopausal symptoms relative to placebo.*

❗ Warning: *Limit to three cups a day. Sage comes in a couple species: common garden sage* (Salvia officinalis) *and Spanish sage* (Salvia lavandulaefolia). *The former contains thujone, a chemical that, in higher doses, can be toxic to the nervous system and stimulate seizures in vulnerable people. Aside from use as a food seasoning, pregnant and nursing women should avoid medicinal doses of garden sage (as it can stimulate uterine contractions and bleeding and also diminish breast milk).*

 Soy Smoothie with Flaxseeds

This may be the best smoothie you've ever tasted—rich and full of flavor.

1 ripe banana, quartered
1 large peach, pitted and sliced (Use frozen peaches if not in season.)
1 cup (170 g) fresh or (255 g) frozen strawberries
1 cup (235 ml) soy milk
½ cup (115 g) soy yogurt
2 tablespoons (40 g) honey
2 tablespoons (14 g) flaxseed meal

PREPARATION AND USE:
In a blender, puree the fruit with the soy milk, yogurt, and honey until smooth. Add the flax seed and give it a final blend. Pour and sip.

YIELD: ABOUT 4 CUPS (946 ML)

❓ How it works: *Flaxseeds contain lignans, which are phytoestrogens (estrogen-like substances in plants). Two out of 3 studies using flaxseeds show a reduction in menopausal symptoms.*

Note: Buy packaged flaxseed meal or grind the seeds in small batches in a coffee grinder or food mill. Store in the refrigerator.

Savory and Grounding Lentil Soup

This soup is rich and soothing and delicious with a loaf of French bread. It refrigerates well so you can enjoy it for several days.

1½ cups (288 g) dried lentils
2 tablespoons (28 ml) vegetable oil
1 onion, diced
3 garlic cloves, minced
1 can (14.5 ounces, or 411 g) diced tomatoes
2 carrots, peeled and diced
2 celery stalks, diced
1 quart (946 ml) vegetable stock
2 sage leaves, or 1 teaspoon (1 g) dried sage
2 bay leaves
½ teaspoon ground cumin
Sea salt and freshly ground black pepper

PREPARATION AND USE:

Rinse the lentils and then soak them in water for at least 1 hour.

Pour the oil into a large saucepan over medium heat. Sauté the onion and garlic for about 2 minutes. Add the tomatoes, carrots, and celery and sauté for 3 to 5 minutes more. Pour in the stock and add the sage, bay leaves, cumin, and salt and pepper to taste. Stir in the lentils and bring to a boil. Lower the heat to low and simmer for 20 minutes. Remove the bay and sage leaves before serving.

YIELD: 6 SERVINGS

❓ **How it works:** *Legumes other than soy contain phytoestrogens. Soy just happens to have the highest content and the most research study.*

When Simple Doesn't Work

A number of herbs may relieve some perimenopausal symptoms. The best researched is black cohosh (Actaea racemosa), with the majority of studies on concentrated extracts producing positive results. Black cohosh seems to be safe for women at risk for uterine or breast cancer. Two studies show benefit for the combination of black cohosh and St. John's wort (Hypericum perforatum). Several studies support use of the South American herb maca (Lepidium meyenii). The research on extracts of red clover (Trifolium pretense) is mixed. Check with your doctor before mixing herbs and prescription medications.

Some nonhormonal medications can reduce symptoms such as hot flashes. They include the antidepressant venlafaxine (Effexor), antidepressants called selective-serotonin reuptake inhibitors (paroxetine, fluoxetine, and citalopram), and the antiseizure medication gabapentin.

For women interested in using hormone replacement therapy, a variety of options are available. Estrogen (both estradiol and Premarin from pregnant mares) come in pills. Estradiol is also available in skin patches, vaginal rings, vaginal tablets, and vaginal creams. Natural and synthetic versions of progesterone come in capsules and vaginal gels.

🍃 Salad Pepper-Uppers

We love the crunchy pick-me-up these seeds add to a salad.

Handful of pomegranate arils or sesame seeds

PREPARATION AND USE:
Sprinkle the arils or seeds over salads or soups.

YIELD: 1 SERVING

❓ **How it works:** *Both pomegranate arils and sesame seeds have phytoestrogens, the chemical that makes soy a menopausal favorite. A 2012 study showed mild benefits for a pomegranate seed oil taken for twelve weeks (though the effects didn't reach the threshold for statistical significance in reducing hot flashes and other menopausal symptoms). The authors called for further studies on pomegranate. Pomegranate does contain a number of healthful nutrients, flavonoids, and omega-3 fatty acids.*

🍃 Take It Outside

The biggest long-term risks of menopause are osteoporosis and heart disease. Staying in motion fights both.

You
A good pair of shoes
Athletic gear or vehicles of your choice
The great outdoors or a roomy area

PREPARATION AND USE:
Walk, jog, dance, cycle, rake leaves, jump rope, or dance. You're aiming for moderate aerobic exercise, which means you have enough breath to talk but not sing. The goal is 30 to 60 minutes a day of physical activity, though you can break the exercise into 10-minute chunks.

YIELD: 1 FULFILLING TIME

❓ **How it works:** *Studies indicate that regular, moderate aerobic exercise reduces hot flashes. It also keeps the heart strong. All the activities listed in this recipe are weight-bearing exercises, the type key to maintaining bones.*

🍃 Breathe Through It

This remedy is for hot flash relief, and it helps in any stressful situation.

You
A quiet place
A comfortable chair or rug

PREPARATION AND USE:
Sit in a comfortable position. Close your eyes. Concentrate on your breathing, making each inhalation slow and deep, from the diaphragm. Breathe out as slowly, letting all the air out of your lungs before the next breath. Moderate your breath to inhale and exhale six times per minute. Repeat for 15 minutes and a total of 90 breaths.

YIELD: 1 SESSION

❓ **How it works:** *A recent study found that slow, deep, diaphragmatic breathing (six breaths per minute for 15 minutes once or twice a day) reduces hot flashes. Such breathing quiets the fight-or-flight response and increases relaxation. You can also experiment with slow, deep breathing in the midst of a hot flash.*

Yoga Stretch

This flowing exercise stretches your entire body, wakes up your spine, and calms and focuses your brain.

You
Loose, stretchable clothing or yoga wear
A floor or flat ground

PREPARATION AND USE:
Stand with both feet firmly planted on the ground, about hip distance apart. Distribute your weight evenly on your feet (front to back, side to side).

Extend your arms at your sides, fingertips pointing down. Align the back of your head and shoulders over your heels. Feel your shoulder blades slide down your back. Raise your arms over your head on an inhalation. Pause.

Holding your core muscles steady, exhale as you slowly swan dive forward. If your fingertips don't touch your toes, bend your knees. Inhaling, put your palms on your shins. Straighten your arms so that your back makes a table-top (with torso at a 90-degree angle to your legs). Exhaling, reach again toward your toes. Let your head and neck go. On an inhale, core solid, lift your arms and your torso back to standing (arms over head). Exhaling, bring your palms together in front of your heart. Close your eyes and breathe. Notice a difference?

YIELD: 1 STRETCH

❓ **How it works:** *Recent studies show that yoga (which combines physical postures with meditation and breathing exercises) reduces some menopausal symptoms, though it may be more beneficial for associated psychological complaints and insomnia than hot flashes. If you haven't tried it, check to see whether beginner's yoga classes are offered in your neighborhood.*

When to Call the Doctor

Doctors continue to prescribe hormones and other medications to women going through menopause. There's no question that they work. If you're feeling tired, fuzzy-headed, sweaty, and otherwise uncomfortable, make an appointment. You may find that a low dose of estrogen and progesterone is well worth the small, individual risk.

It's also a good idea to call if you have any unusual gynecological symptoms such as the resumption of spotting or menstrual bleeding after menopause.

Do keep up on regular gynecological exams as recommended by your doctor.

Lifestyle Tip

Stop smoking and limit alcohol consumption. Studies show that both can affect hot flashes.

Chapter 48

Menstrual Cramps

More than half of young women's monthly periods come with pain. In one study, 20 percent of female college students had cramps that were severe enough to cause them to miss class.

Doctors aren't exactly sure what causes cramps. A prominent theory is that the pain has to do with rising levels of inflammatory chemicals in the uterus. These chemicals cause the uterus to contract and the local blood vessels to constrict, thus diminishing blood flow. These chemicals tend to rise in all women during the latter half of the cycle. But some research shows that these levels are higher in women who experience more pain.

Other causes of discomfort include endometriosis (a condition in which uterine lining tissue grows in other areas of the body), uterine fibroids (benign tumors), and pelvic infections.

The good news is that monthly cramps usually diminish with age. That's cold comfort if you're doubled over in pain now. But there are some therapies and recipes for relief. Natural therapies can help reduce cramps, but work best if started before the pain begins or right at the start of mild symptoms. Once pain becomes severe, it's often better to take an over-the-counter or prescription pain reliever.

History

Given that, throughout history, many herbalists were women, it's not surprising that a number of medicinal plants have been used to manage menstrual discomfort. In traditional Chinese medicine, dong quai *(Angelica sinensis)* was used. Indeed, root extracts open constricted arteries, relax smooth muscle, and decrease inflammation. Another Asian favorite is ginger *(Zingiber officinale)*, which reduces pain and inflammation. North American natives brewed teas from black haw *(Viburnum prunifolium)* and its botanical sister crampbark *(Viburnum opulus)*. Early American physicians recommended teas and tinctures *(alcoholic extracts)* to relieve monthly cramping. Lab studies show both plants relax uterine muscle. Other herbs still favored by natural healers include black cohosh *(Actaeus racemosa)*, wild yam *(Dioscorea villosa)*, and raspberry leaf *(Rubus idaeus)*.

Warm Monthly Relief

2 cups (480 g) Epsom salts
5 to 10 drops peppermint essential oil

PREPARATION AND USE:
As you run a warm bath, mix in the Epsom salts until they dissolve. Swish in peppermint drops. Soak.

YIELD: 1 SOOTHING SOAK

❓ **How it works:** *Heat increases blood flow and relaxes muscles (and the uterus is a mainly made of smooth muscle). One of the theoretic problems with cramps is vasoconstriction (constricted arteries). Increased circulation might also help flush out inflammatory chemicals. Years of tradition and, now, scientific papers do show that heat works and can be as effective as over-the-counter pain relievers. Epsom salts are magnesium sulfate, and magnesium helps muscles relax. Peppermint relaxes intestinal smooth muscle. Scientists have yet to examine its effects on uterine muscle.*

Lifestyle Tip

Beat the cramps with direct heat: try placing a hot water bottle or a heating pad on your abdomen for quick relief. Place a towel or clean cloth between the heat source and your skin to keep from burning.

Lifestyle Tip

Nuts, especially Brazil nuts and almonds, are a great vitamin E delivery vehicle. Mix them up for a quick and healthy snack or sprinkle them over your lunchtime salad.

Castor Oil Pack

2 cups (475 ml) hot water (or enough to fill a hot water bottle)
½ cup (120 ml) castor oil
2 to 3 drops lavender or peppermint essential oil

PREPARATION AND USE:
Heat the water to your desired temperature and pour into a hot water bottle. In a large bowl, mix the castor oil and lavender or peppermint oil. Fold a piece of flannel or woolen cloth into two or three layers. Dip the folded cloth into castor oil mixture. Lie down and apply the soaked cloth to your abdomen. Cover with a sheet of plastic wrap or a plastic bag laid flat. Place the hot water bottle on top of the plastic. Lay the large towel over the hot water bottle and tuck it under each side of your body to hold in warmth. Keep the pack in place for at least 30 minutes. Repeat daily, as long as cramps persist.

YIELD: 1 APPLICATION

❓ **How it works:** *Castor oil has been known to relax the uterine muscles involved in cramping. Lavender relaxes smooth muscles and mental tension. Peppermint relaxes smooth muscle and acts as an analgesic.*

Sweet Spice Tea

2 cups (475 ml) water
2 teaspoons (4 g) aniseeds
1 teaspoon (2 g) celery seeds
1 tablespoon (2 g) dried peppermint leaves
¼ teaspoon saffron
Honey or stevia (optional)

PREPARATION AND USE:

Boil the water. Place the aniseeds, celery seeds, peppermint, and saffron in a teapot or bowl. Pour in the boiling water. Let steep for 15 to 20 minutes. Strain. Sweeten to taste, if desired.

YIELD: 2 SERVINGS

❓ How it works: *One study found that when women with a history of menstrual cramps took a special, concentrated extract of saffron, celery seeds, and aniseeds three times a day, their severe discomfort diminished in intensity and duration. Peppermint is included in this recipe for its muscle-relaxing qualities.*

Note: The spice saffron is made from dried stigmas (threadlike female parts of the flower) of a species of crocus *(Crocus sativus)*. One gram costs about fifteen dollars.

Tea for Ginger Tummies

This general soother works especially well for menstrual cramps.

2 cups (475 ml) water
2 teaspoons (5 g) grated fresh ginger
1 tablespoon (20 g) honey

PREPARATION AND USE:

Boil the water. Place the ginger in a teapot. Add the boiling water and allow the ginger to steep for 15 minutes. Stir in the honey. Sip.

YIELD: 1 SERVING

❓ How it works: *Ginger reduces pain and inflammation. One study found that a special ginger extract taken four times a day eased pain as effectively as ibuprofen.*

Omega Time

In one study, Danish women who regularly ate fish had milder menstrual symptoms.

1 tablespoon (15 ml) olive oil
¼ teaspoon dried ginger, or 1 teaspoon
   (3 g) grated fresh
2 salmon steaks
Salt and freshly ground black pepper
Pinch of curry powder
Lemon slices, for garnish

PREPARATION AND USE:

Mix the olive oil and ginger.

Set the oven to broil, and place the fish on a broiler pan. Mix the olive oil and ginger. Baste the salmon on both sides with the oil mixture. Season with salt and pepper on both sides.

Broil until the fish is opaque, 4 to 5 minutes for each side. Add a final pinch of pepper and the curry powder. Garnish with lemon slices.

YIELD: 2 SERVINGS

❓ How it works: *Salmon is rich in omega-3s. These anti-inflammatory fatty acids that counter the small chemicals that cause uterine cramps. An Italian study found that young women who consumed more fish, fruit, and eggs (and less wine) were less likely to have cramps. Ginger and curry powder have anti-inflammatory properties.*

Olive-Topia Tapenade

¼ cup (25 g) pitted black olives, chopped finely
1½ teaspoons (5 g) minced fresh garlic
Olive oil
Pinch of sea salt
Small loaf of crusty French bread

PREPARATION AND USE:

Preheat the oven to 350°F (180°C, or gas mark 4).

Combine the chopped olives and garlic in a small bowl and mix fully. Drizzle with enough olive oil to bind the mixture. Stir in a pinch of sea salt. Cut the bread in 1-inch (2.5 cm) slices. Spread with the tapenade and briefly heat in the oven until just warm. Savor!

YIELD: 4 SERVINGS

❓ How it works: *Black olives are rich in vitamin E. Two studies have shown diminution of menstrual pain with supplements containing 400 to 500 IU of the vitamin a day.*

When Simple Doesn't Work

Try ibuprofen or naproxen and take as directed. Going a step further, you may also want to try acupuncture or chiropractic manipulation. Studies suggest that both treatments can reduce menstrual pain.

Decramping Almond Spread

2 cups (290 g) raw almonds

PREPARATION AND USE:

Preheat the oven to 300°F (150°C, or gas mark 2).

Spread the nuts on a dry baking sheet. Roast in the oven for 30 minutes. Let cool fully. In a food processor, grind the nuts on the top setting until they are of granular consistency. Scrape the sides of the processor bowl. Grind the nuts again, for about 2 minutes, until the nut oils release. The spread is ready when the nut oils have turned the powder to a creamy consistency. Put the spread into an airtight glass jar and keep refrigerated. It will last for about three weeks.

YIELD: 8 SERVINGS

How it works: *Almonds, cashews, and other nuts are high in magnesium as well as other nutrients, including vitamin E and omega-3s. Three studies show that magnesium supplements reduced menstrual pain.*

Quick and Soothing Breakfast

¼ cup (20 g) instant oats
¼ cup (60 g) Greek yogurt
⅓ cup (80 ml) water
Stevia or honey
Handful of almonds and/or apricots

PREPARATION AND USE:

Mix the oats, yogurt, and water together in a microwave-safe bowl.

Microwave on high for about 1 minute. Stir and then heat for an additional minute or until it reaches a good consistency. Stir in sweetener, as needed. Top with almonds or apricots.

YIELD: 1 SERVING

How it works: *One study showed that college students who consumed more dairy products had a reduced chance of having cramps. And eating yogurt has many other health benefits, including maintaining bone strength and optimizing your immune system. The vitamin E in almonds and apricots support the dairy's soothing qualities (see the Olive-Topia Tapenade, page 369, for another E-rich recipe).*

Work It Out: Sublime Stretches

You
A quiet place
A mat or rug or other clean, comfortable surface

PREPARATION AND USE:

Stretch 1—Cobra Pose: Lie face down on a clean, comfortable surface. Press your toenails into the floor. Tighten your legs. Tuck in your tailbone (opposite of arching your back). Place your hands close to your sides at nipple level. Pull your elbows in (like cricket wings). With firm core (including abdominal muscles), begin to straighten your arms. Go only as far as is comfortable. You're creating a gentle bend in your upper spine. Inhale and exhale deeply five times.

Lower. Repeat three to five times. When you finish, push back so that your bottom touches (or nearly touches) your heels and your forehead rests on the ground. Let your belly fall between your parted knees. This position is called "child's pose." Rest here for as long as you like.

Stretch 2—Cat-Cow: Get onto all fours—knees under hips, hands under shoulders, and arms straight without locking at the elbow. On an inhalation, let your belly fall, your back sway, and your buttocks and head rise (the "cow" part of the pose). On a slow exhalation, arch your back

370   **500 Time-Tested Home Remedies and the Science Behind Them**

like a cat. Tuck your tailbone down and tuck your head as though you are looking toward your belly button. Repeat as many times as feels good.

YIELD: 1 SESSION

❓ **How it works:** *Regular exercise can reduce menstrual cramps. A recent study showed that these two yoga postures practiced over two monthly cycles eased cramping in young women.*

◗ Take the Pressure Off Chinese Acupressure

Your two hands
A quiet place
A comfortable chair

PREPARATION AND USE:

Sit in a comfortable position. Cross your right leg over your left.

On the right leg, locate the acupressure spot called Spleen 6 (abbreviated SP6)—it is 4 finger widths above your inner ankle bone, just behind the shin bone. With your thumb, press on SP6 (if you feel tenderness, you are probably on the correct spot). Press for 6 seconds, and then release for 2 seconds. Keep this up for 5 minutes. Switch to your left leg and repeat the pressure. Repeat once again on each leg. Feel better.

YIELD: 1 SESSION

❓ **How it works:** *According to ancient Chinese medicine, pressure on sp6 helps relax the uterus and cervix. Nine out of ten studies found acupressure (using fingers or other blunt objects to stimulate acupuncture points) effective in taming menstrual cramps.*

❗ **Warning:** *When you find the correct point, it will feel tender. Often, the pain subsides at the point (and in your womb) as you continue to press. If you feel outright pain, back off.*

When to Call the Doctor

Any time you experience severe pain, you should see your doctor. It's also a good idea to make an appointment if cramping is new for you. In that case, you want to find out if there's an underlying, treatable cause, such as endometriosis, fibroids, ovarian cysts or tumors, or infection. Bladder infection could generate pain in the same region as the uterus, though it's usually also accompanied by frequent, urgent, painful urination. Pelvic inflammatory disease (PID) is a serious, treatable infection of the uterus and fallopian tubes. Signs and symptoms of PID include lower abdominal pain with or without intercourse, foul-smelling vaginal discharge, irregular menstrual bleeding, and fever. If you have any doubts about the cause of pelvic pain, call your doctor's office.

Chapter

49

Morning Sickness

Nausea and vomiting are one of the most common complaints during a woman's pregnancy—and perhaps the first time that cracks appear in her romantic notions of motherhood. In fact, 50 to 90 percent of women have queasiness during the first trimester (the first thirteen weeks). Symptoms usually begin at the end of the first month, peak during the third month, and dissipate by week 14. Of all the races, white women are most commonly affected.

Up to 3 percent of women develop severe and persistent nausea and vomiting. This condition, called *hyperemesis gravidarum*, may require hospitalization to maintain nutrition and hydration. A number of factors are thought to cause nausea and vomiting in pregnancy. They include hormonal shifts, heightened sense of smell, psychological challenges, and genetics.

Fortunately, most women have mild symptoms. Although those symptoms may be miserable for you, the good news is that nausea and vomiting during pregnancy doesn't stunt your fetus's growth.

History

Pregnancy often comes with a nausea that can make even those with the strongest stomachs lurch at the smell of food. Reportedly, nineteenth-century English novelist Charlotte Brontë had such a severe case that she couldn't keep anything down and died in early pregnancy. The earliest known descriptions of expectant mothers' malaise of nausea and vomiting go back to 2000 BCE. Throughout history, herbs such as ginger *(Zingiber officinale)*, chamomile *(Matricaria recutita)*, lemon balm *(Melissa officinalis)*, peppermint *(Mentha x piperita)*, and raspberry leaf *(Rubus idaeus)* have been made into soothing teas. Nineteenth-century Eclectic physicians, who used both traditional herbal and conventional treatments, recommended menthol vapors. Tragically, the prescribed use of the drug thalidomide for morning sickness in the 1950s led to the birth of some ten thousand babies with stunted or absent arms or legs. Since then, the low-risk approach of few or no prescription drugs during pregnancy has remained in effect.

These recipes are especially focused on morning sickness; look in Chapter 51, on nausea and vomiting, to find additional and related recipes.

 ## Morning Bedside Snack

Rice cakes, crackers, or dry toast
Peanut, cashew, or almond butter, or tahini
Glass of water

PREPARATION AND USE:

Prepare your snack the night before. (Or ask your partner to serve you in bed.) Spread the nut butter on the cakes or crackers and leave them on a plate at your bedside. (If nut butters suddenly seem loathsome, leave them off.)

Before you do as much as lift your head from the pillow, nibble your snack. Sip the water. Take your time. Get up slowly.

YIELD: 1 SNACK

❷ How it works: *Low blood sugar often triggers nausea and vomiting during pregnancy. Your goal is to prevent low blood sugar. Carbohydrates, especially refined carbohydrates, quickly raise blood sugar. While you sleep, you're fasting. That's why you want to break that fast as soon as possible. Try to eat a small meal every 2 hours.*

Lifestyle Tip

Take time to relax and to get enough sleep. Many women find that stress and exhaustion worsens symptoms.

 ## B₆ Boost

1 cup (30 g) spinach, rinsed and drained
¼ cup (56 g) diced, boiled potato
1 tablespoon (15 ml) olive oil
1 tablespoon (15 ml) balsamic vinegar
¼ cup (36 g) sunflower seeds
1 can (6 ounces, or 168 g) tuna or 6 ounces (170 g) cooked chicken breast (optional)
1 hard-boiled large egg, sliced
1 slice whole wheat bread, toasted

PREPARATION AND USE:

Toss the spinach and potato in a salad bowl. Whisk the oil and vinegar in a small bowl. Drizzle the vinaigrette into the salad and toss again. Toss in the sunflower seeds. If the smell of tuna or chicken doesn't make you gag, add as much as you want. Top with slices of egg. Nibble the toast as you eat the salad.

YIELD: 1 SERVING

❷ How it works: *Several studies have shown that vitamin B₆ supplements reduce nausea in pregnancy. Spinach, sunflower seeds, potatoes, tuna, chicken, and whole grains are all good sources of B₆. Other sources include nuts, peas, and beans. Eggs offer high protein, which takes longer to digest, so it stays in your system longer. All of these foods contain valuable nutrients.*

Note: Use additional oil and vinegar, if desired, but keep their ratio 1:1.

Veggified Rice with Garlic and Ginger

1¾ cups (410 ml) water
1 garlic clove, minced
Pinch of salt
¾ cup (143 g) uncooked brown rice
1 broccoli floret, sliced
1 carrot, diced
½ red bell pepper, seeded and diced
½ onion, diced
½ teaspoon fresh minced fresh ginger

PREPARATION AND USE:

Add the garlic and salt to the water and bring to a boil. Stir in the rice and bring to a boil again. Lower the heat to low, cover, and simmer for about 30 minutes. Stir the vegetables into the fully cooked rice. Sprinkle in the ginger and fluff the mixture. Remove from the heat and keep covered for 15 minutes, allowing the ginger flavor and its benefits to permeate the rice.

YIELD: 4 SERVINGS

❷ **How it works:** *The carbohydrates in rice help settle the stomach. Carrots, broccoli, and peppers are filled with vitamin B$_6$, and ginger is a vetted antinausea agent (see the Nausea-Quelling Ginger Tea, page 375).*

Note: Eating garlic is safe during pregnancy. However, if the smell or taste of garlic makes you queasy, leave it out.

Fact or Myth?

TAKE IT EASY DURING PREGNANCY AND TRY NOT TO EXERCISE.

Myth. Get outside and move. Fresh air and exercise can definitely help morning sickness and overall health—both yours and the baby's. If you're not used to exercising, start slow. Walking is great exercise for everyone. Be sure to drink water afterward.

Comforting Potato-Cauli Mash

2 boiled potatoes, peeled
1 garlic clove, minced
½ head cauliflower, steamed until easily pierced with a fork
Freshly ground black pepper

PREPARATION AND USE:

With a potato masher, mash the still-warm potatoes in a medium-size bowl. Mash in the minced garlic. In a separate bowl, mash the warm cauliflower. Mix together the potatoes and cauliflower. Add the pepper and enjoy while still warm.

YIELD: 2 SERVINGS

❷ **How it works:** *Potatoes and cauliflower are rich in vitamin B$_6$. The warming food is also comforting to the stomach.*

Steady-on Afternoon Snack

1 tablespoon (16 g) organic peanut butter
   (with no added salt or sugar)
1 organic apple, cored and sliced

PREPARATION AND USE:

Spread the apple slices with the peanut butter
and enjoy.

YIELD: 1 SNACK

❓ **How it works:** *Apples contain both simple
and complex carbohydrates. Peanut butter contains protein and fats. The combination can help
keep your blood sugar steady and avoid nausea.*

Recipe Variation: Put slices of high-protein
cheese or dollops of cottage cheese on crackers.

Nausea-Quelling Ginger Tea

2 cups (475 ml) water
1 teaspoon (3 g) grated fresh ginger, or
   ½ teaspoon dried
Honey or agave nectar

PREPARATION AND USE:

Bring the water to a boil in a small saucepan.
Lower the heat to low. Add the ginger. Simmer for
5 minutes. Cover and steep for 15 minutes. Strain.
Add sweetener, as desired. Sip over the course
of the day.

YIELD: 2 SERVINGS

❓ **How it works:** *A half-dozen studies support
the use of ginger for nausea and vomiting during
pregnancy. One study in pregnant women found
that ginger was nearly as effective as the antinausea drug metoclopramide (Reglan) and another
found it was as effective as dimenhydrinate
(Dramamine). Study doses have not exceeded
1 gram a day (usually divided into four doses)
of encapsulated ginger nor have they continued
past the first trimester.*

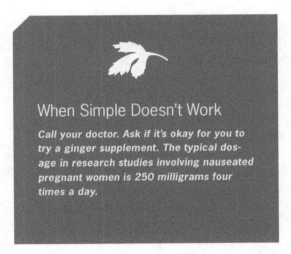

When Simple Doesn't Work

*Call your doctor. Ask if it's okay for you to
try a ginger supplement. The typical dosage in research studies involving nauseated
pregnant women is 250 milligrams four
times a day.*

Lifestyle Tip

**Shun strong smells. That might mean
avoiding restaurants that use lots of spices
and fry their foods, such as fast-food diners and Indian and Chinese restaurants.
Artificial fragrances in personal care products can also be problematic. Don't feel
shy about asking friends and co-workers to
refrain from wearing perfume around you.
And definitely invite smokers to leave your
airspace.**

Homemade Lemon Ginger Ale

Ginger ale is a longstanding stomach settler. But it needs to be made with real ginger. Start with the Nausea-Quelling Ginger Tea recipe (page 375), and add the following ingredients. Experiment with how much honey and lemon you like.

2 cups Nausea-Quelling Ginger Tea (page 375, but use twice the amount of ginger)

1 cup (235 ml) carbonated water (Sparkling mineral water works well.)

2 to 3 teaspoons (10 to 15 ml) fresh lemon juice

2 to 3 tablespoons (40 to 60 g) honey

PREPARATION AND USE:

Make the ginger tea as directed. Stir in the carbonated water, lemon, and honey. Sip.

YIELD: 3 SERVINGS

❓ How it works: *As noted previously, ginger reduces nausea and vomiting during pregnancy. The honey and fresh lemon juice provide potassium, which vomiting can deplete. Lemon contains antioxidant, immune-boosting flavonoids and vitamin C. Honey also provides sugars.*

Press Away Nausea

You

A quiet place

PREPARATION AND USE:

Locate the two large tendons on the inside of your wrist that run between your palm and your elbow. Find the groove between them, about three finger widths from the top crease at the base of your palm. In acupressure, this point is called Pericadium-6 (PC6), or neiguan. With your middle and index finger, press firmly on the groove for 90-second intervals for about 10 minutes.

YIELD: 1 APPLICATION

❓ How it works: *According to ancient Chinese medicine, pressure on PC6 opens and relaxes the chest and affects the stomach and digestive tract to help relieve nausea. Studies show that acupressure at this point can control nausea and vomiting during pregnancy.*

Note: You can buy wristbands that impart pressure at that precise point in drugstores, health stores, and boating stores. Studies on acupressure for pregnancy-induced nausea have used wristbands.

Manipulate Aromas

Strong odors often trigger nausea and vomiting. During my second pregnancy, I couldn't shop at mainstream supermarkets, which seemed suddenly to reek of popcorn, chewing gum, and synthetic fragrances. As an antidote, carry this instant scent-reliever in your bag. ~ LBW

4 drops spearmint essential oil

PREPARATION AND USE:

Place a cotton ball in a 1-ounce (28 ml) bottle. Drop in the spearmint essential oil. Cap. Open and inhale the scent as needed. If you have an aromatherapy diffuser, you can use it to deliver scents into the air.

YIELD: MULTIPLE APPLICATIONS

❓ How it works: *Some plant aromas have actually been studied as treatments for nausea and vomiting. For instance, essential oils of peppermint, spearmint, ginger, and cardamom reduce postoperative nausea. Although nurse midwives commonly recommend aromatherapy to pregnant women, studies have not yet evaluated effectiveness. The most important thing is that the essential oil smells good to you.*

Note: Pregnant women can apply essential oils during pregnancy, but should cut the concentration in half. If a recipe calls for 10 drops of essential oil blended into a carrier oil, use 5 drops instead. Kathi Keville and Mindy Green, authors of *Aromatherapy: A Complete Guide to the Healing Art*, recommend that pregnant women stick to essential oils derived from flowers. Examples include rose, ylang-ylang, German and Roman chamomile, and citrus (bergamot, mandarin, orange, lemon, lime, and neroli). Spearmint and sandalwood are also okay.

 ## Scented, Soothing Spearmint and Chamomile Tea

Chamomile and spearmint are easy to grow. But you can also find them in bulk in natural food stores and in tea bag form.

2 cups (475 ml) water
2 teaspoons (1 g) dried spearmint leaves
2 teaspoons (1 g) dried chamomile flowers

PREPARATION AND USE:
Boil the water. Add the spearmint and chamomile. Steep, covered, for 15 minutes. Strain and sip.

YIELD: 2 SERVINGS

❷ How it works: *Spearmint's soothing aroma and chamomile's antispasmodic qualities also may help quell rising nausea.*

Note: Alternatively, boil 2 cups (475 ml) of water and dunk in one spearmint tea bag and one chamomile tea bag.

Lifestyle Tip

Nibble watermelon. Getting enough fluids is vital during pregnancy and can help dispel queasiness. Watermelon is a delicious water-delivery system. It contains energy-boosting carbohydrates, electrolytes (mineral salts), carotenoids, potassium, vitamin B6 (previously noted as taming nausea of pregnancy), and other B vitamins. Also, it's relatively low in calories and contains fiber, which can counteract pregnancy-associated constipation.

When to Call the Doctor

- *You have any questions about your pregnancy.*

- *Simple home remedies fail to relieve nausea and vomiting*

- *You feel nauseated all day.*

- *You vomit more than three times a day and can't keep down food and fluids.*

- *You lose more than 2 pounds (905 g).*

- *You vomit blood.*

- *Nausea and vomiting continue longer than four months.*

Chapter 50

Musculoskeletal Pain: Arthritis, Joint Swelling, and Sprains

Pain is a useful sensory perception. Without it, you might continue walking after a tack punctured your foot. Or, you might arise from a skiing accident and continue downhill with a ruptured ligament. Pain alerts you to injury and forces you to lie low until you recover.

Chronic pain is another story. If you have arthritis (joint degeneration), you're well aware of the problem. Not using the joint can actually further the deterioration. Yet the ache holds you back. In this case, a visual cue—perhaps a change in the color of your fingernails—seems kinder and equally helpful. When it's time to rest, your fingernails would glow a fire engine red.

A number of maladies can cause discomfort in muscles and joints. We're going to focus on two things: traumatic injuries and osteoarthritis.

Mechanical trauma can hurt all elements of the musculoskeletal system: muscles, the tendons that attach muscle to bone, the ligaments that hold the joints together, the joints, and the bones.

To a lesser extent, overuse can injure the musculoskeletal system. Many people who use a computer keyboard have experienced tendinitis (tendon inflammation). "Weekend warriors"—relatively inactive people who decide to jog 10 miles (16 kilometers) or play three sets of tennis on Saturday—also know the signs and symptoms.

After a rigorous workout, it's not uncommon to experience muscle soreness the next day. Unless the pain is severe, consider this discomfort a sign of weakness leaving your body. What's happened is that high-intensity workouts cause microscopic tears in muscle fibers. The muscle then rebuilds and gains bulk. The repair process makes it stronger.

Strains and sprains are ailments that occur at any age. **Strains** occur when a muscle or the tendon that attaches it to the bone becomes pulled or twisted. They can occur suddenly (such as from shoveling snow) or over a longer period from overuse.

Sprains occur when the ligaments holding a joint in place become stretched or torn. Usually a fall or twisting motion forces the joint out of its normal alignment. Wrists, ankles, thumbs, and knees are common sprain locations.

Both sprains and strains produce pain, swelling, and sometimes bruising. Symptoms can be mild or so severe as to interfere with normal movement. Severe sprains can be difficult to distinguish from a bone fracture. The treatment is different. That's why getting a physician diagnosis is a good idea.

Arthritis (joint inflammation) is more likely to cause pain and loss of function with age. According to the Centers for Disease Control and Prevention, about 50 million adults (one in five) have received a diagnosis. There are more than one hundred types of arthritis. Osteoarthritis is the most common. Wear and tear causes it. Being overweight, obesity, and traumatic injuries raise the risk of getting it. Another relatively common arthritis, rheumatoid arthritis, is an autoimmune disorder, wherein the body's immune system attacks the joint. Symptoms of that condition can begin in childhood.

Arthritis symptoms include stiffness, pain, aching, and joint swelling. Symptoms of osteoarthritis often improve with movement. Physical activity improves most kinds of arthritis. Medications and physical therapy can also help.

History

Even the dinosaurs had arthritis, so their bones tell us. Evidence of arthritis in humans goes back more than five thousand years. The bones of the famous well-preserved mummy Otzi the Iceman (a.k.a. Frozen Fritz), found in a glacier of the Alps and dated to about 3300 BCE, showed osteoarthritis in his joints. What we don't know is how arthritis sufferers of long ago treated their pains.

We do know, however, that an alpine plant, *Arnica montana*, used in pagan and medieval rituals, was by the 1500s being praised by the Italian physician and botanist Pietro Andrea Mattioli for healing muscle aches and pains. In North America, Native Americans used indigenous species of arnica to soothe aches and muscle injuries. Over the centuries, arnica found its way not only into folk medicines in Europe and America but also gained the endorsement of the European Scientific Cooperative on Phytotherapy for its anti-inflammatory and analgesic properties, including for sprains and muscle and joint pain. A 2008 study confirmed that a topical arnica gel worked as well as ibuprofen for arthritis of the hand.

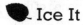

Ice It

*I learned this method from a physical therapist
when I had "tennis elbow." It really helped. ~ LBW*

Water
Small paper cups

PREPARATION AND USE:

Pour water into 6 small paper cups and set them
on a shelf in the freezer. Once the water has
frozen, remove a cup. Starting at the top of the
cup, peel away a strip of paper wide enough to
expose the ice. The remaining paper protects
your fingers from the cold. Briskly massage the
inflamed area with the ice for 3 to 5 minutes.
(Do not hold the ice stationary on the same spot;
doing so can eventually freeze tissue, damaging
it.) If it's a tendon, passing the ice across the fiber
(perpendicular to its length) enhances mobility.

YIELD: 6 APPLICATIONS

❓ How it works: *The cold reduces
inflammation.*

Lifestyle Tip

**A number of gadgets can reduce the stress
on your joints. Rubber grips on gardening
tools, pens, and kitchen appliances increase comfort. Try placing a rubber band
around twist-off tops for jars, bottles, and
tubes (e.g., toothpaste) to make it easier
to open them. Long-handled grippers can
help you grab objects.**

Avo-Kale Arthritis Arrester

1½ cups (100 g) washed, chopped kale,
    divided
⅛ teaspoon salt
Juice of 1 lime
1 avocado, pitted, peeled, and cut into chunks
1 tomato, chopped and seeded
1 carrot, grated
¼ cup (25 g) pitted and chopped green olives
1 garlic clove, minced
¼ cup (36 g) cashews
2 tablespoons (8 g) chopped fresh flat-leaf
    parsley or (2 g) cilantro leaves
Freshly ground black pepper

PREPARATION AND USE:

In a large bowl, sprinkle 1 cup (67 g) of the kale
with the salt and massage the kale leaves for a
minute or so until they begin to wilt. Transfer the
kale to a colander to rinse off the salt and then return the kale to the bowl. Drizzle in the lime juice
and massage again so that the kale is covered
with the juice. Add the avocado, gently tossing
it with the kale while maintaining the avocado's
chunkiness.

Mix in the remaining kale, along with the
tomato, carrot, olives, garlic, and cashews.
Sprinkle in the parsley, add the pepper, and toss
gently. Taste and adjust seasonings or lime juice
as needed. Divide between two plates and serve.

YIELD: 2 SERVINGS

❓ How it works: *Brightly colored fruits and
vegetables, such as kale, avocado, tomato, carrot, and green olives, indicate the presence of
antioxidant and anti-inflammatory flavonoids
and carotenoids. The oil in avocados—called the
"unsaponifiable fractions"—has been found to
improve pain and disability of osteoarthritis.*

RICE: Rest, Ice, Compression, Elevation

This treatment applies to acute injuries involving tendons and ligaments, such as ankle sprains. This method also works for injuries to arms and legs.

A clean cloth

An ice pack (a commercial ice pack, bag of
    frozen peas, or plastic bag of crushed ice
    all work)

Pillows

An elastic wrap (optional)

PREPARATION AND USE:

Wet a clean cloth under the tap and wring it out. Wrap the cloth around the ice pack and apply it to the injured area. Slide pillows under your arm or leg—enough so that, when you recline, the injured area is above the level of your heart. After 10 minutes, remove the ice pack. Wait 10 minutes. Ice for another 10 minutes. Remove.

If you've injured an ankle, knee or wrist, stabilize that joint with an elastic wrap. Start below the joint and wind upward until you're a couple finger widths above that joint. The goal is to provide support without impeding circulation: The bandage should be loose enough that you can insert your index finger under the wrap.

In 2 hours, repeat the process. Continue the regimen for three days.

YIELD: 1 APPLICATION

❓ How it works: *Rest allows you to heal. Cold reduces swelling, pain, and inflammation. Elevation encourages fluids that have leaked into the tissues to return to the circulation. Compression stabilizes the ligaments so that, as you move about, you don't further stretch them. It also eases pain. A 2006 study published in the* British Journal of Sports Medicine *found that the interval method of icing—10 minutes on, 10 minutes off, and 10 minutes on—led to greater improvements in people with ankle sprains than icing for 20 consecutive minutes.*

Lifestyle Tip

If you have arthritis, stay active. Inactivity and extreme activity (e.g., repeatedly running marathons) both raise the risk of osteoarthritis. Moderation in all things seems to be the key.

Turmeric-Ginger Inflammation Fighter

I rely on these antioxidant, anti-inflammatory, pain-relieving spices to counter the inevitable aches and pains of a an active lifestyle and—let's face it—an aging body. ~ LBW

1 tablespoon (6 g) minced fresh ginger,
  or 1½ teaspoons (3 g) dried
1 teaspoon (2 g) ground turmeric
½ teaspoon ground cumin
⅛ teaspoon freshly ground black pepper
¼ teaspoon cayenne pepper
1 cup (235 ml) vegetable or chicken stock
1 tablespoon (15 ml) sesame oil
½ cup (80 g) chopped onion
2 cups (142 g) broccoli florets
1 cup (130 g) thinly sliced carrot
1 seeded and diced red bell pepper
1 cup (70 g) sliced shiitake mushrooms
1 cup (230 g) cubed tofu
2 cups (134 g) washed and torn kale, packed
2 garlic cloves, minced
2 tablespoons (2 g) fresh cilantro leaves, for
  garnish
4 cups (780 g) cooked brown rice (optional)

PREPARATION AND USE:

In a small bowl, mix the ginger, turmeric, cumin, black and cayenne pepper, and stock.

Heat the sesame oil in a skillet or wok over medium heat. Sauté the onion for 3 to 5 minutes until soft. Add the herb-laced stock and stir for 3 minutes. Add the broccoli, carrot, bell pepper, mushrooms, and tofu. Cover the pan. Simmer the vegetables for 3 to 5 minutes until the broccoli turns a brilliant green. Add the kale and garlic. Cook over low heat for 1 to 2 more minutes. Garnish with cilantro leaves. Serve alone or over brown rice.

YIELD: SERVES 4

❓ How it works: *Brightly colored vegetables contain antioxidant and anti-inflammatory flavonoids and carotenoids. Turmeric, the spice that makes curry yellow, contains the potent anti-inflammatory chemical curcumin. Studies show specially prepared curcumin supplements have helped ease arthritis pain. Ginger, which belongs to the same plant family as turmeric, decreases pain and inflammation. In one study, 250 milligrams four times a day of a ginger extract diminished pain from knee osteoarthritis, but only after three months of continuous use.*

Lifestyle Tip

Consider magnets. For people with osteoarthritis in the hip or knee, a few studies have shown that wearing magnets helped relieve joint pain more effectively than a placebo. However, it's hard to know whether the magnetic bracelets, necklaces, and pads on the retail market are as strong as those used in studies. There is interest in magnet therapy because the body has natural electromagnetic fields that researchers think may react positively to magnets. For instance, muscle contractions induced by signals from the nervous system are linked to magnetic activity. There is not yet enough information on exactly how magnets work to relieve pain, but researchers note that such products seem to do no harm.

Muscle-Boosting Beet and Tart Cherry Tonic

1 cup (155 g) fresh tart cherries, stemmed, pitted, and halved, or (245 g) frozen or canned cherries

2 apples, peeled, cored, and cut into chunks

¼ cup (60 ml) beet juice, or 1 small beet peeled and chopped

3 to 4 ice cubes

PREPARATION AND USE:

Put the cherries and apples into a blender. Add the beet juice or chopped beet and ice. Blend. Drink for a muscle tune-up.

YIELD: 2 SMALL SERVINGS OR 1 LARGE SERVING

❓ How it works: *Cherries contain a number of antioxidant and anti-inflammatory flavonoids. Studies have shown that tart cherry juice prevents weakness and pain that might otherwise follow a bout of intense exercise. Another trial found that consuming cherry juice (relative to a placebo juice) five days before a marathon and continuing for the day of the event and two days afterward reduced muscle inflammation and promoted recovery.*

Eating cherries also helps. Two studies found that eating forty-five cherries a day decreased blood levels of the body's inflammatory chemicals. Another showed that people with gout who ate cherries had fewer attacks of painful arthritis. Researchers have shown that drinking beet juice may improve athlete performance by enhancing the efficiency of skeletal muscles' use of oxygen. As a side benefit, blood pressure was also reduced.

Note: Beet juice is available at natural food stores or online. As a quick alternative, add 1 cup (235 ml) of pomegranate juice to 1 cup (245 g) of canned tart cherries and blend. Yum!

Fact or Myth?

RUNNING INCREASES YOUR RISK OF KNEE OSTEOARTHRITIS.

The answer is a qualified no. In otherwise healthy people who have good form, moderate running doesn't seem to raise the risk of knee arthritis. Actually, obesity is much harder on knees and other joints. However, high-intensity running, particularly when combined with spinning and twisting movements, may lead to arthritis.

Lifestyle Tip

Stretch three times a week. Slowly move your joints through their complete range of motion. Doing so helps to maintain flexibility and reduces the risk of injury.

Muscle Approach by Poach

32 ounces (946 ml) extra-virgin olive oil, with or without flavoring
2 garlic cloves, crushed
1 teaspoon (2 g) freshly ground black pepper
1 teaspoon (3 g) paprika
2 tablespoons (8 g) fresh chopped fresh dill
3 bay leaves
4 salmon steaks (4 ounces, or 115 g)

PREPARATION AND USE:

Preheat the oven to 300°F (150°C, or gas mark 2).

Fill a baking pan halfway with water and place on the lower rack of the oven (this will keep the fish moist).

Pour the oil into a cast-iron skillet on the stove. Heat the oil over low heat, stirring in the garlic, pepper, paprika, dill, and bay leaves until the oil simmers. Add the salmon and spoon the herbed oil over the steaks, ensuring that they are fully covered by the oil. Allow the oil to return to a simmer. Remove the pan from the stove and place in the oven on the middle rack, above the pan of water. Bake for about 15 minutes. The salmon is ready when it flakes with a fork. Do not overcook.

YIELD: 4 SERVINGS

❓ How it works: *Extra-virgin olive oil and cold-water fish, both part of the Mediterranean diet, contain fats with anti-inflammatory effects. The Mediterranean diet reduces inflammation and may be helpful in people with rheumatoid arthritis. Fish oil supplements also reduce morning stiffness associated with rheumatoid arthritis.*

Açai Smoothie

⅓ cup (80 ml) açai berry juice
⅓ cup (75 g) plain Greek yogurt
1 banana, chopped
½ cup (128 g) frozen strawberries
1 cup (235 ml) almond milk

PREPARATION AND USE:

Combine all the ingredients in a blender and blend until smooth. Enjoy.

YIELD: 1 SERVING

❓ How it works: *Açai grows in the Amazon. In addition to its nutritional value, the fruit possesses anti-inflammatory and antioxidant properties. A pilot study involving people with pain and limited range of motion (mainly from arthritis) showed that a particular açai juice significantly improved symptoms.*

Lifestyle Tip

Try the Castor Oil Pack on page 367. This time you can increase the concentration of the essential oils (8 to 10 drops of lavender, peppermint, or ginger essential oil) to ½ cup (120 ml) of castor oil. Apply to sore muscles and joints.

Anti-Inflammatory Pineapple-Ginger Salsa

1 cup (165 g) fresh pineapple chunks
1 tablespoon (6 g) minced fresh ginger
1 teaspoon (5 ml) fresh lemon juice

PREPARATION AND USE:

In a blender or food processor, blend the pineapple and ginger so that the pineapple still has a chunky appearance. Stir in the lemon juice.

Enjoy on freshly baked or roasted fish or chicken.

YIELD: 12 PORTIONS

❓ How it works: *Pineapple contains an enzyme called bromelain, which, when taken as a supplement, reduces inflammation and pain associated with arthritis and traumatic injury. Some studies combine bromelain with other enzymes or the herb turmeric. Studies have not evaluated the possible benefits of eating pineapple, though it is also rich in antioxidant substances such as vitamin C. Dietary intake of vitamin C appears to protect against progression of osteoarthritis. Ginger contains anti-inflammatory and analgesic substances. Extracts modestly relieve pain in osteoarthritis.*

Herbal Pain-Relieving Poultice

1 tablespoon (15 g) *Aloe vera* gel
1 tablespoon (15 ml) olive oil
2 teaspoons (4 g) ground turmeric
2 teaspoons (4 g) ground ginger
1 teaspoon (2 g) cayenne pepper

PREPARATION AND USE:

In a small bowl, blend all the ingredients into a paste. Spread the paste over the affected knee, elbow, or other area. Hold it in place with cheesecloth or plastic wrap. Wash your hands with soap and water. Remove the paste in 30 minutes.

YIELD: 1 APPLICATION

❓ How it works: *Aloe has anti-inflammatory and pain-relieving properties. It absorbs quickly into skin, pulling other ingredients along with it. A 2012 study found that topical virgin olive oil was superior to an ointment containing the anti-inflammatory drug piroxicam. People with knee osteoarthritis applied 1 gram of the olive oil (or piroxicam) three times a day for four weeks. Turmeric and ginger are traditional Indian analgesic and anti-inflammatory agents. Scientific studies back that up. Although studies investigate internal use, the herbs are traditionally used topically. Cayenne contains capsaicin, which acts as a counterirritant. That means it initially causes a mild burning sensation, then silences local pain nerves. Studies show that topical capsaicin reduces pain from osteoarthritis, rheumatoid arthritis, and back pain.*

Note: Turmeric is used to dye fabrics yellow. It will stain clothing and temporarily tinge your skin yellow. The cayenne can burn sensitive areas; avoid touching your eyes after handling cayenne.

When Simple Doesn't Work

- *Over-the-counter analgesic and anti-inflammatory drugs, such as ibuprofen and naproxen, can relieve symptoms. Take with food to minimize stomach irritation. Acetaminophen reduces pain but not inflammation.*

- *Physical therapy effectively manages many musculoskeletal ailments. These professionals have techniques for reducing pain and swelling, improving range of motion, and strengthening muscles.*

- *Acupuncture has been shown to be effective in treating pain associated with carpal tunnel syndrome, arthritis, low back pain, and sprains.*

- *Chiropractic manipulation spells relief for many people with back pain.*

- *A number of studies indicate that two supplements, glucosamine sulfate and SAMe (s-adenosylmethionine), improve symptoms related to osteoarthritis. A 2005 analysis of 20 human trials on glucosamine sulfate showed a collective improvement in pain and function. Most studies focus on people with knee osteoarthritis. SAMe compares favorably relative to placebo treatment. One study found this supplement to be as effective, though slower to take effect, than the anti-inflammatory medicine celecoxib.*

- *Comfrey (Symphytum officinale) is an herb with anti-inflammatory, analgesic, and wound-healing effects. A study involving 203 people with ankle sprains found that a cream containing 10 percent comfrey significantly reduced pain and improved function compared to an inactive cream. Look in your natural food store for creams or ointments containing this plant. Because this herb contains chemicals with the potential to harm the liver, it is not intended for internal use.*

- *Concentrated extracts of four herbs have proved effective in reducing pain and improving function in people with osteoarthritis: boswellia (Boswellia serrata, also called Indian frankincense), devil's claw (Harpagophytum procumbens), ginger (Zingiber officinale), and turmeric (Curcuma longa). As mentioned previously, turmeric contains a potent antioxidant and anti-inflammatory compound called curcumin. Taken as a concentrated extract, it can improve symptoms of osteoarthritis. You may find a combination of these herbs in supplement form. Concentrated extracts of willow bark have been shown to reduce back pain.*

Cooling Muscle Balm

2 tablespoons (30 g) *Aloe vera* gel
8 to 10 drops peppermint essential oil

PREPARATION AND USE:
Blend the aloe and oil in a small, clean bowl. Massage the mixture into sore muscles. Wash your hands afterward and avoid getting it in your eyes.

YIELD: 1 APPLICATION

❓ How it works: *Peppermint contains menthol, which, when applied topically, causes a cooling sensation and is thought to inhibit pain receptors.*

❗ Warning: *Some people are sensitive to peppermint essential oil. If you develop skin irritation, discontinue use.*

Note: Apply to a small area first to adjust the amount of the peppermint to your liking.

Lifestyle Tip

Listen to your body: If you awaken feeling stiff and sore from a workout, you need to decide whether to take a day off from the gym. If the discomfort is mild and dissipates as you start moving, continue with your usual exercise regime. If your muscles are screaming at you, take a break. Stick with walking and stretching. If the pain is coming from a tendon or ligament, rest is best.

Bathe Away Muscle Aches

Whenever I overdo an exercise workout, my first step is a hot bath with Epsom salts and plant essential oils. ~ LBW

2 cups (480 g) Epsom salts
10 to 12 drops peppermint essential oil (or ginger, cedarwood, cypress, or rosemary essential oil or a blend of these)

PREPARATION AND USE:
Blend the salts and the essential oils in a bowl. While a warm bath is running, stir in the mixture. Swish the water with your hand to dissolve it. Step in and soak until your skin puckers. Drink a glass or two of water afterward.

YIELD: 1 APPLICATION

❓ How it works: *Epsom salt baths are traditionally used for muscle aches. How they work is unclear. Epsom salts contain magnesium sulfate. Magnesium helps relax muscles. Two Italian studies using a mud-bath treatment high in calcium, sulfate, and magnesium salts produced relief from arthritis. With the exception of ginger and peppermint, science has yet to evaluate the effectiveness of these herbs on musculoskeletal pain. However, herbal baths have a long history of use to relieve aches and pains.*

Note: Alternatively, stand in a hot shower. This is a quick and effective way to relieve muscle aches. Apply the cooling muscle balm afterward.

Roll Away Back Pain

I learned this simple exercise to relieve tight muscles in neck, back, and shoulders from Kristine Whittle, Denver yoga instructor, massage therapist, and assistant director of the dance company Control Group. I now use it almost daily. ~ LBW

2 tennis balls
1 clean athletic sock

PREPARATION AND USE:
Stuff a tennis ball, followed by the other, into the sock. Knot the top of the sock as close to the second ball as possible. Lie on your back. Place the sock of balls at the top of your spine, so that one ball rests on either side of your vertebra. Relax your muscles against the pressure of the balls. To create more pressure, try lifting your hips. Very slowly, slide your back upward (or the balls downward), so that the two balls glide along your spine. Whenever you find a tight area, stop, breathe deeply and slowly, and wait for the muscles to relax. Proceed all the way down to your sacrum.

If you have neck tightness, try placing the balls at the occiput (the bony back of your neck, just above the spine). You can also turn on your side and position the balls to massage tight gluteal muscles. When I experience tension headaches, I get into the yoga position called "child's pose" (page 371) and let my forehead rest on the balls.

YIELD: 1 SESSION

❓ How it works: *The balls act in the similar way as a skilled massage therapist's fingers, compressing and releasing tight muscles to encourage relaxation and improved blood flow.*

When to Call the Doctor

- *You sustain a moderate or serious injury of any kind.*
- *An injury results in severe pain, limited movement at a joint, or inability to bear weight.*
- *You may have hurt your head or neck.*
- *You suspect you broke a bone.*
- *A mild strain or sprain has not improved after three days of home care.*
- *You habitually have muscle tenderness and fatigue.*
- *A joint or group of joints is increasingly painful.*
- *Low back pain has limited your ability to function.*
- *In addition to pain, the area around the joint(s) is reddened, hot, and swollen.*
- *Overuse has led to pain whenever you repeat a particular motion.*

Chapter 51

Nausea and Vomiting

Nausea and vomiting are common and stem from multiple causes. Like diarrhea, vomiting represents a nonspecific defense to rid the body of noxious substances. Culprits include alcohol intoxication, injudicious eating, food allergies and intolerances, food poisoning, microbes that infect the gastrointestinal tract, and chemotherapy. Sometimes there isn't anything nasty to expel. Take, for example, motion sickness and morning sickness in pregnancy. Migraine headaches can produce nausea, and the headache may subside after a bout of vomiting.

Regardless of the cause, the symptoms are certainly unpleasant. Here are some tips for managing the situation:

- Rest your stomach. Let your stomach empty itself before you put anything in. A good rule of thumb is to wait 8 hours before attempting solid foods.

- After 1 to 2 hours, begin drinking small amounts of clear fluids. Stretching the stomach may cause reflex vomiting, so even if you're thirsty, start with sips. Children may need to be given fluids by the spoonful. (If your child is under twelve months of age, call your pediatrician for advice.)

- If those first fluids do cause vomiting, wait another hour or two before trying again.

- Stay hydrated. That can be difficult when you can only drink tiny amounts—but keep at it. Sip frequently. Dehydration causes nausea, which may lead to vomiting, which increases your fluid losses. Dehydration also increases body temperature, which further increases fluid losses. And it can give you a headache.

- Don't rely on plain water as your main rehydration fluid. You've lost electrolytes and other bodily chemicals.

- Steer clear of dairy products for at least twenty-four hours.

- After 8 hours of clear liquids (and no more vomiting), try bland foods such as pasta, rice, saltine crackers, bananas, applesauce, and cooked carrots.

History

Throughout the ages, Arabic, Indian, and Asian healers have prized ginger for relieving nausea and vomiting caused by illness and seasickness. As one sixteenth-century physician put it: "Ginger does good for a bad stomach." Research later confirmed that ginger reduces nausea and vomiting from many causes.

RECIPES TO PREVENT AND TREAT NAUSEA AND VOMITING

Rice Water

3 cups (710 ml) water
⅛ teaspoon (0.75 g) salt
¼ cup (49 g) uncooked white rice
1 tablespoon (9 g) raisins
1 teaspoon (3 g) grated fresh ginger
Honey, to taste

PREPARATION AND USE:

In a medium-size saucepan, combine water, salt, and rice. Bring to a boil. Lower the heat. Stir in the raisins and ginger, and then cover. Cook over low heat for an hour. Pour through a strainer into a mug. Set aside the rice and raisins for when you're keeping down clear liquids. Allow the rice water to cool. Add honey or salt as desired, and sip.

YIELD: 1 SERVING

❓ **How it works:** *This traditional Asian remedy can help replace the water, sugars, and salts your body has lost. Ginger is the best-researched antinausea agent.*

Note: For a nutritious soup, add ½ cup (120 ml) vegetable or chicken stock to the rice water and ½ cup (93 g) of the strained rice.

Fact or Myth?

CHEMOTHERAPY ALWAYS CAUSES NAUSEA AND VOMITING.

Myth. Although nausea may occur—depending on the type of chemo patients receive—premedication for cancer patients includes many antinausea drugs that have been found to be effective.

Lifestyle Tip

Breathe and visualize. Close your eyes and breathe slowly in and out, imagining yourself well and thriving and back on top of the world.

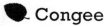 # Congee

This rice porridge is traditionally used in Asian countries.

1½ quarts (1.4 L) water
1 cup (185 g) uncooked long-grain white rice
1 teaspoon (6 g) salt

PREPARATION AND USE:

In a large pot, mix the water and rice. Bring the mixture to a boil. Cover, tilting the lid to release steam. Lower the heat to its lowest setting. Cook for 4 hours, stirring occasionally, until the rice is very soft and creamy. Stir in the salt.

YIELD: MULTIPLE SERVINGS, DEPENDING ON SIZE. EAT A LITTLE AT A TIME, AS THE STOMACH ALLOWS.

❓ **How it works:** *This soft rice is easy to digest and returns water and salt to the depleted system.*

 # Soup-er Broth

This soup is nourishing, tasty, and easy to digest.

2 cups (475 ml) water
2 chicken bouillon cubes
2 teaspoons (4 g) minced fresh ginger
Pinch of ground cinnamon

PREPARATION AND USE:

In a small saucepan, boil the water with the bouillon cubes, stirring until dissolved. Add the ginger and cook over low heat for 30 minutes. Strain out the ginger. Serve with a pinch of cinnamon.

YIELD: 2 SERVINGS

❓ **How it works:** *Bouillon broth returns salt and other nutrients to the depleted system. Ginger and cinnamon can also help settle the stomach.*

Fact or Myth?

NAUSEA AND VOMITING GO ALONG WITH THE FLU.

Myth: Some people refer to the nausea, vomiting, and diarrhea of infectious gastroenteritis (inflammation of the stomach and intestines) as "stomach flu." However, influenza viruses, which cause flu, infect the respiratory system and only rarely affect the gut. Different viruses, as well as bacteria and protozoa, cause infectious gastroenteritis.

Lifestyle Tip

When traveling:

- Before you take a car, boat, plane, or bus trip, eat a small amount of starch—toast or saltines are a good bet.

- If you're in a car or bus, it helps to sit in the front seat and keep the window open. Look straight ahead, not out to the sides as the scenery whooshes by.

- If you're in a plane, make sure the vent air is blowing directly on you to keep you cooled down.

- On a boat, stay on deck. If you have to go below, stay in the middle of the boat where it's most stable.

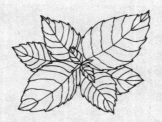

Spotlight: **Ginger**

For thousands of years, people have treasured ginger as food and medicine. Records indicate use in ancient Greece, China, and India. This tropical plant is in the same botanical family as turmeric and cardamom.

Ginger has multiple uses. It reduces pain and inflammation, making it valuable in managing arthritis, headache, and menstrual cramps. It has a warming effect and stimulates circulation. It inhibits rhinovirus (which can cause the common cold), such bacteria as *Salmonella* (that cause diarrhea), and protozoa, such as *Trichomonas*. In the intestinal tract, it reduces gas and painful spasms and may prevent stomach ulcers caused by nonsteroidal anti-inflammatory drugs, such as aspirin and ibuprofen.

The best-researched use of ginger is in combating nausea and vomiting. Several studies confirm its ability to quell pregnancy-induced and postoperative nausea. The studies on ginger to prevent motion sickness are mixed. One study showed ginger to be as effective, though with fewer side effects, as dimenhydrinate (Dramamine). Some studies indicate that, when added to antinausea medications, it further reduces nausea and vomiting from chemotherapy.

You can take it in whatever form appeals: as tea, soup, or capsules (up to 250 milligrams four times a day if you're pregnant; 500 milligrams three times a day if you're not). If you chose a carbonated beverage, make sure it's made from real ginger, or make your own (see Homemade Lemon Ginger Ale, on page 376). You can also nibble crystallized ginger.

To counter motion sickness, 1 gram of dried, powdered, encapsulated ginger is usually taken 30 minutes to 2 hours before travel. In a recent study on the use of ginger to thwart postoperative nausea, the dose was 500 milligrams 30 minutes before surgery and 500 milligrams 2 hours after surgery. Otherwise, ginger is usually not recommended during the seven to ten days leading up to surgery because of its effect on blood clotting. Discuss the use of ginger with your surgeon or anesthesiologist before trying it.

Zingy Minty Nausea Fighter

I like this tea because the ginger and mint work together to fight nausea. ~ LBW

2 cups (475 ml) water
2 teaspoons (1 g) dried peppermint or spear-
    mint leaves, or 1 tablespoon (6 g) fresh
1 teaspoon (3 g) grated fresh ginger, or
    ⅛ teaspoon dried
1 teaspoon (7 g) honey

PREPARATION AND USE:

In a saucepan, bring the water to a boil. Add the peppermint and ginger. Turn off the heat, cover, and steep for 15 minutes. Strain out the herbs. Stir in the honey. Sip frequently.

YIELD: 2 SERVINGS

❓ How it works: *The prime antinausea agent ginger combines with mint, which also reduces nausea and generally helps settle the stomach.*

❗ Warning: *Do not give honey to children under twelve months of age. Use molasses, pure maple syrup, or raw sugar instead.*

Note: Alternatively, use tea bags instead of fresh leaves. Also, you can double the recipe and set aside to sip continuously throughout the day.

Stomach-Settling Tea

This tea can be particularly comforting if you're feeling chilled.

2 cups (475 ml) water
1 teaspoon (2 g) dried ginger, or 2 teaspoons
    (5 g) grated fresh
¾ teaspoon aniseeds
¼ teaspoon ground cardamom
Honey

PREPARATION AND USE:

In a small saucepan, bring water to a boil. Turn heat to low. Add spices and stir. Simmer for 5 minutes. Cover and steep for 20 minutes. Strain. Add honey, if desired. Sip slowly.

YIELD: 2 SERVINGS

❓ How it works: *Ginger combats nausea. Anise and cardamom reduce intestinal spasm if your nausea is accompanied by diarrhea.*

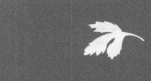

When Simple Doesn't Work

Severe nausea and vomiting, such as that associated with cancer chemotherapy, can require prescription medications. Regardless of the cause, severe, repeated vomiting may require intravenous fluids to correct dehydration.

Rehydrate and Restore

This recipe is adapted from the Rehydration Project, a global organization that fights dehydration through simple, accessible treatments. It predicts that this and other home-based solutions can help save the lives of some 2 million children each year.

1 level teaspoon (6 g) salt
8 level teaspoons (22 g) sugar
5 cups (1.2 L) clean water (If unsure, boil and then cool.)
½ cup (120 ml) orange juice, or ¼ cup (56 g) mashed banana

PREPARATION AND USE:
Stir the salt and sugar into the water until fully dissolved. Whisk in the orange juice or banana until fully blended. Take slowly, by the teaspoonful (5 ml), ingesting as much as possible after a vomiting or diarrheal episode. If another episode takes place, wait 10 minutes and then begin taking the solution again.

YIELD: MULTIPLE APPLICATIONS

❷ **How it works:** *Starch, sugar, sodium, and potassium return vital nutrients to the body after depletion by vomiting, diarrhea, or other loss of fluids. They also help the body retain essential fluids and salts when another episode takes place.*

Note: Store in a cool place. This solution is good for about twenty-four hours. After that time, prepare a fresh one. Take additional liquids to help restore hydration.

Cool Head Luke

I find this remedy particularly soothing when I have a headache related to nausea. ~ LBW

6 ice cubes

PREPARATION AND USE:
Fill a sandwich-size resealable plastic bag with ice cubes. Wrap in a clean towel or T-shirt. Lie down in a quiet place. Apply the pack to your forehead, temples, or the back of your neck.

YIELD: 1 APPLICATION

❷ **How it works:** *No one knows why a cool pack makes you feel better if you've been vomiting. It just seems to work for some people.*

Stomach-Soothing Scent

Diffusing pleasant-smelling plant essential oils can calm nausea.

2 to 3 drops peppermint essential oil

PREPARATION AND USE:
Drop the essential oil onto a clean, cold washcloth, and then place on your forehead as you lie prone. Close your eyes and breathe in the scent.

YIELD: 1 APPLICATION

❷ **How it works:** *Studies show that inhaling essential oils of peppermint, spearmint, or ginger can reduce nausea and vomiting. In a 2012 study of pregnant women needing C-sections, inhaling peppermint essential oil reduced postoperative nausea. A 2013 study found that spearmint and peppermint essential oils (combined with standard antinausea medications) significantly reduced nausea and vomiting in cancer patients receiving chemotherapy. The volunteers received capsules containing only sugar, sugar plus 2 drops of peppermint essential oil, or sugar plus 2 drops of spearmint essential oil.*

Note: Alternatively: Ideally, you should get a diffuser for essential oils, available in a health food store or online. Some are inexpensive; others may cost fifty dollars and up. Also, if you have a collection of plant essential oils, feel free to choose any scent that makes you feel less queasy.

 ## Soothing Stomach Rub

This recipe is an immediate soother, adapted from Aromatherapy: A Complete Guide to the Healing Art *by Kathi Keville and Mindy Green.*

2 tablespoons (30 ml) olive or other carrier oil
6 drops German chamomile essential oil
2 drops ginger essential oil
4 drops peppermint essential oil

PREPARATION AND USE:
Combine all the ingredients in a clean jar. Cap and shake. Gently massage a small amount into your belly.

YIELD: 1 APPLICATION

❓ **How it works:** *The pleasant scent helps calm nausea. The massaging motion is soothing and imparts the antinausea effects of ginger and peppermint. German chamomile adds an antispasmodic effect to reduce cramping. The essential oils can cross the skin into your bloodstream and provide benefits as you inhale the aromas.*

Lifestyle Tip

Suck a peppermint. It has a cooling sensation on the stomach and can help calm nausea.

When to Call the Doctor

- *Vomiting hasn't stopped within 12 hours.*

- *Eight hours after symptoms begin, you (or your child) cannot keep down any fluids.*

- *Signs of dehydration occur: dry lips and mouth, crying without tears, no urination within 8 hours, or sunken eyes. (Small children can become easily dehydrated.)*

- *You develop a fever higher than 103°F (39.4°C).*

- *You vomit blood. (Old blood can resemble coffee grounds.)*

- *You have severe pain.*

- *You experience cyclic episodes of nausea and vomiting.*

- *Persistent vertigo accompanies nausea and vomiting.*

- *You have recurrent episodes of severe head or eye pain with nausea and vomiting.*

- *You've had a head injury and have vomited more than once.*

- *Nausea and vomiting coincides with the start of a new medication.*

- *You frequently have a burning sensation behind your breastbone.*

- *Severe anxiety precedes nausea and vomiting.*

- *You have a serious chronic condition, such as diabetes, liver disease, or kidney disease.*

Chapter 52

Premenstrual Syndrome

A comic rendition of how fierce a woman suffering from premenstrual syndrome (PMS) can be was well portrayed in the 1990s sitcom *Mad About You*, when the protagonist's younger sister was allowed to go home alone in New York City—armed with PMS and a stun gun.

The moods that sometimes result from PMS can indeed be formidable. Yet, during their reproductive years, some 80 percent of young women have to cope with premenstrual syndrome (PMS). In up to 8 percent, PMS is incapacitating. Happily, for most women, symptoms are mild.

PMS describes a cluster of symptoms that gang up on a woman in the days before her periods only to ebb at the onset of menstrual flow. They include fluid retention, abdominal bloating, headaches, breast tenderness, low back pain, constipation or diarrhea, fatigue, insomnia, sugar cravings, forgetfulness, irritability, decreased self-esteem, social withdrawal, anxiety, and mild depression.

PMS symptoms can cluster into subgroups, depending upon whether the predominant complaint is fluid retention, carbohydrate cravings, anxiety, or depression. A severe form of PMS called premenstrual dysphoric disorder (PMDD) causes marked psychological symptoms: irritability, mood swings, depressed mood, and nervous tension.

The cause of PMS remains a medical mystery. Clearly, monthly oscillations in reproductive hormones have something to do with it. Risk factors include psychological stress, being overweight, and smoking.

Doctors sometimes prescribe hormonal contraceptives to smooth out the normal fluctuations in estrogen and progesterone and, occasionally, diuretics to reduce fluid retention and breast tenderness. Antidepressants, either given continuously or only during the last two weeks of the monthly cycle, are helpful for PMDD and when psychological symptoms predominate the PMS picture.

History

Although PMS wasn't an established syndrome 2,500 years ago, ancient healers did recognize menstrual difficulties. Greek physicians Hippocrates and Dioscorides and Roman naturalist Pliny the Elder mention the benefits of chaste tree *(Vitex agnus-castus)* in easing menstrual difficulties. Hippocrates recommended that women drink "dark wine in which the leaves of the chaste tree have been steeped." In the mistaken belief that the berries suppressed sexual desire—hence the name "chaste tree"—monks added the ground fruits to their meals. (Because the fruits look and taste somewhat like peppercorns, another common name was "monk's pepper.")

Chaste tree's value for treating menstrual problems continued through the Middle Ages and into the present. Herbalists traditionally prepare chaste tree berries as a tincture (extract made with water and alcohol). In the mid-1900s, both animal and clinical studies confirmed the effectiveness of *Vitex* preparations in balancing hormonal problems associated with gynecological disorders. More recent studies show that chaste tree extracts offer relief for symptoms of PMS. In Germany, the Commission E monograph on chaste tree fruits supports use of chaste tree fruits as a safe, effective, low-priced remedy for PMS.

Fact or Myth?

CHOCOLATE JUST MAKES PMS WORSE.

Myth—when eaten in moderation. A moderate amount of dark chocolate actually has health benefits. Avoid milk chocolate and other candy bars laden with sugar and fats, which will only make you feel worse. A small piece of dark chocolate as dessert is fine.

RECIPES TO PREVENT AND TREAT PMS

◖ Pre-Attack Snack Mix

¼ cup (36 g) raw almonds
¼ cup (25 g) raw walnut halves
¼ cup (35 g) raisins
¼ cup (21 g) banana chips
¼ cup (21 g) dried apple slices or
   (32.5 g) apricots
¼ cup (44 g) carob chips

PREPARATION AND USE:
Preheat the oven to 350°F (180°C, or gas mark 4).

Mix the nuts and spread on a baking sheet. Toast for about 10 minutes, stirring after 5 minutes. Remove from the oven, let cool, and pour into a bowl. Toss in the dried fruit and carob chips. Store in an airtight container.

YIELD: 6 SERVINGS

❷ How it works: *Low blood sugar (hypoglycemia) is thought to account for at least some PMS symptoms. Keeping your blood sugar steady with healthy snacks can also help you resist sugar cravings.*

Lifestyle Tip

Drink water. Extra fluids will help flush your system. Drink at least eight 8-ounce (235 ml) glasses a day or add more water-laden fruits and veggies, such as watermelon and cucumbers, to your diet.

Crunchy Blood Sugar Balance

1 apple
1 celery stalk
1 to 2 tablespoons (16 to 32 g) peanut butter

PREPARATION AND USE:
Slice the apple, with its peel, into multiple pieces. Slice the celery width-wise, so you retain the dip in the center. Put a dab of peanut butter in each piece of celery and each apple slice. Crunch away.

YIELD: 1 SERVING

❓ How it works: *As stated previously, hypoglycemia is thought to account for at least some PMS symptoms. Keep your blood sugar steady with healthy snacks like this one. In addition, the fiber in the apple and celery will avert constipation, a PMS plague.*

Note: Keep your peanut butter servings to dabs, as it is high in calories and easy to overdo.

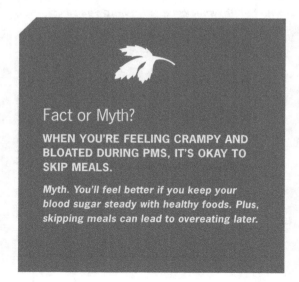

Fact or Myth?

WHEN YOU'RE FEELING CRAMPY AND BLOATED DURING PMS, IT'S OKAY TO SKIP MEALS.

Myth. You'll feel better if you keep your blood sugar steady with healthy foods. Plus, skipping meals can lead to overeating later.

Lifestyle Tip

Chill on the caffeine and alcohol, which may aggravate some of PMS symptoms.

 PMS Super Salad

1 cup (47 g) torn romaine lettuce
1 cup (28 g) torn red leaf lettuce
½ cup (50 g) torn escarole
½ cup (10 g) torn arugula
⅓ red onion, sliced thinly
½ red bell pepper, seeded and sliced thinly
4 cherry tomatoes
2 tablespoons (30 ml) olive oil
1½ teaspoons (8 ml) balsamic vinegar
1 tablespoon (15 ml) fresh lemon juice
Pinch of freshly ground black pepper

PREPARATION AND USE:
Toss together the leafy greens. Add the onion, bell pepper, and tomatoes. In a separate small bowl, beat together the oil, vinegar, and lemon juice to make a vinaigrette. Add a pinch of black pepper. Drizzle over the greens and toss. Serve.

YIELD: 2 LARGE OR 4 SMALL SERVINGS

❓ How it works: *Some health experts believe that high-fiber, low-fat diets may reduce PMS symptoms. In theory, such diets improve elimination of estrogen. The fats to avoid are hydrogenated (trans) fats (in many processed foods) and fat subjected to high heat (present in chips and other fried foods). Healthy fats include monounsaturated fats (e.g., olive oil) and polyunsaturated fats (flaxseed oil, fish oil, evening primrose oil, borage seed oil, and black currant seed oil), which benefit you by reducing inflammation.*

Juice It Away

1 cup (235 ml) low-sodium tomato or V8 juice
1 cup (30 g) torn baby spinach, rinsed and drained
1 cup (67 g) torn kale
Salt-free herbal seasoning, such as
    ½ teaspoon (0.5 g) herbes de Provence
Freshly ground black pepper

PREPARATION AND USE:

Pour the tomato juice into a blender. Gradually add the spinach and kale, mincing it a little at a time so the leaves don't clog the blades. Once minced, blend at high speed to fully pulverize the greens into a liquid. Add more tomato juice if the mixture is too thick. Pour in a tall glass and season to taste with salt-free seasoning and black pepper.

YIELD: 2 SERVINGS (ABOUT 2 CUPS [475 ML])

❓ How it works: *In addition to providing fiber, dark green leafy vegetables contain calcium and magnesium. Low levels of these two minerals are one of the postulated theories about the cause of PMS.*

Friendly Fat Salmon-Flax-Avocado Melt

1 can salmon, (4.5 ounces, or 127.5 g) drained
¼ cup (30 g) diced celery
1 tablespoon (10 g) minced red onion
1 teaspoon (4 g) coarsely ground flaxseeds
1 tablespoon (15 g) low-fat plain yogurt
1 teaspoon (5 ml) wine vinegar
Freshly ground black pepper
2 slices whole wheat bread
½ avocado, peeled, pitted, and sliced

PREPARATION AND USE:

In a bowl, mix together the salmon, celery, onion, flaxseeds, yogurt, and vinegar. Top each slice of bread with half of the salmon mixture.

Spray a skillet lightly with canola oil cooking spray. Cook the open-faced sandwiches over low heat for about 5 minutes until the bread is toasty. Top each sandwich with the avocado slices.

YIELD: 2 SERVINGS

❓ How it works: *Some studies have shown that the omega-3 fatty acids found in fish oils, avocado, nuts, flaxseeds, and olive oil can help reduce bloating and discomfort associated with PMS. One recent study showed that women who ate 25 grams of flaxseeds every day had reduced premenstrual breast pain. A possible explanation is that flaxseeds contain lignans, which act as phytoestrogens (natural estrogen-like substances).*

Milk-It Ginger-Sesame Smoothie

1 large banana, cut into pieces
1½ cups (355 ml) calcium-fortified soy milk
1 tablespoon (6 g) minced fresh ginger
1 tablespoon (8 g) crushed sesame seeds
   or crushed almonds
3 ice cubes

PREPARATION AND USE:

Place the banana, soy milk, ginger, and sesame seeds in a blender and blend. Add the ice cubes for a final blending.

YIELD: TWO 8-OUNCE (235 ML) SERVINGS OR ONE 16-OUNCE (475 ML) SERVING

? How it works: *Some studies suggest that calcium supplementation eases PMS symptoms. Sesame seeds contain a whopping 120 milligrams calcium per 1-tablespoon (8 g) serving. Also, higher dietary intake of vitamin D may be helpful perhaps, in part, because it increases calcium absorption.*

B-Rich Burritos

3 cups (516 g) cooked pinto beans
1 cup (260 g) salsa
3 tablespoons (30 g) chopped onion
1 cup (195 g) cooked brown rice
1 ripe avocado, pitted, peeled, and sliced
8 tortillas, preferably whole wheat

PREPARATION AND USE:

Mix together the beans, salsa, onion, and rice. Fill each tortilla with about 3 tablespoons (185 g) of the mixture. Top with avocado.

YIELD: 8 SERVINGS

? How it works: *Several of the B vitamins, including B_6, are needed to make brain chemicals, some of which influence mood and may have to do with PMS. A recent study found that women who consume more B vitamins from food sources had a lower risk of PMS. Beans, lentils, whole grains, avocados, and bananas are good sources.*

Lifestyle Tip

Reduce the sugar and salt in your snacks and meals. This will help decrease bloating, especially in hands and feet. Snack on fruits and veggies instead.

Nutty Rice Regulator

This delicious and textured recipe delivers the magnesium and B vitamins that can help block PMS.

1½ cups (292 g) uncooked brown rice
1 cup (100 g) crushed almonds
1 cup (240 g) canned chickpeas, drained and rinsed
2½ cups (570 ml) water
1 tablespoon (15 ml) olive oil
1 teaspoon (1 g) salt-free herbal seasoning
2 garlic cloves, crushed

PREPARATION AND USE:

Preheat the oven to 375°F (190°C, or gas mark 5).

Stir together the rice, almonds, and chickpeas, and pour into a medium-size glass baking dish. In a saucepan, bring the water, olive oil, and seasoning to a boil. Pour the boiling water over the rice mixture and stir. Stir in the crushed garlic. Cover the dish tightly with aluminum foil. Bake for 1 hour on the oven's middle rack.

YIELD: 6 TO 8 SERVINGS

❓ How it works: *Brown rice and almonds are among the foods highest in magnesium content, supplying a hearty 100 milligrams per serving. Supplemental magnesium has been shown to help with mood swings and fluid retention during PMS. Chickpeas are high in B vitamins, which also help reduce PMS.*

When Simple Doesn't Work

- *A recent analysis concluded that acupuncture produces promising results in women with PMS.*

- *Chaste tree berry (Vitex agnus-castus) extracts have been shown in a half-dozen studies to safely and effectively reduce PMS.*

- *St. John's wort (Hypericum perforatum) extracts appear to help manage psychological symptoms associated with PMS and PMDD. The herb is safe but does have some precautions: (1) It can increase sun sensitivity. If you're fair-skinned, cover up or use sunscreen. (2) It should not be combined with prescription antidepressants. (3) Concentrated extracts speed the breakdown of a number of medications, including hormonal contraceptives. In the case of hormonal contraceptives, breakthrough bleeding and pregnancy can occur.*

Weight-Walking PMS Relief

There's nothing better than setting out for a healthy hike with a couple weights and a pal. Smooth, moderate walking will bring fresh air into your lungs, weights will tone your arms, and being with a friend will boost your spirits.

You
2 weights (2 pounds, or 905 g)
Walking shoes
A friend, similarly outfitted

PREPARATION AND USE:
With a friend, determine your 2-mile (3.2 km) walk. Walk with head up, shoulders back, breathing the fresh air deeply. As you walk, pump the weights at a comfortable pace, alternating left and right. Talk and get things off your chest.

In no time, you'll be feeling toned and brighter.

YIELD: 1 SESSION

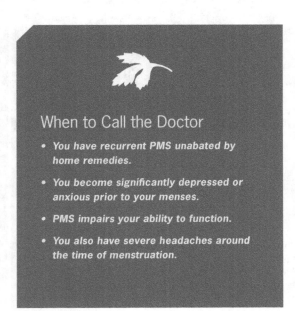

When to Call the Doctor

- **You have recurrent PMS unabated by home remedies.**

- **You become significantly depressed or anxious prior to your menses.**

- **PMS impairs your ability to function.**

- **You also have severe headaches around the time of menstruation.**

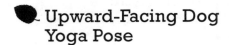 **How it works:** *Exercise can reduce PMS. It also helps manage risk factors such as obesity and stress. Exercise releases endorphins that enhance your well-being and can help you fight the low self-esteem and the general depressive feelings of PMS.*

Upward-Facing Dog Yoga Pose

You
A yoga mat or soft carpet

PREPARATION AND USE:
Lie facedown on the floor. Stretch your legs behind you, with the tops of your feet against the floor. Plant your palms on the floor beside your waist. Bend your elbows slightly, with your forearms perpendicular to the floor. Inhale and press your palms firmly into the floor and slightly back. Straighten your arms and lift up your torso, also lifting your legs a few inches (centimeters) off the floor. Keep your thighs firm and turned inward. Keep your arms firm with your elbows facing directly backward. Press your tailbone forward, lifting your pubis toward the navel. Keep your buttocks firm. Exhale. Inhale, lifting through the top of the sternum and tipping head back slightly. Hold for 30 seconds, inhaling and exhaling easily. Release back to the floor. Repeat as you are comfortable.

YIELD: 1 SESSION

How it works: *Yoga provides physical activity and relaxation training. Preliminary research suggests it reduces stress in women with PMS.*

Chapter 53

Prostate Health

The prostate is a walnut-size gland that encircles the urethra just below the bladder. Glandular tissue contributes fluid to the semen; muscles within the prostate help expel semen during ejaculation.

Disorders of the prostate are relatively common. More than 30 million men suffer from prostate conditions, such as prostatitis, benign prostatic hyperplasia, and prostate cancer. The first is more common in younger men; the last two become more common with age.

Prostatitis (prostate inflammation) affects about half of men sometime during their lifetime. Bacteria can infect the prostate gland. The prostate is also susceptible to acute and chronic noninfectious inflammation, though the underlying cause is poorly understood.

The symptoms of acute bacterial prostatitis include frequent and painful urination, pain in the low back or behind the testicles, painful ejaculation, aching muscles, fever, chills, and fatigue. Chronic bacterial infection can cause mild symptoms or none at all. Noninfectious prostatitis mainly causes pelvic pain, as well as pain with ejaculation and urination.

Bacterial prostatitis is treated with antibiotics. Treatment of noninfectious prostatitis is more challenging. Pain relievers, a class of medication called beta-blockers, and physical therapy may help.

Benign prostatic hyperplasia, also called benign prostatic hypertrophy (BPH), affects mostly older men. About half of fifty- to sixty-year-old men develop BPH. Between ages eighty and ninety that proportion rises to nearly 90 percent. This noncancerous enlargement of the prostate encroaches on the urethra, decreasing the ability of urine to easily flow from the bladder. Symptoms include increased frequency and urgency of urination, nighttime urination, a weak urine stream, an inability to fully empty the bladder, and difficulty stopping and starting urination.

The underlying cause is an age-related rise in prostate levels of dihydrotestosterone (DHT) as well as estrogen, which stimulate cells to multiply.

Prescription medications can reduce prostate size and improve urine flow. Severe cases may require surgery.

Some herbs may be helpful in cases of mild BPH. These include extracts of the African plant pygeum *(Pygeum africanum)*, saw palmetto *(Serenoa repens)*, and nettle root *(Urtica dioica)*. Several studies show that supplemental beta-sitosterol (a plant chemical structurally similar to cholesterol) reduces BPH symptoms. These botanical treatments mainly reduce symptoms, but without shrinking the size of the prostate. Reported side effects for these supplements are minor and rare.

Excluding skin cancer, **prostate cancer** is the most commonly diagnosed cancer in men. Each year, some 230,000 men learn they have it. For most men, the prognosis is good with adequate treatment. Risks include family history, older age, black race, obesity, and higher consumption of meat and high-fat dairy products.

Until it spreads to other tissues, prostate cancer causes no symptoms unless it narrows the urethra (making urination more difficult) or releases blood into the urine. That's why annual physical exams are important. Specifically, a doctor or nurse performs a digital rectal exam, which allows the examiner to estimate the size and texture of the prostate gland.

Controversy exists about screening tests using prostate specific antigen (PSA), a protein unique to the prostate. The problem is that, in addition to prostate cancer, other prostate conditions (prostatitis and benign prostatic hyperpla-

sia) increase levels of this protein. That means that many men with benign causes of elevated PSA levels are subjected to prostate biopsies and needless anxiety. Furthermore, most cases of prostate cancer progress relatively slowly.

When the U.S. Preventive Services Task Force reviewed studies on PSA testing in 2012, it concluded that the harms related to testing outweighed the potential benefits. Nevertheless, PSA testing is the best screening tool currently available. The American Urologic Association (AUA) does not recommend PSA screening for men younger than age forty. For men ages forty to fifty-four, PSA testing is only recommended for those at higher risk for prostate cancer—African Americans and those with a family history of prostate cancer. For men between ages fifty-five and sixty-nine, the AUA recommends shared decision-making between the man and his doctor. In other words, discuss this test with your doctor.

Treatments vary from watchful waiting (for mild cases), to chemotherapy, radiation therapy, hormonal treatments, and removal of the prostate gland.

History

The enlarged prostate has taken a lot of abuse over the centuries. It has been lanced, punctured (often fatally), punched (a kind of procedure), and worse to try to facilitate the outflow of urine from the obstructed urethra. Electric current and even castration were also tried before being abandoned in the nineteenth century. In the twentieth century, urologists turned to less invasive procedures. Today they use lasers, heat, and other forms of energy to shrink the enlarged gland to restore urine flow and relieve urinary tract problems.

Herbal treatment for an enlarged prostate has also had a long—if less draconian—tradition. In the 1700s, Europeans learned about the use of the bark of the African tree pygeum (*Pygeum africanum*) to treat bladder and urinary problems. It took another two hundred years for medicinal pygeum extracts to be introduced in France.

Native Americans of the southeastern United States used the berries of saw palmetto (*Serenoa repens*) for urinary complaints, passing their knowledge along to the American Eclectic physicians, who recommended extracts in the early twentieth century. Today, along with the root of stinging nettle (*Urtica dioica*), saw palmetto and pygeum are widely used, often in combination, in the United States and Europe. Research on saw palmetto used alone has been inconsistent, although some studies show it might be as effective as the prescription medication Proscar. Studies on pygeum have been more consistently positive. Lab studies indicate that pygeum extracts also suppress prostate cancer.

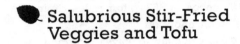

Salubrious Stir-Fried Veggies and Tofu

1 cup (248 g) firm tofu, cubed
1½ teaspoons (8 ml) soy sauce
3 tablespoons (45 ml) olive oil, divided
3 cups (400 g) combination of any of the following: chopped red bell pepper, asparagus, onion, broccoli, and mushrooms
3 garlic cloves, minced
1½ teaspoons (4 g) grated fresh ginger
Freshly ground black pepper

PREPARATION AND USE:

In a bowl, toss together tofu, soy sauce, and 1 tablespoon (15 ml) of the olive oil.

Heat a skillet over medium-high and sauté the coated tofu about 3 minutes until it begins to brown. Transfer the tofu to a bowl and set aside. Into the hot skillet place the remaining olive oil, veggies, garlic, and ginger. Sauté the mix for about 6 minutes. Add the tofu and combine it with the vegetables. Add black pepper to taste. Enjoy the veggies in a bowl or over brown rice.

YIELD: 3 TO 4 SERVINGS

❓ **How it works:** *Traditional Asian diets are associated with a reduced likelihood of BPH and prostate cancer. These diets include regular consumption of vegetables, soy, and green tea, all of which contain substances that restrain prostate growth. On the other hand, diets high in fats, carbohydrates, and red meat seem to increase the risk.*

Super Tomatillo-Pumpkin Seed Salad Dressing

1 can (13 ounces, or 368 g) tomatillos, drained
½ white onion, chopped
¼ cup (4 g) fresh cilantro leaves, chopped
¼ cup (32 g) roasted pumpkin seeds
1 jalapeño pepper, seeded and chopped
1 garlic clove
1 tablespoon (15 ml) fresh lime juice
Water
Salt

PREPARATION AND USE:

Purée the tomatillos, onion, cilantro, pumpkin seeds, jalapeño, garlic, and lime juice in a blender until coarse. Pour in a bowl and add just enough water to give it a saucelike consistency. Add salt to taste. Drizzle over broiled chicken or fish.

YIELD: 4 SERVINGS

❓ **How it works:** *Pumpkin seeds contain healthy oil, fiber, carotenes (which are antioxidant and promote immune function), vitamin E, and zinc. Pumpkin seed oil extracts, with or without saw palmetto, can reduce BPH symptoms. Zinc seems to inhibit proliferation of prostate cancer cells. Low zinc can occur in men with BPH and prostate cancer. Zinc is also needed for sperm production.*

Lifestyle Tip

Avoid tobacco smoke. It causes cancer in multiple organ systems.

Green Tea for Guys

Drinking green tea with your meal aids digestion.

2 green tea bags
Handful of fresh mint
Fresh lime juice
Honey, to taste

PREPARATION AND USE:

Bring the water to a boil in a saucepan and then turn off the heat. Add the tea and mint and steep, covered, for about 10 minutes. Pour into cups, straining out the mint. Stir in the lime juice and honey. Enjoy hot or cold.

YIELD: 2 SERVINGS

❓ **How it works:** *Habitual consumption of green tea correlates with reduced cancer risk. Lab studies show that green tea polyphenols impair the ability of prostate cancer cells to divide and trigger the death of these cells.*

Powerful Pomegranate Smoothie

2 cups (400 g) plain nonfat Greek yogurt
8 ounces (235 ml) pure pomegranate juice
1 banana, peeled, cut into chunks, and frozen
½ cup (128 g) sliced strawberries, frozen

PREPARATION AND USE:

Pour the yogurt and juice into a blender. Add the fruit and blend until smooth. Enjoy!

YIELD: 2 SERVINGS

❓ **How it works:** *Pomegranate juice inhibits the development of prostate cancer and the progression of already existent prostate cancer. Compounds in pomegranate cause prostate cancer cells to die and decrease the migration of these cells. A study in men with prostate cancer resulted in none of the patients progressing to advanced stages while drinking 8 ounces (235 ml) of pomegranate juice a day. Pomegranate also slowed the rise in blood levels of PSA.*

Lifestyle Tip

Follow a whole-foods diet—one high in vegetables and fruits with moderate intake of animal foods. In addition to age and family history, other risk factors for developing BPH include diabetes, obesity, high blood pressure, or heart disease. Consuming lots of carbohydrates (especially refined carbohydrates and added sugar) and fats is also a risk. In general, excessive calorie intake promotes unhealthy weight gain, elevated blood sugar levels, and resistance to the actions of insulin (the hormone that stimulates sugar to enter cells), which causes insulin levels to rise. Insulin seems to promote prostatic growth.

Broiled Tomatoes with Beneficial Garlic

3 large round tomatoes (not Roma or plum)
3 large garlic cloves
2 teaspoons (2 g) crushed dried thyme leaves
Freshly ground black pepper
¼ cup (60 ml) olive oil
1 tablespoon (10 g) crushed garlic
Warm, crusty loaf of whole-grain bread

PREPARATION AND USE:

Preheat the oven to broil.

Cut each tomato in half across its equator. Place the tomato halves face up on a baking sheet. Slice the garlic cloves lengthwise to make six pieces and insert a piece into each of the tomatoes. Sprinkle each tomato half with thyme and pepper. Drizzle with oil. Broil for about 10 minutes. After broiling, dot the tomatoes with the crushed garlic (broiling tends to deactivate benefits of the inserted garlic). Serve with warm, crusty bread.

YIELD: 6 SERVINGS

❓ How it works: *Studies in the early part of the twenty-first century linked high intake of tomato products (and the lycopene they contain) with a lower risk of prostate cancer. A few years later, however, the correlation failed to hold up. Nevertheless, tomatoes and other plant foods contain a host of nutrients beneficial to health. One study found that garlic extracts improve urine flow in men with BPH and prostate cancer. Garlic also enhances immune function and has anti-prostate-cancer activity.*

Recipe Variation: For a more pizzalike dish, mash the soft, warm tomatoes over the sliced-open loaf and top with ¼ cup (38 g) of goat cheese.

Fact or Myth?

MEN WHO TAKE SUPPLEMENTS OF BETA-CAROTENE ENJOY A DECREASED RISK OF PROSTATE CANCER.

Myth. Initial studies indicated a protective effect for a different carotene, lycopene. However, subsequent studies yielded mixed results, with either some protection or no effect. Beta-carotene supplements, however, may actually increase the risk. Vitamin E supplements have also been linked to an increased risk of prostate cancer.

Lifestyle Tip

Catch some rays. Prostate cancer is more common at higher latitudes, where the skin produces no vitamin D in response to UV radiation during the winter months. Lower levels of vitamin D may also explain why black men are more at risk for aggressive prostate cancer than are white men (who require less UV exposure to make vitamin D). If you're thinking of taking vitamin D supplements, talk to your doctor first.

Antioxidant Orange Cranberry Muffins

2 cups (180 g) oat flour

2 teaspoons (9 g) baking powder

1 cup (110 g) chopped pecans or (120 g) walnuts

2 teaspoons (5 g) flaxseed meal

½ cup (120 ml) canola oil

1 cup (235 ml) fresh orange juice

3 tablespoons (60 g) honey or agave nectar

1 cup (120 g) coarsely chopped dried cranberries

PREPARATION AND USE:

Preheat the oven to 350°F (180°C, or gas mark 4).

Grease a twelve-compartment muffin tin or line it with paper liners.

In a large bowl, mix the oat flour, baking powder, pecans, and flaxseed meal. Pour the oil, orange juice, and honey into the flour mixture and stir until just moistened. Fold in the cranberries. Do not overmix. Spoon the batter into the prepared muffin tin. Bake for about 25 minutes, or until a toothpick inserted into the center of a muffin comes out clean. Transfer the muffin tin to a cooling rack and cool for 5 minutes.

YIELD: 10 TO 12 MUFFINS

❓ **How it works:** *Cranberry contains potent antioxidant and anti-inflammatory substances, which helps prevent bacterial urinary tract infections in women. One study found that dried, powdered cranberries (500 milligrams three times a day for six months) ameliorated symptoms in men with chronic nonbacterial prostatitis. A test-tube study found that cranberry extract inhibited growth of human prostate cancer cells.*

When Simple Doesn't Work

One study demonstrated improved success in antibiotic treatment of chronic bacterial prostatitis with the addition of a supplement containing the antioxidant quercetin and the herbs saw palmetto, nettles, and curcumin (the active ingredient in turmeric). Ask your doctor about the herbs noted in the introduction to this chapter, which have minor or rare side effects and may help reduce symptoms without actually shrinking the size of the prostate, as well as about the supplement beta-sitosterol.

You may also discuss with your doctor prostatic massage, in which the doctor inserts a gloved, lubricated finger into the rectum and presses gently on the prostate. Frequent massage may help open ducts that are blocked in the prostate and help improve circulation. However, if you have acute bacterial prostatitis, massage could spread infection through the body. Warning: Do not try this at home without first discussing with your physician.

The Big Q Baked Onion

The big Q—quercetin—is a prostate protector. You'll find quercetin in onions, citrus fruits, apples, parsley, sage, tea, red wine, and olive oil.

2 Vidalia onions
Olive oil
¼ cup (7 g) whole fresh rosemary leaves
Freshly ground black pepper

PREPARATION AND USE:
Preheat the oven to 350°F (180°C, or gas mark 4).

Place two squares of aluminum foil, each large enough to wrap an onion, on a baking sheet. Leave the skins on the Vidalias and cut out the stems, making an indentation about an inch (2.5 cm) deep and wide on each onion. Place each onion on a foil square. Baste each onion indentation with olive oil. Sprinkle pepper into the indentation and fill it with whole rosemary leaves. Enclose each onion in the foil and pinch the top together. Bake for about 1 hour. The onions should be tender and easy to pierce with a fork. Remove them from the aluminum foil and peel before serving.

YIELD: 2 TO 4 SERVINGS

❓ How it works: *Quercetin—an antioxidant found in many plants—and other flavonoids seem to protect against several cancers, including prostate cancer. In one study, supplemental quercetin (500 milligrams twice daily for one month) reduced symptoms of chronic non-bacterial prostatitis. In onions, the quercetin is concentrated in the skin, so keep the skin intact while baking and remove afterward. In addition to onions, quercetin comes in flavonoid-rich fruits, such as grapes, dark cherries, blackberries, bilberries, and blueberries.*

Muscle-Toning Kegel Exercises

These exercises improve the tone of the pelvic floor muscles and may reduce urinary symptoms of prostatitis and improve urinary continence after surgical removal of the prostate.

You
A rug or comfortable pad

PREPARATION AND USE:
First, locate the pelvic floor muscles, which are below the bladder; the easiest time to identify them is during urination. (You use the same muscles to stop yourself from passing gas.)

Partway through urination, purposely contract those muscles to stop the flow of urine without holding your breath or tensing the other muscles in your abdomen, legs, or buttocks. When you successfully interrupt the flow, you have located the correct muscles. Also, the contraction causes your testicles and base of your penis to rise. From now on, perform Kegels when you're not urinating. Doing it while urinating may weaken, rather than strengthen, pelvic floor muscles.

Next: With an empty bladder, lie flat on your back on the rug or pad. Counting to five, slowly contract the pelvic floor muscles you have located above. Counting to five again, slowly relax the pelvic floor muscles.

Repeat this pair of movements ten times for one full set. Practice three full sets daily. Gradually, within a month, work up to counting to ten as you contract and relax the muscles. Work up to five sets daily. As your muscles become stronger, do the exercise in a standing position. This will increase your muscle control.

YIELD: MULTIPLE SESSIONS

How it works: *In men, urinary incontinence can be caused by a weak urinary sphincter that may result from surgery for prostate cancer, an overactive bladder, or a bladder that doesn't contract. By toning the pelvic floor muscles beneath the bladder, Kegel exercises can help you improve—or in some cases completely regain—bladder control. They help control urination and curb dribbling and incontinence.*

Note: Focus only on tensing the pelvic floor muscles. Try to keep your other muscles—abdomen, legs, and buttocks—relaxed during Kegels. If a month has passed and the symptoms haven't improved, it may be a sign that you're not exercising the right muscles. Ask your doctor for help locating them.

Soothing Sitz Bath

A bathtub
You

PREPARATION AND USE:
Run enough warm bath water to cover your hips and buttocks. Relax in the tub for 10 to 15 minutes.

YIELD: 1 SESSION

 How it works: *Warm water increases circulation. Although sitz baths are a traditional treatment for prostatitis, research studies to determine effectiveness are lacking.*

When to Call the Doctor

- *You have symptoms of prostatitis. Fever, chills, and nausea are associated with acute bacterial prostatitis. Chronic bacterial prostatitis can cause blood in semen or urine.*

- *You have symptoms of BPH: frequent and painful urination, pain in the low back, pelvis, or behind the testicles, painful ejaculation, aching muscles, fever, chills, and fatigue. Get a proper diagnosis, even if you want to try a dietary supplement such as saw palmetto. Symptoms of BPH can overlap with those of prostate cancer.*

- *You develop trouble urinating, blood in urine or semen, discomfort in the pelvic area, or bone pain.*

- *Discuss screening tests for prostate cancer with your doctor.*

Chapter 54

Psoriasis

Psoriasis is a common, chronic skin condition. The immune system generates inflammation in the skin, as well as other bodily tissues. Inflammatory chemicals spur excessive multiplication of cells in the epidermis, or outer layer of skin. Normally, new cells continually form at the base of the epidermis and move to the top, where they slough off. In psoriasis, new cell production outpaces the shedding of old cells, leading to a pileup at the surface, like an unraked lawn in autumn.

These raised patches on the skin are called plaques. The pink or red patches are sometimes itchy and topped by silvery scales. There may be one patch or many. The scalp, elbows, buttocks, and knees are most commonly affected.

Although scientists have yet to pinpoint the exact cause, both genetic and environmental factors contribute to psoriasis. Although often chronic, psoriasis waxes and wanes. Triggers include stress, physical trauma (a cut, scratch, or scrape), sunburn, tobacco smoke, infections, low blood calcium levels, some medications, and perhaps diet. Some people with psoriasis are sensitive to gluten, a protein found in wheat and other grains, and a gluten-free diet seems to help them. Consult your doctor about the role diet may play in treating psoriasis.

Inflammation can affect other parts of the body. Fingernails and toenails may become pitted and discolored. Up to 10 percent of people with skin plaques develop psoriatic arthritis, a potentially debilitating condition requiring strong medications.

History

The treatment of psoriasis in ancient times was not for the faint of heart. In ancient Egypt, according to some reports, cat feces were applied topically to the red skin lesions. Other treatments believed to be in the ancients' arsenal include urine, wasp droppings in sycamore milk, and a soup made from vipers. In the eighteenth and nineteenth centuries, dermatologists applied Fowler's solution, a poisonous compound made from arsenic, to psoriatic plaques.

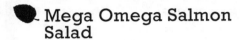

Mega Omega Salmon Salad

1 pound (455 g) salmon fillet or 4 salmon
   steaks, preferably wild
¼ cup (60 ml) fresh lemon juice
Salt and freshly ground black pepper
2 onions, diced
1 tablespoon (15 ml) olive oil
1 tablespoon (15 ml) balsamic vinegar
1 tablespoon (4 g) minced fresh dill
Sliced cucumber, capers, and fresh parsley,
   for garnish

PREPARATION AND USE:

Preheat the oven to 375°F (190°C, or gas mark 5).

   Place the salmon in a baking dish and brush
the fish with the lemon juice. Sprinkle with salt
and pepper. Bake for 20 minutes. Remove from
the oven and let cool.

   Skin and debone the fish, and then slice the
salmon into chunks and toss into a large bowl
along with the onion. In a separate bowl, combine
the oil, vinegar, and dill. Pour over the salmon
chunks and toss. Add salt and pepper to taste.
Refrigerate for 20 minutes. Garnish the final
dish with cucumbers, capers, and parsley.
Serve chilled.

YIELD: 4 SERVINGS

❷ **How it works:** *Salmon is high in omega-3
fatty acids, which have anti-inflammatory effects. The eicosapentaenoic acid (EPA) in fish oil
may be particularly valuable. A few studies have
shown benefits from oral and topical preparations of EPA.*

Lifestyle Tip

**Expose yourself. Phototherapy with ul-
traviolet light B (UVB) is a conventional
treatment for psoriasis. Sunlight contains
both UVB and UVA. The National Psoriasis
Foundation recommends repeated, short
exposure to sunlight—5 to 10 minutes of
midday sun a day. Once you finish your
brief sunbath, avoid sun damage by applying sunscreen, covering with hat and clothing, or seeking shade.**

Fish Oil Skin Soother

Fish oil capsule

PREPARATION AND USE:

Puncture a capsule. Smooth inside liquid over
affected skin.

YIELD: 1 CAPSULE PER APPLICATION

❷ **How it works:** *As noted previously, preliminary research indicates that topical applications
of the EPA (eicosapentaenoic acid) in fish oil
may improve psoriasis symptoms.*

Lifestyle Tip

**Dab on tea tree oil with gauze or a clean
cloth. New research suggests that the
essential oil of tea tree may counter
psoriasis, perhaps because of its anti-
inflammatory properties.**

Aloe Skin Soother

1 *Aloe vera* plant

PREPARATION AND USE:
Select an aloe leaf and split it open lengthwise with a clean knife. Scoop out the gel. With clean fingers, smooth the gel over the affected area.

YIELD: 1 APPLICATION

❓ How it works: *Topical aloe gel reduces the redness, inflammation, and flakiness of psoriasis. One study found an aloe cream slightly more effective than a topical steroid.*

Note: Alternatively, buy commercially packaged aloe that's 99 to 100 percent aloe gel.

Vitamin D Treatment

Oil-based vitamin D3 supplement

PREPARATION AND USE:
Take your dosage by mouth. The Institute of Medicine recommends 600 IU a day for people from age one to seventy. Consult with your doctor about proper dosing.

YIELD: 1 APPLICATION

❓ How it works: *Studies show people with psoriasis often have low levels of vitamin D, which favorably alters the immune system. Oral and topical derivatives of vitamin D3 can improve symptoms. In fact, the prescription ointment calcipotril is a synthetic derivative of vitamin D.*

Note: Alternatively, you can puncture the oil-based capsule (more than one, as needed) and apply to your skin.

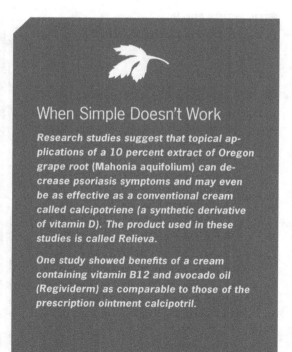

When Simple Doesn't Work

Research studies suggest that topical applications of a 10 percent extract of Oregon grape root (Mahonia aquifolium) can decrease psoriasis symptoms and may even be as effective as a conventional cream called calcipotriene (a synthetic derivative of vitamin D). The product used in these studies is called Relieva.

One study showed benefits of a cream containing vitamin B12 and avocado oil (Regividerm) as comparable to those of the prescription ointment calcipotril.

Do the Avocado Mash

1 ripe avocado, cut in half and pitted
Warm water

PREPARATION AND USE:

Scoop out the fruit into a clean bowl. Mash and apply to patches of psoriasis. Allow to dry. Wash with warm water and pat dry with a clean towel.

YIELD: 1 APPLICATION FOR ONE LARGE OR SEVERAL SMALL AREAS

❓ **How it works:** *Avocado contains monoun-saturated and polyunsaturated fats. In one study, a cream containing avocado oil improved psoriasis.*

Calming Capsaicin Rub

1 chile pepper

PREPARATION AND USE:

Wash the pepper. Cut lengthwise and remove the seeds. Rub a small piece over psoriatic skin. Be sure to wash your hands thoroughly with soap and water before touching your eyes, nose, genitals, or any cuts or scrapes.

YIELD: 1 APPLICATION

❓ **How it works:** *Chile peppers produce the hot-tasting powder cayenne. Capsaicin is a key ingredient in cayenne. Capsaicin depletes substance P, a chemical involved in pain transmission. Substance P also contributes to itching. Frequent applications of capsaicin cream can reduce itching associated with psoriasis.*

❗ **Warning:** *With either product, expect to feel temporary heat before itching decreases.*

Note: Alternatively, buy a commercially prepared cream that contains capsaicin.

Chamomile Compress

1 cup (235 ml) water
1 German chamomile tea bag

PREPARATION AND USE:

Boil the water and drop in the tea bag. Remove from the heat and let cool. Remove the tea bag. Dunk a piece of gauze or clean cloth into the tea. Apply to the affected area.

YIELD: 1 APPLICATION

❓ **How it works:** *German chamomile (Matricaria recutita) reduces inflammation, inhibits bacteria, and speeds wound healing.*

❗ **Warning:** *If you're allergic to chamomile, skip this recipe. If you're allergic to ragweed or other plants in the same family, first try this recipe on a small test area, wait twenty-four hours, and stop if inflammation occurs.*

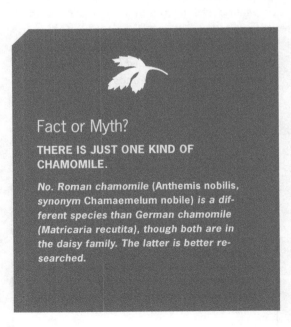

Fact or Myth?

THERE IS JUST ONE KIND OF CHAMOMILE.

No. Roman chamomile (Anthemis nobilis, synonym Chamaemelum nobile) is a different species than German chamomile (Matricaria recutita), though both are in the daisy family. The latter is better researched.

Turmeric and Aloe Paste

1 tablespoon (7 g) ground turmeric
Aloe Vera gel

PREPARATION AND USE:

Put the turmeric in a small bowl. Mix in just enough aloe gel to make a paste. Dot onto patches of the inflamed skin. Let the paste dry for about 15 minutes. Wash away.

YIELD: 1 APPLICATION

❓ How it works: *Turmeric contains the potent anti-inflammatory chemical curcumin. Lab studies show that it has antipsoriasis activity when used both externally and internally. Anecdotal reports suggest that it reduces symptoms when taken internally through capsules or added as a spice to food. Aloe has its own benefits and can help move other chemicals across the skin.*

❗ Warning: *Some people develop contact dermatitis (skin rash) from turmeric. Try a small test patch first and wait several hours before applying again. Also, wear old clothing when using this treatment! Turmeric, which is also used as a textile dye, can stain clothes and temporarily yellow your skin.*

Lifestyle Tip

Keep a container of ground cayenne pepper on your table next to the salt and pepper; add a pinch to vegetable sautés, salads, and bean dishes to spice them up—and get the benefit of capsaicin's psoriasis-soothing qualities at the same time.

Lifestyle Tip

Try this breathing exercise to reduce stress, which can trigger an outbreak. Find a quiet place. Sit in a relaxed position and close your eyes. Let your muscles melt. Breathe slowly and deeply. As you breathe in, imagine yourself bringing peace into your body, filling every pore. As you breathe out, expel the anxiety and negative feelings. Repeat four times.

When to Call the Doctor

- *You have symptoms and signs of psoriasis but have yet to receive a diagnosis.*

- *Treatment has failed to control the condition.*

- *Prescribed medications have caused undesirable side effects.*

- *You develop signs of a skin bacterial infection: localized redness, swelling, increased warmth, tenderness, and yellowish discharge.*

- *You develop signs of psoriatic arthritis: pain, swelling, and decreased mobility at the joints.*

Chapter 55

Sinusitis

In the classic Broadway hit *Guys and Dolls*, night-club singer Miss Adelaide sings of her romantic disappoinments and the annoyance that comes when sinusitis complicates a cold—postnasal drip and "a sinus that's really a pip." In fact, one study found that more than 80 percent of people with the common cold had signs of sinusitis, or sinus inflammation, on CT scans.

Here's what happens: Viral respiratory infections, as well as allergies and air pollutants such as tobacco smoke, inflame the upper respiratory membranes. The resultant swelling and excess mucus blocks the tiny openings that connect the normally air-filled sinuses with the nasal cavities. The mucus normally made by the cells lining the sinuses starts to accumulate, generating a sense of pressure. If bacteria have become trapped within the sinuses, they start to multiply, leading to symptoms of acute bacterial sinusitis.

Most of the time, respiratory viruses cause sinusitis. Symptoms include mild fatigue, pressure, and discomfort in the affected sinus. (There are four pairs of sinuses in your face.) With a cold, nasal mucus typically changes from clear and watery to yellowish and thick.

So, when do you start worrying that the infection has become bacterial? Cold symptoms, including sinus congestion, should resolve within ten days. If the infection lingers, that's a sign of bacterial infection or other problems. Also, symptoms are usually worse, including sinus pain (usually worsened by leaning down), fatigue, fever, bad breath, and green or brownish nasal discharge. Postnasal drip can irritate the throat and cause nighttime cough. Another pattern is recurrence of symptoms after they seemed to have gotten better. Otherwise, acute sinusitis often resolves without treatment. Simple home remedies can help relieve symptoms.

History

The treatment of sinusitis can be traced back some four thousand years to the Chinese and later the Egyptians. More recently, from the mid-nineteenth century until about 1940, a medical group in the United States known as the Eclectic physicians treated sinusitis using medicinal plants. Among other herbs, this group recommended echinacea (*E. purpurea, E. angustifolia*, and other species) teas and tinctures for sinusitis, colds, and other infections. Traditionally, herbal practitioners also recommend other American plant natives, such as Oregon grape (*Mahonia aquifolium*) and goldenseal (*Hydrastis candensis*), to combat sinus infection.

RECIPES TO PREVENT AND TREAT SINUSITIS

 Sinus Tea

2 peppermint tea bags
1 cup (235 ml) water

PREPARATION AND USE:
Boil the water and pour it into a cup. Add the tea bags (two, to make it strong). Steep for 10 minutes, covering the top with a saucer to keep peppermint's essential oils from escaping. Inhale the aroma through your nose as you sip.

YIELD: 1 SERVING

? How it works: *Staying hydrated by drinking lots of warm, clear liquids helps keep respiratory mucus thin and easy to expel. Peppermint provides a sense of decongestion.*

 Pepperminty Steam Inhalation

2 cups (475 ml) water
2 to 3 drops peppermint essential oil

PREPARATION AND USE:
Boil the water in a large pot. Pour into a bowl. Add the peppermint oil. Leaning over, drape a towel over your head to trap the vapors. Inhale through your nose for about 1 minute. Repeat four or five times a day.

YIELD: 1 APPLICATION

? How it works: *Peppermint has anti-inflammatory, analgesic, antibacterial, and subtle antihistamine effects. By breathing in through your nose, your sinuses get the peppermint's immediate effect.*

! Warning: *If you want to try this with a child, use only 1 drop of essential oil. Stay with your child to ensure that small hands don't touch hot objects or tip over the bowl.*

Note: Don't lean over so far that the steam feels too hot. If you have asthma, inhale steam without any essential oils, which may trigger airway spasms in vulnerable people. If plain steam causes no problems, cautiously inhale the steam with only 1 drop of essential oil. Stop if it makes you cough or wheeze.

Fact or Myth?

OVER-THE-COUNTER SINUS MEDICATIONS ARE USUALLY THE MOST EFFICIENT TREATMENTS FOR A SINUS INFECTION.

Myth. Most products on the market contain a combination of antihistamines, decongestants, and pain relievers (usually acetaminophen). Studies have not proven that antihistamines and decongestants help. Both have side effects. Because antihistamines thicken the mucus, some experts suspect they may actually increase the risk of sinusitis developing. If you have a headache, pain relievers can make you more comfortable. Be careful not to exceed the maximum daily dosage of 3,000 milligrams. The danger comes in taking more than one medicine containing acetaminophen (e.g., Tylenol and a combination sinus medicine). In higher doses, acetaminophen can injure the liver.

Warm Washcloth Relief

Hot water

PREPARATION AND USE:

Dampen a washcloth with hot water—not too hot to the touch. Wring out excess moisture. Apply to the affected sinus area. Remove when no longer hot. Repeat several times a day.

YIELD: 1 APPLICATION

❷ How it works: *The heat breaks up the congestion and soothes inflamed mucous membranes.*

When Simple Doesn't Work

A product containing cowslip, gentian, elderflowers, verbena, and sorrel (SinuComp and Sinupret) has been shown to reduce symptoms of acute and chronic sinusitis. Preliminary evidence also suggests that serrapeptase (an enzyme isolated from silkworms) reduces symptoms of chronic sinusitis. It may generally improve chronic airway disease by increasing the clearance of mucus. Serrapeptase is sold as a dietary supplement.

Emerging studies also support extracts made from the root of South African geranium (Pelargonium sidoides) for symptoms of sinusitis, as well as sore throat, the common cold, and bronchitis. The product used in studies is called Umckaloabo.

Nostril Cleanse

½ cup (120 ml) sterile water (see warnings)

¼ teaspoon salt (without iodine or preservatives)

¼ teaspoon baking soda

PREPARATION AND USE:

Have ready a ceramic neti pot or clean creamer bowl (see warnings). Mix sterile water, salt, and baking soda in a clean neti pot. Leaning over the sink, angle your head so that one nostril is down and one is up, with your forehead slightly higher than your chin. Insert the spout of the neti pot into the top nostril. Pour. Water will drain out of the downward-facing nostril. (If a nostril is completely blocked, quit.) Switch sides. *Gently* blow your nose. Discard any excess solution. Wash the neti pot in hot, soapy water or the dishwasher. Repeat two to three times a day, making a fresh batch each time.

YIELD: 1 APPLICATION

❓ How it works: *The salt solution helps remove excess mucus and microbes clinging to nasal passages. It does not clean out the sinuses. However, some studies show that nasal irrigation helps manage acute and chronic sinusitis.*

⚠ Warning: *Sterile water is essential. Two deaths have been reported from people using tap water contaminated with amoebas. Health experts maintain that nasal washes are safe—as long as you use sterile water. Either boil the tap water for 1 minute (3 minutes if you live above 6,600 feet [2 km]) or buy distilled or sterilized water. Allow boiled water to cool before attempting nasal irrigation.*

Use a ceramic, not plastic, neti pot, which resembles Aladdin's lamp. These are available in most natural food stores and from online retailers. Most nasal irrigation pots sold in drug stores are plastic, which are difficult to sterilize.

Note: Avoid nighttime sinus rinses; remain upright for a couple of hours to encourage drainage.

Lifestyle Tip

Turn on the shower and close the bathroom door for a sauna. The steam opens airways and loosens the mucus in your sinuses as it relaxes you.

Sinus-Clearing Spicy Soup

1 cup (235 ml) vegetable or chicken stock
1 garlic clove, minced
⅛ teaspoon cayenne pepper

PREPARATION AND USE:
Pour the stock into a small pan. Heat until steaming. Stir in the garlic and cayenne and serve immediately.

YIELD: 1 SERVING

❓ How it works: *Ever notice that spicy foods make your nose run, making the thin, watery mucus easier to expel? Cayenne peppers contain capsaicin. Spicy plants, such as horseradish and mustard, contain allyl isothiocyanate. Both plant chemicals stimulate mucous membranes to make copious, thin mucus. Spicy foods, such as cayenne peppers and garlic, are also generally antimicrobial. Garlic also enhances immune function; cayenne can help reduce pain.*

Lifestyle Tip

Blow your nose the right way: Close one nostril by pressing with your finger and blow gently to clear the other nostril. Blowing too hard will force the phlegm into your ear, causing an earache. And blow your nose regularly—don't sniff the infected mucus back into your nose and sinuses.

Horseradish "Gum"

1 teaspoon (5 g) prepared horseradish

PREPARATION AND USE:
Put the horseradish your mouth. Chew, allowing the aromas to work as a decongestant. Spit out any remaining substance.

YIELD: 1 APPLICATION

❓ How it works: *Horseradish, sometimes called "stingnose," contains chemicals that irritate mucous membranes. In response, your upper respiratory passages release thin, copious mucus, thereby helping you clear your nasal passages. Horseradish is also antibacterial and has anti-inflammatory properties.*

When to Call the Doctor

If you have any concerns that you have bacterial sinusitis, contact your doctor. The research on whether antibiotics make much difference is inconclusive. Many doctors prescribe on a case-by-case basis. If you develop high fever, confusion, or swelling around your eyes or over your sinuses, seek immediate treatment. You may have developed a serious complication. Also call your doctor's office if you have persistent (lasting longer than two weeks) or recurring symptoms of sinusitis.

Chapter 56

Sore Throat

You know that scratchy feeling that gets worse when you try to swallow. Sometimes a raw throat is the first sign of the common cold or other respiratory infection. Other agents can irritate the throat, too: hot liquids, chemicals, smoke, allergies, postnasal drip from sinusitis, and even sleeping with your mouth open at night.

Viruses—particularly those associated with the common cold—are far and away the most common infectious cause. Normally, other respiratory symptoms, such as runny nose and sneezing, accompany the throat pain. Viral sore throat should resolve on its own within a few days.

Another viral illness that starts with a sore throat is mononucleosis, a condition that typically strikes teens and young adults. In addition to severe sore throat, signs and symptoms include extreme fatigue, malaise, decreased appetite, chills, fever, body aches, swollen lymph nodes in the neck, enlarged spleen, and sensitivity to light. The Epstein-Barr virus is the cause. It spreads from close contact with infected saliva or respiratory mucus—hence the illness's nickname "the kissing disease."

Bacteria can also infect the throat, particularly *Streptococcus pyogenes*, the cause of strep throat. The onset of sore throat is sudden, with pain on swallowing, tender and swollen lymph nodes in the neck, fever, headache, and possibly nausea and vomiting (especially in children). Unless you have the bad luck of also having a cold, a runny nose, sneezing, and cough are absent. Doctors treat strep throat with antibiotics.

History

Through the ages, teas and gargles have been used to soothe sore throats. Thyme and sage teas have a long history of use in Europe, as does licorice tea in India (along with many others). A saltwater gargle has been a common treatment for sore throat worldwide for centuries. According to the ancients, the best medicine for a sore throat was chamomile tea with lemon and honey. In eastern North America, Native American tribes used the powdered bark of the slippery elm tree, mixed with fats or oils, to ease sore throats.

Listerine Gargle

Listerine is named for Joseph Lister, the English surgeon who introduced antiseptic techniques in surgery. The mixture below is warm and soothing.

1 cup (235 ml) hot (but not scalding) tap water
1 teaspoon (6 g) salt
1 tablespoon (15 ml) Listerine, or 1 drop either
   eucalyptus or tea tree essential oil

PREPARATION AND USE:

Mix the water, salt, and Listerine. If using essential oil rather than Listerine (in which case you're eliminating such things as preservatives, saccharin, alcohol, sorbitol, and artificial coloring), mix the ingredients in a small jar and shake well to disperse the essential oil. Gargle and spit out. Continue until you finish the cup. Repeat four to five times a day, making a hot, fresh batch each time.

YIELD: 1 APPLICATION

❓ How it works: *Listerine's antiseptic ingredients are thymol (which comes from thyme, oregano, and a couple of other mint-family herbs), menthol (from peppermint), and eucalyptol (from eucalyptus). It also contains water, ethanol (alcohol), sweetener, coloring, and preservatives. Tea tree oil is antimicrobial, with activity against a number of bacteria, including strep bacteria, and viruses, including influenza virus. Likewise, eucalyptus essential oil is antibacterial (including against strep) and some respiratory viruses. If you have time, use plant essential oils or make the gargle using dried herbs as described in the recipes that follow.*

Recipe Variation: Try gargling with a capful of straight Listerine for a throat wash (if you don't mind the sweeteners and alcohol).

Fact or Myth?

WHEN YOU FEEL A SORE THROAT COMING ON, TAKE EXTRA DOSES OF VITAMIN C AND IT WILL HEAL QUICKLY.

Maybe. Accumulated research has failed to support the use of vitamin C in preventing the common cold (which typically causes sore throat). The exception is people performing extreme exercise, especially in very cold weather. Extra vitamin C started after a cold begins may shorten symptom duration. Also, eating five or more daily servings of fruits and vegetables (which naturally contain vitamin C and other beneficial chemicals) strengthens the immune system.

Sage and Thyme Gargle

1 cup (235 ml) water
1 tablespoon (3 g) dried thyme
2 teaspoons (2 g) dried sage
1 teaspoon (6 g) salt

PREPARATION AND USE:

Bring the water to a boil in a small pan. Stir in the thyme and sage. Cover and steep for 20 minutes. Strain. Reheat, if necessary. (You want the water as hot as you can stand it without burning.) Add the salt and stir. Gargle and spit out. Continue until you finish the cup. Repeat four to five times a day, making a hot, fresh batch each time.

YIELD: 1 APPLICATION

❓ How it works: *Sage and thyme are antioxidant and antimicrobial.*

423

Lemon-Honey Ginger Tea

A pinch of cayenne adds healing agents—and punch.

2 cups (475 ml) water
2 tablespoons (12 g) minced fresh ginger,
    or 4 teaspoons (7 g) dried
1 tablespoon (20 g) honey
1 tablespoon (15 ml) fresh lemon juice
⅛ teaspoon cayenne pepper,
    or to taste

PREPARATION AND USE:

Bring the water to a boil in a nonreactive pot. Add the ginger. Turn off the heat. Cover and steep 15 minutes. Strain. Stir in the honey, lemon juice, and cayenne.

YIELD: 2 SERVINGS

❓ How it works: *Ginger is antiviral, antibacterial, antioxidant, anti-inflammatory, and warming. Lemon inhibits some bacteria, is antioxidant, and provides bioflavonoids and vitamin C. Honey moistens irritated mucous membranes, soothes inflammation, and discourages bacterial growth. (Manuka honey, which comes from bees that extract nectar from the manuka flower in New Zealand, is active against strep bacteria.) Cayenne is antioxidant, anti-inflammatory, analgesic (despite the burn), and active against some bacteria.*

❗ Warning: *Do not give honey to children under twelve months of age because of the small risk of botulism.*

Sore Throat Tea

Down this tangy throat soother while the honey is still warm.

1 cup (235 ml) water
1 tablespoon (2 g) fresh thyme leaves
1 tablespoon (4 g) fresh oregano leaves
1 tablespoon (3 g) fresh sage leaves
Honey

PREPARATION AND USE:

Boil the water in the bottom of a double boiler. Place the other ingredients in the top of the double boiler. Gently heat the honey mixture for 30 to 60 minutes. Strain through a tea strainer. (You'll get about ¼ cup [60 ml] or less.) Drink right away while still warm.

YIELD: ABOUT ¼ CUP (60 ML), JUST ENOUGH TO COAT THE THROAT

❓ How it works: *Honey is antibacterial, soothing, and moistening. The three herbs are antimicrobial. With heat, you've infused the honey with the herb's healing chemicals.*

Lifestyle Tip

Cranberry juice is a great gargle and an even better drink. It contains salicylic acid (the backbone chemical of aspirin), which eases inflammation and pain in the throat.

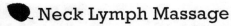 Neck Lymph Massage

Perform this yourself or ask a partner to help so that you can completely relax.

1 teaspoon (5 ml) olive, apricot, almond,
    or sesame oil
3 drops peppermint essential oil

PREPARATION AND USE:

Wash your hands. Pour your preferred carrier oil into your palm. Add the peppermint essential oil. Blend with a fingertip. Massage into your neck, focusing on the area under the jaw (where you may feel tender lymph nodes) and the muscle that runs parallel to your trachea (windpipe). Stroke downward from the base of your jaw toward your collarbones. Avoid contact with your eyes. Wash your hands well after you finish.

YIELD: 1 APPLICATION

❓ How it works: *Massage can increase local circulation of blood and lymph (an immune system fluid). Peppermint is analgesic and antimicrobial against some viruses and bacteria.*

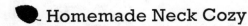 Homemade Neck Cozy

3 cups (about 540 g) rice, dried lentils, millet,
    barley, or other microwave-safe grain
10 drops lavender, peppermint, eucalyptus,
    or other essential oil

PREPARATION AND USE:

Pour the grain into a bowl, sprinkle the essential oil over it, and mix.

Pour the scented grain into a clean tube sock. Leave enough room to knot the open end of the sock. (You can also sew it closed.) Microwave on high for 60 to 90 seconds.

Check the temperature: It should feel pleasantly warm to the touch but not scalding hot. Wrap the sock around your neck. Ideally, you should do this after the neck massage described in the previous recipe. Sip warm tea and relax.

YIELD: 1 APPLICATION

❓ How it works: *Heat increases local circulation, which increases the delivery of immune cells and the removal of wastes. It also feels good. The essential oils are antimicrobial, smell nice, and help clear a stuffy nose that accompanies your sore throat.*

When Simple Doesn't Work

Many grocery stores stock teas by Traditional Medicinals. One is Throat Coat, which contains licorice, marsh mallow, slippery elm, cinnamon, wild cherry, and sweet orange. Collectively, these herbs coat and soothe irritated membranes, enhance immune function, and discourage microbes. In one study, this tea was superior to a placebo beverage in reducing pain in people with sore throats. Former president Bill Clinton is said to have used it to combat hoarseness on the campaign trail.

🌰 Apple-Cinnamon Toddy

While you reap the benefits of the apple and spices, the warm liquid helps soothe an irritated throat and loosen congestion.

1 quart (946 ml) apple juice or cider
1 quart (946 ml) water (to dilute the sugar in the juice)
1 cinnamon stick
3 or 4 whole cloves
½ teaspoon ground ginger
Fresh lemon juice

PREPARATION AND USE:
Pour the juice and water into a large pan. Add the spices. Heat until just beginning to boil. Turn the heat to low, stirring occasionally. Simmer for 30 minutes. Strain out the cinnamon stick and cloves. Enjoy each cup with a squirt of lemon juice.

YIELD: 4 SERVINGS

❓ **How it works:** *You're delivering warmth and antimicrobial plant chemicals to your throat, which both soothe and heal it. Ginger is especially warming, antiviral, anti-inflammatory, and pain relieving.*

When to Call the Doctor

- *Sore throat pain persists for more than three days.*

- *Throat pain is severe. The throat and tonsils often look fiery red with whitish deposits in the crevices of the tonsils. Strep throat can cause significant illness and complications. (The only way to know for sure whether you have it is to get a "strep test," which entails swabbing the back of the throat and testing for strep bacteria.) See the doctor to make sure you don't have strep throat.*

- *Severe throat pain is accompanied by extreme fatigue and other whole-body symptoms. You might have mononucleosis or another condition that warrants physician monitoring.*

- *You have difficulty swallowing.*

- *You have any other questions about your health.*

Chapter 57

Stress and Anxiety

Perhaps you've had the dream. You're about to make an important presentation. Everything seems perfect—until you look down and realize you're not wearing any pants.

Sometimes anxiety bubbles up in our sleep. Or it manifests as muscle tension—the clenched jaw, furrowed brow, and tight shoulders. Anxiety can cause headaches, stomach upset, worried thoughts, insomnia, and other symptoms. Psychological stress is the most common cause of transient and low-level anxiety.

Unfortunately, stress is all too common in America. Surveys show that about one-third of people feel routinely overwhelmed by stress. Worse, many stressed people use unhealthy means to manage it. Experts in the field have called stress overload a public health crisis.

Paradoxically, the stress response damages health but is essential to survival. It's supremely designed to help us survive physical stressors. Confrontation with a saber-toothed tiger (or other threat) inspires alarm. Ancient brain areas activate the sympathetic nervous system (fight-or-flight response) and two adrenal hormones: epinephrine (adrenaline) and cortisol (related to the drug cortisone).

The end result is increased blood sugar, heart rate, breathing rate, and blood pressure. Dilation of arteries to the brain, heart, and muscles ensures the delivery of oxygen and glucose-rich blood. Blood vessels to other organs constrict and activity of those organs (e.g., the intestinal tract) declines. Basically, a crisis is not the time to digest lunch.

The biological situation is perfect—if you are fighting or fleeing a predator. It's not so good if you're caught in a traffic jam and late for an important date. All that palpitating will only hurt your health.

Chronic stress overload raises the risk for a number of conditions that commonly plague Americans. They include high blood pressure, atherosclerosis, heart disease, diabetes, immune system dysfunction, increased sensitivity to pain, and fatigue. Chronic stress contributes to stomach ulcers, indigestion, and irritable bowel syndrome. It throws a wet blanket over sexual desire and can interfere with menstrual cycles. It makes us crave high-calorie food and store fat in our abdomens. It disrupts sleep, impairs learning and memory, and renders us irritable and moody. Over the long haul, stress accelerates aging.

Stressful events can also trigger mood disorders in people who are vulnerable. Having the occasional bout of nervousness is normal. Anxiety disorders are not, although they're common. According to the National Institute of Mental Health, in any given year, 18 percent of adults have symptoms of an anxiety disorder, though only a third receive treatment. Children suffer, too. Anxiety disorders include generalized anxiety disorder, obsessive compulsive disorder, panic disorder, social phobias, specific phobias, and posttraumatic stress disorder. Without proper treatment, these conditions can be chronic and disabling.

History

Calming herbs—chamomile, lavender, skullcap, lemon balm, and more—have long been used to ease stress-induced anxiety. Although not as strong as prescription drugs on the market today, they do help and have far fewer side effects.

A different category of herbs is the adaptogens, a term coined in 1947 by Russian pharmacologist N. V. Lazarev. Adaptogens are nontoxic substances that help the body cope with stress. Historical use of such herbs preceded Lazarev by a few thousand years. Traditional Chinese medicine practitioners revered ginseng *(Panax ginseng)*, astragalus *(Astragalus membranaceus)*, and schisandra *(S. chinensis)* for revitalizing the body. Native Americans used American ginseng *(Panax quinquefolius)*. In ancient India, Ayurvedic practitioners used ashwaganda *(Withania somnifera)* and bacopa *(Bacopa monnieri)* for three thousand years to relieve stress and tension.

Rhodiola *(R. rosea)* and eleuthero *(Eleutherococcus senticosus)*, also used by the ancients, have seen renewed interest from Russian scientists over the last half-century. Emerging scientific study shows these herbs counter stress on a cellular level, in lab studies, and in humans coping with challenges.

RECIPES TO PREVENT AND MANAGE STRESS AND ANXIETY

De-Stress Journal

You
A journal
A pen

PREPARATION AND USE:

Write about one incident in your recent past that made you feel stressed. Record your thoughts, emotions, and bodily sensations: Did you feel angry and blame others? Helpless? Resigned to the situation? Did you feel tightness, pain, or tension in your body? If so, where?

Record the steps you took to address the stress: Did you light a cigarette? Have a drink? Go outside? Call a friend? Slam doors?

Next, record daily stressful incidents and your reactions for a week. At the end of the week, review the journal and identify your patterns of reaction. Zero in on one or two reactions that you feel are especially harmful to your mental or physical health and that you want to change.

YIELD: DAILY SESSION

Lifestyle Tip

Avoid turning to alcohol, sedatives, tobacco, and junk food for stress relief. They might bring you a fleeting release. However, all of these substances actually aggravate stress. Substitute such habits with healthier alternatives, such as those suggested in the remedies in this chapter.

❓ How it works: *The purpose of this exercise is to recognize how you respond to stress. The way we react to daily hassles becomes ingrained and automatic. The goal isn't to avoid stress altogether (which would be impossible and not even truly desirable), but to respond in ways that serve you. Awareness is the first step toward changing unhealthy habits and maximizing the skills that are working for you.*

Just Breathe

You
A quiet place

PREPARATION AND USE:

Set aside 10 minutes in a quiet place. Sit or recline. Do a body scan to identify where you're holding tension. Inhale to a slow count of four. Hold for four counts. Exhale for six counts. Repeat. With each breath, imagine your mind slowing and the breath helping to dissolve those areas of tension.

YIELD: 1 SESSION

❓ How it works: *For millennia, practitioners from around the globe have prescribed breathing exercises. Slow, deep breaths give you control over the so-called autonomic (involuntary) nervous system, increasing parasympathetic (rest and digest) nervous system activity and dialing down the sympathetic nervous system. Research confirms that it works. Counting also distracts your mind from worried thoughts. Dwelling on unfortunate episodes and forecasting doom make things worse. If you visualize yourself sitting in an exam hall or standing before an audience, trembling, tongue-tied, and dumbstruck—you'll undoubtedly tense up.*

Lifestyle Tip

Simplify. A common reason for stress is overscheduling. If something makes you feel stressed and has little value, let it go. That "something" could be relatively trivial (housecleaning or canceling a dinner party) or more fundamental (disconnecting from a dysfunctional relationship, resigning from a committee, or quitting a stressful job).

Lifestyle Tip

Take short breaks during work—regardless of whether such labor involves running a corporation, studying for exams, gardening, or caring for children. A good rule of thumb is a 5- to 10-minute break every hour. Doing so will actually improve productivity, along with mental and physical health. If your job is sedentary, do something physical. If your job involves manual labor, rest.

Also, it's important to compartmentalize your job, especially if you work at home. In other words, try to avoid taking work home for nights and weekends. Some people respond to stress by becoming workaholics. Overwork comes at the expense of social life, relaxation, sleep, and personal health. Plus, it raises the risk for burnout. Symptoms include apathy, fatigue, irritability, and declining productivity.

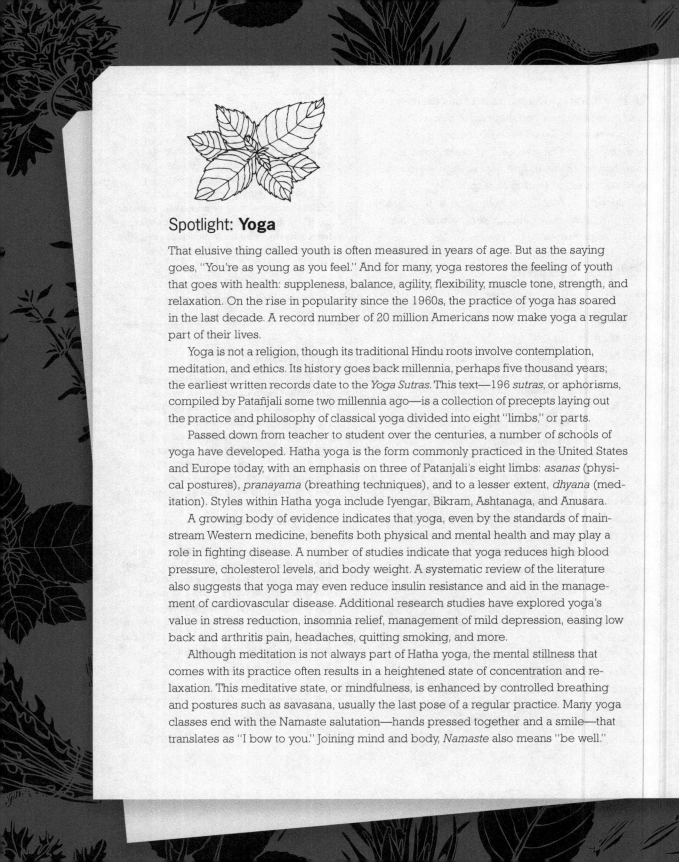

Spotlight: **Yoga**

That elusive thing called youth is often measured in years of age. But as the saying goes, "You're as young as you feel." And for many, yoga restores the feeling of youth that goes with health: suppleness, balance, agility, flexibility, muscle tone, strength, and relaxation. On the rise in popularity since the 1960s, the practice of yoga has soared in the last decade. A record number of 20 million Americans now make yoga a regular part of their lives.

Yoga is not a religion, though its traditional Hindu roots involve contemplation, meditation, and ethics. Its history goes back millennia, perhaps five thousand years; the earliest written records date to the *Yoga Sutras*. This text—196 *sutras*, or aphorisms, compiled by Patañjali some two millennia ago—is a collection of precepts laying out the practice and philosophy of classical yoga divided into eight "limbs," or parts.

Passed down from teacher to student over the centuries, a number of schools of yoga have developed. Hatha yoga is the form commonly practiced in the United States and Europe today, with an emphasis on three of Patanjali's eight limbs: *asanas* (physical postures), *pranayama* (breathing techniques), and to a lesser extent, *dhyana* (meditation). Styles within Hatha yoga include Iyengar, Bikram, Ashtanaga, and Anusara.

A growing body of evidence indicates that yoga, even by the standards of mainstream Western medicine, benefits both physical and mental health and may play a role in fighting disease. A number of studies indicate that yoga reduces high blood pressure, cholesterol levels, and body weight. A systematic review of the literature also suggests that yoga may even reduce insulin resistance and aid in the management of cardiovascular disease. Additional research studies have explored yoga's value in stress reduction, insomnia relief, management of mild depression, easing low back and arthritis pain, headaches, quitting smoking, and more.

Although meditation is not always part of Hatha yoga, the mental stillness that comes with its practice often results in a heightened state of concentration and relaxation. This meditative state, or mindfulness, is enhanced by controlled breathing and postures such as savasana, usually the last pose of a regular practice. Many yoga classes end with the Namaste salutation—hands pressed together and a smile—that translates as "I bow to you." Joining mind and body, *Namaste* also means "be well."

Visualize Confidence

You

A quiet place

PREPARATION AND USE:

In a quiet place, visualize a forthcoming situation that you think will cause you stress: a presentation, a discussion with an estranged loved one, or an exam. Visualize the optimal way you can address this challenge. Imagine yourself feeling calm and focused and others responding positively to you. Prepare for the event, and then let it go (do not let your mind return to it). Enter the situation with confidence and address it as you have visualized. You will be surprised at the outcome. And, keep in mind that it's normal to feel performance anxiety.

YIELD: 1 SESSION

❷ How it works: *By imagining the strongest outcome for a challenging situation, you can prepare for and enter it with confidence and calm. Even if the results aren't exactly what you've envisioned, they will likely be more successful than if you'd anticipated conflict and defeat. Addressing a situation with a positive outlook usually brings positive results.*

Progressive Relaxation

You'll find a similar recipe in Chapter 46, on insomnia. You can also try this variation.

You

A soft rug or mattress

PREPARATION AND USE:

Lie flat on your back on a soft rug or mattress. Feel the floor or mattress receiving your weight. Scan your body for tension. Start breathing slowly and deeply.

Starting with your feet, contract the muscles and let them go. Gradually work your way up your body, to your calves, thighs, buttocks, abs, arms, hands, face, and scalp, sequentially contracting each muscle group and letting go. Silently say, "Let go" or "Relax" on the release. Feel warmth flooding each muscle group. Feel your full body relax.

YIELD: 1 SESSION

❷ How it works: *Multiple studies show that progressive relaxation (also called progressive muscle relaxation) ameliorates stress and anxiety. Herbert Benson, MD, a Harvard professor and founder of the Mind/Body Medical Institute at Massachusetts General Hospital in Boston, termed this state the "relaxation response." Just as your body knows how to mount a stress response, it also knows (though it may need a reminder) how to recover with the relaxation response.*

Person-to-Person Mindfulness

A friend or family member
Your complete focus

PREPARATION AND USE:

Set aside 10 minutes to sit quietly and focus completely on the other person and what that person has to say. Concentrate fully on your companion's mood and delivery and why the message is important to that person.

Refrain from criticizing or judging. Appreciate the person as an individual and feel privileged to be in that person's presence. End by thanking the person for sharing those thoughts and for bringing a new outlook to you.

YIELD: 1 SESSION

❷ **How it works:** *By concentrating completely on another individual and that person's importance, you will come away enlightened and refreshed by new discoveries. Mindfulness, the deliberate attention to the present moment, has its roots in Eastern thought. Jon Kabat-Zinn, Ph.D., developed a formal program called Mindfulness-Based Stress Reduction (MBSR) at the University of Massachusetts Medical Center. Multiple studies show that MSBR reduces measurements of stress and anxiety. By practicing mindful exercises, you will learn to engage with the world around you, turning your attention away from negative, depressive, and anxious thinking.*

Note: Practice this and other mindfulness exercises in this chapter for at least a month and reassess. Determine how you've become more aware of your world, calmer, and more appreciative.

Super Senses Mindfulness

You
An apple or other piece of fruit

PREPARATION AND USE:

Sit quietly. Hold the apple, polish it, smell it, feel its contours, look carefully at its color, its blemishes, and its beauty. Anticipate eating it. Bite into the apple. Slowly, deliberately chew it, savoring the burst of flavor. Don't swallow it immediately, but try to identify the different kinds of tastes and scents you are experiencing. What thoughts are going through your mind? Does eating this apple remind you of pleasant memories?

YIELD: 1 SESSION

❷ **How it works:** *This mindfulness exercise stimulates the senses, guiding you to more deeply appreciate the world right in front of you and the simple things that make it up.*

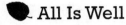

All Is Well

This "mantra" can help burst a fit of panicky thinking. If you find yourself freaking out, find a quiet and safe place, close your eyes, and practice this.

You

PREPARATION AND USE:

Sit in a quiet place (or close your eyes if you cannot leave a crowded room). Repeat silently or out loud, as the surroundings allow, "All is well."

One minute of practice in a crowded room can deliver calm. Five minutes in a quiet room where you sit in solitude will bring peace and well-being that will remain with you throughout the day.

YIELD: 1 SESSION

❓ How it works: *Doing this exercise helps break useless negative ruminating and anticipatory angst. Most of the time, the present moment is tolerable. Worrying spoils the present moment and has no power to change the past or future.*

Lifestyle Tip

Schedule time for you. First, decide what you need to do to restore balance and feel more relaxed. Put that thing on your calendar, whether it's meditating, exercising, getting a massage, napping, or creating art or music. Now that it's on your calendar, it's an appointment. If something else comes up (unless it's an emergency), say, "I'm sorry but I have an appointment scheduled at that time." You'll be a better worker, friend, partner, and parent if you do.

Hypnotize Yourself

You
A chair

PREPARATION AND USE:

Sit in a chair and close your eyes. Imagine yourself walking down a flight of stairs. As you descend, it becomes darker and pleasantly warm.

Maybe you smell roses. Tell yourself that with each downward step you are becoming more relaxed. Once you feel calm, imagine yourself turning around and mentally climbing back up. With each step tell yourself that you are becoming more ready to cope with the challenge that awaits you. Once you get to the top, say to yourself, "I am calm and capable. I am refreshed and ready." Keep your eyes closed until you feel centered. Open them and feel refreshed.

YIELD: 1 SESSION

❓ How it works: *Research shows that self-hypnosis can ameliorate stress. Through self-hypnosis using visualization and imagery techniques, you imagine yourself effectively managing the stress systems in your life. Practicing such techniques on a frequent schedule can help you cope with those stressors on a daily basis.*

Lifestyle Tip

Get enough sleep. Sleep deprivation activates stress hormones and also makes it harder to cope with everyday hassles.

Moving Meditation: Parting the Clouds

This movement is part of the ancient Chinese practice of qigong (pronounced chi kung*). Qi is the Chinese term for body energy.*

You
Comfortable clothes
A quiet place

PREPARATION AND USE:

Stand with your legs comfortably apart, knees relaxed. Hold your hands loosely in front of your chest, the backs of your hands lightly touching at the knuckles to form a V. Breathing in deeply, slowly stretch your hands and arms up over your head, "to heaven." Exhaling, part your hands with your fingers fully open and slowly bring your arms down, "from heaven to earth," in a circular motion on either side of your body, opening your chest. Bend your knees as you complete the circle.

Bring the backs of your hands together again into a V in front of your chest and straighten your legs to a standing position. Repeat this circular motion eight times. When the last circle is complete, bring your palms to rest, one on top of the other, on your belly.

Close your eyes and breathe in deeply, enjoying the refreshing energy. When you feel fully centered, slowly open your eyes. Lightly tickle your skin—your hands, arms, scalp, face, ears, and the rest of your body—as if you are brushing away all stress. Enjoy an energized day.

YIELD: 1 SESSION

❷ How it works: *The aim of qigong is to promote the flow of energy through meditation, physical movement, and breathing exercises. Qigong, yoga, and tai chi are all forms of moving meditation. All help reduce psychological distress. Physical exercise is a great outlet for frustration.*

When Simple Doesn't Work

Humans have long relied upon adaptogens, such as Asian and American ginseng, astragalus, schisandra, eleuthero, ashwagandha, and rhodiola, as described earlier in the chapter. In lab studies, extracts of such plants have actions such as normalizing levels of the stress hormone cortisol and protecting against ailments associated with chronic stress. Clinical trials show that rhodiola fights stress-related fatigue and reduces cortisol levels in people with burnout and also improves mental function and relieves symptoms of depression and anxiety.

Psychological stress is a common cause of anxiety. The best-researched herb for anxiety is the South Pacific native, kava kava (Piper methysticum). A number of clinical trials have shown that concentrated kava extracts countered anxiety better than a placebo and on par with some conventional anti-anxiety drugs—but with fewer side effects. Although adverse effects haven't been reported in studies, more than one hundred case reports have linked kava extracts to liver damage. In many cases, people were also drinking alcohol or taking medications that can injure liver. Some people, however, may have unusual responses to kava.

Interestingly, a 2013 study in people with generalized anxiety disorder (a condition marked by chronic and excessive worry about everyday things) found that six weeks of two doses of kava (providing 120 milligrams a day, or 240 milligrams a day of active chemicals called kavalactones) reduced anxiety, improved sexual function (unlike many antidepressants used to treat anxiety), and produced no significant adverse effects—including alterations in blood tests for liver function.

Ingestion of this herb is not recommended for children, pregnant or nursing women, people with liver disease, heavy drinkers, and people on medication that can harm the liver. The drug that most commonly harms the liver is acetaminophen (Tylenol). People who habitually consume kava extracts should also ask their doctor about blood tests to monitor liver function. Also, people allergic to pepper may also be allergic to kava, which belongs to the same plant family.

Other research-backed anti-anxiety herbs include passionflower (Passiflora incarnata), German chamomile (Matricaria recutita), hawthorn (Crataegus oxycantha), and California poppy (Eschscholzia californica).

Nerve-Calming Aroma Relief

Choosing to surround yourself with a scent will link you with situations in which you've felt peaceful.

Essential oil of your favorite aroma (choose from lavender, chamomile, rose, jasmine, bergamot, or neroli)

PREPARATION AND USE:
Fill a bathtub with warm water. Drop in 10 to 12 drops of your choice of essential oil. Disperse the oil with your hand. Luxuriate.

YIELD: 1 APPLICATION

❷ **How it works:** *Aromas are relayed to those ancient brain areas that trigger the stress response. Emerging research shows that some plant essential oils reduce objective and subjective measurements of stress and anxiety. Examples include German and Roman chamomile, lavender, rose, and jasmine.*

Note: Other options for aroma use: Diffuse it or add it to lotion, using 10 to 12 drops per ounce (28 ml).

Destressing Aroma Inhaler

Your favorite essential oil

PREPARATION AND USE:
Drop a few drops of your favorite oil on a cotton ball. Place the ball in a clean jar and cap it. Open the jar and inhale the aroma when you are in any stressful situation.

YIELD: MULTIPLE APPLICATIONS

❷ **How it works:** *Some plant essential oils help reduce stress and feelings of anxiety. Carry this inhaler with you for immediate stress relief.*

Relaxing Beauty Visualization

You

PREPARATION AND USE:
Create a script for imaging a peaceful, relaxing, safe place: for instance, you are lying on a beach, lulled by sounds of surf, palm fronds, and seagulls. You smell salt, seaweed, and sunblock. You hear and feel the water. The sunlight glints off the ocean. The orange sunset blazes at the end of the day.

Close your eyes and run this vision through your mind. Gradually feel yourself relaxing.

YIELD: 1 SESSION

❷ **How it works:** *When we're worried, we often paint a bleak picture in our mind. But you can change that mental movie. Doing so has the power to turn down the fight-or-flight response. Studies do show that positive imagery can reduce stress.*

When to Call the Doctor

Sometimes stress symptoms become intolerable and rob our lives of beauty and joy. A host of health professionals can help: medical doctors (including psychiatrists), psychologists, social workers, body workers, and more. Get help if you notice you have some combination of the following stress-induced symptoms on a regular basis:

- *tight, painful muscles, particularly in the neck, shoulders, jaw, and temples*
- *frequent headaches*
- *teeth clenching or grinding*
- *trembling hands, racing heart, or sweaty palms*
- *belly pain*
- *insomnia (difficulty falling or staying asleep)*
- *mental tension and nervousness*

In addition, you should seek help if you have symptoms of an anxiety disorder. Following are some of the warning signs. The key is they occur most days of the week and interfere with quality of life and function.

- *constant worrying*
- *perpetually feeling restless and keyed up*
- *difficulty concentrating*
- *insomnia*
- *muscle tension*
- *rapid breathing with tingling feelings in the hands and feet*
- *social withdrawal*
- *nightmares and flashbacks (posttraumatic stress disorder)*
- *dread of interacting with strangers (social phobia)*
- *preoccupation with order and symmetry, germs, or unpleasant images that is relieved by rituals (obsessive-compulsive disorder)*
- *intense fear of things that don't bother most people (enclosed spaces, heights, spiders, etc.)*
- *repeated panic attacks (trembling, racing heart, shortness of breath, hyperventilation, sweating, and feelings of doom)*

Rethink the Situation

A pad of paper
A pen

PREPARATION AND USE:

Sit quietly. Write down all your worried thoughts. Now, with the objectivity and detachment of a scientist or doctor, question those thoughts: How realistic are they? Could you view the situation in a different way? Could you see it as a challenge or opportunity, something that inspires eagerness, confidence, and hope? How do you have control in this situation? If yes, how can you work that control to your advantage? If no, how can learn to accept the situation?

YIELD: 1 SESSION

❷ How it works: *Of all the animals, we humans excel at thinking our way into a stressed-out frenzy. Our big brain is capable of both* rumination *(turning a thought over and over in our heads) and* anticipation *(forecasting into the future about what may come). The process described above is reappraisal or reframing. Using our higher brain areas, we have the power to either ramp up the stress response or turn it off. You can choose how to react. Repeated studies show that when people feel a reasonable sense of control they feel less stressed. Remind yourself that you, as a human, are programmed to adapt.*

Lifestyle Tip

Control caffeine intake. An excess of caffeine mimics the symptoms of anxiety.

Lifestyle Tip

Work it out. Moderate exercise is a great antidote to stress and mild anxiety. Regular exercisers report feeling less stressed.

 ## Sereni-Tea

1 cup (26 g) dried lemon balm leaves
¼ cup (6 g) dried German chamomile flowers
2 tablespoons (3 g) dried lavender flowers
2 tablespoons (3 g) dried rosebuds or petals
¼ cup (6 g) dried passionflower
2 cups (475 ml) water
Stevia or honey (optional)

PREPARATION AND USE:

Mix the dried herbs and place them in a clean jar. Boil the water in a pot. Remove from the heat. Add 2 tablespoons (3 g) of the mixture and cover. Steep 15 minutes. Strain and serve. Add stevia or honey if you want it sweeter. Sip and relax.

YIELD: 2 SMALL SERVINGS

❷ How it works: *All of these herbs calm the nervous system. Most of the herbs have been studied in the laboratory. One study found a special extract of German chamomile helped people with generalized anxiety disorder.*

Note: All measurements are for dried plants. If you use fresh, double the amounts.

If you don't have access to bulk herbs, buy chamomile tea bags or a tea blend of some of these herbs. Other calming herbs include hops, skullcap, and valerian. All act as gentle sedatives. Reserve stronger herbs, such as hops and valerian, until closer to bedtime.

Chapter 58

Ulcers

As commonplace as they seem, stomach ulcers have caused pain, illness, and even premature death. Take Charles Darwin, who attributed his constant stomach problems to seasickness. Doctors now suspect he was infected with the ulcer-causing bacterium *Helicobacter pylori*. Stomach ulcers, combined with a parasitic infection that damaged his heart, contributed to his ill chronic health and death at age seventy-three.

By definition, an *ulcer* is an erosion on any bodily surface—the skin or the mucous membranes that line hollow organs. When people use the word, they're usually referring to peptic ulcers, in which case the craterlike sores occur in the stomach or duodenum (first part of the small intestine). However, ulcers can occur anywhere along the gastrointestinal tract, from mouth to anus.

Let's start with the mouth. **Canker sores** (also called aphthous ulcers) are the most common problem. These small, but painful sores usually heal within seven to ten days. Genetic vulnerability seems to play a role. Triggers include food allergies, stress, smoking, trauma (from braces, dentures, hot foods, or hard toothbrushes), certain medications, toothpastes containing sodium lauryl sulfate, and nutrient deficiencies (vitamin C, vitamin B_{12}, folic acid, and iron).

A different entity altogether, **fever blisters** (also called cold sores) occur on the lips, are caused by herpes simplex virus, and are very contagious (see page 162).

A more serious condition is **inflammatory bowel disease**. This category includes ulcerative colitis and Crohn's disease. In ulcerative colitis, the inflammation and ulcers stay within the colon (large intestine). In Crohn's disease, the entire gastrointestinal tract is vulnerable to ulceration. Both conditions require careful medical management.

Back to gastric (stomach) ulcers. The problem often begins with **gastritis**, inflammation of the stomach. Causes include alcohol abuse, nonsteroidal anti-inflammatory drugs (aspirin, ibuprofen, naproxen), and infection with the bacterium *Helicobacter pylori*. The condition may lack symptoms or produce upper abdominal pain, nausea, and vomiting. If an ulcer develops, signs of bleeding include black, tarry stools, red blood in the stool, or bloody vomitus.

H. pylori is now considered the main cause of **peptic ulcers**. The bacterium is present in the majority of people with ulcers. However, only 20 percent of people infected with *H. pylori* develop ulcers. Clearly, other factors contribute.

Stress, even if it doesn't directly cause peptic ulcers, does increase vulnerability by inhibiting the production of the mucus that normally coats and protects the stomach, reducing blood flow to the gut, impairing wound healing, and depressing the immune system. Other controllable risk factors include tobacco use, sleep deprivation, nonsteroidal anti-inflammatory drugs, and low intake of fruits and vegetables.

Medical treatment of peptic ulcer involves antacids to neutralize existing stomach acid and medications to inhibit acid secretion. Complications of ulcers include profuse bleeding, perforation (the ulcer chews through the wall of the stomach or duodenum), and intestinal obstruction.

History

Symptoms of peptic ulcer disease have been described since ancient times. For centuries, physicians and herbalists soothed stomach irritations and ulcers with a staple of herbal medicine, slippery elm *(Ulmus rubra)*. (Adding a pint of boiling water to a paste made from cold water and a teaspoon [5 g] of slippery elm powder was one recipe.) In *De Materia Medica*, first-century BCE physician and botanist Dioscorides also praised the resin of the mastic gum tree *(Pistachia lentiscus* 'Chia') for treating stomach disorders. (As recently as 2001, researchers confirmed the efficacy of this treatment.)

Then, more than a hundred years ago, the presence of bacteria was discovered in the human stomach—a place previously considered too acidic for bacterial life. In the 1980s, Australian physicians Robin Warren, M.D., and Barry Marshall, M.D., linked the presence of *H. pylori* to gastritis and ulcers. Marshall actually swallowed some of the bacteria to prove that they did indeed inflame the stomach. In 2005, Marshall and Warren were awarded a Nobel Prize. Medical treatment shifted from asking patients about their stress levels (though stress increases vulnerability to ulcers) to prescribing antibiotics to kill *H. pylori*.

Fact or Myth?

COFFEE CAUSES ULCERS.

That's a controversial issue. Although coffee and other caffeine-containing beverages stimulate secretion of stomach acid, they don't seem to cause ulcers. Furthermore, decaffeinated coffee also releases stomach acid. Nevertheless, if coffee worsens your symptoms or your doctor recommends you quit, follow that advice.

Lifestyle Tip

Exercise. Although extreme exercise can increase the risk of gastritis and peptic ulcers, moderate, regular physical activity has a protective effect on the gut and also relieves stress. A bit of advice: Wait a good 30 minutes after eating before you engage in aerobic exercise to allow your food to digest.

Cabbage Juice Relief

Cabbage juice is a long-standing folk medicine against peptic ulcers. During the early 1950s, Garnett Cheney, MD, conducted research on "vitamin U," an antiulcer factor in raw cabbage juice.

½ head white cabbage, washed and chopped coarsely (no hearts)
About 2 cups (475 ml) water

PREPARATION AND USE:

Fill a blender with the cabbage. Add water to the two-thirds mark. Blend on high speed until fully blended, about a minute. Strain or press the mixture. (A medium-size French press works well to strain out the juice.) Drink ½ cup (120 ml) up to three times a day. Store the unused portion in the refrigerator. Discard after twenty-four hours.

YIELD: 12 OUNCES (355 ML) CABBAGE JUICE

❷ How it works: *In the 1950s, Cheney and colleagues conducted a study on San Quentin Prison inmates that demonstrated improved healing of peptic ulcers from concentrated cabbage juice relative to a placebo beverage. Volunteers received 50 milliliters (just under 2 ounces, or ¼ cup) a day for twenty-one days. Later research showed that the fresh juice of white cabbage stimulates the immune system and contains glutamine, an amino acid that may improve the stomach's protective lining.*

Note: If you have a juicer, you can simply juice a white cabbage. For another effective recipe, see the Oatmeal and Slippery Elm Porridge (page 307).

For another effective recipe, see the Oatmeal and Slippery Elm Porridge (page 307).

Lifestyle Tip

For mouth ulcers, make a solution that's half water and half hydrogen peroxide. Dab the solution onto the sore. Next coat the area with milk of magnesia. Repeat three or four times a day. MedlinePlus, the National Library of Medicine's website for consumer health information, recommends this remedy for soothing relief.

Breakfast Boost

Studies show that fasting during Ramadan increases stomach acidity and increases the odds of ulcer reactivation. Aside from religious fasting, many people skip breakfast. This simple, healthful breakfast boost has ingredients that inhibit H. pylori bacteria.

1 large banana, frozen and sliced
1 cup (255 g) frozen sliced strawberries
1 cup (230 g) vanilla yogurt
3 tablespoons (36 g) psyllium powder
1 to 2 cups (235 to 475 ml) cranberry or cranapple juice

PREPARATION AND USE:

In a blender, blend together the bananas, strawberries, and yogurt. Blend in the psyllium powder. Add the juice to your desired consistency and amount.

YIELD: 2 SERVINGS

❷ How it works: *A bacterium common in fermented dairy products* (Lactobacillus acidophilus) *produces fatty acids that suppress H. pylori. In test-tube studies, cranberry extract and honey inhibit H. pylori.*

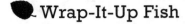

Wrap-It-Up Fish

2 long sheets (about 13 x 18-inches
   [33 x 45.5 cm]) phyllo pastry
1 tablespoon (15 ml) olive oil
½ zucchini, chopped
8 broccoli florets, halved
1 garlic clove, minced
1 salmon fillet (8 ounces, or 225 g), skin
   removed
1 tablespoon (10 ml) vegetable stock
1 teaspoon (10 g) chopped dill

PREPARATION AND USE:

Preheat the oven to 350°F (180°C, or gas mark 4).

   Lightly spray a large baking sheet with cooking spray. Spread out one phyllo sheet on the prepared baking sheet. Lightly brush the phyllo sheet with olive oil. Place the second sheet on top of the first and lightly brush with olive oil. Cover the top layer of phyllo with a layer of zucchini and broccoli. Sprinkle with the garlic. Lay the salmon on top. Spoon the vegetable stock over the salmon. Sprinkle the dill on top. Fold up the phyllo pastry, envelope style, to cover the salmon and pinch together the edges. Lightly brush the outside of the packet with olive oil. Bake for 20 minutes.

YIELD: 2 SERVINGS

❷ **How it works:** *Some polyunsaturated fatty acids, including the kind in fish oil, evening primrose oil, flaxseed oil, and black currant seed oil, are anti-inflammatory and inhibit H. pylori. A type of fatty acid prominent in oily fish, such as salmon, may be particularly helpful. In test-tube studies, garlic inhibits H. pylori.*

Mouth Ulcer Paste

1 teaspoon (5 g) baking soda
Water

PREPARATION AND USE:

In a small, clean dish, mix together the baking soda and as much water as needed to form a paste. With a cotton swab, apply to each sore to your desired thickness. Create a fresh batch and apply three times a day.

YIELD: 1 APPLICATION

❷ **How it works:** *The baking soda paste covers the sore to protect it from irritants. The Mayo Clinic recommends this mixture to ease pain and help healing.*

Alternate: For a quick rinse, mix 1 cup (235 ml) of warm water, ¼ teaspoon of baking soda, and ⅛ teaspoon of salt. Rinse several times a day using a new batch each time. Then rinse with a plain cup (235 ml) of water.

Slippery Elm Mouth Ulcer Relief

1 tablespoon (15 g) *Aloe vera* gel
1 teaspoon (5 g) powdered slippery elm bark

PREPARATION AND USE:

Put both ingredients in a small, clean jar and blend with a chopstick. Dot on mouth ulcers as needed. Cap the jar when not in use.

YIELD: MULTIPLE APPLICATIONS

❷ **How it works:** Aloe vera *gel decreases inflammation, stimulates the immune system, and enhances wound healing. Preliminary studies show that topical aloe gel decreases the pain of aphthous ulcers and speeds healing. The inner bark of slippery elm (Ulmus rubra) contains mucilaginous substances that coat and soothe irritated membranes.*

Note: Use either 99 percent aloe gel or fresh aloe gel gently scraped from the inner leaf of an *Aloe vera* plant (we recommend growing one in an indoor pot). You can find powdered slipper elm bark at natural food stores and herb retailers.

Aloe Minty Ulcer Relief

1 tablespoon (15 g) 99 percent *Aloe Vera* gel
1 drop peppermint essential oil

PREPARATION AND USE:

Put the aloe gel in a small, clean jar. Add 1 drop of peppermint essential oil. Blend with a chopstick. Cap tightly. Using a clean finger, dot on mouth ulcers as needed.

YIELD: MULTIPLE APPLICATIONS

❓ **How it works:** *As noted earlier, preliminary research suggests that aloe gel reduces mouth ulcer discomfort and hastens healing. Applied topically, the menthol in peppermint essential oil decreases pain.*

Note: Alternatively, cut off the end of a leaf from a fresh *Aloe vera* plant. Slice the piece lengthwise. Scoop out a little gel with your finger and dot directly on mouth ulcers.

When Simple Doesn't Work

Long used as a remedy for ulcers in the intestinal tract, licorice root is anti-inflammatory and mucilaginous. Long-term use of whole root extracts aren't feasible because a chemical called glycyrrhizin stimulates retention of salt and water and loss of potassium, which can elevate blood pressure and raise the risk of irregular heartbeat. The good news is that glycyrrhizin can be removed without losing benefits for aphthous and peptic ulcers. The product is called deglycyrrhizinated (DGL) licorice and is available at natural food stores. Discuss its use with your physician. If you have low potassium levels or liver or kidney disease, this supplement may not be appropriate.

Preliminary research has shown that Aloe vera gel taken by mouth improved ulcerative colitis. In one study, patients started with 25 to 50 milliliters twice a day and, as tolerated, worked up to 100 milliliters twice a day for four weeks. The product used was one intended for internal use that was diluted 50 percent. If you have ulcerative colitis, discuss use of dietary supplements with your doctor.

Positively Pleasing Ulcer Potion

6 cups (1.4 L) water
¼ cup (25 g) fresh ginger slices
6 chamomile tea bags
1 tablespoon (3 g) chopped fresh sage
3 cups (700 ml) pure cranberry juice
Honey (optional)

PREPARATION AND USE:

Boil the water in a large pot. Add the ginger, tea bags, and sage; steep for 10 minutes. Strain into a pitcher. Stir in the juice. Add honey, if desired. Drink throughout the day.

YIELD: 8 SERVINGS

❓ How it works: *In test-tube studies, chamomile and sage inhibit* H. pylori. *Cranberry and honey are inhibitors as well. Animal studies indicate that ginger reduces the concentration of* H. pylori *and inflammation in the stomach and protects against stress-induced ulcers. Whether these plants are similarly helpful in humans isn't yet known. However, they all have other health benefits and taste great.*

Lifestyle Tip

Get enough sleep. Chronic sleep deprivation raises your risk of peptic ulcer disease and worsens inflammatory bowel disease. See Chapter 46, on insomnia, for tips on sleeping better.

Lifestyle Tip

Stay away from tobacco. Tobacco decreases blood flow to the gut, worsening ulcerative conditions.

When to Call the Doctor

Make an appointment if:

- *You suspect you have a gastritis, peptic ulcer, or inflammatory bowel disease.*

- *You notice black stools (and are not taking iron supplements).*

- *You have already been diagnosed with an ulcer and have recurrent symptoms.*

Seek emergency care if:

- *You have bright red blood in your stool (not related to hemorrhoids).*

- *You vomit blood (old blood can have a coffee-grounds appearance).*

- *You have severe abdominal pain.*

- *You have a history of ulcers and become faint.*

Chapter 59

Vaginal Yeast Infections (Yeast Vaginitis)

Vaginitis means inflammation of the vagina. A number of things can irritate the vagina: infections with bacteria, fungi, and protozoa; harsh chemicals in personal care products; and even the loss of estrogen after menopause.

Yeast, a type of fungus, normally colonize the vagina though in small numbers relative to health-promoting bacteria such as lactobacilli. An overgrowth of certain types of yeast, such as *Candida albicans*, produces vaginal yeast infections (also called yeast vaginitis or vaginal candidiasis). Usually the labia and clitoris are also inflamed. About 75 percent of women have at least one episode in their lifetime; 5 to 10 percent have recurrent attacks.

The following factors raise the risk of yeast vaginitis:

- Antibiotics kill the "friendly" bacteria that normally defend the vagina.
- Douches and some vaginal "hygiene" sprays can irritate the vagina and disrupt the microbial ecology.
- Cancer chemotherapy, cortisone-like medications, and HIV infection suppress the immune system, allowing disease-causing microbes to flourish.
- Diabetes mellitus raises glucose (sugar) levels in bodily fluids, allowing feasting yeast to proliferate.
- Other factors include receptive oral sex (cunnilingus), pregnancy (because of hormonal shifts), and some contraceptives (contraceptive sponges, hormonal contraceptives, and intrauterine devices).

Symptoms include itching, burning, a thick white discharge, and discomfort during intercourse. Health professionals diagnose the condition with visual inspection and microscopic examination of the discharge. Treatment centers on intravaginal antifungal creams and suppositories. Oral antifungal drugs may be prescribed for more severe cases.

Before you try home remedies or over-the-counter antifungal creams, we recommend you get a medical diagnosis. Women correctly self-diagnose yeast vaginitis only about half the time. Other pathogens that don't respond to antifungal drugs—some with potentially serious complications—can cause similar symptoms or may coexist with the yeast overgrowth.

Home management is only appropriate if you're sure you have yeast and your symptoms are mild. If you're pregnant, do not try any home remedies (with the exception of eating yogurt) without consulting your physician.

History

For millennia, gynecological problems, such as vaginal yeast infections, were largely left to midwives or to the sufferers themselves to treat. A famous nineteenth-century drawing by Jacques-Pierre Maygnier helps to explain why. A physician kneels in front of a fully clothed woman, his hands up her long dress, his face turned away so he cannot see her genitalia. This historic taboo against the examination of female genitalia by male doctors inhibited the science of gynecology for centuries.

Nevertheless, medical attempts to doctor "female" problems persisted through the ages. The first female gynecologist in ancient Greece is believed to have been Agnodice (ca. fourth century BCE) who disguised herself as a man in order to practice. Midwives also practiced in ancient Greece specializing in traditional ailments for women as did the few female doctors. Midwifery flourished throughout the ancient world in Egypt, Byzantium, Mesopotamia, Athens, and Rome as well as in early America. (The first hospital for women in America was not established until 1855.)

Lifestyle Tip

If you have diabetes, work with your health practitioner to control your blood sugar. When blood sugar is abnormally high, so is the sugar in vaginal secretions, which feeds the yeast. Even if you don't have diabetes, avoid sweetened beverages, alcoholic drinks (which contain carbohydrates), refined carbohydrates, and other sweets, which can promote the growth of yeast.

The historical record has little enough to say about treating vaginal yeast infections, but the benefits of vinegar, honey, and garlic, for example, have been commonplace for centuries. And the gynecologic benefits are well-known, too: vinegar douches for infections; honey as a contraceptive in the time of Cleopatra; and garlic as a cure-all for scores of ailments, including infections. Hence, it is probably safe to assume that through the centuries, midwives and others divined the usefulness of these ancient medicines in treating vaginal yeast infections as well.

Healing Honeyed Yogurt

1 cup (235 ml) water
2 tablespoons (40 g) raw (unprocessed) honey
2 tablespoons (30 g) plain, active-culture
  yogurt

PREPARATION AND USE:

Boil the water in a kettle or saucepan. Allow it to cool so that it's very warm but not scalding.

Place the honey in a bowl. Raw honey can be very thick, so add just enough of the warm water (no more than 1 to 2 teaspoons [5 to 10 ml]) so that you can blend the honey with the yogurt. Add the yogurt and blend thoroughly with a clean spoon. Transfer the mixture to a clean jar.

With clean fingers, apply about 1 teaspoon (11.5 g) to the vagina and vulva. (Don't double-dip. If you have a clean vaginal applicator, you can spoon the mixture into it and apply it that way.) Repeat two times a day for seven days. We recommend you wear a panty liner. Store the jar in the refrigerator between applications. Toss after one week.

YIELD: TWELVE 1-TEASPOON (11.5 G) APPLICATIONS

❷ How it works: *Raw honey has antifungal activity. Yogurt contains* Lactobacilli, *which is the type of bacteria normally found in the vagina. These friendly bacteria promote healthy immune system function and lower pH (more acidic environments are hostile to fungi). In a study published in 2012 in the* **Archives of Obstetrics and Gynecology,** *researchers created a blend of distilled water, local honey, and yogurt and then assigned pregnant women with yeast vaginitis to use the honey-yogurt blend or topical antifungal cream. Both were effective, but the honey-yogurt blend more so.*

Note: Raw honey hasn't been processed or heated, thus retaining all active ingredients.

Fact or Myth?

YEAST VAGINITIS IS A SEXUALLY TRANSMITTED INFECTION.

Not necessarily. Men can pick it up from their female partners, though they less often develop symptoms. However, women who have never had sexual intercourse can develop yeast vaginitis. Yeast, which already exist in the vagina, simply grow out of control.

Lifestyle Tip

Change tampons or pads frequently during menstruation.

When Simple Doesn't Work

Some antifungal creams, such as miconazole and clotrimazole, are available over the counter.

Boric acid suppositories have also been successfully used, though the method is less well researched than antifungal creams. Boric acid is antiseptic and inhibits fungi. Some products are available over-the-counter. Most studies have used 600 milligrams of boric acid in a gelatin capsule inserted into the vagina. Boric acid is toxic if eaten, should not be used long term in the vagina, and should not be used at all by pregnant women. Side effects include watery discharge, redness, and mild burning.

Probiotic supplements have preventive value. Some studies show that oral or intravaginal capsules or suppositories containing certain strains of lactobacilli (Lactobacillus acidophilus, L. rhamnosus GR-1, L. fermentum RC-14, L. crispatus, and L. reuteri) help reduce recurrences of yeast vaginitis and bacterial vaginosis (caused by imbalances in vaginal bacteria).

Products made from the juice of fresh Echinacea pupurea have been shown to be useful add-on therapies to an antifungal cream to prevent vaginal yeast infections. They also improve immune system function during an acute infection.

Doctors use topical antifungal agents to prevent recurrences. Combining the cream with oral echinacea (a product made from the juice of the above-ground parts of the plant preserved in alcohol) significantly increased the effectiveness.

Lifestyle Tip

When you bathe, use a hypoallergenic soap and rinse well with clear water. Avoid commercial vaginal sprays and douches. Harsh soaps and vaginal sprays may inflame the vagina and disrupt the normal microbial ecology. Frequent douching may remove friendly bacteria from the vagina, allowing an overgrowth of disease-causing microorganisms. The pressure from douching may also propel microorganisms into the uterus and fallopian tubes. Remember that the vagina cleans itself by secreting mucus.

 Intravaginal Yogurt

Plain, active-culture yogurt

PREPARATION AND USE:
Apply to the vagina and vulva two or three times a day.

YIELD: MULTIPLE APPLICATIONS

❷ **How it works:** *Yogurt contains* lactobacilli, *which protect against yeast vaginitis. Despite a long folk tradition, clinical trials have not evaluated intravaginal yogurt used alone for women with recurrent yeast infections. Such use may have more potential value as a preventive rather than a treatment for an active yeast infection.* Lactobacilli *do, however, interfere with the ability of disease-causing bacteria to colonize the vagina.*

🍃 Garlic Suppository

1 garlic clove, peeled

PREPARATION AND USE:

Wrap the clove in a single layer of sterile gauze and twist, to create a "tail" that's 1 to 2 inches (2.5 to 5 cm) long. (If you have no irritation after the first application, you can gently nick the clove next time.) Insert the gauze-covered clove into the vagina, leaving a small piece of the tail-end of the gauze at the vaginal entrance. (Adding a bit of K-Y Jelly or other lubricant to the end can ease the insertion). Remove after 1 hour. Repeat three times a day.

YIELD: 1 APPLICATION

❓ **How it works:** *Garlic is antimicrobial, with activity against fungi. However, no clinical trials have evaluated this folk remedy.*

❗ **Warning:** *Prolonged use of topical garlic can irritate skin and mucous membranes. Some people are allergic. Discontinue use if irritation occurs.*

🍃 Yogurt and Berries Breakfast Treat

1 cup (230 g) plain nonfat, active-culture yogurt (We like Greek yogurt, which has a satisfying thickness even when low in fat.)

¼ cup (36 g) fresh berries (or other favorite fruit)

PREPARATION AND USE:

Scoop the yogurt into a bowl. Top with the berries. Spoon into your mouth and enjoy.

YIELD: 1 SERVING

❓ **How it works:** *Yogurt contains probiotics, live microorganisms (mainly bacteria), that promote human health. Regularly eating yogurt seems to help prevent yeast infections. Active-culture yogurt contains bacteria normally found in the intestinal tract and vagina. These organisms promote healthy immune function.*

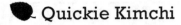 ## Quickie Kimchi

1 head savoy cabbage

1 cup (110 g) grated carrot

¼ cup (60 g) sea salt

½ teaspoon minced fresh garlic

4 scallions, chopped

1 teaspoon (5 ml) Asian fish sauce

1 tablespoon (13 g) sugar

½ teaspoon ground ginger

2 teaspoons (5.2 g) chili powder, or to taste

PREPARATION AND USE:

Trim the bottom of the cabbage, slice it lengthwise, and cut each half into chunks. Mix together the cabbage chunks and carrot in a large glass bowl. Toss with the salt to coat the vegetable mixture.

Cover the bowl securely with plastic wrap and allow to sit at room temperature for 5 to 6 hours. Transfer the mixture from the bowl to a colander, rinse off the salt, and then drain the vegetable mixture, thoroughly, pressing out all the liquid. Return the mixture to the rinsed bowl and stir in all the remaining ingredients, except the chili powder.

When all the ingredients are combined, add the chili powder and stir well to coat. You can knead it in by hand, but wear plastic gloves to protect your fingers from the heat.

Transfer the mixture to a clean 24-ounce (710 ml) glass jar. Cap the lid tightly. Set the jar in a cool, dry place for four days. Refrigerate, then serve. Refrigerated, the mixture keeps for about four weeks.

YIELD: 4 SERVINGS

❷ How it works: *Fermented foods contain probiotics. The intestines are the source of fungi that infect the vagina (and also of the bacteria that cause bladder infections and a non–sexually transmitted vaginal infection called bacterial vaginosis). Disruption in the microbial ecology of the gut (due to antibiotics and other causes) can promote fungal overgrowth in the vagina. Although oral probiotics are unlikely to treat an active yeast infection, regular consumption may help prevent them.*

Note: Also see the Simply (Probiotic) Sauerkraut (page 329).

 ## Antiyeast Bath

1 cup (235 ml) apple cider vinegar

PREPARATION AND USE:

As you run a warm bath, pour in the apple cider vinegar and disperse it with your hand. Luxuriate for at least 20 minutes as the vinegar works to inhibit yeast growth.

YIELD: 1 APPLICATION

❷ How it works: *Vinegar can help arrest the growth of* **Candida albicans,** *a common cause of yeast infections. All three essential oil alternatives are antifungal.*

Recipe Variation: Add essential oils to your bath, along with the vinegar: tea tree oil, eucalyptus, or lavender.

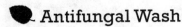 **Antifungal Wash**

2 cups (475 ml) water
1 tablespoon (6 g) green tea
1 tablespoon (3 g) dried rosemary or
   (2 g) sage
1 tablespoon (15 ml) apple cider vinegar
1 drop tea tree essential oil

PREPARATION AND USE:

Boil the water. Add the tea and rosemary. Cover
and steep 15 to 20 minutes.

Strain into a jar. Add the vinegar and oil and
shake well to disperse the oil. Moisten a tampon
with the mixture and insert into the vagina. After
15 minutes, remove the tampon. Wear a panty
liner.

YIELD: 1 APPLICATION

❓ How it works: *Some natural medicine practitioners use diluted tea tree oil to manage vaginitis. Tea tree essential oil is antimicrobial against
a number of organisms, including* Candida albicans. *Ensure that it is diluted as local irritation
and allergic reactions are possible. Tea tree essential oil is very strong and should only be applied externally; it can be toxic if ingested. Tea
(*Camellia sinensis*), rosemary, and sage are also
active against* Candida *yeast. Vinegar contains
acetic acid, which discourages yeast overgrowth.*

❗ Warning: *Do not douche or insert tampons
while pregnant.*

Note: This formula has not been tested in any
clinical trial.

Alternatively, you can very gently douche with
this mixture. Although it's okay to do so if you
have a yeast infection, do not continue douching
on a regular basis. Doing so can disrupt the normal ecology of vaginal microbes. Be sure to wear
a panty liner.

Lifestyle Tip

Refrain from sex until the infection clears.

When to Call the Doctor

- *This the first time you have had vaginal
  irritation and discharge. It's important to
  get a proper diagnosis.*

- *The infection hasn't cleared after you finish a round of antifungal cream.*

- *Two days of home treatment have not
  improved symptoms or symptoms have
  worsened.*

- *You have recurrent episodes of vaginitis.*

- *You have multiple sexual partners and
  now have vaginal discharge. Sexually
  transmitted bacteria can lead to pelvic
  inflammatory disease (infection of the
  uterus and fallopian tubes). If not treated
  immediately, it can lead to infertility and
  ectopic (out of place) pregnancy.*

- *You have not been consistently using a
  condom during intercourse. (If you're in
  a long-standing and strictly monogamous
  relationship, ignore this one.)*

Chapter 60

Weight Management

Which would you rather have: (a) the Fountain of Youth or (b) a body like Halle Berry (or Daniel Craig, if you're a guy)? It's a tough choice. We're betting that most red-blooded Americans would go with (b). Here's why: One, humans like instant gratification. Two, being lean and healthy correlates with better health and longevity. Three, many Americans desperately want to lose weight.

Only one-third of Americans boast a "normal" weight for their height. About a third are overweight but not obese; more than a third are obese. Over the past three decades, the proportion of obese adults has doubled from 15 percent to nearly 36 percent. The number of overweight children has tripled. More than 30 percent of children and adolescents are overweight or obese. "Globesity" is a word coined to reflect the worldwide epidemic of obesity.

Before we go further, we'd like to point out that body fat has benefits. It forms cell membranes, fills out the contours of your face, insulates you from the cold, and cushions your bones and organs. Excessive fat, however, especially when it's deposited in your abdomen, undermines health. This so-called visceral fat releases inflammatory chemicals and a number of proteins.

The net result of excess body weight is an increased risk for high blood pressure, atherosclerosis, heart disease, type-2 diabetes, metabolic syndrome (a clustering of risk factors for cardiovascular disease and diabetes), gallstones, gastroesophageal reflux disease (heartburn), and certain cancers. Excess fat in the throat can lead to obstructive sleep apnea, a condition marked by recurrent bouts of snoring and breath-holding, which leads to extreme daytime sleepiness and raises the risk for heart attack and stroke. Increased body weight causes low back pain and arthritis.

On the other hand, losing unhealthy body fat has benefits—even if you don't reach an "ideal" body weight. Dropping just 10 pounds (4.5 kg) can lower blood pressure, cholesterol, and triglycerides (blood fat).

Changing habits that have become somewhat automatic can challenge the best of us. But it's entirely possible. Remind yourself of the changes you've willingly and successfully taken on: starting a new job, moving house, adopting a pet, getting married, or having a child. Doubtless you've already made countless transformative shifts.

History

"Pleasingly plump," "zaftig," even "Ruben-esque" were compliments, not insults, in Western cultures up until the twentieth century. Curvaceous early-twentieth-century-movie actress and sex symbol Lillian Russell tipped the scales at 200 pounds (90.7 kilos). Even King Louis XVI is believed to have added padding to convey strength and virility. Large meant healthy and prosperous.

Over the past century, attitudes have shifted dramatically, along with views on health, weight, and diet. Ironically, while our attitudes were doing a 180-degree turn, our habits were moving in the opposite direction. The Western world became more industrialized, more sedentary, and more well fed. Or at least more fed—as food became more readily available, more processed, more pre- and commercially prepared, more varied, and more caloric. Portion sizes also grew, and most of those extra calories came from a deluge of carbohydrates, including sugary drinks and snacks, refined grains, starches, and fast food. As we consumed more calories and burned fewer, we ballooned. And so did our health problems.

The twenty-first century ushered in new definitions of healthy weights. Doctors had generally used weight-for-height tables to set standards for men and women. But in the late 1990s, the body mass index (BMI), a formula for measuring body fat devised in the nineteenth century, took on greater significance. In 1998, the National Institutes of Health and the Centers for Disease Control and Prevention used the BMI to reassess weight standards—lowering the cutoff of normal weight from BMI 27.8 to BMI 25. Some 29 million Americans previously defined as healthy were redefined as overweight.

Today, national initiatives abound: First Lady Michelle Obama's "Let's Move" campaign; Strive for Five (fruits and veggies daily); heart-healthy options, such as the Mediterranean diet; and NBC's reality TV show *The Biggest Loser.* Yet the fat war continues to be a leading public health problem. Although there is some evidence that rates of obesity may have plateaued, we remain one nation, overweight.

RECIPES FOR WEIGHT MANAGEMENT

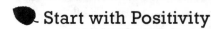 **Start with Positivity**

You
A pencil
Paper

PREPARATION AND USE:
Write down three physical attributes and three psychological attributes that you like about yourself. Post these positive attributes where you can see them.

YIELD: BOUNTIFUL—ESPECIALLY IF REPEATED ON A REGULAR BASIS

❷ **How it works:** *Americans labor under an impossible paradox. The majority of us are overweight or obese, yet we discriminate against overweight and obese people. The social stigma takes a huge toll. It's difficult to feel capable of change without starting with self-love. You are enough as you are right now. Everyone has room for improvement. Just because someone carries less body fat doesn't make him or her a better person than you.*

Breaking the Morning Fast

1 to 2 teaspoons (5 to 10 ml) olive oil
½ cup (35 g) sliced mushrooms (your
  favorite type)
2 large eggs
1 tablespoon (15 ml) nonfat milk
¼ teaspoon dried thyme
¼ teaspoon dried tarragon
¼ teaspoon dried basil, or 2 fresh leaves as
  garnish
½ cup (15 g) baby spinach, rinsed and drained
Pinch of cracked pepper

PREPARATION AND USE:
Pour the oil into an omelet or medium-size pan over medium heat (you'll need enough to prevent the mushrooms from sticking). Add the mushrooms and sauté for 3 to 5 minutes until soft.

While the mushrooms are cooking, whisk together the eggs, milk, and dried herbs in a small bowl.

When the mushrooms are browned, transfer them to a plate. No need to wash the omelet pan. Return it to the stove and add the egg mixture. Turn the heat to medium-high and cook one side of the omelet. Once the eggs solidify on one side,

about 2 minutes, flip and layer with the mushrooms and the spinach.

Cook for another 1 to 2 minutes, so the bottom side of the omelet sets. Fold the cooked eggs over the top of the vegetables. Add cracked pepper to taste. Serve, garnished with the fresh basil leaves if you have omitted the dried basil.

For a beverage, pass on the orange juice (or at least cut it by 50 percent with water). Instead, drink warm water with fresh lemon, green tea, or coffee.

YIELD: 1 SERVING

❷ **How it works:** *Certain studies show that eating breakfast protects against being overweight. For many people, a good breakfast satisfies the hunger of the overnight fast and maintains energy until lunch (and prevents famished overeating midday). The high protein content of eggs fends off hunger longer than does a high-carbohydrate breakfast, such as a bagel with jam. The vegetables contain fiber, which creates a sense of fullness with few calories and many nutrients.*

Chickie-Veg Sauté

2 tablespoons (30 ml) olive oil

2 chicken breasts, skinned

½ cup (120 ml) chicken or vegetable stock, plus more as needed

2 teaspoons (2 g) herbes de Provence, divided

2 teaspoons (4 g) chopped scallion

Paprika

Freshly ground black pepper

1 cup (70 g) mushrooms, sliced

1 cup (150 g) red bell pepper, seeded and sliced

1 cup (120 g) zucchini, sliced

1 garlic clove, chopped

PREPARATION AND USE:

Pour the oil into a large skillet over medium heat and then place chicken breasts in the pan and sauté for 5 minutes on each side. Add the stock, cover the skillet, and cook over low heat for about 10 minutes until the chicken is done in the center. Remove the chicken, sprinkle with half of the herbes de Provence, scallion, and paprika and black pepper to taste, and transfer to a plate. Cover to keep warm.

Add the vegetables, garlic, and rest of the herbes de Provence to the pan and sauté in the existing broth, pouring in more stock as needed to keep the vegetables moist. Cook over medium heat until tender, about 5 minutes. Add the vegetables to the chicken and serve.

YIELD: 2 SERVINGS

❷ **How it works:** *Dietary fat, including that found in olive oil, satisfies hunger. But a little goes a long way. Fats have more than twice the calories, gram per gram, as carbohydrates and protein. Avoid deep-fat frying. Instead, bake, broil, roast, or cook with water or broth to poach, braise, steam, or stew.*

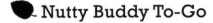

Nutty Buddy To-Go

1 cup (145 g) raw almonds
1 cup (100 g) walnuts
1 teaspoon (6 g) sea salt
½ cup (80 g) dried cherries or (75 g) golden raisins

PREPARATION AND USE:

Preheat the oven to 350°F (180°C, or gas mark 4).

Place the nuts on a baking sheet and toss with the salt. Spread the nuts across the sheet evenly. Roast for 30 minutes. Remove from the oven and let cool. Mix the roasted nuts with the raisins. Place in bags in small containers and keep in your purse, car, backpack, or office for snacks.

YIELD: 2 TO 3 SERVINGS

❷ **How it works:** *Having good food on hand keeps you from snacking on junk food. Several studies indicate that people who regularly eat nuts tend to be leaner. Dried fruits, such as cherries and raisins, provide fiber and energy-maintaining carbohydrates. Nuts are satisfying and their fiber slows down their energy absorption. Walnuts are high in healthy omega-3, fatty acids, and almonds are rich in fiber, protein, calcium, and iron. However, dried fruit and nuts are relatively high in calories. Simple math dictates that adding calories to the diet results in weight gain. The goal is to substitute small amounts of nuts for less healthy snacks such as chips and candy.*

Note: Raw vegetables are also a good choice because they are relatively low in calories but high in fiber. Instead of fruit, pack snackable vegetables, such as baby carrots, sugar snap peas, and grape tomatoes.

Sweet Potato Chips

Ditch the white potatoes and white bread. Forget the French fries and chips and baked potatoes topped with sour cream and cheese. Starchy and refined foods tend to promote weight gain. Instead, opt for nutritious substitutes, such as sweet potatoes.

2 medium-size sweet potatoes
1 tablespoon (15 ml) olive oil
Pinch of sea salt (optional)
½ cup (115 g) plain nonfat Greek yogurt
Fresh lime wedges (optional)

PREPARATION AND USE:

Preheat the oven to 400°F (200°C, or gas mark 6).

Scrub the sweet potatoes thoroughly and slice them into thin pieces. Place them on a baking sheet, drizzle with the olive oil, add the salt, if using, and toss. Bake for about 20 minutes. The centers should still be soft and the rims crispy. Serve warm with Greek yogurt as a dip or topped with squeezes from a fresh lime wedge.

YIELD: 4 SERVINGS

❷ **How it works:** *Substituting a sweet potato for a white baked potato (or chips) or a piece of white bread is satisfying and rich in fiber, vitamin A, beta-carotene, and potassium. In addition, people who consume more fruits and vegetables have a lower risk of weight gain. Long-term studies show that people who substitute fruits, vegetables, and whole grains for chips and white bread lose weight—even when they hadn't intended to do so.*

● Super-Easy Super-Size Green Salad

For the salad:

3 cups (165 g) Boston or Bibb lettuce, red lettuce, and endive—or your favorite mix

½ cucumber, peeled and sliced

½ red bell pepper, seeded and sliced

½ cup (75 g) strawberries, halved

½ cup (55 g) slivered almonds

For the dressing:

2 tablespoons (30 ml) olive oil

1 tablespoon (15 ml) fresh lemon juice

1 tablespoon (15 ml) balsamic vinegar

1 teaspoon (7 g) honey

¼ cup (16 g) fresh dill, or 1 tablespoon (3 g) dried

PREPARATION AND USE:

Make the salad: Combine the salad ingredients in a large bowl and toss.

Prepare the dressing: In a separate bowl, whisk together the dressing ingredients. Drizzle over the salad and toss.

YIELD: 2 TO 3 SERVINGS

❷ How it works: *The volume of food in our stomachs signals satiety. Leafy greens take up space and contain valuable nutrients but few calories. The goal is to make that volume both low in calories and high in nutrients. Vegetables fit the bill—as long as you steer clear of calorie-packed, creamy salad dressings and sauces. Try lightly dressing greens with olive oil and vinegar (plus or minus the herbs).*

Lifestyle Tip

Eat only when you're hungry and, even then, eat only real food: fruits, vegetables, meat, poultry, fish, nuts, and seeds. Avoid processed food. To do so, shop the periphery of the grocery store. Eschew most items that come in bags and boxes. If they're not in the house, you can't be tempted by them.

● Go for Yogurt

Greek yogurt, called for in this recipe, has a rich, satisfying consistency.

1 cup (230 g) plain nonfat Greek yogurt

1 apple or pear, cored and chopped

¼ cup (33 g) fresh berries

Pinch of ground cinnamon

PREPARATION AND USE:

Put the yogurt into a small bowl. Add the apple and berries and mix. Top with a pinch of cinnamon. Enjoy.

YIELD: 1 SERVING

❷ How it works: *Adding nonfat or low-fat yogurt to the diet is associated with weight loss. Yogurt may be beneficial because it favorably alters intestinal bacteria. Fascinating lab research suggests that gut microbes influence weight. Fruit contains satisfying sweetness and fiber, which creates a sense of fullness. A study of overweight women who ate an apple or pear (versus oatmeal cookies) three times a day found that they lost an average of 2.7 pounds (1.2 kg) over twelve weeks.*

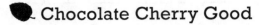

Chocolate Cherry Good

1 cup (155 g) cherries, sliced and pitted
2 squares (1 ounce, or 28 g) thinly sliced dark
chocolate
2 tablespoons (30 g) plain nonfat Greek yogurt

PREPARATION AND USE:

Divide the cherries between two dessert dishes.
Add a tablespoon (15 g) of Greek yogurt to each
plate. Sprinkle the top of each with a square's
worth of dark chocolate. Enjoy!

YIELD: 2 SERVINGS

❷ How it works: *A 2011 study published in the*
Journal of the American Dietetic Association
found that a reduced-calorie diet that allowed a
daily sweet (a chocolate or nonchocolate snack)
led to reductions in weight, fat mass, and waist
and hip circumference.

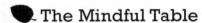

The Mindful Table

Many of us eat without savoring the experience.
We eat at our desks, in our cars, and before the
television set—everywhere but the dining room
table. With sudden surprise, we notice our fingers
scraping the bottom of the cookie bag.

Your favorite dishes and utensils
A bright napkin
Candles (optional)

PREPARATION AND USE:

Set a colorful or soothing place setting at the
table, away from the television. Light candles.
Sit down. Focus on the napkin as you drape it
across your lap. Look at the food on your plate
and give thanks for it. Breathe in the good scents
of the meal.

As you eat, chew slowly, counting to seven
with each bite before swallowing.

Put down your fork between bites and savor
the taste. Focus on the distinctive flavor of each
food. Then focus on the contrast between all the
foods on your plate.

Take your time, working to double the time it
usually takes you to eat a meal.

Give thanks at the end of the meal.

YIELD: 1 SESSION

❷ How it works: *People who eat hastily tend to*
gain more weight than do those who eat slowly.
Enjoy your food.

Lifestyle Tip

**Eat fresh fruit rather than fruit juice or
dried fruit. Because they are higher in
water (and are therefore more filling), ⅔
cup (100 g) of juicy grapes slakes hunger
better than ¼ cup (35 g) of raisins, even
though both pack 100 calories. Fruit juice
is packed with sugar naturally contained in
fruit but without the hunger-satisfying fiber.**

🍵 Lemongrass Green Tea

This is the green tea version of a time-honored refreshing Thai drink that often accompanies afternoon and evening meals.

½ cup (33 g) chopped fresh lemongrass
  (see Preparation and Use)
3 cups (710 ml) water, divided
2 teaspoons (4 g) loose green tea
Stevia

PREPARATION AND USE:
Trim the tough bottoms of the lemongrass stalks by 2 to 6 inches (5 to 15 cm). Cut the lemongrass tops into ½-inch (1.3 cm) chunks to fill ½ cup (33 g). Set aside.

Bring 2 cups (475 ml) of water to a boil in a saucepan and lower the heat to a simmer. Add the lemongrass and stevia to taste, stirring to dissolve. Cover and simmer for 20 minutes. Add the green tea. Remove from the heat and steep 3 minutes.

In a blender, blend the mixture so that the lemongrass pieces are finely minced. Strain the tea into a pitcher, removing the tea and lemongrass particles. Discard these.

You should have a little more than 1 cup (235 ml) left. Add remaining cup (235 ml) of water. Stir in additional stevia to taste. If you prefer your drinks cold, serve over ice.

YIELD: 2 SERVINGS

❓ **How it works:** *Green tea contains caffeine (though not as much as coffee) and substances called green tea polyphenols. Some, but not all, studies indicate that concentrated green tea extracts that concentrate the polyphenols lead to weight loss. Lemongrass (Cymbopogon citratus), which is native to India and Southeast Asia, creates a zingy taste. Stevia-based sweeteners are made from extracts of the leaves of Stevia rebaudiana, a South American plant used for centuries as a sweetener. Gram for gram, it's much sweeter than table sugar and contains no calories.*

Lifestyle Tip

Wear clothes that flatter your figure. These clothes should fit your contours. Many overweight people make the mistake of either wearing clothes that are too tight or that create a tentlike effect. You'll look better and feel better about yourself if your clothes fight correctly. Tailors can help make that happen.

Thai Turmeric Chicken

4 boneless chicken thighs
2 teaspoons (10 ml) Asian fish sauce
1 tablespoon (15 ml) soy sauce
2 teaspoons (14 g) honey
¼ cup (4 g) minced cilantro stems
½ cup (68 g) garlic cloves, peeled
1 teaspoon (2 g) freshly ground white or black pepper
1 teaspoon (2 g) ground turmeric

PREPARATION AND USE:

Skin the chicken (the skin remains in the traditional Thai recipe, but this is healthier), rinse the chicken well, and place it in a medium-size bowl. With a fork, prick the flesh so it can receive the seasonings.

In a small bowl, stir together the fish sauce, soy sauce, and honey. Baste the chicken pieces with the mixture, coating thoroughly.

In a small bowl, crush together the cilantro stems and garlic cloves. Mix in the pepper and turmeric and continue crushing the mixture together to form a paste. Fully baste the chicken with the paste. Cover the bowl and refrigerate for 4 hours.

Preheat the oven to 350°F (180°C, or gas mark 4). Transfer the chicken to an oven-safe pan and place in the oven. Roast the chicken until the centers are just past pink, about 45 minutes. Don't overcook.

YIELD: 2 LARGE OR 4 SMALL SERVINGS

❓ How it works: *Turmeric contains a substance called curcumin whose anti-inflammatory action helps oppose the inflammation associated with obesity. It may also counteract other adverse effects of obesity, such as insulin resistance, high blood levels of glucose, triglycerides, and cholesterol.*

● Veggie Chili Weight-Off

2 tablespoons (30 ml) olive oil
2 cups (320 g) chopped onion
4 garlic cloves, minced
1 tablespoon (3 g) dried oregano
1 red bell pepper, seeded and chopped
1 quart (946 ml) vegetable stock, divided
1 tablespoon (20 g) honey
1 teaspoon (2 g) cayenne pepper
1 tablespoon (15 ml) soy sauce
1 can (15 ounces, or 428 g) each pinto beans, chickpeas, kidney beans, and black beans, all rinsed and drained
1 can (14.5 ounces, or 414 g) diced tomatoes, undrained
1 cup (164 g) frozen corn
1 can (12 ounces, or 355 ml) tomato paste
Freshly ground black pepper

PREPARATION AND USE:

Heat the oil in a large pot over medium-high heat. Add the onion, garlic, oregano, and red pepper; sauté for a few minutes until tender. Add 3 cups (710 ml) of the vegetable stock. Mix in the honey, cayenne, and soy sauce. Stir in the beans, undrained tomatoes, and corn.

In a small bowl, whisk together the remaining cup (235 ml) of vegetable stock and the tomato paste and stir it into the pot.

Bring the chili to a boil. Lower the heat and simmer until heated throughout, about 5 minutes.

Add the black pepper and additional cayenne to taste.

YIELD: EIGHT ¾-CUP (12-OUNCE [340 G]) SERVINGS

❷ How it works: *Beans are rich in fiber, which isn't absorbed from the gut, thereby increasing a sense of fullness. Chile peppers (also called cayenne) contain a substance called capsaicin. Animal studies show that capsaicin enhances fat and energy breakdown, thereby burning calories. Adding cayenne to meals increases thermogenesis, a heat-producing process that burns calories. Other studies show that capsaicin can increase energy expenditure by 50 calories a day.*

Recipe Variation: For a "meatier" texture, add soy burger crumbles to taste after you've mixed the beans together.

Flax Breakfast Bowl

1 apple, cored and chopped (skin on)

1 teaspoon (2 g) minced fresh ginger

¼ cup (30 g) crushed walnuts

1 teaspoon (2 g) ground cinnamon

½ cup (40 g) steel-cut oats

1½ cups (355 ml) water

1 tablespoon (7 g) coarsely ground flaxseeds

1 tablespoon (9 g) raisins

2 tablespoons (30 g) plain nonfat Greek yogurt

PREPARATION AND USE:

Combine all the ingredients, except the flaxseeds, raisins, and yogurt in a small, microwave-safe bowl. Microwave the mixture on high for 2 minutes. Remove from the microwave and stir in the flaxseeds and raisins. Microwave on high for another minute. Let stand for 5 minutes.

Top each serving with 1 tablespoon (15 g) of yogurt.

YIELD: 2 SERVINGS

❓ How it works: *Flaxseeds contain fiber as well as healthy oils. One study found that consuming 2.5 grams of flaxseeds (as a drink or in tablet form) 2 hours before a meal reduced appetite and decreased calories consumed.*

Lifestyle Tip

Manage stress in ways that don't involve food. Psychological stress promotes weight gain for several reasons: The stress hormone cortisol and other stress-induced hormones increase appetite. Moreover, cortisol pushes us toward high-calorie foods. This hormone also promotes deposition of visceral fat. Chronic stress depletes those feel-good chemicals called endorphins and the brain chemical dopamine, which is associated with pleasure. Eating delicious food releases endorphins and dopamine, making us feel better. It's no surprise that recurrent stress promotes compulsive overeating. (See Chapter 57, on stress and anxiety, for more information.)

Lifestyle Tip

Be wary of weight-loss supplements. If the promise sounds too good to be true, it probably is. Some of these products are downright dangerous.

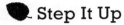 **Step It Up**

See the Lifestyle Tips throughout the book for more ideas on how to move.

You
Comfortable workout clothes
A pair of athletic shoes

PREPARATION AND USE:

For 60 minutes *every day*, walk, jog, ride the elliptical trainer, swim, play tennis, or do a combination of these activities.

YIELD: 1 DAILY SESSION (WORK UP TO 90 MINUTES EACH DAY FOR WEIGHT LOSS.)

❓ **How it works:** *Sedentary lifestyles foster weight gain. Being more physically active directly burns calories. Exercises that build muscle lead to higher metabolic rate at rest. Muscle consumes more calories than body fat. Studies show that regular exercise can overturn genetic predispositions to be overweight. Experts recommend 60 minutes a day of moderate-intensity exercise to prevent weight gain and 90 minutes to lose weight. It's perfectly fine to exercise in 10-minute chunks.*

Exercise has the added benefits of increasing total body function, boosting your self-esteem, and helping you sleep better at night. To shed excess weight, calories expended in exercise need to outnumber the calories in your diet. If exercise piques your appetite, satisfy your hunger with fruits, vegetables, fish, lean meats, and nuts.

When to Call the Doctor

- *You have any concerns about your body weight and eating habits. Your doctor may recommend meeting with a registered dietitian, athletic trainer, or joining a weight-loss group. He or she can also discuss the pros and cons of prescription medications and of bariatric surgery.*

- *You have a chronic condition associated with being overweight or obesity. Such illnesses as diabetes, high blood pressure, and heart disease require close monitoring.*

- *You suspect you have an eating disorder. Warning signs include being preoccupied with food, eating in secret, feeling anxiety about body weight and eating habits, binging (uncontrollable consumption of large amounts of food in one sitting), and using unhealthy means to control body weight, such as vomiting or laxatives.*

Endnotes

Part 1

Andersen LL, Jay K, Andersen CH, et al. Acute effects of massage or active exercise in relieving muscle soreness: Randomized controlled trial. *Journal of Strength and Conditioning Research.* 2013 Mar 21. [Epub ahead of print]

Barnes VA, Orme-Johnson DW. Prevention and treatment of cardiovascular disease in adolescents and adults through the Transcendental Meditation Program: a research review update. *Current Hypertension Reviews.* 2012 Aug;8(3):227–242. www.ncbi. nlm.nih.gov/pmc/articles/pmc3510697/. Accessed April 6, 2013.

Barraza JA, Zak PJ. Empathy toward strangers triggers oxytocin release and subsequent generosity. *Annals of the New York Academy of Sciences.* 2009 Jun;1167:182–189. doi: 10.1111/ j.1749-6632.2009.04504.x.

Baum SJ, Kris-Etherton PM, Willett WC, et al. Fatty acids in cardio-vascular health and disease: a comprehensive update. *Journal of Clinical Lipidology.* 2012 May;6(3):216–234.

Beetz A, Uvnäs-Moberg K, Julius H, Kotrschal K. Psychosocial and psychophysiological effects of human-animal interactions: the possible role of oxytocin. *Frontiers in Psychology.* 2012;3:234. doi: 0.3389/fpsyg.2012.00234.www.ncbi.nlm.nih.gov/pmc/articles/ pmc3408111/. Accessed April 6, 2013.

Bennett MP, Zeller JM, Rosenberg L, McCann J. The effect of mirth-ful laughter on stress and natural killer cell activity. *Alternative Therapies in Health and Medicine.* 2003;9(2):38–45.

Burkett JP, Young LJ. The behavioral, anatomical and pharma-cological parallels between social attachment, love and addic-tion. *Psychopharmacology* (Berlin). 2012 Nov;224(1):1–26. doi: 10.1007/s00213-012-2794-x.

Cacioppo JT, Hawkley LC. Social isolation and health, with an emphasis on underlying mechanisms. *Perspectives in Biology and Medicine.* 2003;46(3 Suppl):S39–52.

Christie W, Moore C. Impact of humor on patients with cancer. *Clinical Journal of Oncology Nursing.* 2005;9(2):211–218.

Denova-Gutiérrez E, Huitrón-Bravo G, Talavera JO, et al. Dietary glycemic index, dietary glycemic load, blood lipids, and coronary heart disease. *Journal of Nutrition and Metabolism.* 2010;2010. pii: 170680. doi: 10.1155/2010/170680. www.ncbi.nlm.nih.gov/pmc/ articles/pmc2911609/. Accessed April 6, 2013.

Dilzer A, Park Y. Implication of conjugated linoleic acid (CLA) in human health. *Critical Reviews in Food and Science Nutrition.* 2012;52(6):488–513.

Ding M. Tai Chi for stroke rehabilitation: a focused review. *American Journal of Physical Medicine and Rehabilitation.* 2012 Dec;91(12):1091–1096. doi: 10.1097/phm.0b013e31826edd21.

Dunbar RI. The social role of touch in humans and primates: behavioural function and neurobiological mechanisms. *Neuroscience Biobehavioral Reviews.* 2010 Feb;34(2):260–268. doi: 10.1016/j.neubiorev.2008.07.001.

Edenfield TM, Saeed SA. An update on mindfulness meditation as a self-help treatment for anxiety and depression. *Psychology Research and Behavioral Management.* 2012;5:131–141. doi: 10.2147/prbm.s34937. www.ncbi.nlm.nih.gov/pmc/articles/ pmc3500142/. Accessed April 6, 2013.

Emmons RA, McCullough ME. Counting blessings versus burdens: an experimental investigation of gratitude and sub-jective well-being in daily life. *Journal of Personality and Social Psychology.* 2003 Feb;84(2):377–389.

Fan C, Zirpoli H, Qi K. n-3 fatty acids modulate adipose tissue inflammation and oxidative stress. *Current Opinion in Clinical Nutrition and Metabolic Care.* 2013 Mar;16(2):124–132. doi: 10.1097/mco.0b013e32835c02c8.

Fike L, Najera C, Dougherty D. Occupational therapists as dog handlers: the collective experience with animal-assisted therapy in Iraq. *U.S. Army Medical Department Journal.* 2012 Apr–Jun:51–54.

Kaada B, Torsteinbø O. Increase of plasma beta-endorphins in connective tissue massage. *General Pharmacology.* 1989;20(4):487–489.

Kemp AH, Quintana DS, Kuhnert RL, Griffiths K, Hickie IB, Guastella AJ. Oxytocin increases heart rate variability in humans at rest: implications for social approach-related motivation and capacity for social engagement. *PLoS One.* 2012;7(8):e44014. doi: 10.1371/journal.pone.0044014.

Kraut R, Lundmark R, Patterson M, Kiesler S, Mukopadhyay T, Scherlis W. Internet paradox: a social technology that reduces social involvement and psychological well-being? *American Psychologist.* 1998; 53(9):1017–1031.

Lee MS, Pittler MH, Ernst E. Tai chi for osteoarthritis: a systematic review. *Clinical Rheumatology.* 2008 Feb;27(2):211–218.

Luchtman DW, Song C. Cognitive enhancement by omega-3 fatty acids from child-hood to old age: findings from animal and clinical studies. *Neuropharmacology.* 2013 Jan;64:550–565. doi: 10.1016/j.neuropharm.2012.07.019. Epub 2012 Jul 27.

Marques-Aleixo I, Oliveira PJ, Moreira PI, Magalhães J, Ascensão A. Physical exercise as a possible strategy for brain protection: evidence from mitochondrial-mediated mechanisms. *Progress in Neurobiology*. 2012 Nov;99(2):149–162. doi: 10.1016/j.pneurobio.2012.08.002.

McGinnis JM, Williams-Russo P, Knickman JR. The case for more active policy attention to health promotion. *Health Affairs* (Millwood). 2002 Mar–Apr;21(2):78–93.

Mishra SI, Scherer RW, Snyder C, Geigle PM, Berlanstein DR, Topaloglu O. Exercise interventions on health-related quality of life for people with cancer during active treatment. Cochrane Database of Systematic Reviews. 2012 Aug 15;8:CD008465. doi: 10.1002/14651858.CD008465.pub2.

Morhenn V, Beavin LE, Zak PJ. Massage increases oxytocin and reduces adrenocorticotropin hormone in humans. *Alternative Therapies in Health and Medicine*. 2012 Nov–Dec;18(6):11–18.

Nadtochiy SM, Redman EK. Mediterranean diet and cardioprotection: the role of nitrite, polyunsaturated fatty acids, and polyphenols. *Nutrition*. 2011 Jul–Aug;27(7–8):733–744. doi: 10.1016/j.nut.2010.12.006. Epub 2011 Mar 30. Review.

Okonta NR. Does yoga therapy reduce blood pressure in patients with hypertension?: an integrative review. *Holistic Nurse Practitioner*. 2012 May–Jun;26(3):137–141. doi: 10.1097/hnp.0b013e31824ef647.

Olff M. Bonding after trauma: on the role of social support and the oxytocin system in traumatic stress. *European Journal of Psychotraumatology*. 2012;3. doi: 10.3402/ejpt.v3i0.18597.

Ponnampalam EN, Mann NJ, Sinclair AJ. Effect of feeding systems on omega-3 fatty acids, conjugated linoleic acid and trans fatty acids in Australian beef cuts: potential impact on human health. *Asian Pacific Journal of Clinical Nutrition*. 2006;15(1):21–29.

Remig V, Franklin B, Margolis S, Kostas G, Nece T, Street JC. Trans fats in America: a review of their use, consumption, health implications, and regulation. *Journal of the American Dietetic Association*. 2010 Apr;110(4):585–592. doi: 10.1016/j.jada.2009.12.024.

Sojcher R, Gould Fogerite S, Perlman A. Evidence and potential mechanisms for mindfulness practices and energy psychology for obesity and binge-eating disorder. *Explore* (NY). 2012 Sep;8(5):271–276. doi: 10.1016/j.explore.2012.06.003.

Sydenham E, Dangour AD, Lim WS. Omega 3 fatty acid for the prevention of cognitive decline and dementia. Cochrane Database of Systematic Reviews. 2012 Jun 13;6:CD005379. doi: 10.1002/14651858.cd005379.pub3.

Takahashi M. Prioritizing sleep for healthy work schedules. *Journal of Physiological Anthropology*. 2012 Mar 13;31:6. doi: 10.1186/1880-6805-31-6. www.ncbi.nlm.nih.gov/pmc/articles/pmc3375037/. Accessed April 10, 2013.

Trezza V, Damsteegt R, Achterberg EJ, Vanderschuren LJ. Nucleus accumbens μ-opioid receptors mediate social reward. *Journal of Neuroscience*. 2011 Apr 27;31(17):6362–6370. doi: 10.1523/jneurosci.5492-10.2011.

Uhlig T. Tai Chi and yoga as complementary therapies in rheumatologic conditions. *Best Practice and Research Clinical Rheumatology*. 2012 Jun;26(3):387–398. doi: 10.1016/j.berh.2012.05.006.

van den Berg AE, Maas J, Verheij RA, Groenewegen PP. Green space as a buffer between stressful life events and health. *Social Science Medicine*. 2010 Apr;70(8):1203–1210.

van den Eijnden RJ, Meerkerk GJ, Vermulst AA, Spijkerman R, Engels RC. Online communication, compulsive Internet use, and psychosocial well-being among adolescents: a longitudinal study. *Developmental Psychology*. 2008 May;44(3):655–665.

Vayalilkarottu J. Holistic health and well-being: a psycho-spiritual/religious and theological perspective. *Asian Journal of Psychiatry*. 2012 Dec;5(4):347–350. doi: 10.1016/j.ajp.2012.09.010.

Wansink B. *Mindless Eating: Why We Eat More Than We Think*. New York: Bantam; 2010.

Wardhana, Surachmanto ES, Datau EA. The role of omega-3 fatty acids contained in olive oil on chronic inflammation. *Acta Medica Indonesiana*. 2011 Apr;43(2):138–143. www.ncbi.nlm.nih.gov/pubmed/21785178. Accessed June 27, 2013.

Weisenberg M, Raz T, Hener T. The influence of film-induced mood on pain perception. *Pain*. 1998;76(3):365–375.

Zschucke E, Gaudlitz K, Ströhle A. Exercise and physical activity in mental disorders: clinical and experimental evidence. *Journal of Preventive Medicine and Public Health*. 2013 January;46 (Suppl 1):S12–21. Published online 2013 January 30. doi: 10.3961/jpmph.2013.46.S.S12 www.ncbi.nlm.nih.gov/pubmed/23412549. Accessed April 6, 2013.

Chapter 7 Acne

Halvorsen JA, Dalgard F, Thoresen M, Bertness E, Lien L. Is the association between acne and mental distress influenced by diet? Results from a cross-sectional population study among 3775 late adolescents in Oslo, Norway. *BMC Public Health*. 2009 Sep 16;9:340.

Ilknur T, Demirta Olum, Biçak MU, Ozkan S., Glycolic acid peels versus amino fruit acid peels for acne. *Journal of Cosmetic and Laser Therapy*. 2010 Oct;12(5):242–245.

Kwon HH, Yoon JY, Hong JS, Jung JY, Park MS, Suh DH. Clinical and histological effect of a low glycaemic load diet in treatment of acne vulgaris in Korean patients: a randomized, controlled trial. *Acta Dermato-Venereologica*. 2012 May;92(3):241–246. doi: 10.2340/00015555-1346.

Ozdemir O. Any benefits of probiotics in allergic disorders? *Allergy and Asthma Proceedings.* 2010 Mar;31(2):103–111.

Tom WL, Barrio VR. New insights into adolescent acne. *Current Opinion in Pediatrics.* 2008 Aug;20(4):436–440.

Wei B, Pang Y, Zhu H, et al. The epidemiology of adolescent acne in North East China. *Journal of the European Academy of Dermatology and Venereology.* 2010 Aug;24(8):953–957.

Woo SI, Kim JY, Lee YJ, Kim NS, Hahn YS. Effect of Lactobacillus sakei supplementation in children with atopic eczema-dermatitis syndrome. *Annals of Allergy, Asthma, and Immunology.* 2010 Apr;104(4):343–348.

Chapter 8 Allergic Skin Reactions

Abrams Motz V, Bowers CP, Mull Young L, Kinder DH. The effectiveness of jewelweed, Impatiens capensis, the related cultivar I. balsamina and the component, lawsone in preventing post poison ivy exposure contact dermatitis. *Journal of Ethnopharmacology.* 2012 Aug 30;143(1):314–318. doi: 10.1016/j.jep.2012.06.038.

Bakhshaee M, Jabbari F, Hoseini S, et al. Effect of silymarin in the treatment of allergic rhinitis. *Otolaryngology—Head and Neck Surgery.* 2011;145:904–909.

Chandrashekhar VM, Halagali KS, Nidavani RB, et al. Anti-allergic activity of German chamomile (Matricaria recutita L.) in mast cell mediated allergy model. *Journal of Ethnopharmacology.* 2011 Sep 1;137(1):336–340.

Isolauri E, Salminen S.; Nutrition, Allergy, Mucosal Immunology, and Intestinal Microbiota (NAMI) Research Group. Probiotics: Use in allergic disorders: a Nutrition, Allergy, Mucosal Immunology, and Intestinal Microbiota (NAMI) Research Group Report. *Journal of Clinical Gastroenterology.* 2008 Jul;42(Suppl 2):S91–96. doi: 10.1097/mcg.0b013e3181639a98.

Kim J, Lee I, Park S, Choue R. Effects of Scutellariae radix and Aloe vera gel extracts on immunoglobulin E and cytokine levels in atopic dermatitis NC/Nga mice. *Journal of Ethnopharmacology.* 2010 Nov 11;132(2):529–532.

MacArtain P, Gill C, Brooks M, et al. Nutritional value of edible seaweeds. *Nutrition Reviews.* 2007;65(12):535–543. http://li123-4.members.linode.com/files/nutritional%20value%20of%20edible%20seaweeds.pdf. Accessed April 8, 2013.

Marchisio P, Varricchio A, Baggi E, et al. Hypertonic saline is more effective than normal saline in seasonal allergic rhinitis in children. *International Journal of Immunopathology and Pharmacology.* 2012 Jul–Sep;25(3):721–730.

Mittman, P. Randomized, double-blind study of freeze-dried Urtica dioica in the treatment of allergic rhinitis. *Planta Medica.* 1990;56:44–47.

Miyake Y, Tanaka K, Okubo H, Sasaki S, Arakawa M. Dietary meat and fat intake and prevalence of rhinoconjunctivitis in pregnant Japanese women: baseline data from the Kyushu Okinawa Maternal and Child Health Study. *Nutrition Journal.* 2012 Mar 27;11:19.

Miyake Y, Sasaki S, Ohya Y, et al; Osaka Maternal and Child Health Study Group. Dietary intake of seaweed and minerals and prevalence of allergic rhinitis in Japanese pregnant females: baseline data from the Osaka Maternal and Child Health Study. *Annals of Epidemiology.* 2006 Aug;16(8):614–621.

Ozdemir O. Any benefits of probiotics in allergic disorders? *Allergy and Asthma Proceedings.* 2010 Mar;31(2):103–111.

Pazyar N, Yaghoobi R, Kazerouni A, Feily A. Oatmeal in dermatology: a brief review. *Indian Journal of Dermatology, Venereology, and Leprology.* 2012 Mar–Apr;78(2):142–145. www.ijdvl.com/article.asp?issn=0378-6323;year=2012;volume=78;issue=2;spage=142;epage=145;aulast=pazyar. Accessed April 8, 2013.

Saarinen K, Jantunen J, Haahtela T. Birch pollen honey for birch pollen allergy—a randomized controlled pilot study. *International Archives of Allergy and Immunology.* 2011;155(2):160–166.

Woo SI, Kim JY, Lee YJ, Kim NS, Hahn YS. Effect of Lactobacillus sakei supplementation in children with atopic eczema-dermatitis syndrome. *Annals of Allergy, Asthma, and Immunology.* 2010 Apr;104(4):343–348.

Chapter 9 Asthma

Coelho-de-Souza LN, Leal-Cardoso JH, de Abreu Matos FJ, Lahlou S, Magalhães PJ. Relaxant effects of the essential oil of Eucalyptus tereticornis and its main constituent 1,8-cineole on guinea-pig tracheal smooth muscle. *Planta Medica.* 2005 Dec;71(12):1173–1175.

Flohr C, Yeo L. Atopic dermatitis and the hygiene hypothesis revisited. *Current Problems in Dermatology.* 2011;41:1–34.

Houssen ME, Ragab A, Mesbah A, et al. Natural anti-inflammatory products and leukotriene inhibitors as complementary therapy for bronchial asthma. *Clinical Biochemistry.* 2010 Jul;43(10–11):887–890.

Huntley A, White AR, Ernst E. Relaxation therapies for asthma: a systematic review. *Thorax.* 2002 Feb;57(2):127–131. www.ncbi.nlm.nih.gov/pmc/articles/pmc1746244/?tool=pubmed. Accessed April 8, 2013.

Juergens UR, Dethlefsen U, Steinkamp G, Gillissen A, Repges R, Vetter H. Anti-inflammatory activity of 1.8-cineol (eucalyptol) in bronchial asthma: a double-blind placebo-controlled trial. *Respiratory Medicine.* 2003 Mar;97(3):250–256.

Kramer A, Bekeschus S, Bröker BM, et al. Maintaining health by balancing microbial exposure and prevention of infection: the hygiene hypothesis versus the hypothesis of early immune challenge. *Journal of Hospital Infection.* 2013 Feb;83(Suppl 1):S29–34. doi: 10.1016/s0195-6701(13)60007-9.

Marra F, Lynd L, Coombes M, et al. Does antibiotic exposure during infancy lead to development of asthma?: a systematic review and metaanalysis. *Chest*. 2006 Mar;129(3):610–618. http://chestjournal.chestpubs.org/content/129/3/610.long. Accessed April 8, 2013.

Neuman I, Nahum H, Ben-Amotz A. Prevention of exercise-induced asthma by a natural isomer mixture of beta-carotene. *Annals of Allergy, Asthma, and Immunology*. 1999;82:549–553.

Nilani P, Kasthuribai N, Duraisamy B, et al. In vitro antioxidant activity of selected antiasthmatic herbal constituents. *Ancient Science of Life*. 2009 Apr;28(4):3–6.

Peat JK, Mihrshahi S, Kemp AS, et al. Three-year outcomes of dietary fatty acid modification and house dust mite reduction in the Childhood Asthma Prevention Study. *Journal of Allergy and Clinical Immunology*. 2004;114:807–813.

Posadzki P, Ernst E. Yoga for asthma? a systematic review of randomized clinical trials. *Journal of Asthma*. 2011;48(6):632–639. doi: 10.3109/02770903.2011.584358. Epub 2011 May 31.

Renz-Polster H, David MR, Buist AS, et al. Caesarean section delivery and the risk of allergic disorders in childhood. *Clinical and Experimental Allergy*. 2005 Nov;35(11):1466–1472.

Schubert R, Kitz R, Beermann C, et al. Effect of n-3 polyunsaturated fatty acids in asthma after low-dose allergen challenge. International *Archives of Allergy and Immunology*. 2009;148:321–329.

Chapter 10 Athlete's Foot

Carvalhinho S, Costa AM, Coelho AC, Martins E, Sampaio A. Susceptibilies of Candida albicans mouth isolates to antifungal agents, essentials oils and mouth rinses. *Mycopathologia*. 2012 Jul;174(1):69–76. doi: 10.1007/s11046-012-9520-4.

de Oliveira Pereira F, Mendes JM, de Oliveira Lima E. Investigation on mechanism of antifungal activity of eugenol against Trichophyton rubrum. *Medical Mycology*. 2012 Nov 27. [Epub ahead of print] Abstract at www.ncbi.nlm.nih.gov/pubmed/23181601.

Inouye S, Uchida K, Nishiyama Y, Hasumi Y, Yamaguchi H, Abe S. Combined effect of heat, essential oils and salt on fungicidal activity against Trichophyton mentagrophytes in a foot bath. *Nihon Ishinkin Gakkai Zasshi*. 2007;48(1):27–36.

Lanzotti V, Barile E, Antignani V, Bonanomi G, Scala F. Antifungal saponins from bulbs of garlic, Allium sativum L. var. Voghiera. *Phytochemistry*. 2012 Jun;78:126–134. doi: 10.1016/j.phytochem.2012.03.009.

Ledezma E, Marcano K, Jorquera A, et al. Efficacy of ajoene in the treatment of tinea pedis: a double-blind and comparative study with terbinafine. *Journal of the American Academy of Dermatology*. 2000 Nov;43(5 Pt 1):829–832.

Khattak S, Saeed-ur-Rehman, Ullah Shah H, Ahmad W, Ahmad M. Biological effects of indigenous medicinal plants Curcuma longa and Alpinia galanga. *Fitoterapia*. 2005 Mar;76(2):254–257.

Kuwaki S, Ohhira I, Takahata M, Murata Y, Tada M. Antifungal activity of the fermentation product of herbs by lactic acid bacteria against tinea. *Journal of Bioscience and Bioengineering*. 2002;94(5):401–405.

Ogbolu DO, Oni AA, Daini OA, Oloko AP. In vitro antimicrobial properties of coconut oil on Candida species in Ibadan, Nigeria. *Journal of Medicinal Food*. 2007 Jun;10(2):384–387.

Pattnaik S, Subramanyam VR, Kole C. Antibacterial and antifungal activity of ten essential oils in vitro. *Microbios*. 1996;86(349):237–246.

Romero-Cerecero O, Zamilpa A, Jiménez-Ferrer E, Tortoriello J. Therapeutic effectiveness of Ageratina pichinchensis on the treatment of chronic interdigital tinea pedis: a randomized, double-blind clinical trial. *Journal of Alternative and Complementary Medicine*. June 2012;18(6):607–611.

Satchell AC, Saurajen A, Bell C, Barnetson RS. Treatment of interdigital tinea pedis with 25% and 50% tea tree oil solution: a randomized, placebo-controlled, blinded study. *Australasian Journal of Dermatology*. 2002;43:175–178.

Chapter 11 Bad Breath

Al-Zahrani MS, Zawawi KH, Austah ON, Al-Ghamdi HS. Self reported halitosis in relation to glycated hemoglobin level in diabetic patients. *Open Dentistry Journal*. 2011;5:154–157.

Bollen CM, Beikler T. Halitosis: the multidisciplinary approach. *International Journal of Oral Science*. 2012 Jun;4(2):55–63. doi: 10.1038/ijos.2012.39/. www.ncbi.nlm.nih.gov/pmc/articles/pmc3412664/. Accessed April 1, 2013.

Kamaraj DR, Bhushan KS, Laxman VK, Mathew J. Detection of odoriferous subgingival and tongue microbiota in diabetic and nondiabetic patients with oral malodor using polymerase chain reaction. *Indian Journal of Dental Research*. 2011 Mar–Apr;22(2):260–265. doi: 10.4103/0970-9290.84301.

Loesche WJ, Kazor C. Microbiology and treatment of halitosis. *Periodontology*. 2000;28:256–279.

Quirynen M, Avontroodt P, Soers C, Zhao H, Pauwels M, van Steenberghe D. Impact of tongue cleansers on microbial load and taste. *Journal of Clinical Periodontology*. 2004 Jul;31(7):506–510.

Chapter 12 Bites and Stings

Atkinson PRT, Boyle A, Hartin D, McAuley D. Is hot water immersion an effective treatment for marine envenomation? *Emergency Medicine Journal.* 2006;23(7):503–508. www.ncbi.nlm.nih.gov/pmc/articles/pmc2579537/#ref19. Accessed April 12, 2013.

Barua CC, Pal SK, Roy JD, et al. Studies on the anti-inflammatory properties of Plantago erosa leaf extract in rodents. *Journal of Ethnopharmacology.* 2011 Mar 8;134(1):62–66. doi: 10.1016/j.jep.2010.11.044.

Dendane T, Abidi K, Madani N, et al. Reversible myocarditis after black widow spider envenomation. *Case Reports in Medicine.* 2012;2012: 794540. doi: 10.1155/2012/794540. www.ncbi.nlm.nih.gov/pmc/articles/pmc3272799/. Accessed April 10, 2013.

Dorai AA. Wound care with traditional, complementary and alternative medicine. *Indian Journal of Plastic Surgery.* 2012;45(2):418–424. www.ncbi.nlm.nih.gov/pmc/articles/pmc3495394/. Accessed April 10, 2013.

Medscape. Coral snake envenomation. emedicine. http://emedicine.medscape.com/article/771701-overview#a0199. Accessed April 10, 2013.

Meyer PK. Stingray injuries. *Wilderness & Environmental Medicine.* 1997 Feb;8(1):24–28.

Zubair M, Ekholm A, Nybom H, Renvert S, Widen C, Rumpunen K. Effects of Plantago major L. leaf extracts on oral epithelial cells in a scratch assay. *Journal of Ethnopharmacology.* 2012;141(3):825–830. doi: 10.1016/j.jep.2012.03.016.

Chapter 13 Bladder Infections

Afshar K, Stothers L, Scott H, MacNeily AE. Cranberry juice for the prevention of pediatric urinary tract infection: a randomized controlled trial. *Journal of Urology.* 2012 Oct;188(4 Suppl):1584–1587. doi: 10.1016/j.juro.2012.02.031.

Basu A, Du M, Leyva MJ, et al. Blueberries decrease cardiovascular risk factors in obese men and women with metabolic syndrome. *Journal of Nutrition.* 2010 Sep;140(9):1582–1587. doi: 10.3945/jn.110.124701.

Clare BA, Conroy RS, Spelman K. The diuretic effect in human subjects of an extract of Taraxacum officinale folium over a single day. *Journal of Alternative and Complementary Medicine.* 2009 Aug;15(8):929–934. doi: 10.1089/acm.2008.0152.

Colgan R, Williams M. Diagnosis and treatment of acute uncomplicated cystitis. *American Family Physician.* 2011;84(7):771–776.

Gull I, Saeed M, Shaukat H, Aslam SM, Samra ZQ, Athar AM. Inhibitory effect of Allium sativum and Zingiber officinale extracts on clinically important drug resistant pathogenic bacteria. *Annals of Clinical Microbiology and Antimicrobials.* 2012 Apr 27;11:8.

Takahashi S, Hamasuna R, Yasuda M, et al. A randomized clinical trial to evaluate the preventive effect of cranberry juice (UR65) for

patients with recurrent urinary tract infection. *Journal of Infection and Chemotherapy.* 2013 Feb;19(1):112–117. doi: 10.1007/s10156-012-0467-7.

Uehara S, Monden K, Nomoto K, Seno Y, Kariyama R, Kumon H. A pilot study evaluating the safety and effectiveness of Lactobacillus vaginal suppositories in patients with recurrent urinary tract infection. *International Journal of Antimicrobial Agents.* 2006 Aug;28(Suppl 1):S30–34.

Chapter 14 Body Odor

Albrecht J, Demmel M, Schöpf V, et al. Smelling chemosensory signals of males in anxious versus nonanxious condition increases state anxiety of female subjects. *Chemical Senses.* 2011 Jan;36(1):19–27. doi: 10.1093/chemse/bjq087.

Exley C, Charles LM, Barr L, Martin C, Polwart A, Darbre PD. Aluminium in human breast tissue. *Journal of Inorganic Biochemistry.* 2007;101:1344–1346. doi: 10.1016/j.jinorgbio.2007.06.005.

Graves AB, White E, Koepsell TD, Reifler BV, van Belle G, Larson EB. The association between aluminum-containing products and Alzheimer's disease. *Journal of Clinical Epidemiology.* 1990;43(1):35–44.

Kippenberger S, Havlik J, Bernd A, Thaçi D, Kaufmann R, Meissner M. 'Nosing around' the human skin: what information is concealed in skin odour? *Experimental Dermatology.* 2012 Sep;21(9):655–659. doi: 10.1111/j.1600-0625.2012.01545.x.

Martin A. Antibacterial chemical raises safety issues. The *New York Times.* August 19, 2011. www.nytimes.com/2011/08/20/business/triclosan-an-antibacterial-chemical-in-consumer-products-raises-safety-issues.html?pagewanted=all&_r=0. Accessed April 22, 2013.

McGrath KG. An earlier age of breast cancer diagnosis related to more frequent use of antiperspirants/deodorants and underarm shaving. *European Journal of Cancer Prevention.* 2003 Dec;12(6):479–485.

Milinksi M, Croy I, Hummel T. Boehm T. Major histocompatibility complex peptide ligands as olfactory cues in human body odour assessment. *Proceedings of the Royal Society: Biological Sciences.* 2013 March 22;280(1755):20122889. doi: 10.1098/rspb.2012.2889. www.ncbi.nlm.nih.gov/pmc/articles/pmc3574394/. Accessed April 22, 2013.

Namer M, Luporsi E, Gligorov J, Lokiec F, Spielmann M. The use of deodorants/antiperspirants does not constitute a risk factor for breast cancer. *Bulletin du Cancer.* 2008 Sep;95(9):871–880. doi: 10.1684/bdc.2008.0679.

Shirasu M, Touhara K. The scent of disease: volatile organic compounds of the human body related to disease and disorder. *Journal of Biochemistry.* 2011 Sep;150(3):257–266. doi: 10.1093/jb/mvr090.

Chapter 15 Bone Health

Castelo-Branco C, Cancelo Hidalgo MJ. Isoflavones: effects on bone health. *Climacteric.* 2011 Apr;14(2):204–211.

Cofrades S, López-Lopez I, Bravo L, et al. Nutritional and antioxidant properties of different brown and red spanish edible seaweeds. *Food Science and Technology International.* 2010 Oct;16(5):361–370.

Frassetto LA, Todd KM, Morris RC Jr, Sebastian A. Worldwide incidence of hip fracture in elderly women: relation to consumption of animal and vegetable foods. *Journals of Gerontology.* Series A, Biological Sciences and Medical Sciences. 2000 Oct;55(10):M585–592.

U.S. Department of Agriculture. Agricultural Research Service. 2012. USDA National Nutrient Database for Standard Reference, Release 25. Available at http://ndb.nal.usda.gov/ndb/foods/show/2946?fg=&man=&lfacet=&format=&count=&max=25&offset=&sort=&qlookup=dandelion. Accessed June 28, 2013.

Hegarty V, May H, Khaw K. Tea drinking and bone mineral density in older women. *American Journal of Clinical Nutrition.* 2000;71(4):1003–1007.

Devine A, Hodgson JM, Dick IM, Prince RL. Tea drinking is associated with benefits on bone density in older women. *American Journal of Clinical Nutrition.* 2007;86(4):1243–1247.

Prynne CJ, Mishra GD, O'Connell MA, et al. Fruit and vegetable intakes and bone mineral status: a cross-sectional study in 5 age and sex cohorts. *American Journal of Clinical Nutrition.* 2006;83:1420–1428.

Taku K, Melby MK, Kurzer MS, Mizuno S, Watanabe S, Ishimi Y. Effects of soy isoflavone supplements on bone turnover markers in menopausal women: systematic review and meta-analysis of randomized controlled trials. *Bone.* 2010 Aug;47(2):413–423.

Tsapakis EM, Gamie Z, Tran GT, et al. The adverse skeletal effects of selective serotonin reuptake inhibitors. *European Psychiatry.* 2011 Feb 2. [Epub ahead of print]

Watson, S. Proposed recommendations question the value of calcium, vitamin D supplements. Harvard Health Publications. Harvard Medical School. Posted June 27, 2012. www.health.harvard.edu/blog/proposed-recommendations-question-the-value-of-calcium-vitamin-d-supplements-201206274921. Accessed April 6, 2013.

Chapter 16 Brain Health

Annweiler C, Rolland Y, Schott AM, et al. Higher vitamin D dietary intake is associated with lower risk of Alzheimer's disease: a 7-year follow-up. *Journals of Gerontology.* Series A, Biological Sciences and Medical Sciences. 2012 Nov;67(11):1205–1211. doi: 10.1093/gerona/gls107.

Bedrosian TA, Nelson RJ. Pro: Alzheimer's disease and circadian dysfunction: chicken or egg? *Alzheimer's Research and Therapy.* 2012 Aug 13;4(4):25.

Biasibetti R, Tramontina AC, Costa AP, et al. Green tea (-)epigallocatechin-3-gallate reverses oxidative stress and reduces acetylcholinesterase activity in a streptozotocin-induced model of dementia. *Behavioural Brain Research.* 2013 Jan 1;236(1):186–193. doi: 10.1016/j.bbr.2012.08.039. Epub 2012 Sep 1.

Brautigam MR, Blommaert FA, Verleye G, et al. Treatment of age-related memory complaints with Gingko biloba extract: a randomized double blind placebo-controlled study. *Phytomedicine.* 1998;5:425–434.

Cao C, Loewenstein DA, Lin X, et al. High blood caffeine levels in MCI linked to lack of progression to dementia. *Journal of Alzheimer's Disease.* 2012;30:559–572.

Chaplin K, Smith AP. Breakfast and snacks: associations with cognitive failures, minor injuries, accidents and stress. *Nutrients.* 2011 May;3(5):515–528. doi: 10.3390/nu3050515.

Craft S. Insulin resistance and Alzheimer's disease pathogenesis: potential mechanisms and implications for treatment. *Current Alzheimer's Research.* 2007 Apr;4(2):147–152.

Downey LA, Kean J, Nemeh F, et al. An acute, double-blind, placebo-controlled crossover study of 320 mg and 640 mg doses of a special extract of Bacopa monnieri (CDRI 08) on sustained cognitive performance. *Phytotherapy Research.* 2012 Dec 19. doi: 10.1002/ptr.4864.

Erickson KI, Voss MW, Prakash RS, et al. Exercise training increases size of hippocampus and improves memory. *Proceedings of the National Academy of the Sciences of the United States of America.* 2011;108(7):3017–3022. www.ncbi.nlm.nih.gov/pmc/articles/pmc3041121/. Accessed April 23, 2013.

Fiocco AJ, Shatenstein B, Ferland G, et al. Sodium intake and physical activity impact cognitive maintenance in older adults: the NuAge Study. *Neurobiology of Aging.* 2011;33(4):829.e21–28. doi: 10.1016/j.neurobiolaging.2011.07.004.

Francis ST, Head K, Morris PG, Macdonald IA. The effect of flavanol-rich cocoa on the fMRI response to a cognitive task in healthy young people. *Journal of Cardiovascular Pharmacology.* 2006;47(Suppl 2):S215–220.

Freedman ND, Park Y, Abnet CC, et al. Association of coffee drinking with total and cause-specific mortality. *New England Journal of Medicine.* 2012;366:1891–1904.

Gao X, Cassidy A, Scwazschild MA, Rimm EB, Ascherio A. Habitual intake of dietary flavonoids and risk of Parkinson's disease. *Neurology.* 2012;78(15):1138–1145.

Gao S, Jin Y, Unverzagt FW, Liang C, et al. Selenium level and depressive symptoms in a rural elderly Chinese cohort. *BMC Psychiatry.* 2012 Jul 3;12:72. doi: 10.1186/1471-244x-12-72.

Hall CB, Lipton RB, Sliwinski M, Katz MJ, Derby CA, Verghese J. Cognitive activities delay onset of memory decline in persons who develop dementia. *Neurology.* 2009 Aug 4;73(5):356–361. doi: 10.1212/wnl.0b013e3181b04ae3. www.ncbi.nlm.nih.gov/pmc/articles/pmc2725932/. Accessed April 23, 2013.

Holwerda TJ, Deeg DJ, Beekman AT, et al. Feelings of loneliness, but not social isolation, predict dementia onset: results from the Amsterdam Study of the Elderly (AMSTEL). *Journal of Neurology, Neurosurgery, and Psychiatry.* 2012 Dec 10. doi:10.1136/jnnp-2012-302755.

Huxley R, Lee CM, Barzi F, et al. Coffee, decaffeinated coffee, and tea consumption in relation to incident type-2 diabetes mellitus: a systematic review with meta-analysis. *Archives of Internal Medicine.* 2009;169:2053–2063.

Kennedy DO, Dodd FL, Robertson BC, et al. Monoterpenoid extract of sage (Salvia lavandulaefolia) with cholinesterase inhibiting properties improves cognitive performance and mood in healthy adults. *Journal of Psychopharmacology.* 2011 Aug;25(8):1088–1100. doi: 10.1177/0269881110385594.

Kennedy DO, Pace S, Haskell C, Okello EJ, Milne A, Scholey AB. Effects of cholinesterase inhibiting sage (Salvia officinalis) on mood, anxiety and performance on a psychological stressor battery. *Neuropsychopharmacology.* 2006 Apr;31(4):845–852.

Kennedy DO, Wake G, Savelev S, et al. Modulation of mood and cognitive performance following acute administration of single doses of Melissa officinalis (Lemon balm) with human CNS nicotinic and muscarinic receptor-binding properties. *Neuropsychopharmacology.* 2003 Oct;28(10):1871–1881.

Kritz-Silverstein D, Lopez LB, Barrett Connor E. High dietary and plasma levels of the omega-3 fatty acid docosahexaenoic acid are associated with decreased dementia risk: the Rancho Bernardo study. *Journal of Nutrition Health and Aging.* 2011;15(1):25–31.

Larsson SC, Virtamo J, Wolk A. Chocolate consumption and risk of stroke in women. *Journal of the American College of Cardiology.* 2011;58:1828–1829.

Lee Y, Back JH, Kim J, et al. Systematic review of health behavioral risks and cognitive health in older adults. International *Psychogeriatrics.* 2010 Mar;22(2):174–187.

Llewellyn DJ, Lang IA, Langa KM, et al. Vitamin D and risk of cognitive decline in elderly persons. *Archives of Internal Medicine.* 2010 Jul 12;170(13):1135–1141.

Mandel SA, Weinreb O, Amit T, Youdim MB. Molecular mechanisms of the neuroprotective/neurorescue action of multi-target green tea polyphenols. *Frontiers in Bioscience* (Scholar Edition). 2012 Jan 1;4:581–598.

Moss M, Cook J, Wesnes K, Duckett P. Aromas of rosemary and lavender essential oils differentially affect cognition and mood in healthy adults. *International Journal of Neuroscience.* 2003 Jan;113(1):15–38.

Moss L, Rouse M, Wesnes KA, Moss M. Differential effects of the aromas of Salvia species on memory and mood. *Human Psychopharmacology.* 2010 Jul;25(5):388–396.

Nagamatsu LS, Chan A, Davis JC, et al. Physical activity improves verbal and spatial memory in older adults with probable mild cognitive impairment: a 6-month randomized controlled trial. *Journal of Aging Research.* 2013;2013:861893. doi: 10.1155/2013/861893. www.ncbi.nlm.nih.gov/pmc/articles/pmc3595715/. Accessed April 23, 2013.

Ono K, Condron MM, Ho L, et al. Effects of grape seed-derived polyphenols on amyloid beta-protein self-assembly and cytotoxicity. *Journal of Biological Chemistry.* 2008 Nov 21;283(47):32176–32187.

Neale, T. Exercise Prevents Dementia in Some Seniors, MedPage Today. November 10, 2012. www.medpagetoday.com/cardiology/dementia/35685?utm_content=&utm_medium=email&utm_campaign=dailyheadlines&utm_source=wc&xid=nl_dhe_2012-11-02&eun=g454574d0r&userid=454574&email=jill.mays@gmail.com&mu_id=5550658.

Pavlik V, Massman P, Barber R, Doody R. Differences in the association of peripheral insulin and cognitive function in non-diabetic Alzheimer's disease cases and normal controls. *Journal of Alzheimer's Disease.* 2013 Jan 1;34(2):449–456. doi: 10.3233/jad-121999. www.ncbi.nlm.nih.gov/pubmed/23241558. Accessed April 22, 2013.

Pengelly A, Snow J, Mills SY, Scholey A, Wesnes K, Butler LR. Short-term study on the effects of rosemary on cognitive function in an elderly population. *Journal of Medicinal Food.* 2012 Jan;15(1):10–7. doi: 10.1089/jmf.2011.0005.

Pillai JA, Hall CB, Dickson DW, Buschke H, Lipton RB, Verghese J. Association of crossword puzzle participation with memory decline in persons who develop dementia. *Journal of the International Neuropsychological Society.* 2011 Nov;17(6):1006–1013. doi: 10.1017/s1355617711001111.

Poulose SM, Fisher DR, Larson J, et al. Anthocyanin-rich açai (Euterpe oleracea Mart.) fruit pulp fractions attenuate inflammatory stress signaling in mouse brain BV-2 microglial cells. *Journal of Agricultural and Food Chemistry.* 2012 Feb 1;60(4):1084–1093. doi: 10.1021/jf203989k.

Rai GS, Shovlin C, Wesnes KA. A double-blind, placebo-controlled study of Ginkgo biloba extract ('tanakan') in elderly outpatients with mild to moderate memory impairment. *Current Medical Research and Opinion.* 1991;12:350–355.

Solfrizzi V, Panza F, Frisardi V, et al. Diet and Alzheimer's disease risk factors or prevention: the current evidence. *Expert Review of Neurotherapeutics.* 2011 May;11(5):677–708. doi: 10.1586/ern.11.56.

Stough C, Downey LA, Lloyd J, et al. Examining the nootropic effects of a special extract of Bacopa monniera on human cognitive functioning: 90 day double-blind placebo-controlled randomized trial. *Phytotherapy Research.* 2008 Dec;22(12):1629–1634.

Singh Y, Sharma R, Talwar A. Immediate and long-term effects of meditation on acute stress reactivity, cognitive functions, and intelligence. *Alternative Therapies in Health and Medicine.* 2012 Nov–Dec;18(6):46–53.

Slinin Y, Paudel M, Taylor BC. Association between serum 25(OH) vitamin D and the risk of cognitive decline in older women. *Journals of Gerontology.* Series A, Biological Sciences and Medical Sciences. 2012 Oct;67(10):1092–1098.

Soni M, Kos K, Lang IA, Jones K, Melzer D, Llewellyn DJ. Vitamin D and cognitive function. *Scandinavian Journal of Clinical and Laboratory Investigation Supplement.* 2012 Apr;243:79–82. doi: 10.3109/00365513.2012.681969.

Shytle RD, Tan J, Bickford PC, et al. Optimized turmeric extract reduces Beta-amyloid and phosphorylated Tau protein burden in Alzheimer's transgenic mice. *Current Alzheimer Research.* 2012 May;9(4):500–506.

Sydenham E, Dangour AD, Lim WS. Omega 3 fatty acid for the prevention of cognitive decline and dementia. Cochrane Database of Systematic Reviews. 2012 Jun 13;6:CD005379. doi: 10.1002/14651858.cd005379.pub3.

Tangney CC, Kwasny MJ, Li H, et al. Adherence to a Mediterranean-type dietary pattern and cognitive decline in a community population. *American Journal of Clinical Nutrition.* 2010;93(3):601–607. doi: 10.3945/ajcn.110.007369.

Tildesley NT, Kennedy DO, Perry EK, et al. Positive modulation of mood and cognitive performance following administration of acute doses of Salvia lavandulaefolia essential oil to healthy young volunteers. *Physiology and Behavior.* 2005 Jan 17;83(5):699–709.

Vemuri P, Weigand SD, Przybelski SA, et al. Cognitive reserve and Alzheimer's disease biomarkers are independent determinants of cognition. *Brain.* 2011;134(Pt 5):1479–1492. doi: 10.1093/brain/awr049. www.ncbi.nlm.nih.gov/pmc/articles/pmc3097887/. Accessed April 23, 2013.

Verdelho A, Madureira S, Ferro JM, et al. Physical activity prevents progression for cognitive impairment and vascular dementia: results from the LADIS (Leukoaraiosis and Disability) study. *Stroke.* 2012;43(12):331–335. doi: 10.1161/strokeaha.112.661793.

Watson GS, Craft S. Insulin resistance, inflammation, and cognition in Alzheimer's disease: lessons for multiple sclerosis. *Journal of Neurological Sciences.* 2006 Jun 15;245(1–2):21–33.

Wu JN, Ho SC, Zhou C, et al. Coffee consumption and risk of coronary heart diseases: a meta-analysis of 21 prospective cohort studies. *International Journal of Cardiology.* 2009;137:216–225.

Chapter 17 Breast Tenderness

Alvir JM, Thys-Jacobs S. Premenstrual and menstrual symptom clusters and response to calcium treatment. *Psychopharmacology Bulletin.* 1991;27(2):145–148.

Carmichael AR. Can Vitex Agnus Castus be used for the treatment of mastalgia? What is the current evidence? *Evidence-Based Complementary and Alternative Medicine.* 2008 Sep;5(3):247–250. doi: 10.1093/ecam/nem074. www.ncbi.nlm.nih.gov/pmc/articles/pmc2529385/. Accessed April 6, 2013.

Halaska M, Beles P, Gorkow C, Sieder C. Treatment of cyclical mastalgia with a solution containing a Vitex agnus castus extract: results of a placebo-controlled double-blind study. *Breast.* 1999;8:175–181.

Ingram DM, Hickling C, West L, Mahe LJ, Dunbar PM. A double-blind randomized controlled trial of isoflavones in the treatment of cyclical mastalgia. *Breast.* 2002 Apr;11(2):170–174.

McFadyen IJ, Chetty U, Setchell KDR, et al. A randomized double blind, cross over trial of soya protein for the treatment of cyclical breast pain. *Breast.* 2000;9:271–276.

Prilepskaya VN, Ledina AV, Tagiyeva AV, Revazova FS. Vitex agnus castus: successful treatment of moderate to severe premenstrual syndrome. *Maturitas.* 2006;55(Suppl 1):S55–63.

Pruthi S, Wahner-Roedler DL, Torkelson, CJ, et al. Vitamin E and evening primrose oil for management of cyclical mastalgia: a randomized pilot study. *Alternative Medicine Reviews.* 2010 Apr;15(1):59–67. www.altmedrev.com/publications/15/1/59.pdf. Accessed April 6, 2013.

Singleton G. Premenstrual disorders in adolescent females: integrative management. *Australian Family Physician.* 2006;36(8):629–630. www.racgp.org.au/afp/200708/17823. Accessed April 6, 2013.

Walker AF, De Souza MC, Vickers MF, Abeyasekera S, Collins ML, Trinca LA. Magnesium supplementation alleviates premenstrual symptoms of fluid retention. *Journal of Women's Health.* 1998 Nov;7(9):1157–1165.

Chapter 18 Bruises

Arsić I, Zugić A, Tadić V, et al. Estimation of dermatological application of creams with St. John's wort oil extracts. *Molecules.* 2011 Dec 28;17(1):275–294. doi: 10.3390/molecules17010275.

Korting HC, Schafer-Korting M, Hart H, et al. Anti-inflammatory activity of hamamelis distillate applied topically to the skin. Influence of vehicle and dose. *European Journal of Clinical Pharmacology.* 1993;44:315–318.

Leu S, Havey J, White LE, et al. Accelerated resolution of laser-induced bruising with topical 20% arnica: a rater-blinded randomized controlled trial. *British Journal of Dermatology*. 2010 Sep;163(3):557–563. doi: 10.1111/j.1365-2133.2010.09813.x.

Masson M. Bromelain in blunt injuries of the locomotor system. A study of observed applications in general practice. *Fortschritte der Medizin*. 1995;113(19):303–306.

Reddy AV, Chan K, Jones JI, Vassallo M, Auger M. Spontaneous bruising in an elderly woman. *Postgraduate Medical Journal*. 1998 May;74(871):273–275.

Schulz V, Hansel R, Tyler VE. *Rational Phytotherapy: A Physician's Guide to Herbal Medicine*. Terry C. Telger, transl. 3rd ed. Berlin, Germany: Springer; 1998.

Staiger C. Comfrey: a clinical overview. *Phytotherapy Research*. 2012 Oct;26(10):1441–1448. doi: 10.1002/ptr.4612.

Wolff HH, Kieser M. Hamamelis in children with skin disorders and skin injuries: results of an observational study. *European Journal of Pediatrics*. 2007 Sep;166(9):943–948.

Chapter 19 Burns
Chan EW, Soh EY, Tie PP, Law YP. Antioxidant and antibacterial properties of green, black, and herbal teas of Camellia sinensis. *Pharmacognosy Research*. 2011 Oct;3(4):266–272. doi: 10.4103/0974-8490.89748.

Fronza M, Heinzmann B, Hamburger M, Laufer S, Merfort I. Determination of the wound healing effect of Calendula extracts using the scratch assay with 3T3 fibroblasts. *Journal of Ethnopharmacology*. 2009 Dec 10;126(3):463–467. doi: 10.1016/j.jep.2009.09.014.

Hajhashemi V, Ghannadi A, Sharif B. Anti-inflammatory and analgesic properties of the leaf extracts and essential oil of Lavandula angustifolia Mill. *Journal of Ethnopharmacology*. 2003;89:67–71.

Jarrahi M, Vafaei AA, Taherian AA, Miladi H, Rashidi Pour A. Evaluation of topical Matricaria chamomilla extract activity on linear incisional wound healing in albino rats. *Natural Product Research*. 2010 May;24(8):697–702. doi: 10.1080/14786410701654875.

Jenkins R, Cooper R. Improving antibiotic activity against wound pathogens with manuka honey in vitro. *PLoS One*. 2012;7(9):e45600. doi: 10.1371/journal.pone.0045600.

Jeon HY, Kim JK, Kim WG, Lee SJ. Effects of oral epigallocatechin gallate supplementation on the minimal erythema dose and UV-induced skin damage. *Skin Pharmacology and Physiology*. 2009;22(3):137–141. doi: 10.1159/000201562. Epub 2009 Feb 12.

Maenthaisong R, Chaiyakunapruk N, Niruntraporn S, Kongkaew C. The efficacy of aloe vera used for burn wound healing: a systematic review. *Burns*. 2007 Sep;33(6):713–718.

Mandal MD, Mandal S. Honey: its medicinal property and antibacterial activity. *Asian Pacific Journal of Tropical Biomedicine*. 2011 Apr;1(2):154–160. doi: 10.1016/s2221-1691(11)60016-6. www.ncbi.nlm.nih.gov/pmc/articles/pmc3609166/. Accessed April 29, 2013.

Mumcuoglu KY. Clinical applications for maggots in wound care. *American Journal of Clinical Dermatology*. 2001;2(4):219–227.

Sevin A, Oztaş P, Senen D, et al. Effects of polyphenols on skin damage due to ultraviolet A rays: an experimental study on rats. *Journal of the European Academy of Dermatology and Venereology*. 2007 May;21(5):650–66.

Sheikhan F, Jahdi F, Khoei EM, et al. Episiotomy pain relief: use of lavender oil essence in primiparous Iranian women. *Complementary Therapies in Clinical Practice*. 2012 Feb;18(1):66–70. doi: 10.1016/j.ctcp.2011.02.003.

Turkmen A, Graham K, McGrouther DA. Therapeutic applications of the larvae for wound debridement. *Journal of Plastic, Reconstructive, and Aesthetic Surgery*. 2010 Jan;63(1):184–188. doi: 10.1016/j.bjps.2008.08.070.

Chapter 20 Cancer Prevention
Adhami VM, Khan N, Mukhtar H. Cancer chemoprevention by pomegranate: laboratory and clinical evidence. *Nutrition and Cancer*. 2009;61(6):811–815.

Afaq F, Zaid MA, Khan N, Dreher M, Mukhtar H. Protective effect of pomegranate-derived products on UVB-mediated damage in human reconstituted skin. *Experimental Dermatology*. 2009;18:553–561.

American Institute for Cancer Research. "Cancer Experts on Garlic: Chop, then Stop." June 18, 2007. www.aicr.org/site/news2?abbr=pr_&page=newsarticle&id=12154.

Anand P, Sundaram C, et al. Curcumin and cancer: an "old-age" disease with an "age-old" solution. *Cancer Letters*. 2008 Aug 18;267(1):133–164.

Azqueta A, Collins AR. Carotenoids and DNA damage. *Mutation Research*. 2012 May 1;733(1–2):4–13.

Bergman Jungestrom M, Thompson LU, Dabrosin C. Flaxseed and its lignans inhibit estradiol-induced growth, angiogenesis, and secretion of vascular endothelial growth factor in human breast cancer xenografts in vivo. *Clinical Cancer Research*. 2007 Feb 1;13(3):1061–1067.

Boeing H, Bechthold A, Bub A, et al. Critical review: vegetables and fruit in the prevention of chronic diseases. *European Journal of Nutrition*. 2012 Jun 9. [Epub ahead of print]

Borchers AT, Keen CL, Gershwin ME. Mushrooms, tumors, and immunity: an update. *Experimental Biology and Medicine* (Maywood). 2004;229:393–406.

Brennan SF, Cantwell MM, Cardwell CR, Velentzis LS, Woodside JV. Dietary patterns and breast cancer risk: a systematic review and meta-analysis. *American Journal of Clinical Nutrition*. 2010;91(5):1294–1302. http://ajcn.nutrition.org/content/91/5/1294.long. Accessed April 24, 2013.

Cashman JR, Ghirmai S, Abel KJ, Fiala M. Immune defects in Alzheimer's disease: new medications development. *BMC Neuroscience*. 2008 Dec 3;9(Suppl 2):S13.

Chandran B, Goel A. A randomized, pilot study to assess the efficacy and safety of curcumin in patients with active rheumatoid arthritis. *Phytotherapy Research*. 2012;26:1719–1725.

Chen J, Power KA, Mann J, Cheng A, Thompson LU. Flaxseed alone or in combination with tamoxifen inhibits MCF-7 breast tumor growth in ovariectomized athymic mice with high circulating levels of estrogen. *Experimental Biology and Medicine* (Maywood). 2007 Sep;232(8):1071–1080.

Costa G, Haus E, Stevens R. Shift work and cancer—considerations on rationale, mechanisms, and epidemiology. *Scandinavian Journal of Work, Environment, and Health*. 2010 Mar;36(2):163–179.

Dai J, Patel JD, Mumper RJ. Characterization of blackberry extract and its antiproliferative and anti-inflammatory properties. *Journal of Medicinal Food*. 2007 Jun;10(2):258–265.

Danbara N, Yuri T, Tsujita-Kyutoku M, et al. Enterolactone induces apoptosis and inhibits growth of Colo 201 human colon cancer cells both in vitro and in vivo. *Anticancer Research*. 2005 May–Jun;25(3B):2269–2276.

Deep G, Agarwal R. Antimetastatic efficacy of silibinin: molecular mechanisms and therapeutic potential against cancer. *Cancer Metastasis Reviews*. 2010 Sep;29(3):447–463.

Demark-Wahnefried W, Polascik TJ, George SL, et al. Flaxseed supplementation (not dietary fat restriction) reduces prostate cancer proliferation rates in men presurgery. *Cancer Epidemiology, Biomarkers, and Prevention*. 2008 Dec;17(12):3577–3587.

Deodhar SD, Sethi R, Srimal RC. Preliminary study on antirheumatic activity of curcumin (diferuloyl methane). *Indian Journal of Medical Research*. 1980;71:632–634.

Do MH, Lee SS, Jung PJ, Lee MH. Intake of fruits, vegetables, and soy foods in relation to breast cancer risk in Korean women: a case-control study. Nutrition and Cancer. 2007;57(1):20–27.

Doll R, Peto R, Boreham J, Sutherland I. Mortality in relation to smoking: 50 years' observations on male British doctors. *BMJ*. 2004;328(7455):1519–1527.

Dong JY, Qin LQ. Soy isoflavones consumption and risk of breast cancer incidence or recurrence: a meta-analysis of prospective studies. *Breast Cancer Research and Treatment*. 2011 Jan;125(2):315–323.

Durak I, Biri H, Devrim E, Sözen S, Avci A. Aqueous extract of Urtica dioica makes significant inhibition on adenosine deaminase activity in prostate tissue from patients with prostate cancer. *Cancer Biology and Therapy*. 2004 Sep;3(9):855–857.

Edinger MS, Koff WJ. Effect of the consumption of tomato paste on plasma prostate-specific antigen levels in patients with benign prostate hyperplasia. *Brazilian Journal of Medical and Biological Research*. 2006 Aug;39(8):1115–1119.

Ellinger S, Ellinger J, Stehle P. Tomatoes, tomato products and lycopene in the prevention and treatment of prostate cancer: do we have the evidence from intervention studies? *Current Opinion in Clinical Nutrition and Metabolic Care*. 2006 Nov;9(6):722–727.

Giacosa A, Barale R, Bavaresco L, et al. Cancer prevention in Europe: the Mediterranean diet as a protective choice. *European Journal of Cancer Prevention*. 2013 Jan;22(1):90–95. doi: 10.1097/cej.0b013e328354d2d7.

Goodman MT, Wilkens LR, Hankin JH, et al. Association of soy and fiber consumption with the risk of endometrial cancer. *American Journal of Epidemiology*. 1997 Aug 15;146(4):294–306.

Haniadka R, Rajeev AG, Palatty PL, Arora R, Baliga MS. Zingiber officinale (Ginger) as an anti-emetic. Cancer Chemotherapy: A Review. *Journal of Alternative and Complementary Medicine*. 2012 May;18(5):440–444.

Hassan MM, Bondy ML, Wolff RA, et al. Risk factors for pancreatic cancer: case-control study. *American Journal of Gastroenterology*. 2007 Aug 31. [Epub ahead of print]

Jee SH, Ohrr H, et al. Fasting serum glucose level and cancer risk in Korean men and women. *JAMA*. 2005 Jan 12;293(2):194–202.

Kakuta Y, Nakaya N, Nagase S, et al. Case-control study of green tea consumption and the risk of endometrial endometrioid adenocarcinoma. *Cancer Causes & Control*. 2009 Jul;20(5):617–24.

Kamat AM, Lamm DL. Chemoprevention of bladder cancer. *Urologic Clinics of North America*. 2002 Feb;29(1):157–168.

Khan N, Afaq F, Saleem M, Ahmad N, Mukhtar H. Targeting multiple signaling pathways by green tea polyphenol-epigallocatechin-3-gallate. *Cancer Research*. 2006 Mar 1;66(5):2500–2505.

Kodama N, Komuta K, Nanba H. Can maitake MD-fraction aid cancer patients? *Alternative Medicine Review*. 2002 Jun;7(3):236–239.

Kuptniratsaikul V, Thanakhumtorn S, Chinswangwatanakul P, et al. Efficacy and safety of Curcuma domestica extracts in patients with knee osteoarthritis. *Journal of Alternative and Complementary Medicine*. 2009;15:891–897.

Li Y, Wicha MS, Schwartz SJ, Sun D. Implications of cancer stem cell theory for cancer chemoprevention by natural dietary compounds. *Journal of Nutritional Biochemistry*. 2011 Sep;22(9):799–806. doi: 10.1016/j.jnutbio.2010.11.001.

473

Myung SK, Ju W, Choi HJ, Kim SC; Korean Meta-Analysis (KORMA) Study Group. Soy intake and risk of endocrine-related gynaeco-logical cancer: a meta-analysis. *BJOG*. 2009 Dec;116(13):1697–1705.

Nagel JM, Brinkoetter M, Magkos F, et al. Dietary walnuts inhibit colorectal cancer growth in mice by suppressing angiogenesis. *Nutrition*. 2012 Jan;28(1):67–75.

Nagle CM, Olsen CM, Bain CJ, Whiteman DC, Green AC, Webb PM. Tea consumption and risk of ovarian cancer. *Cancer Causes & Control*. 2010 Sep;21(9):1485–1491.

Nechuta SJ, Caan BJ, Chen WY, et al. Soy food intake after diag-nosis of breast cancer and survival: an in-depth analysis of com-bined evidence from cohort studies of US and Chinese women. *American Journal of Clinical Nutrition*. 2012 May 30. [Epub ahead of print]

Neto CC. Cranberry and blueberry: evidence for protective effects against cancer and vascular diseases. *Molecular Nutrition and Food Research*. 2007 Jun;51(6):652–664.

Ollberding NJ, Lim U, Wilkens LR, et al. Legume, soy, tofu, and isoflavone intake and endometrial cancer risk in postmenopausal women in the multiethnic cohort study. *Journal of the National Cancer Institute*. 2012 Jan 4;104(1):67–76.

Pan A, Sun Q, Bernstein AM, et al. Red meat consumption and mortality: results from 2 prospective cohort studies. *Archives of Internal Medicine*. 2012 Apr 9;172(7):555–563. doi: 10.1001/archinternmed.2011.2287. Epub 2012 Mar 12.

Patel S, Goyal A. Recent developments in mushrooms as anti-cancer therapeutics: a review. *3 Biotech*. 2012 Mar;2(1):1–15. Epub 2011 Nov 25. www.ncbi.nlm.nih.gov/pmc/articles/pmc3339609/?tool=pubmed. Accessed June 12, 2012.

Pereira MM, Haniadka R, Chacko PP, Palatty PL, Baliga MS. Zingiber officinale Roscoe (ginger) as an adjuvant in cancer treat-ment: a review. *Journal of BUON*. 2011 Jul–Sep;16(3):414–424.

Peto R, Darby S, Deo H, et al. Smoking, smoking cessation, and lung cancer in the U.K. since 1950: Combination of national statis-tics with two case-control studies. *BMJ*. 2000;321(7257):323–329.

Prucksunand C, Indrasukhsri B, Leethochawalit M, Hungspreugs K. Phase II clinical trial on effect of the long turmeric (Curcuma longa Linn) on healing of peptic ulcer. *Southeast Asian Journal of Tropical Medicine and Public Health*. 2001 Mar;32(1):208–215.

Rao AV, Rao LG. Carotenoids and human health. *Pharmacological Research*. 2007 Mar;55(3):207–216.

Reiche EM, Nunes SO, Morimoto HK. Stress, depression, the immune system, and cancer. *Lancet Oncology*. 2004 Oct;5(10):617–625.

Rosanoff A, Weaver CM, Rude RK. Suboptimal magnesium status in the United States: are the health consequences under-estimated? *Nutrition Reviews*. 2012 Mar;70(3):153–164. doi: 10.1111/j.1753-4887.2011.00465.x.

Sagar SM, Yance D, Wong RK. Natural health products that inhibit angiogenesis: a potential source for investigational new agents to treat cancer-Part 2. *Current Oncology*. 2006 Jun;13(3):99–107.

Sakauchi F, Khan MM, Mori M, et al; JACC Study Group. Dietary habits and risk of ovarian cancer death in a large-scale cohort study (JACC study) in Japan. *Nutriton and Cancer*. 2007;57(2):138–145.

Setiawan VW, Monroe KR, Goodman MT, et al. Alcohol con-sumption and endometrial cancer risk: the multiethnic cohort. *International Journal of Cancer*. 2007 Aug 31. [Epub ahead of print]

Shanmugam MK, Kannaiyan R, Sethi G. Targeting cell signaling and apoptotic pathways by dietary agents: role in the prevention and treatment of cancer. *Nutrition and Cancer*. 2011;63(2):161–173. doi: 10.1080/01635581.2011.523502. http://dx.doi.org/10.1080/01635581.2011.523502.

Shin A, Kim J, Lim SY, Kim G, Sung MK, Lee ES, Ro J. Dietary mush-room intake and the risk of breast cancer based on hormone receptor status. *Nutrition and Cancer*. 2010;62(4):476–483.

Shukla Y, Kalra N. Cancer chemoprevention with garlic and its constituents. *Cancer Letters*. 2007 Mar 18;247(2):167–181.

Shukla Y, Singh M. Cancer preventive properties of ginger: a brief review. *Food and Chemical Toxicology*. 2007 May;45(5):683–690. Epub 2006 Nov 12.

Siddiqui IA, Saleem M, Adhami VM, Asim M, Mukhtar H. Tea bev-erage in chemoprevention and chemotherapy of prostate cancer. *Acta Pharmacologica Sinica*. 2007 Sep;28(9):1392–1408.

Sigstedt SC, Hooten CJ, Callewaert MC, et al. Evaluation of aque-ous extracts of Taraxacum officinale on growth and invasion of breast and prostate cancer cells. *International Journal of Oncology*. 2008 May;32(5):1085–1090.

Singletary KW, Jung KJ, Giusti M. Anthocyanin-rich grape extract blocks breast cell DNA damage. *Journal of Medicinal Food*. 2007 Jun;10(2):244–251.

Sun Z, Zhu Y, Wang PP, et al. Reported intake of selected micro-nutrients and risk of colorectal cancer: results from a large population-based case-control study in Newfoundland, Labrador and Ontario, Canada. *Anticancer Research*. 2012 Feb;32(2):687–696.

Talalay P, Fahey JW. Phytochemicals from cruciferous plants protect against cancer by modulating carcinogen metabolism. *Journal of Nutrition*. 2001 Nov;131(11 Suppl):3027S–3033S.

Tsugane S, Sasazuki S. Diet and the risk of gastric cancer: review of epidemiological evidence. *Gastric Cancer*. 2007;10(2):75–83. Epub 2007 Jun 25. Review.

Vas CJ, Pinto C, Panikker D, et al. Prevalence of dementia in an urban Indian population. *International Psychogeriatrics*. 2001 Dec;13(4):439–450.

Wang CY, Wang SY, Yin JJ, Parry J, Yu LL. Enhancing antioxidant, antiproliferation, and free radical scavenging activities in strawberries with essential oils. *Journal of Agricultural and Food Chemistry*. 2007 Aug 8;55(16):6527–6532.

Xu T, Beelman RB, Lambert JD. The cancer preventive effects of edible mushrooms. *Anticancer Agents in Medicinal Chemistry*. 2012 Dec;12(10):1255–1263.

Yan L, Spitznagel EL, Bosland MC. Soy consumption and colorectal cancer risk in humans: a meta-analysis. *Cancer Epidemiology, Biomarkers, and Prevention*. 2010 Jan;19(1):148–158.

Yang F, Lim GP, Begum AN, et al. Curcumin inhibits formation of amyloid beta oligomers and fibrils, binds plaques, and reduces amyloid in vivo. *Journal of Biological Chemistry*. 2005 Feb 18;280(7):5892–5901.

Zafra-Stone S, Yasmin T, Bagchi M, et al. Berry anthocyanins as novel antioxidants in human health and disease prevention. *Molecular Nutrition and Food Research*. 2007 Jun;51(6):675–683.

Zaineddin AK, Buck K, Vrieling A, et al. The association between dietary lignans, phytoestrogen-rich foods, and fiber intake and postmenopausal breast cancer risk: a german case-control study. *Nutrition and Cancer*. 2012 May 16. [Epub ahead of print]

Chapter 21 Cholesterol Management

Aprikian O, Duclos V, Guyot S, et al. Apple pectin and a polyphenol-rich apple concentrate are more effective together than separately on cecal fermentations and plasma lipids in rats. *Journal of Nutrition*. 2003 Jun;133(6):1860–1865.

Basu A, Lyons TJ. Strawberries, blueberries, and cranberries in the metabolic syndrome: clinical perspectives. *Journal of Agricultural and Food Chemistry*. 2011;60:5687.

Geleijnse JM, Launer LJ, van der Kuip DA, et al. Inverse association of tea and flavonoid intakes with incident myocardial infarction: the Rotterdam Study. *American Journal of Clinical Nutrition*. 2002;75:880–886.

Khan A, Safdar M, Ali Khan MM, Khattak KN, Anderson RA. Cinnamon improves glucose and lipids of people with type-2 diabetes. *Diabetes Care*. 2003 Dec;26(12):3215–3218.

Mani UV, Mani I, Biswas M, Kumar SN. An open-label study on the effect of flax seed powder (Linum usitatissimum) supplementation in the management of diabetes mellitus. *Journal of Dietary Supplements*. 2011 Sep;8(3):257–265. doi: 10.3109/19390211.2011.593615.

Manjunatha H, Srinivasan K. Hypolipidemic and antioxidant effects of dietary curcumin and capsaicin in induced hypercholesterolemic rats. *Lipids*. 2007 Dec;42(12):1133–1142.

Tinahones FJ, Rubio MA, Garrido-Sánchez L, et al. Green tea reduces LDL oxidability and improves vascular function. *Journal of the American College of Nutrition*. 2008 Apr;27(2):209–213.

Chapter 22 Colds

Benmalek Y, Yahia OA, Belkebir A, Fardeau ML. Anti-microbial and anti-oxidant activities of Illicium verum, Crataegus oxyacantha ssp monogyna and Allium cepa red and white varieties. *Bioengineered*. 2013 Apr 11;4(4).

Brinkeborn RM, Shah DV, Degenring FH. Echinaforce and other Echinacea fresh plant preparations in the treatment of the common cold: a randomized, placebo controlled, double-blind clinical trial. *Phytomedicine*. 1999;6:1–6.

Chakraborty B, Sengupta M. Boosting of nonspecific host response by aromatic spices turmeric and ginger in immunocompromised mice. *Cellular Immunology*. 2012 Nov;280(1):92–100. doi: 10.1016/j.cellimm.2012.11.014.

Charan J, Goyal JP, Saxena D, Yadav P. Vitamin D for prevention of respiratory tract infections: a systematic review and meta-analysis. *Journal of Pharmacology and Pharmacotherapeutics*. 2012 Oct;3(4):300–303. doi: 10.4103/0976-500x.103685. www.ncbi.nlm.nih.gov/pmc/articles/pmc3543548/. Accessed April 12, 2013.

Elaissi A, Rouis Z, Salem NA, et al. Chemical composition of 8 eucalyptus species' essential oils and the evaluation of their antibacterial, antifungal and antiviral activities. *BMC Complementary and Alternative Medicine*. 2012 Jun 28;12:81. doi: 10.1186/1472-6882-12-81.

Gabrielian ES, Shukarian AK, Goukasova GI, et al. Andrographis paniculata in the symptomatic treatment of uncomplicated upper respiratory tract infection: systematic review of randomized controlled trials. *Journal of Clinical Pharmacology and Therapeutics*. 2004 Feb;29(1):37–45.

Hemilä H. Vitamin C supplementation and respiratory infections: a systematic review. *Military Medicine*. 2004 Nov;169(11):920–925.

Josling P. Preventing the common cold with a garlic supplement: a double-blind, placebo-controlled survey. *Advances in Therapy*. 2001 Jul–Aug;18(4):189–193.

Kubra IR, Rao LJ. An impression on current developments in the technology, chemistry, and biological activities of ginger (Zingiber officinale Roscoe). *Critical Reviews in Food Science and Nutrition*. 2012;52(8):651–688. doi: 10.1080/10408398.2010.505689.

Lee HJ, Hyun EA, Yoon WJ, et al. In vitro anti-inflammatory and anti-oxidative effects of Cinnamomum camphora extracts. *Journal of Ethnopharmacology*. 2006;103:208–216.

Lindenmuth GF, Lindenmuth EB. The efficacy of echinacea compound herbal tea preparation on the severity and duration of upper respiratory and flu symptoms: a randomized, double-blind, placebo-controlled study. *Journal of Alternative and Complementary Medicine*. 2000;6:327–334.

Meltzer EO, Hamilos DL. Rhinosinusitis diagnosis and management for the clinician: a synopsis of recent consensus guidelines. *Mayo Clinic Proceedings*. 2011;86(5):427–443. doi: 10.4065/mcp.2010.0392. www.ncbi.nlm.nih.gov/pmc/articles/pmc3084646/. Accessed April 12, 2013.

Popova M, Molimard P, Courau S, et al. Beneficial effects of probiotics in upper respiratory tract infections and their mechanical actions to antagonize pathogens. *Journal of Applied Microbiology*. 2012 Dec;113(6):1305–1318. doi: 10.1111/j.1365-2672.2012.05394.x.

Rennard BO, Ertl RF, Gossman GL, Robbins RA, Rennard SI. Chicken soup inhibits neutrophil chemotaxis in vitro. *Chest*. 2000 Oct;118(4):1150–1157.

Saketkhoo K, Januszkiewicz A, Sackner MA. Effects of drinking hot water, cold water, and chicken soup on nasal mucus velocity and nasal airflow resistance. *Chest*. 1978 Oct;74(4):408–410.

Saunders PR, Smith F, Schusky RW. Echinacea purpurea L. in children: safety, tolerability, compliance, and clinical effectiveness in upper respiratory tract infections. *Canadian Journal of Physiology and Pharmacology*. 2007 Nov;85(11):1195–1199.

Science M, Johnstone J, Roth DE, Guyatt G, Loeb M. Zinc for the treatment of the common cold: a systematic review and meta-analysis of randomized controlled trials. *CMAJ: Canadian Medical Association Journal*. 2012 Jul 10;184(10):E551–561. doi: 10.1503/cmaj.111990. www.ncbi.nlm.nih.gov/pmc/articles/pmc3394849/. Accessed April 12, 2013.

Suekawa M, Ishige A, Yuasa K, et al. Pharmacological studies on ginger. I. Pharmacological actions of pungent constitutents, (6)-gingerol and (6)-shogaol. *Journal of Pharmacobio-dynamics*. 1984;7:836–848.

Taylor JA, Weber W, Standish L, et al. Efficacy and safety of echinacea in treating upper respiratory tract infections in children: a randomized controlled trial. *JAMA*. 2003 Dec 3;290(21):2824–2830.

Upton R, ed. Astragalus Root: analytical, quality control, and therapeutic monograph. Santa Cruz, CA: *American Herbal Pharmacopoeia*. 1999:1–25.

Wagner H. A double blind, placebo-controlled study of Andrographis paniculata fixed combination Kan Jang in the treatment of acute upper respiratory tract infections including sinusitis. *Phytomedicine*. 2002 Oct;9(7):589–597.

Wayse V, Yousafzai A, Mogale K, Filteau S. Association of subclinical vitamin D deficiency with severe acute lower respiratory infection in Indian children under 5 years. *European Journal of Clinical Nutrition*. 2004;58:563–567.

Weber W, Taylor JA, Stoep AV, Weiss NS, Standish LJ, Calabrese C. Echinacea purpurea for prevention of upper respiratory tract infections in children. *Journal of Alternative and Complementary Medicine*. 2005 Dec;11(6):1021–1026.

Chapter 23 Cold Sores

Al-Waili NS. Topical honey application vs. acyclovir for the treatment of recurrent herpes simplex lesions. *Medical Science Monitor*. 2004 Aug;10(8):MT94–98.

Arens M, Travis S. Zinc salts inactivate clinical isolates of herpes simplex virus in vitro. *Journal of Clinical Microbiology*. 2000;38:1758–1762.

Griffith RS, Walsh DE, Myrmel KH, et al. Success of L-lysine therapy in frequently recurrent herpes simplex infection: treatment and prophylaxis. *Dermatologica*. 1987;175:183–190.

Hoheisel O. The effects of Herstat (3% propolis ointment ACF) application in cold sores: a double-blind placebo-controlled clinical trial. *Journal of Clinical Research*. 2001;4:65–75.

Kneist W, Hempel B, Borelli S. [Clinical, double-blind trial of topical zinc sulfate for herpes labialis recidivans]. *Arzneimittel-Forschung*. 1995;45:624–626.

Koytchev R, Alken RG, Dundarov S. Balm mint extract (Lo-701) for topical treatment of recurring herpes labialis. *Phytomedicine*. 1999 Oct;6(4):225–230.

Nolkemper S, Reichling J, Stintzing FC, Carle R, Schnitzler P. Antiviral effect of aqueous extracts from species of the Lamiaceae family against Herpes simplex virus type 1 and type 2 in vitro. *Planta Medica*. 2006 Dec;72(15):1378–1382.

Schnitzler P, Schön K, Reichling J. Antiviral activity of Australian tea tree oil and eucalyptus oil against herpes simplex virus in cell culture. *Pharmazie*. 2001 Apr;56(4):343–347.

Schnitzler P, Schuhmacher A, Astani A, Reichling J. Melissa officinalis oil affects infectivity of enveloped herpes viruses. *Phytomedicine*. 2008 Sep;15(9):734–740. doi: 10.1016/j.phymed.2008.04.018.

Schuhmacher A, Reichling J, Schnitzler P. Virucidal effect of peppermint oil on the enveloped viruses herpes simplex virus type 1 and type 2 in vitro. *Phytomedicine*. 2003;10(6–7):504–510.

Steinmann J, Buer J, Pietschmann T, Steinmann E. Anti-infective properties of epigallocatechin-3-gallate (EGCG), a component of green tea. *British Journal of Pharmacology*. 2013 Mar;168(5):1059–1073. doi: 10.1111/bph.12009.

Szmeja Z, Kulczynski B, Konopacki K. [Clinical usefulness of the preparation Herpestat in the treatment of Herpes labialis]. *Otolaryngoogia Polska*. 1987;41:183–188.

Uchakin PN, Parish DC, Dane FC, et al. Fatigue in medical residents leads to reactivation of herpes virus latency. *Interdisciplinary Perspectives on Infectious Diseases.* 2011:571340. Article ID 571340. doi:10.1155/2011/571340. www.hindawi.com/journals/ipid/2011/571340/. Accessed April 24, 2013.

Vogler BK, Ernst E. Aloe vera: a systematic review of its clinical effectiveness. *British Journal of General Practice.* 1999 Oct;49(447):823–828.

Chapter 24 Colic

Al Dhaheri W, Diksic D, Ben-Shoshan M. IgE-mediated cow milk allergy and infantile colic: diagnostic and management challenges. *BMJ Case Reports.* 2013 Feb 6;2013. pii: bcr2012007182. doi: 10.1136/bcr-2012-007182.

Blumenthal I. The gripe water story. *Journal of the Royal Society of Medicine.* 2000;93(4):172–174.

Huhtala V, Lehtonen L, Heinonen R, Korvenranta H. Infant massage compared with crib vibrator in the treatment of colicky infants. *Pediatrics.* 2000 Jun;105(6):E84.

Keefe MR, Kajrlsen KA, Lobo ML, Kotzer AM, Dudley WN. Reducing parenting stress in families with irritable infants. *Nursing Research.* 2006 May–Jun;55(3):198–205.

Mhaske S, Mhaske S, Badrinarayan S, Zade R, Shirsath U. Role of protein rich maternal diet in infantile colic. *Journal of the Indian Medical Association.* 2012 May;110(5):317–318.

Savino F, Cresi F, Castagno E, Silvestro L, Oggero R. A randomized double-blind placebo-controlled trial of a standardized extract of Matricariae recutita, Foeniculum vulgare and Melissa officinalis (ColiMil) in the treatment of breastfed colicky infants. *Phytotherapy Research.* 2005 Apr;19(4):335–340.

Savino F, Oggero R. Management of infantile colics. *Minerva Pediatrica.* 1996 Jul–Aug;48(7–8):313–319.

Savino F, Pelle E, Palumeri E, Oggero R, Miniero R. Lactobacillus reuteri (American Type Culture Collection Strain 55730) versus simethicone in the treatment of infantile colic: a prospective randomized study. *Pediatrics.* 2007;119(1):e124–130.

Weizman, Z, et al. Efficacy of herbal tea preparation in infantile colic. *Journal of Pediatrics.* 1993;122:650–652.

Chapter 25 Constipation

Badiali D, Corazziari E, Habib FI, et al. Effect of wheat bran in treatment of chronic nonorganic constipation: a double-blind controlled trial. *Digestive Diseases and Sciences.* 1995;40:349–356.

Bekkali NL, Bongers ME, Van den Berg MM, Liem O, Benninga MA. The role of a probiotics mixture in the treatment of childhood constipation: a pilot study. *Nutrition Journal.* 2007 Aug 4;6:17.

de Milliano I, Tabbers MM, van der Post JA, Benninga MA. Is a multispecies probiotic mixture effective in constipation during pregnancy?: a pilot study. *Nutrition Journal.* 2012 Oct 4;11(1):80. [Epub ahead of print]

De Schryver AM, Keulemans YC, Peters HP, et al. Effects of regular physical activity on defecation pattern in middle-aged patients complaining of chronic constipation. *Scandinavian Journal of Gastroenterology.* 2005 Apr;40(4):422–429.

Drummond L, Gearry RB. Kiwifruit modulation of gastrointestinal motility. *Advances in Food and Nutrition Research.* 2013;68:219–232. doi: 10.1016/b978-0-12-394294-4.00012-2.

McRorie JW, Daggy BP, Morel JG, et al. Psyllium is superior to docusate sodium for treatment of chronic constipation. *Alimentary Pharmacology and Therapeutics.* 1998;12:491–497.

Tabbers MM, Chmielewska A, Roseboom MG, et al. Effect of the consumption of a fermented dairy product containing Bifidobacterium lactis DN-173 010 on constipation in childhood: a multicentre randomised controlled trial (NTRTC:1571). *BMC Pediatrics.* 2009 Mar 18;9:22.

Trottier M, Erebara A, Bozzo P. Treating constipation during pregnancy. *Canadian Family Physician.* 2012 Aug;58(8):836–838. www.ncbi.nlm.nih.gov/pmc/articles/pmc3418980/. Accessed April 18, 2013.

Wald A. Is chronic use of stimulant laxatives harmful to the colon? *Journal of Clinical Gastroenterology.* 2003 May–Jun;36(5):386–389.

Chapter 26 Coughs and Bronchitis

Bladt S, Wagner H. From Zulu medicine to the European phytomedicine Umckaloabo. *Phytomedicine.* 2007;14(Suppl 1):2–4.

Cohen HA, Rozen J, Kristal H, et al. Effect of honey on nocturnal cough and sleep quality: a double-blind, randomized, placebo-controlled study. *Pediatrics.* 2012 Sep;130(3):465–471.

Lawson LD, Gardner CD. Composition, stability, and bioavailability of garlic products used in a clinical trial. *Journal of Agricultural and Food Chemistry.* 2005 Aug 10;53(16):6254–6261. www.ncbi.nlm.nih.gov/pmc/articles/pmc2584604/. Accessed April 19, 2013.

Linder JA, Sim I. Antibiotic treatment of acute bronchitis in smokers: a systematic review. *Journal of General Internal Medicine.* 2002;17(3):230–234. www.ncbi.nlm.nih.gov/pmc/articles/pmc1495016/. Accessed April 19, 2013.

Matthys H, Eisebitt R, Seith B, Heger M. Efficacy and safety of an extract of Pelargonium sidoides (EPs 7630) in adults with acute bronchitis: a randomised, doubleblind, placebo-controlled trial. *Phytomedicine.* 2003;10(Suppl 4):7–17.

Paul IM, Beiler J, McMonagle A, Shaffer ML, Duda L, Berlin CM Jr. Effect of honey, dextromethorphan, and no treatment on nocturnal cough and sleep quality for coughing children and their parents. *Archives of Pediatric and Adolescent Medicine.* 2007;161(12):1140–1146.

Sadlon AE, Lamson DW. Immune-modifying and antimicrobial effects of Eucalyptus oil and simple inhalation devices. *Alternative Medicine Review.* 2010 Apr;15(1):33–47. www.altmedrev.com/publications/15/1/33.pdf. Accessed April 19, 2013.

Timmer A, Günther J, Rücker G, Motschall E, Antes G, Kern WV. Pelargonium sidoides extract for acute respiratory tract infections. *Cochrane Database of Systematic Reviews*. 2008;(3):CD006323.

Chapter 27 Cuts and Scrapes

Banu A, Sathyanarayana B, Chattannavar G. Efficacy of fresh Aloe vera gel against multi-drug resistant bacteria in infected leg ulcers. *Australasian Medical Journal*. 2012;5(6):305–309. doi: 10.4066/amj.2012.1301.

Castro FC, Magre A, Cherpinski R, et al. Effects of microcurrent application alone or in combination with topical Hypericum perforatum L. and Arnica montana L. on surgically induced wound healing in Wistar rats. *Homeopathy*. 2012 Jul;101(3):147–153. doi: 10.1016/j.homp.2012.05.006.

Dat AD, Poon F, Pham KB, Doust J. Aloe vera for treating acute and chronic wounds. *Cochrane Database of Systematic Reviews*. 2012 Feb 15;2:CD008762. doi: 10.1002/14651858.cd008762.pub2.

Gee RH, Charles A, Taylor N, Darbre PD. Oestrogenic and androgenic activity of triclosan in breast cancer cells. *Journal of Applied Toxicology*. 2008 Jan;28(1):78–91.

Kragh JF Jr, Walters TJ, Baer DG, et al. Survival with emergency tourniquet use to stop bleeding in major limb trauma. *Annals of Surgery*. 2009 Jan;249(1):1–7. doi: 10.1097/sla.0b013e31818842ba.

Müller P, Alber DG, Turnbull L, et al. Synergism between Medihoney and rifampicin against methicillin-resistant Staphylococcus aureus (MRSA). *PLoS One*. 2013;8(2):e57679. doi: 10.1371/journal.pone.0057679. Epub 2013 Feb 28.

Parente LM, Lino Júnior Rde S, Tresvenzol LM, et al. Wound healing and anti-inflammatory effect in animal models of Calendula officinalis L. growing in Brazil. *Evidence-Based Complementary and Alternative Medicine*. 2012;2012:375671. doi: 10.1155/2012/375671.

Pazyar N, Yaghoobi R, Bagherani N, Kazerouni A. A review of applications of tea tree oil in dermatology. *International Journal of Dermatology*. 2013 Jul;52(7):784–790. doi: 10.1111/j.1365-4632.2012.05654.x.

Silva N, Alves S, Gonçalves A, Amaral JS, Poeta P. Antimicrobial activity of essential oils from mediterranean aromatic plants against several foodborne and spoilage bacteria. *Food Science and Technology International*. 2013 Feb 26. www.ncbi.nlm.nih.gov/pubmed/23444311. [Epub ahead of print]

Süntar IP, Akkol EK, Yilmazer D, et al. Investigations on the in vivo wound healing potential of Hypericum perforatum L. *Journal of Ethnopharmacology*. 2010 Feb 3;127(2):468–477. doi: 10.1016/j.jep.2009.10.011.

Visavadia BG, Honeysett J, Danford MH. Manuka honey dressing: an effective treatment for chronic wound infections. *British Journal of Oral and Maxillofacial Surgery*. 2008 Jan;46(1):55–56.

Zampieri N, Zuin V, Burro R, Ottolenghi A, Camoglio FS. A prospective study in children: pre- and post-surgery use of vitamin E in surgical incisions. *Journal of Plastic, Reconstructive, and Aesthetic Surgery*. 2010 Sep;63(9):1474–1478. doi: 10.1016/j.bjps.2009.08.018.

Zhai Z, Haney DM, Wu L, et al. Alcohol extract of Echinacea pallida reverses stress-delayed wound healing in mice. *Phytomedicine*. 2009 Jun;16(6–7):669–678. doi: 10.1016/j.phymed.2009.02.010.

Chapter 28 Dandruff

Gaitanis G, Magiatis P, Hantschke M, Bassukas ID, Velegraki A. The Malassezia genus in skin and systemic diseases. *Clinical Microbiology Reviews*. 2012 Jan;25(1):106–141. doi: 10.1128/cmr.00021-11.

Hammer KA, Carson CF, Riley TV. In vitro activities of ketoconazole, econazole, miconazole, and Melaleuca alternifolia (tea tree) oil against Malassezia species. *Antimicrobial Agents and Chemotherapy*. 2000 Feb;44(2):467–469.

Ouwehand AC, Batsman A, Salminen S. Probiotics for the skin: a new area of potential application. *Letters in Applied Microbiology*. 2003;36(5):327–331. http://onlinelibrary.wiley.com/doi/10.1046/j.1472-765X.2003.01319.x/full. Accessed April 6, 2013.

Ro BI, Dawson TL. The role of sebaceous gland activity and scalp microfloral metabolism in the etiology of seborrheic dermatitis and dandruff. *Journal of Investigative Dermatology*. Symposium Proceedings. 2005 Dec;10(3):194–197.

Satchell AC, Saurajen A, Bell C, Barnetson RS. Treatment of dandruff with 5% tea tree oil shampoo. *Journal of the American Academy of Dermatology*. 2002;47:852–855.

Chapter 29 Depression

Akhondzadeh Basti A, Moshiri E, Noorbala AA, Jamshidi AH, Abbasi SH, Akhondzadeh S. Comparison of petal of Crocus sativus L. and fluoxetine in the treatment of depressed outpatients: a pilot double-blind randomized trial. *Progress in Neuropsychopharmacology & Biological Psychiatry*. 2007 Mar 30;31(2):439–442.

Cheung RY, Park IJ. Anger suppression, interdependent self-construal, and depression among Asian American and European American college students. *Cultural Diversity & Ethnic Minority Psychology*. 2010 Oct;16(4):517–525.

Cho EA, Oh HE. Effects of laughter therapy on depression, quality of life, resilience and immune responses in breast cancer survivors. *Journal of Korean Academy of Nursing*. 2011 Jun;41(3):285–293. doi: 10.4040/jkan.2011.41.3.285.

Conrad P, Adams C. The effects of clinical aromatherapy for anxiety and depression in the high risk postpartum woman—a pilot study. *Complementary Therapies in Clinical Practice*. 2012 Aug;18(3):164–168. doi: 10.1016/j.ctcp.2012.05.002.

Dirmaier J, Steinmann M, Krattenmacher T, Watzke B, Barghaan D, Koch U, et al. Non-pharmacological treatment of depressive disorders: a review of evidence-based treatment options. *Reviews on Recent Clinical Trials.* 2012 May;7(2):141–149.

Emmons RA, McCullough ME. Counting blessings versus burdens: an experimental investigation of gratitude and subjective well-being in daily life. *Journal of Personality and Social Psychology.* 2003 Feb;84(2):377–389.

Garcion E, Wion-Bardot N, Montero-Menei C, Berger F, Didier W. New clues about vitamin D functions in the nervous system. *Trends in Endocrinololgy and Metabolism.* 2002;13:100.

Hoffman BM, Babyak MA, Craighead WE, et al. Exercise and pharmacotherapy in patients with major depression: one-year follow-up of the SMILE study. *Psychosomatic Medicine.* 2011 Feb–Mar;73(2):127–133.

Jacka FN, Pasco JA, Mykletun A, et al. Association of Western and traditional diets with depression and anxiety in women. *American Journal of Psychiatry.* 2010 Mar;167(3):305–311. doi: 10.1176/appi.ajp.2009.09060881.

Kasper S, Caraci F, Forti B, Drago F, Aguglia E. Efficacy and tolerability of Hypericum extract for the treatment of mild to moderate depression. *European Neuropsychopharmacology.* 2010 Nov;20(11):747–765.

Lambert NM, Fincham FD, Stillman TF. Gratitude and depressive symptoms: the role of positive reframing and positive emotion. *Cognition and Emotion.* 2011. doi:10.1080/02699931.2011.595393.

Lucas M, Mirzaei F, O'Reilly EJ, et al. Dietary intake of n-3 and n-6 fatty acids and the risk of clinical depression in women: a 10-y prospective follow-up study. *American Journal of Clinical Nutrition.* 2011;93:1337–1343.

Lucas M, Mirzaei F, Pan A, et al. Coffee, caffeine, and risk of depression among women. *Archives of Internal Medicine.* 2011;171:1571–1578.

Mora-Ripoll R. Potential health benefits of simulated laughter: a narrative review of the literature and recommendations for future research. *Complementary Therapies in Medicine.* 2011 Jun;19(3):170–177.

Morris DW, Trivedi MH, Rush AJ. Folate and unipolar depression. *Journal of Alternative and Complementary Medicine.* 2008 Apr;14(3):277–285.

Muzik M, Hamilton SE, Lisa Rosenblum K, Waxler E, Hadi Z. Mindfulness yoga during pregnancy for psychiatrically at-risk women: preliminary results from a pilot feasibility study. *Complementary Therapies in Clinical Practice.* 2012 Nov;18(4):235–240. doi: 10.1016/j.ctcp.2012.06.006.

Niu K, Hozawa A, Kuriyama S, et al. Green tea consumption is associated with depressive symptoms in the elderly. *American Journal of Clinical Nutrition.* 2009 Dec;90(6):1615–22.

Norwood SJ, Bowker A, Buchholz A, Henderson KA, Goldfield G, Flament MF. Self-silencing and anger regulation as predictors of disordered eating among adolescent females. *Eating Behaviors.* 2011 Apr;12(2):112–118.

Panossian A, Wikman G, Sarris J. Rosenroot (Rhodiola rosea): traditional use, chemical composition, pharmacology and clinical efficacy. *Phytomedicine.* 2010 Jun;17(7):481–493.

Papakostas GI, Mischoulon D, Shyu I, et al. S-adenosyl methionine (SAMe) augmentation of serotonin reuptake inhibitors for antidepressant nonresponders with major depressive disorder: a double-blind, randomized clinical trial. *American Journal of Psychiatry.* 2010;167:942–948.

Salgado-Delgado R, Tapia Osorio A, Saderi N, Escobar C. Disruption of circadian rhythms: a crucial factor in the etiology of depression. *Depression Research Treatment.* 2011;2011:839743.

Sánchez-Villegas A, Delgado-Rodríguez M, Alonso A, Schlatter J, Lahortiga F, Serra Majem L, et al. Association of the Mediterranean dietary pattern with the incidence of depression: the Seguimiento Universidad de Navarra/University of Navarra follow-up (SUN) cohort. *Archives of General Psychiatry.* 2009 Oct;66(10):1090–1098.

Seol GH, Shim HS, Kim PJ, et al. Antidepressant-like effect of Salvia sclarea is explained by modulation of dopamine activities in rats. *Journal of Ethnopharmacology.* 2010 Jul 6;130(1):187–190. doi: 10.1016/j.jep.2010.04.035.

Shahidi M, Mojtahed A, Modabbernia A, Mojtahed M, Shafiabady A, Delavar A, et al. Laughter yoga versus group exercise program in elderly depressed women: a randomized controlled trial. *International Journal of Geriatric Psychiatry.* 2011 Mar;26(3):322–327. doi: 10.1002/gps.2545.

Su KP, Huang SY, Chiu CC, Shen WW. Omega-3 fatty acids in major depressive disorder. A preliminary double-blind, placebo-controlled trial. *Eurorpean Neuropsychopharmacology.* 2003;13:267–271.

Uebelacker LA, Epstein-Lubow G, Gaudiano BA, Tremont G, Battle CL, Miller IW. Hatha yoga for depression: critical review of the evidence for efficacy, plausible mechanisms of action, and directions for future research. *Journal of Psychiatric Practice.* 2010 Jan;16(1):22–33. doi: 10.1097/01.pra.0000367775.88388.96.

Chapter 30 Diabetes Prevention

Ahuja KD, Robertson IK, Geraghty DP, Ball MJ. Effects of chili consumption on postprandial glucose, insulin, and energy metabolism. *American Journal of Clinical Nutrition.* 2006 Jul;84(1):63–69.

Alberti G, Zimmet P, Shaw J, Bloomgarden Z, Kaufman F, Silink M; Consensus Workshop Group. Type-2 diabetes in the young: the evolving epidemic: the international diabetes federation consensus workshop. *Diabetes Care.* 2004;27(7):1798–1811.

Bacardi-Gascon M, Duenas-Mena D, Jimenez-Cruz A. Lowering effect on postprandial glycemic response of nopales added to Mexican breakfasts. *Diabetes Care*. 2007;30:1264–1265.

Baker WL, Gutierrez-Williams G, White CM, et al. Effect of cinnamon on glucose control and lipid parameters. *Diabetes Care*. 2008;31:41–43.

Basch E, Ulbricht C, Kuo G, Szapary P, Smith M. Therapeutic applications of fenugreek. *Alternative Medicine Review*. 2003 Feb;8(1):20–27. Review.

Cooper AJ, Sharp SJ, Lentjes MA, et al. A prospective study of the association between quantity and variety of fruit and vegetable intake and incident type-2 diabetes. *Diabetes Care*. 2012 Jun;35(6):1293–1300. www.ncbi.nlm.nih.gov/pmc/articles/pmc3357245/?tool=pubmed. Accessed July 10, 2012.

Frati-Munari AC, Altamirano-Bustamante E, Rodríguez-Bárcenas N, et al. Hypoglycemic action of Opuntia streptacantha Lemaire: study using raw extracts. *Archivos de investigación médica* (Mexico). 1989;20:321–325.

Guevara-Cruz M, Tovar AR, Aguilar-Salinas CA, et al. A dietary pattern including nopal, chia seed, soy protein, and oat reduces serum triglycerides and glucose intolerance in patients with metabolic syndrome. *Journal of Nutrition*. 2012 Jan;142(1):64–69. doi: 10.3945/jn.111.147447. http://jn.nutrition.org/content/142/1/64.long. Accessed May 2, 2013.

Hsu CH, Liao YL, Lin SC, et al. The mushroom Agaricus Blazei Murill in combination with metformin and gliclazide improves insulin resistance in type-2 diabetes: a randomized, double-blinded, and placebo-controlled clinical trial. *Journal of Alternative and Complementary Medicine*. 2007;13:97–102.

Hyson DA. A comprehensive review of apples and apple components and their relationship to human health. *Advances in Nutrition*. 2011 Sep;2(5):408–420. doi: 10.3945/an.111.000513. http://0-www.ncbi.nlm.nih.gov.skyline.ucdenver.edu/pmc/articles/pmc3183591/. Accessed May 2, 2013.

Larsson SC, Wolk A. Magnesium intake and risk of type-2 diabetes: a meta-analysis. *Journal of Internal Medicine*. 2007;262:208–214.

Pan A, Sun J, Chen Y, et al. Effects of a flaxseed-derived lignan supplement in type 2 diabetic patients: a randomized, double-blind, cross-over trial. *PLoS One*. 2007;2:e1148.

Rosenzweig S, Reibel DK, Greeson JM, et al. Mindfulness-based stress reduction is associated with improved glycemic control in type-2 diabetes mellitus: a pilot study. *Alternative Therapies in Health and Medicine*. 2007 Sep–Oct;13(5):36–38.

Salazar-Martinez E, Willett WC, Ascherio A, et al. Coffee consumption and risk for type-2 diabetes mellitus. *Annals of Internal Medicine*. 2004;140:1–8.

Shivanna N, Naika M, Khanum F, Kaul VK. Antioxidant, anti-diabetic and renal protective properties of Stevia rebaudiana. *Journal of Diabetes and its Complications*. 2013 Mar–Apr;27(2):103–113. doi: 10.1016/j.jdiacomp.2012.10.001.

Sierra M, Garcia JJ, Fernandez N, et al. Therapeutic effects of psyllium in type 2 diabetic patients. *European Journal of Clinical Nutrition*. 2002;56:830–842.

Song Y, Manson JE, Buring JE, Liu S. Dietary magnesium intake in relation to plasma insulin levels and risk of type-2 diabetes in women. *Diabetes Care*. 2004;27:59–65.

Song Y, Manson JE, Buring JE, Sesso HD, Liu S. Associations of dietary flavonoids with risk of type-2 diabetes, and markers of insulin resistance and systemic inflammation in women: a prospective study and cross-sectional analysis. *Journal of the American College of Nutrition*. 2005 Oct;24(5):376–384.

Tapola N, Karvonen H, Niskanen L, Mikola M, Sarkkinen E. Glycemic responses of oat bran products in type 2 diabetic patients. *Nutrition Metabolism and Cardiovascular Diseases*. 2005 Aug;15(4):255–261.

Uribe M, Dibildox M, Malpica S, et al. Beneficial effect of vegetable protein diet supplemented with psyllium plantago in patients with hepatic encephalopathy and diabetes mellitus (abstract). *Gastroenterology*. 1985;88:901–907.

Volpe SL. Magnesium, the metabolic syndrome, insulin resistance, and type-2 diabetes mellitus. *Critical Reviews in Food Science and Nutrition*. 2008 Mar;48(3):293–300. doi: 10.1080/10408390701326235.

Wood PJ, Braaten JT, Scott FW, Riedel KD, Wolynetz MS, Collins MW. Effect of dose and modification of viscous properties of oat gum on plasma glucose and insulin following an oral glucose load. *British Journal of Nutrition*. 1994;72:731–734.

Chapter 31 Diaper Rash

Banu A, Sathyanarayana B, Chattannavar G. Efficacy of fresh Aloe vera gel against multi-drug resistant bacteria in infected leg ulcers. *Australasian Medical Journal*. 2012;5(6):305–309. doi: 10.4066/amj.2012.1301.

Bernardes I, Felipe Rodrigues MP, Bacelli GK, Munin E, Alves LP, Costa MS. Aloe vera extract reduces both growth and germ tube formation by Candida albicans. *Mycoses*. 2012 May;55(3):257–261. doi: 10.1111/j.1439-0507.2011.02079.x.

Efstratiou E, Hussain AI, Nigam PS, Moore JE, Ayub MA, Rao JR. Antimicrobial activity of Calendula officinalis petal extracts against fungi, as well as Gram-negative and Gram-positive clinical pathogens. *Complementary Therapies in Clinical Practice*. 2012 Aug;18(3):173–176. doi: 10.1016/j.ctcp.2012.02.003.

Hutter JA, Salman M, Stavinoha WB, et al. Antiinflammatory C-glucosyl chromone from Aloe barbadensis. *Journal of Natural Products*. 1996;59:541–543.

Intahphuak S, Khonsung P, Panthong A. Anti-inflammatory, analgesic, and antipyretic activities of virgin coconut oil. *Pharmaceutical Biology*. 2010 Feb;48(2):151–157. doi: 10.3109/13880200903062614.

Panahi Y, Sharif MR, Sharif A, et al. A randomized comparative trial on the therapeutic efficacy of topical aloe vera and Calendula officinalis on diaper dermatitis in children. *Scientific World Journal*. 2012;2012:810234. doi: 10.1100/2012/810234.

Parente LM, Lino Júnior Rde S, Tresvenzol LM, et al. Wound healing and anti-inflammatory effect in animal models of Calendula officinalis L. growing in Brazil. *Evidence-Based Complementary and Alternative Medicine*. 2012;2012:375671. doi: 10.1155/2012/375671.

Chapter 32 Diarrhea

Bengmark S. Ecological control of the gastrointestinal tract: the role of probiotic flora. *Gut* 1998;42:2–7. As cited in Guarner F, Malagelada JR. Gut flora in health and diseases. *The Lancet* 2003;61(9371):512–519.

Ejemot RI, Ehiri JE, Meremikwu MM, Critchley JA. Hand washing for preventing diarrhoea. *Cochrane Database of Systematic Reviews*. 2008 Jan 23;(1):CD004265. doi: 10.1002/14651858. cd004265.pub2.

Gull I, Saeed M, Shaukat H, Aslam SM, Samra ZQ, Athar AM. Inhibitory effect of Allium sativum and Zingiber officinale extracts on clinically important drug resistant pathogenic bacteria. *Annals of Clinical Microbiology and Antimicrobials*. 2012 Apr 27;11:8.

Hilton E, Rindos P, Isenberg HD. Lactobacillus GG Vaginal Suppositories and Vaginitis. *Journal of Clinical Microbiology*. 1995;33:1433.

Johnson HD, Sholcosky D, Gabello K, Ragni R, Ogonosky N. Sex differences in public restroom handwashing behavior associated with visual behavior prompts. *Perceptual and Motor Skills*. 2003 Dec;97(3 Pt 1):805–10.

Karuppiah P, Rajaram S. Antibacterial effect of Allium sativum cloves and Zingiber officinale rhizomes against multiple-drug resistant clinical pathogens. *Asian Pacific Journal of Tropical Biomedicine*. 2012 Aug;2(8):597–601. doi: 10.1016/ s2221-1691(12)60104-x.

Larsson PG, Stray-Pedersen B, Ryttig KR, Larsen S. Human lactobacilli as supplementation of clindamycin to patients with bacterial vaginosis reduce the recurrence rate: a 6-month, double-blind, randomized, placebo-controlled study. *BMC Women's Health*. 2008;8:3.

Lee HS, Ahn YJ. Growth-inhibiting effects of Cinnamomum cassia bark-derived materials on human intestinal bacteria. *Journal of Agricultural and Food Chemistry*. 1998;46:8–12.

Leyer GJ, Li S, Mubasher ME, et al. Probiotic effects on cold and influenza-like symptom incidence and duration in children. *Pediatrics*. 2009;124:e172–179.

Liu L, Johnson HL, Cousens S, Perin J, Scott S, Lawn JE, et al; Child Health Epidemiology Reference Group of WHO and UNICEF. Global, regional, and national causes of child mortality: an updated systematic analysis for 2010 with time trends since 2000. *The Lancet*. 2012 Jun 9;379(9832):2151–2161. doi: 10.1016/s0140-6736(12)60560-1.

McFarland LV. Meta-analysis of probiotics for the prevention of antibiotic associated diarrhea and the treatment of Clostridium difficile disease. *American Journal of Gastroenterology*. 2006;101:812–822.

McFarland LV. Meta-analysis of probiotics for the prevention of traveler's diarrhea. *Travel Medicine and Infecious Disease*. 2007 Mar;5(2):97–105. Epub 2005 Dec 5.

Niedzielin K, Kordecki H, Birkenfeld B. A controlled, double-blind, randomized study on the efficacy of Lactobacillus plantarum 299V in patients with irritable bowel syndrome. *European Journal of Gastroenterology and Hepatology*. 2001;13:1143–1147.

Parent D, Bossens M, Bayot D, et al. Therapy of bacterial vaginosis using exogenously-applied Lactobacilli acidophili and a low dose of estriol: a placebo-controlled multicentric clinical trial. *Arzneimittelforschung*. 1996;46:68–73.

Savino F, Pelle E, Palumeri E, et al. Lactobacillus reuteri (American Type Culture Collection Strain 55730) versus simethicone in the treatment of infantile colic: a prospective randomized study. *Pediatrics*. 2007;119:e124–130.

Shornikova AV, Casas IA, Mykkanen H, et al. Bacteriotherapy with Lactobacillus reuteri in rotavirus gastroenteritis. *Pediatric Infectious Disease Journal*. 1997;16:1103–1107.

Si W, Gong J, Tsao R, Kalab M, Yang R, Yin Y. Bioassay-guided purification and identification of antimicrobial components in Chinese green tea extract. *Journal of Chromatography*. A. 2006 Sep 1;1125(2):204–210.

Touhami M, Boudraa G, Mary JY, et al. Clinical consequences of replacing milk with yogurt in persistent infantile diarrhea. *Annales des Pédiatrie* (Paris). 1992;39:79–86.

Volman JJ, Mensink RP, Buurman WA, Plat J. In vivo effects of dietary (1→3), (1→4)-Beta-D-glucans from oat on mucosal immune responses in man and mice. *Scandinavian Journal of Gastroenterology*. 2011 May;46(5):603–10.

Chapter 33 Dry Skin

Agero AL, Verallo-Rowell VM. A randomized double-blind controlled trial comparing extra virgin coconut oil with mineral oil as a moisturizer for mild to moderate xerosis. *Dermatitis*. 2004 Sep;15(3):109–116.

Casetti F, Wölfle U, Gehring W, Schempp CM. Dermocosmetics for dry skin: a new role for botanical extracts. *Skin Pharmacology and Physiology*. 2011;24(6):289–293. doi: 10.1159/000329214.

Ghadially R, Brown BE, Sequeira-Martin SM, Feingold KR, Elias PM. The aged epidermal permeability barrier. Structural, functional, and lipid biochemical abnormalities in humans and a senescent murine model. *Journal of Clinical Investigation*. 1995 May;95(5):2281–2290. doi: 10.1172/jcI117919. www.ncbi.nlm.nih.gov/pmc/articles/pmc295841/. Accessed May 6, 2013.

Kempers S, Katz HI, Wildnauer R, Green B. An evaluation of the effect of an alpha hydroxy acid-blend skin cream in the cosmetic improvement of symptoms of moderate to severe xerosis, epidermolytic hyperkeratosis, and ichthyosis. *Cutis*. 1998;61:347–350.

Pappas A. Epidermal surface lipids. *Dermatoendocrinology*. 2009 Mar–Apr;1(2):72–76. www.ncbi.nlm.nih.gov/pmc/articles/pmc2835894/. Accessed May 6, 2013.

Yarmolinsky L, Zaccai M, Ben-Shabat S, Huleihel M. Anti-herpetic activity of Callissia fragrans and Simmondsia chinensis leaf extracts in vitro. *Open Virology Journal*. 2010;4: 57–62. doi: 10.2174/1874357901004010057.

Chapter 34 Earaches

Coco A, Vernacchio L, Horst M, Anderson A. Management of acute otitis media after publication of the 2004 AAP and AAFP clinical practice guideline. *Pediatrics*. 2010 Feb;125(2):214–220. doi: 10.1542/peds.2009-1115. http://pediatrics.aappublications.org/content/125/2/214.long. Accessed May 9, 2013.

Efstratiou E, Hussain AI, Nigam PS, et al. Antimicrobial activity of Calendula officinalis petal extracts against fungi, as well as Gram-negative and Gram-positive clinical pathogens. *Complementary Therapies in Clinical Practice*. 2012 Aug;18(3):173–176. doi: 10.1016/j.ctcp.2012.02.003.

Griffin G, Flynn CA. Antihistamines and/or decongestants for otitis media with effusion (OME) in children. *Cochrane Database of Systematic Reviews*. 2011 Sep 7;(9):CD003423. doi: 10.1002/14651858.cd003423.pub3.

Hao Q, Lu Z, Dong BR, Huang CQ, Wu T. Probiotics for preventing acute upper respiratory tract infections. *Cochrane Database of Systematic Reviews*. 2011 Sep 7;(9):CD006895. doi: 10.1002/14651858.cd006895.pub2.

Hoberman A, Paradise JL, Reynolds EA, Urkin J. Efficacy of Auralgan for treating ear pain in children with acute otitis media. *Archives of Pediatric and Adolescent Medicine*. 1997 Jul;151(7):675–678.

Orhan IE, Kartal M, Gülpinar AR, et al. Assessment of antimicrobial and antiprotozoal activity of the olive oil macerate samples of Hypericum perforatum and their LC-DAD-MS analyses. *Food Chemistry*. 2013 Jun 1;138(2–3):870–875. doi: 10.1016/j.foodchem.2012.11.053.

Sarrell EM, Mandelberg A, Cohen HA. Efficacy of naturopathic extracts in the management of ear pain associated with acute otitis media. *Archives of Pediatric and Adolescent Medicine*. 2001 Jul;155(7):796–799. http://archpedi.jamanetwork.com/article.aspx?articleid=190792. Accessed May 9, 2013.

Turker AU, Camper ND. Biological activity of common mullein, a medicinal plant. *Journal of Ethnopharmacology*. 2002 Oct;82(2–3):117–125.

Chapter 35 Eye Health

Abdel-Aal el-SM, Akhtar H, Zaheer K, Ali R. Dietary sources of lutein and zeaxanthin carotenoids and their role in eye health. *Nutrients*. 2013 Apr 9;5(4):1169–1185. doi: 10.3390/nu5041169. www.mdpi.com/2072-6643/5/4/1169. Accessed May 10, 2013.

Age-Related Eye Disease Study 2 (AREDS2) Research Group. Lutein + zeaxanthin and omega-3 fatty acids for age-related macular degeneration: the Age-Related Eye Disease Study 2 (AREDS2) Randomized Clinical Trial. *JAMA*. 2013 May 5:1–11. doi: 10.1001/jama.2013.4997. [Epub ahead of print]

Bravetti G. Preventive medical treatment of senile cataract with vitamin E and anthocyanosides: clinical evaluation. *Annali di Ottalmologica e Clinica Oculistica*. 1989;115:109. As reported in Head KA. Natural therapies for ocular disorders, part two: cataracts and glaucoma. *Alternative Medicine Review*. 2001 Apr;6(2):141–166.

Brignole-Baudouin F, Baudouin C, Aragona P, et al. A multicentre, double-masked, randomized, controlled trial assessing the effect of oral supplementation of omega-3 and omega-6 fatty acids on a conjunctival inflammatory marker in dry eye patients. *Acta Ophthalmologica*. 2011 Nov;89(7):e591–597. doi: 10.1111/j.1755-3768.2011.02196.x.

Canter PH, Ernst E. Anthocyanosides of Vaccinium myrtillus (bilberry) for night vision—a systematic review of placebo-controlled trials. *Survey of Ophthalmology*. 2004 Jan–Feb;49(1):38–50.

Caselli L. Clinical and electroretinographic study on activity of anthocyanosides. *Archivo di Medicina Interna*. 1985;37:29–35. As reported in Head KA. Natural therapies for ocular disorders, part two: cataracts and glaucoma. *Alternative Medicine Review*. 2001 Apr;6(2):141–166.

Chong EW, Kreis AJ, Wong TY, Simpson JA, Guymer RH. Dietary omega-3 fatty acid and fish intake in the primary prevention of age-related macular degeneration: a systematic review and meta-analysis. *Archives of Ophthalmology*. 2008;126:826–833.

Christen WG, Glynn RJ, Chew EY, et al. Folic acid, pyridoxine, and cyanocobalamin combination treatment and age-related macular degeneration in women. *Archives of Internal Medicine*. 2009;169:335–341.

Christen WG, Manson JE, Glynn RJ. et al. A randomized trial of beta carotene and age-related cataract in US physicians. *Archives of Ophthalmology*. 2003;121(3):372–378.

Dorairaj S, Ritch R, Liebmann JM. Visual improvement in a patient taking ginkgo biloba extract: a case study. *Explore* (NY). 2007 Jul–Aug;3(4):39.

Dornstauder B, Suh M, Kuny S, Gaillard F, Macdonald IM, Clandinin MT, et al. Dietary docosahexaenoic acid supplementation prevents age-related functional losses and A2E accumulation in the retina. *Investigative Ophthalmology and Vision Science*. 2012 Apr 24;53(4):2256–2265. doi: 10.1167/iovs.11-8569.

Fursova AZh, Gesarevich OG, Gonchar AM, et al. [Dietary supplementation with bilberry extract prevents macular degeneration and cataracts in senesce-accelerated OXYS rats]. *Advances in Gerontology*. 2005;16:76–79.

Gupta SK, Halder N, Srivastava S, Trivedi D, Joshi S, Varma SD. Green tea (Camellia sinensis) protects against selenite-induced oxidative stress in experimental cataractogenesis. *Ophthalmic Research*. 2002 Jul–Aug;34(4):258–263.

Heydari B, Kazemi T, Zarban A, Ghahramani S. Correlation of cataract with serum lipids, glucose and antioxidant activities: a case-control study. *West Indian Medical Journal*. 2012 Jun;61(3):230–234.

Ho L, van Leeuwen R, Witteman JC, et al. Reducing the genetic risk of age-related macular degeneration with dietary antioxidants, zinc, and omega-3 fatty acids: the Rotterdam study. *Archives of Ophthalmology*. 2011 Jun;129(6):758–766. doi: 10.1001/archophthalmol.2011.141.

Kangari H, Eftekhari MH, Sardari S, et al. Short-term consumption of oral omega-3 and dry eye syndrome. *Ophthalmology*. 2013 May 1. pii: S0161–6420(13)00337-0. doi: 10.1016/j.ophtha.2013.04.006. [Epub ahead of print]

Liew G, Mitchell P, Wong TY, Rochtchina E, Wang JJ. The association of aspirin use with age-related macular degeneration. *JAMA Internal Medicine*. 2013 Feb 25;173(3):258–264. doi: 10.1001/jamainternmed.2013.1583.

Miyake S, Takahashi N, Sasaki M, Kobayashi S, Tsubota K, Ozawa Y. Vision preservation during retinal inflammation by anthocyanin-rich bilberry extract: cellular and molecular mechanism. *Laboratory Investigation*. 2012 Jan;92(1):102–109. doi: 10.1038/labinvest.2011.132.

Moïse MM, Benjamin LM, Doris TM, Dalida KN, Augustin NO. Role of Mediterranean diet, tropical vegetables rich in antioxidants, and sunlight exposure in blindness, cataract and glaucoma among African type 2 diabetics. *International Journal of Ophthamology*. 2012;5(2):231–237. doi: 10.3980/j.issn.2222-3959.2012.02.23. www.ncbi.nlm.nih.gov/pmc/articles/pmc3359045/. Accessed December 17, 2012.

Perossini M, Guidi G, Chiellini S, Siravo D. [Diabetic and hypertensive retinopathy therapy with Vaccinium myrtillus anthocyanosides (Tegens): a double blind, placebo-controlled clinical trial]. *Annali di ottalmologica e clinica oculistica*. 1987;113:1173–1177.

Scharrer A, Ober M. [Anthocyanosides in the treatment of retinopathies (author's transl)]. *Klinische Monatsblatter fur Augenheilkunde*. 1981 May;178(5):386–389.

Spadea L, Balestrazzi E. Treatment of vascular retinopathies with pycnogenol. *Phytotherapy Research*. 2001;15:219–223.

Steigerwalt RD, Gianni B, Paolo M, et al. Effects of Mirtogenol on ocular blood flow and intraocular hypertension in asymptomatic subjects. *Molecular Vision*. 2008;14:1288–1292.

Vishwanathan R, Chung M, Johnson EJ. A systematic review on zinc for the prevention and treatment of age-related macular degeneration. *Investigative Ophthalmology and Vision Science*. 2013 May 7. pii: iovs.12-11552v1. doi: 10.1167/iovs.12-11552.

Xu JY, Wu LY, Zheng XQ, Lu JL, Wu MY, Liang R. Green tea polyphenols attenuating ultraviolet B-induced damage to human retinal pigment epithelial cells in vitro. *Investigative Ophthalmology and Vision Science*. 2010 Dec;51(12):6665–6670.

Wang LL, Sun Y, Huang K, Zheng L. Curcumin, a potential therapeutic candidate for retinal diseases. *Molecular Nutrition and Food Research*. 2013 Feb 18. doi: 10.1002/mnfr.201200718. [Epub ahead of print]

Wojtowicz JC, Butovich I, Uchiyama E, Aronowicz J, Agee S, McCulley JP. Pilot, prospective, randomized, double-masked, placebo-controlled clinical trial of an omega-3 supplement for dry eye. *Cornea*. 2011 Mar;30(3):308–314. doi: 10.1097/ico.0b013e3181f22e03.

Zafra-Stone S, Yasmin T, Bagchi M, Chatterjee A, Vinson JA, Bagchi D. Berry anthocyanins as novel antioxidants in human health and disease prevention. *Molecular Nutrition and Food Research*. 2007 Jun;51(6):675–683.

Chapter 36 Fatigue

Alm T. Ethnobotany of Rhodiola rosea (Crassulaceae) in Norway. *SIDA*. 2004;21(1):321–344.

Arce M, Michopoulos V, Shepard KN, Ha QC, Wilson ME. Diet choice, cortisol reactivity, and emotional feeding in socially housed rhesus monkey. *Physiology and Behavior*. 2010 November 2;101(4):446–455. doi: 10.1016/j.physbeh.2010.07.010. www.ncbi.nlm.nih.gov/pmc/articles/pmc2949469/. Accessed May 6, 2013.

Bjersing JL, Erlandsson M, Bokarewa MI, Mannerkorpi K. Exercise and obesity in fibromyalgia: beneficial roles of IGF-1 and resistin? *Arthritis Research and Therapy*. 2013 Feb 27;15(1):R34.

Hartz AJ, Bentler S, Noyes R, et al. Randomized controlled trial of Siberian ginseng for chronic fatigue. *Psychological Medicine*. 2004;34:51–61.

Ishaque S, Shamseer L, Bukutu C, Vohra S. Rhodiola rosea for physical and mental fatigue: a systematic review. *BMC Complementary and Alternative Medicine*. 2012;12: 70. doi: 10.1186/1472-6882-12-70. www.ncbi.nlm.nih.gov/pmc/articles/pmc3541197/#b3. Accessed May 6, 2013.

Johansson B, Bjuhr H, Rönnbäck L. Mindfulness-based stress reduction (MBSR) improves long-term mental fatigue after stroke or traumatic brain injury. *Brain Injury*. 2012;26(13–14):1621–1628. doi: 10.3109/02699052.2012.700082.

Panossian A, Wikman G. Evidence-based efficacy of adaptogens in fatigue, and molecular mechanisms related to their stress-protective activity. *Current Clinical Pharmacology*. 2009 Sep;4(3):198–219.

Ross A, Friedmann E, Bevans M, Thomas S. Frequency of yoga practice predicts health: results of a national survey of yoga practitioners. *Evidence-Based Complementary and Alternative Medicine*. 2012;2012:983258. doi: 10.1155/2012/983258. www.ncbi.nlm.nih.gov/pmc/articles/pmc3425136/. Accessed May 6, 2013.

Suh SY, Bae WK, Ahn HY, Choi SE, Jung GC, Yeom CH. Intravenous vitamin C administration reduces fatigue in office workers: a double-blind randomized controlled trial. *Nutrition Journal*. 2012 Jan 20;11:7. doi: 10.1186/1475-2891-11-7.

Varney E, Buckle J. Effect of inhaled essential oils on mental exhaustion and moderate burnout: a small pilot study. *Journal of Alternative and Complementary Medicine*. 2013 Jan;19(1):69–71. doi: 10.1089/acm.2012.0089.

White PD, Goldsmith KA, Johnson AL, et al; PACE trial management group. Comparison of adaptive pacing therapy, cognitive behaviour therapy, graded exercise therapy, and specialist medical care for chronic fatigue syndrome (PACE): a randomised trial. *The Lancet*. 2011 Mar 5;377(9768):823–836. doi: 10.1016/s0140-6736(11)60096-2.

Chapter 37 Hayfever and Seasonal Allergies

Bakhshaee M, Jabbari F, Hoseini S, et al. Effect of silymarin in the treatment of allergic rhinitis. *Otolaryngology—Head and Neck Surgery*. 2011;145:904–909.

Chandrashekhar VM, Halagali KS, Nidavani RB, et al. Anti-allergic activity of German chamomile (Matricaria recutita L.) in mast cell mediated allergy model. *Journal of Ethnopharmacology*. 2011 Sep 1;137(1):336–340.

Johnston CS, Solomon RE, Corte C. Vitamin C depletion is associated with alterations in blood histamine and plasma free carnitine in adults. *Journal of the American College of Nutrition*. 1996;15:586–591.

Käufeler R, Polasek W, Brattström A, Koetter U. Efficacy and safety of butterbur herbal extract Ze 339 in seasonal allergic rhinitis: postmarketing surveillance study. *Advances in Therapy*. 2006 Mar–Apr;23(2):373–384.

Lee DK, Gray RD, Robb FM, Fujihara S, Lipworth BJ. A placebo-controlled evaluation of butterbur and fexofenadine on objective and subjective outcomes in perennial allergic rhinitis. *Clinical and Experimental Allergy*. 2004 Apr;34(4):646–649.

MacArtain P, Gill C, Brooks M, et al. Nutritional value of edible seaweeds. *Nutrition Reviews*. 2007;65(12):535–543. http://li123-4.members.linode.com/files/nutritional%20value%20of%20edible%20seaweeds.pdf. Accessed October 16, 2012.

Marchisio P, Varricchio A, Baggi E, et al. Hypertonic saline is more effective than normal saline in seasonal allergic rhinitis in children. *International Journal of Immunopathology and Pharmacology*. 2012 Jul–Sep;25(3):721–730.

Mittman P. Randomized, double-blind study of freeze-dried Urtica dioica in the treatment of allergic rhinitis. *Planta Medica*. 1990;56:44–47.

Miyake Y, Sasaki S, Ohya Y, et al; Osaka Maternal And Child Health Study Group. Dietary intake of seaweed and minerals and prevalence of allergic rhinitis in Japanese pregnant females: baseline data from the Osaka Maternal and Child Health Study. *Annals of Epidemiology*. 2006 Aug;16(8):614–621.

Miyake Y, Sasaki S, Tanaka K, Ohya Y, Miyamoto S, Matsunaga I, et al; Osaka Maternal and Child Health Study Group. Fish and fat intake and prevalence of allergic rhinitis in Japanese females: the Osaka Maternal and Child Health Study. *Journal of the American College of Nutrition*. 2007 Jun;26(3):279–287.

Otsuka H, Inaba M, Fujikura T, Kunitomo M. Histochemical and functional characteristics of metachromatic cells in the nasal epithelium in allergic rhinitis: studies of nasal scrapings and their dispersed cells. *Journal of Allergy and Clinical Immunology*. 1995 Oct;96(4):528–536.

Saarinen K, Jantunen J, Haahtela T. Birch pollen honey for birch pollen allergy—a randomized controlled pilot study. *International Archives of Allergy and Immunology*. 2011;155(2):160–166.

Schabussova I, Wiedermann U. Lactic acid bacteria as novel adjuvant systems for prevention and treatment of atopic diseases. *Current Opinion in Allergy and Clinical Immunology*. 2008 Dec;8(6):557–564. doi: 10.1097/aci.0b013e328317b88b.

Chapter 38 Headaches: Migraine, Tension, and Sinus

Cady RK, Goldstein J, Nett R, et al. A double-blind placebo-controlled pilot study of sublingual feverfew and ginger (LipiGesic M) in the treatment of migraine. *Headache*. 2011 Jul–Aug;51(7):1078–1086. doi: 10.1111/j.1526-4610.2011.01910.x.

Calhoun, AH, Ford S. Behavioral sleep modification may revert transformed migraine to episodic migraine. *Headache*. 2007 Sep;47(8):1178–1183.

De Marino S, Borbone N, Zollo F, Ianaro A, Di Meglio P, Iorizzi M. New sesquiterpene lactones from Laurus nobilis leaves as inhibitors of nitric oxide production. *Planta Medica*. 2005 Aug;71(8):706–710.

Diamond S, Freitag FG. Cold as an adjunctive therapy for headache. *Postgraduate Medicine*. 1986 Jan;79(1):305–309.

Engstrøm M, Hagen K, Bjørk MH, et al. Sleep quality, arousal and pain thresholds in migraineurs: a blinded controlled polysomnographic study. *Journal of Headache Pain*. 2013 Feb 14;14(1):12. doi: 10.1186/1129-2377-14-12. www.ncbi.nlm.nih.gov/pmc/articles/pmc3620398/. Accessed May 10, 2013.

Ferro EC, Biagini AP, da Silva IE, Silva ML, Silva JR. The combined effect of acupuncture and Tanacetum parthenium on quality of life in women with headache: randomised study. *Acupuncture in Medicine*. 2012 Dec;30(4):252–257. doi: 10.1136/acupmed-2012-010195.

Gobel H, Fresenius J, Heinze A, et al. Effectiveness of Oleum menthae piperitae and paracetamol in therapy of headache of the tension type. *Nervenarzt*. 1996;67:672–681.

Gobel H, Schmidt G, Soyka D. Effect of peppermint and eucalyptus oil preparations on neurophysiological and experimental algesimetric headache parameters. *Cephalalgia*. 1994;14:228–234;discussion 182.

Hsieh LL, Liou HH, Lee LH, Chen TH, Yen AM. Effect of acupressure and trigger points in treating headache: a randomized controlled trial. *American Journal of Chinese Medicine*. 2010;38(1):1–14.

Holroyd KA, O'Donnell FJ, Stensland M, Lipchik GL, Cordingley GE, Carlson BW. Management of chronic tension-type headache with tricyclic antidepressant medication, stress management therapy, and their combination: a randomized controlled trial. *JAMA*. 2001 May 2;285(17):2208–2215.

Kemper KJ. Feverfew (Tanacetum parthenium). Longwood Herbal Task Force. Center for Holistic Pediatric Education and Research. www.longwoodherbal.org/feverfew/feverfew.pdf. Accessed October 31, 2012.

Palatty PL, Haniadka R, Valder B, Arora R, Baliga MS. Ginger in the prevention of nausea and vomiting: a review. *Critical Reviews in Food Science and Nutrition*. 2013;53(7):659–669. doi: 10.1080/10408398.2011.553751.

Sasannejad P, Saeedi M, Shoeibi A, et al. Lavender essential oil in the treatment of migraine headache: a placebo-controlled clinical trial. *European Neurology*. 2012;67(5):288–291.

Silberstein SD, Armellino JJ, Hoffman HD, et al. Treatment of menstruation-associated migraine with the nonprescription combination of acetaminophen, aspirin, and caffeine: results from three randomized, placebo-controlled studies. *Clinical Therapeutics*. 1999;21:475–491.

Singh RK, Martinez A, Baxter P. Head cooling for exercise-induced headache. *Journal of Child Neurology*. 2006 Dec;21(12):1067–1068.

Chapter 39 Heart Health

Ali M, Afzal M. A potent inhibitor of thrombin stimulated platelet thromboxane formation from unprocessed tea. *Prostaglandins, Leukotrienes, and Medicine*. 1987;27:9–13.

Aviram M, Rosenblat M. Pomegranate protection against cardiovascular diseases. *Evidence-Based Complementary and Alternative Medicine*. 2012;2012:382763. doi: 10.1155/2012/382763.

Belin RJ, Greenland P, Martin L, et al. Fish intake and the risk of incident heart failure: the Women's Health Initiative. *Circulation: Heart Failure*. 2011;4:404–413.

Berryman CE, Grieger JA, West SG, et al. Acute consumption of walnuts and walnut components differentially affect postprandial lipemia, endothelial function, oxidative stress, and cholesterol efflux in humans with mild hypercholesterolemia. *Journal of Nutrition*. 2013 Jun;143(6):788–794. doi: 10.3945/jn.112.170993.

Catalgol B, Batirel S, Taga Y, Ozer NK. Resveratrol: French paradox revisited. *Frontiers in Pharmacology*. 2012;3:141. doi: 10.3389/fphar.2012.00141. www.ncbi.nlm.nih.gov/pmc/articles/pmc3398412/. Accessed May 29, 2013.

Eaker ED, Sullivan LM, Kelly-Hayes M, D'Agostino RB Sr, Benjamin EJ. Anger and hostility predict the development of atrial fibrillation in men in the Framingham Offspring Study. *Circulation*. 2004 Mar 16;109(10):1267–1271.

Esmaillzadeh A, Tahbaz F, Gaieni I, et al. Concentrated pomegranate juice improves lipid profiles in diabetic patients with hyperlipidemia. *Journal of Medicinal Food*. 2004;7:305–308.

Estruch R, Ros E, Salas-Salvadó J, et al; PREDIMED Study Investigators. Primary prevention of cardiovascular disease with a Mediterranean diet. *New England Journal of Medicine*. 2013 Apr 4;368(14):1279–290. doi: 10.1056/nejmoa1200303. www.nejm.org/doi/full/10.1056/nejmoa1200303. Accessed May 29, 2013.

Geleijnse JM, Launer LJ, Hofman A, et al. Tea flavonoids may protect against atherosclerosis: the Rotterdam Study. *Archives of Internal Medicine*. 1999;159:2170–2174.

Khan A, Safdar M, Ali Khan MM, Khattak KN, Anderson RA. Cinnamon improves glucose and lipids of people with type-2 diabetes. *Diabetes Care*. 2003 Dec;26(12):3215–3218.

Kokubo Y, Iso H, Ishihara J, Okada K, Inoue M, Tsugane S; Japan Public Health Center–Based Study Group. Association of dietary intake of soy, beans, and isoflavones with risk of cerebral and myocardial infarctions in Japanese populations: the Japan Public Health Center (JPHC)–based study cohort I. *Circulation*. 2007 Nov 27;116(22):2553–2562. http://circ.ahajournals.org/content/116/22/2553.long#ref-3. Accessed May 29, 2013.

Leung LK, Su Y, Chen R, et al. Theaflavins in black tea and catechins in green tea are equally effective antioxidants. *Journal of Nutrition*. 2001;131:2248–2251.

Manson JE, Greenland P, LaCroix AZ, et al. Walking compared with vigorous exercise for the prevention of cardiovascular events in women. *New England Journal of Medicine*. 2002 Sep 5;347(10):716–725. http://www.nejm.org/doi/full/10.1056/nejmoa021067. Accessed May 29, 2013.

McCraty R. Coherence: Bridging personal, social, and global health. *Alternative Therapies in Health and Medicine.* 2010;16 (4):10–24. www.heartmath.org/templates/ihm/downloads/pdf/research/publications/coherence-bridging-personal-social-global-health.pdf. Accessed May 29, 2013.

Mokni M, Limam F, Elkahoui S, et al. Strong cardioprotective effect of resveratrol, a red wine polyphenol, on isolated rat hearts after ischemia/reperfusion injury. *Archives of Biochemistry and Biophysics.* 2007;457:1–6.

Nagai M, Hoshide S, Kario K. Sleep duration as a risk factor for cardiovascular disease: a review of the recent literature. *Current Cardiology Reviews.* 2010 Feb;6(1):54–61. doi: 10.2174/157340310790231635. www.ncbi.nlm.nih.gov/pmc/articles/pmc2845795/. Accessed May 29, 2013.

Nugala B, Namasi A, Emmadi P, Krishna PM. Role of green tea as an antioxidant in periodontal disease: the Asian paradox. *Journal of the Indian Society of Periodontology.* 2012 Jul;16(3):313–316. doi: 10.4103/0972-124x.100902.

Rhodes LE, Darby G, Massey KA, et al. Oral green tea catechin metabolites are incorporated into human skin and protect against UV radiation-induced cutaneous inflammation in association with reduced production of pro-inflammatory eicosanoid 12-hydroxyeicosatetraenoic acid. *British Journal of Nutrition.* 2013 Jan 28:1–10. http://www.ncbi.nlm.nih.gov/pubmed/23351338. [Epub ahead of print]

Ross GW, Abbott RD, Petrovitch H, et al. Association of coffee and caffeine intake with the risk of Parkinson disease. *JAMA.* 2000;283:2674–2679.

Sakuragi S, Sugiyama Y, Takeuchi K. Effects of laughing and weeping on mood and heart rate variability. *Journal of Physiological Anthropology and Applied Human Science.* 2002 May;21(3):159–165.

Smid SD, Maag JL, Musgrave IF. Dietary polyphenol-derived protection against neurotoxic beta-amyloid protein: from molecular to clinical. *Food & Function.* 2012 Aug 24.

Soedamah-Muthu SS, De Neve M, Shelton NJ, Tielemans SM, Stamatakis E. Joint associations of alcohol consumption and physical activity with all-cause and cardiovascular mortality. *American Journal of Cardiology.* 2013 May 3. pii: S0002-9149(13)00901-6. doi: 10.1016/j.amjcard.2013.03.040. [Epub ahead of print]

Sumner MD, Elliott-Eller M, Weidner G, et al. Effects of pomegranate juice consumption on myocardial perfusion in patients with coronary heart disease. *American Journal of Cardiology.* 2005;96:810–814.

Taqvi SI, Shah AJ, Gilani AH. Blood pressure lowering and vasomodulator effects of piperine. *Journal of Cardiovascular Pharmacology.* 2008 Nov;52(5):452–458. doi: 10.1097/fjc.0b013e31818d07c0.

Thompson PL. J-curve revisited: cardiovascular benefits of moderate alcohol use cannot be dismissed. *Medical Journal of Australia.* 2013;198(8):419–422.

Utsugi M, Saijo Y, Yoshioka E, et al. Relationship between two alternative occupational stress models and arterial stiffness: a cross-sectional study among Japanese workers. *International Archives of Occupational and Environmental Health.* 2009 Jan;82(2):175–183.

Vafa M, Mohammadi F, Shidfar F, et al. Effects of cinnamon consumption on glycemic status, lipid profile and body composition in type 2 diabetic patients. *International Journal of Preventive Medicine.* 2012 Aug;3(8):531–536.

Vale S. Psychosocial stress and cardiovascular diseases. *Postgraduate Medicine Journal.* 2005 Jul;81(957):429–435.

Wells R, Outhred T, Heathers JA, Quintana DS, Kemp AH. Matter over mind: a randomised-controlled trial of single-session biofeedback training on performance anxiety and heart rate variability in musicians. *PLoS One.* 2012;7(10):e46597. doi: 10.1371/journal.pone.0046597.

Wu CH, Yang YC, Yao WJ, et al. Epidemiological evidence of increased bone mineral density in habitual tea drinkers. *Archives of Internal Medicine.* 2002;162:1001–1006.

Zheng G, Sayama K, Okubo T, et al. Anti-obesity effects of three major components of green tea, catechins, caffeine and theanine, in mice. *In Vivo.* 2004;18:55–62.

Chapter 40 Heartburn and Gastritis

Abraham NS. Proton pump inhibitors: potential adverse effects. *Current Opinion in Gastroenterology.* 2012 Nov;28(6):615–620. doi: 10.1097/mog.0b013e328358d5b9.

de Oliveira Torres JD, de Souza Pereira R. Which is the best choice for gastroesophageal disorders: Melatonin or proton pump inhibitors? *Journal of Gastrointestinal Pharmacology and Therapeutics.* 2010 Oct 6;1(5):102–106. doi: 10.4292/wjgpt.v1.i5.102. www.ncbi.nlm.nih.gov/pmc/articles/pmc3091156/. Accessed May 11, 2013.

Hawrelak JA, Myers SP. Effects of two natural medicine formulations on irritable bowel syndrome symptoms: a pilot study. *Journal of Alternative and Complementary Medicine.* 2010 Oct;16(10):1065–1071.

Kiefer D. Gastroesophageal reflux disease. Rakel D, ed. *Integrative Medicine.* Saunders, 2007.

Madalinski MH. Does a melatonin supplement alter the course of gastro-esophageal reflux disease? *World Journal of Gastrointestinal Pharmacology and Therapeutics.* 2011 Dec 6;2(6):50–51. doi: 10.4292/wjgpt.v2.i6.50.

Patrick L. Gastroesophageal reflux disease (GERD): a review of conventional and alternative treatments. *Alternative Medicine Review.* 2011;16(2):116–133.

Pereira RS. Regression of gastroesophageal reflux disease symptoms using dietary supplementation with melatonin, vitamins and amino acids: comparison with omeprazole. *Journal of Pineal Research.* 2006;41:195–200.

Singh M, Lee J, Gupta N, et al. Weight loss can lead to resolution of gastroesophageal reflux disease symptoms: a prospective intervention trial. *Obesity* (Silver Spring). 2013 Feb;21(2):284–290. doi: 10.1002/oby.20279.

Chapter 41 Hemorrhoids

[No authors listed] Aesculus hippocastanum (Horse chestnut). Monograph. *Alternative Medicine Review.* 2009 Sep;14(3):278–283. www.altmedrev.com/publications/14/3/278.pdf. Accessed May 13, 2013.

Cesarone MR, Belcaro G, Grossi MG, et al. LINFAVENIX: improvement of signs and symptoms of chronic venous insufficiency and microangiopathy. *Minerva Cardioangiologica.* 2008 Oct;56(5 Suppl):55–61.

Hormann HP, Korting HC. Evidence for the efficacy and safety of topical herbal drugs in dermatology: part I: anti-inflammatory agents. *Phytomedicine.* 1994;1:161–171.

MacKay D. Hemorrhoids and varicose veins: a review of treatment options. *Alternative Medicine Review.* 2001 Apr;6(2):126–140. www.altmedrev.com/publications/6/2/126.pdf. Accessed May 13, 2013.

Misra MC, Parshad R. Randomized clinical trial of micronized flavonoids in the early control of bleeding from acute internal haemorrhoids. *British Journal of Surgery.* 2000;87:868–872.

Pittler MH, Ernst E. Horse chestnut seed extract for chronic venous insufficiency. *Cochrane Database of Systematic Reviews.* 2012 Nov 14;11:CD003230. doi: 10.1002/14651858.cd003230.pub4.

Suter A, Bommer S, Rechner J. Treatment of patients with venous insufficiency with fresh plant horse chestnut seed extract: a review of 5 clinical studies. *Advances in Therapy.* 2006 Jan–Feb;23(1):179–190.

Chapter 42 High Blood Pressure

Apostolidis E, Kwon YI, Shetty K. Potential of cranberry-based herbal synergies for diabetes and hypertension management. *Asia Pacific Journal of Clinical Nutrition.* 2006;15(3):433–441.

Balasuriya N, Rupasinghe HP. Antihypertensive properties of flavonoid-rich apple peel extract. *Food Chemistry.* 2012 Dec 15;135(4):2320–2325. doi: 10.1016/j.foodchem.2012.07.023.

Basu A, Lyons TJ. Strawberries, blueberries, and cranberries in the metabolic syndrome: clinical perspectives. *Journal of Agricultural and Food Chemistry.* 2011 Nov 29. [Epub ahead of print]

Ding, E, Hutfless, S, Ding X, Girotra, S. Chocolate and prevention of cardiovascular disease: a systematic review. *Nutrition & Metabolism.* 2006;3:2. doi:10.1186/1743-7075-3-2. www.nutritionandmetabolism.com/content/3/1/2.

Figueroa A, Wong A, Hooshmand S, Sanchez-Gonzalez MA. Effects of watermelon supplementation on arterial stiffness and wave reflection amplitude in postmenopausal women. *Menopause.* 2013 May;20(5):573–577. doi: 10.1097/gme.0b013e3182733794.

Goldstein CM, Josephson R, Xie S, Hughes JW. Current perspectives on the use of meditation to reduce blood pressure. *International Journal of Hypertension.* 2012;2012:578397. doi: 10.1155/2012/57839. www.ncbi.nlm.nih.gov/pmc/articles/pmc3303565/. Accessed May 13, 2013.

Guo X, Zhou B, Nishimura T, Teramukai S, Fukushima M. Clinical effect of qigong practice on essential hypertension: a meta-analysis of randomized controlled trials. *Journal of Alternative and Complementary Medicine.* 2008 Jan–Feb;14(1):27–37. doi: 10.1089/acm.2007.7213.

Hopkins AL, Lamm MG, Funk JL, Ritenbaugh C. Hibiscus sabdariffa L. in the treatment of hypertension and hyperlipidemia: a comprehensive review of animal and human studies. *Fitoterapia.* 2013 Mar;85:84–94. doi: 10.1016/j.fitote.2013.01.003.

Larson A, Symons J, Jalili T. Therapeutic potential of quercetin to decrease blood pressure: review of efficacy and mechanisms. *Advances in Nutrition.* 2012 Jan;3(1):39–46. doi: 10.3945/an.111.001271. Epub 2012 Jan 5.

Larsson, S, Virtamo J, Wolk A. Chocolate consumption and risk of stroke: a prospective cohort of men and meta-analysis. *Neurology.* 2012 Aug 29. doi: 10.1212/wnl.0b013e31826aacfa. [Epub ahead of print]

Mostofsky E, Levitan E, Wolk A, Mittleman M. Chocolate intake and incidence of heart failure: a population-based, prospective study of middle-aged and elderly women. *Circulation: Heart Failure.* 2010. doi:10.1161/circheartfailure.110.944025.

Palomba D, Ghisi M, Scozzari S, et al. Biofeedback-assisted cardiovascular control in hypertensives exposed to emotional stress: a pilot study. *Applied Psychophysiology and Biofeedback.* 2011 Sep;36(3):185–192. doi: 10.1007/s10484-011-9160-3.

Ravn-Haren G, Dragsted LO, Buch-Andersen T, et al. Intake of whole apples or clear apple juice has contrasting effects on plasma lipids in healthy volunteers. *European Journal of Nutrition.* 2012 Dec 28. [Epub ahead of print]

Sathyapalan T, Campion P, Beckett S, Rigby A, Atkin S. High cocoa polyphenol rich chocolate improves the symptoms of chronic fatigue. *Endocrine Abstracts.* 2006;12:68.

Sheats N, Lin Y, Zhao W, Cheek DE, Lackland DT, Egan BM. Prevalence, treatment, and control of hypertension among African Americans and Caucasians at primary care sites for medically under-served patients. *Ethnicity and Disease.* 2005 Winter;15(1):25–32.

Smith-Spangler CM, Juusola JL, Enns EA, Owens DK, Garber AM. Population strategies to decrease sodium intake and the burden of cardiovascular disease: a cost-effectiveness analysis. *Annals of Internal Medicine.* 2010 Apr 20;152(8):481–487, W170–173. doi: 10.1059/0003-4819-152-8-201004200-00212.

Stowe CB. The effects of pomegranate juice consumption on blood pressure and cardiovascular health. *Complementary Therapies in Clinical Practice.* 2011 May;17(2):113–115. doi: 10.1016/j.ctcp.2010.09.004.

Whelton PK, Buring J, Borhani NO, et al. The effect of potassium supplementation in persons with a high-normal blood pressure. Results from phase 1 of the trials of hypertension prevention (TOHP). *Annals of Epidemiology.* 1995;5:85–95.

Wiseman W, Egan JM, Slemmer JE, et al. Feeding blueberry diets inhibits angiotensin II-converting enzyme (ACE) activity in spontaneously hypertensive stroke-prone rats. *Canadian Journal of Physiology and Pharmacology.* 2011 Jan;89(1):67–71. doi: 10.1139/y10-101.

Chapter 43 Immune System Support

Barak Y. The immune system and happiness. *Autoimmunity Reviews.* 2006 Oct;5(8):523–527.

Bengmark S. Ecological control of the gastrointestinal tract: the role of probiotic flora. *Gut* 1998;42:2–7. As cited in Guarner F, Malagelada JR. Gut flora in health and diseases. *The Lancet.* 2003;61(9371):512–519.

Berggren A, Lazou Ahrén I, Larsson N, Onning G. Randomised, double-blind and placebo-controlled study using new probiotic lactobacilli for strengthening the body immune defense against viral infections. *European Journal of Nutrition.* 2011;50(3):203–210.

Bisen PS, Baghel RK, Sanodiya BS, Thakur GS, Prasad GB. Lentinus edodes: a macrofungus with pharmacological activities. *Current Medicinal Chemistry.* 2010;17(22):2419–2430.

Charnetski CJ, Brennan FX. Sexual frequency and salivary immunoglobulin A (IgA). *Psychological Reports.* 2004 Jun;94 (3 Pt 1):839–844.

Charnetski CJ, Riggers S, Brennan FX. Effect of petting a dog on immune system function. *Psychological Reports.* 2004 Dec;95(3 Pt 2):1087–1091.

Chew BP, Park JS. Carotenoid action on the immune response. *Journal of Nutrition.* 2004;134(1):257S-261S. http://nutrition.highwire.org/content/134/1/257s.full. Accessed May 14, 2013.

Cohen S, Doyle WJ, Skoner DP, Rabin BS, Gwaltney JM Jr. Social ties and susceptibility to the common cold. *JAMA.* 1997 Jun 25;277(24):1940–1944.

Hawkley LC, Cacioppo JT. Loneliness matters: a theoretical and empirical review of consequences and mechanisms. *Annals of Behavioral Medicine.* 2010 Oct;40(2):218–227.

Hinther A, Bromba CM, Wulff JE, Helbing CC. Effects of triclocarban, triclosan, and methyl triclosan on thyroid hormone action and stress in frog and mammalian culture systems. *Environmental Science and Technology.* 2011 Jun 15;45(12):5395–5402. doi: 10.1021/es1041942.

Iciek M, Kwiecień I, Włodek L. Biological properties of garlic and garlic-derived organosulfur compounds. *Environmental and Molecular Mutagenesis.* 2009 Apr;50(3):247–265. doi: 10.1002/em.20474.

Lang PO, Samaras N, Samaras D, Aspinall R. How important is vitamin D in preventing infections? *Osteoporosis International.* 2013 May;24(5):1537–1553. doi: 10.1007/s00198-012-2204-6.

Lee YM. Effect of self-foot reflexology massage on depression, stress responses and immune functions of middle aged women. *Taehan Kanho Hakhoe chi.* 2006 Feb;36(1):179–188.

Lee HS, Ahn YJ. Growth-Inhibiting Effects of Cinnamomum cassia bark–derived materials on human intestinal bacteria. *Journal of Agricultural and Food Chemistry.* 1998;46:8–12.

Li Q, Kawada T. Effect of forest environments on human natural killer (NK) activity. *International Journal of Immunopathology and Pharmacology.* 2011 Jan–Mar;24(1 Suppl):39S–44S.

Nanba H, Kubo K. Effect of Maitake D-fraction on cancer prevention. *Annals of the New York Academy of Sciences.* 1997;833:204–207.

Pae M, Meydani SN, Wu D. The role of nutrition in enhancing immunity in aging. *Aging and Disease.* 2012 Feb;3(1):91–129. www.ncbi.nlm.nih.gov/pmc/articles/pmc3320807/. Accessed May 14, 2013.

Pyo P, Louie B, Rajamahanty S, Choudhury M, Konno S. Possible immunotherapeutic potentiation with D-fraction in prostate cancer cells. *Journal of Hematology and Oncology.* 2008 Dec 4;1:25. doi: 10.1186/1756-8722-1-25. www.ncbi.nlm.nih.gov/pmc/articles/pmc2613393/. Accessed May 14, 2013.

Qin Q, Niu J, Wang Z, Xu W, Qiao Z, Gu Y. Astragalus embranaceus extract activates immune response in macrophages via heparanase. *Molecules.* 2012 Jun 13;17(6):7232–7240. doi: 10.3390/molecules17067232.

Riedel S. Edward Jenner and the history of smallpox and vaccination. *Baylor University Medical Center Proceedings.* 2005;18(1):21–25. www.ncbi.nlm.nih.gov/pmc/articles/pmc1200696/. Accessed May 14, 2013.

Silva N, Alves S, Gonçalves A, Amaral JS, Poeta P. Antimicrobial activity of essential oils from mediterranean aromatic plants against several foodborne and spoilage bacteria. *Food Science and Technology International.* 2013 Feb 26. [Epub ahead of print]

Tanigawa K, Ito Y, Sakai M, Kobayashi Y. Evaluation of quality of life and immune function in cancer patients receiving combined immunotherapy and oral administration of lentinula edodes mycelia extract. *Gan To Kagaku Ryoho.* 2012 Nov;39(12):1779–1781.

Turner RB, Fuls JL, Rodgers ND. Effectiveness of hand sanitizers with and without organic acids for removal of rhinovirus from hands. *Antimicrobial Agents and Chemotherapy*. 2010;54(3):1363–1364.

Wintergerst ES, Maggini S, Hornig DH. Immune-enhancing role of vitamin C and zinc and effect on clinical conditions. *Annals of Nutrition and Metabolism*. 2006;50(2):85–94.

Chapter 44
Indigestion and Irritable Bowel Syndrome

Allescher HD, Wagner H. STW 5/Iberogast: multi-target-action for treatment of functional dyspepsia and irritable bowel syndrome. *Wiener Medizinische Wochenschrift*. 2007;157(13–14):301–307.

Brands MM, Purperhart H, Deckers-Kocken JM. A pilot study of yoga treatment in children with functional abdominal pain and irritable bowel syndrome. *Complementary Therapies in Medicine*. 2011 Jun;19(3):109–114. doi: 10.1016/j.ctim.2011.05.004.

Kligler B, Chaudhary S. Peppermint oil. *American Family Physician*. 2007 Apr 1;75(7):1027–1030.

Mearin F, Calleja JL. Defining functional dyspepsia. *Revista española de enfermedades digestivas*. 2011 Dec;103(12):640–647.

Metabolism: Bitter aperitifs to aid digestion. *Nature*. 2011 Jan;469(7331):446. doi:10.1038/469446d.

Minami S, Suzuki M, Takemura A, et al. Optimal timing of MR sialography by use of a simple method of stimulating the salivary gland: a preliminary report. *Radiological Physics and Technology*. 2008 Jul;1(2):208–213. doi: 10.1007/s12194-008-0030-5.

Sannia A. Phytotherapy with a mixture of dry extracts with hepato-protective effects containing artichoke leaves in the management of functional dyspepsia symptoms. *Minerva gastroenterologica e dietologica*. 2010 Jun;56(2):93–99.

Shah KA, Patel MB, Patel RJ, Parmar PK. Mangifera indica (Mango). *Pharmacognosy Review*. 2010 Jan–Jun;4(7):42–48. doi: 10.4103/0973-7847.65325. www.ncbi.nlm.nih.gov/pmc/articles/pmc3249901/. Accessed May 13, 2013.

Spiller R. Review article: probiotics and prebiotics in irritable bowel syndrome. *Alimentary Pharmacology and Therapeutics*. 2008 Aug 15;28(4):385–396.

Chapter 45 Influenza

Abzug MJ. Nonpolio enteroviruses. In Kliegman RM, Behrman RE, Jenson HB, Stanton BF, eds. *Nelson Textbook of Pediatrics*. 19th ed. Philadelphia, PA: Saunders Elsevier; 2011:chap 242. www.nlm.nih.gov/medlineplus/ency/article/000969.htm. Accessed May 19, 2013.

Barak V, Halperin T, Kalickman I. The effect of Sambucol, a black elderberry-based, natural product, on the production of human cytokines: I. Inflammatory cytokines. *European Cytokine Network*. 2001;12(2):290–296.

Benmalek Y, Yahia OA, Belkebir A, Fardeau ML. Anti-microbial and anti-oxidant activities of Illicium verum, Crataegus oxyacantha ssp monogyna and Allium cepa red and white varieties. *Bioengineered*. 2013 Apr 11;4(4). [Epub ahead of print]

Charan J, Goyal JP, Saxena D, Yadav P. Vitamin D for prevention of respiratory tract infections: a systematic review and meta-analysis. *Journal of Pharmacology and Pharmacotherapeutics*. 2012 Oct;3(4):300–303. doi: 10.4103/0976-500x.103685. www.ncbi.nlm.nih.gov/pmc/articles/pmc3543548/. Accessed May 15, 2013.

Cohen HA, Rozen J, Kristal H, et al. Effect of honey on nocturnal cough and sleep quality: a double-blind, randomized, placebo-controlled study. *Pediatrics*. 2012 Sep;130(3):465–471. doi: 10.1542/peds.2011-3075. Epub 2012 Aug 6. www.ncbi.nlm.nih.gov/pubmed/22869830. Accessed May 19, 2013.

Hirani V. Associations Between vitamin d and self-reported respiratory disease in older people from a nationally representative population survey. *Journal of the American Geriatric Society*. 2013 May 6. doi: 10.1111/jgs.12254. [Epub ahead of print]

Imanishi N, Andoh T, Mantani N, et al. Macrophage-mediated inhibitory effect of Zingiber officinale Rosc, a traditional oriental herbal medicine, on the growth of influenza A/Aichi/2/68 virus. *The American Journal of Chinese Medicine*. 2006;34(1):157–169. www.ncbi.nlm.nih.gov/pubmed/?term=zingiber+influenza. Accessed May 19, 2013.

Jeong SC, Koyyalamudi SR, Pang G. Dietary intake of Agaricus bisporus white button mushroom accelerates salivary immunoglobulin A secretion in healthy volunteers. *Nutrition*. 2012 May;28(5):527–531. doi: 10.1016/j.nut.2011.08.005.

Knight WE, Rickard PhD NS. Relaxing music prevents stress-induced increases in subjective anxiety, systolic blood pressure, and heart rate in healthy males and females. *Journal of Music Therapy*. 2001 Winter;38(4):254–272. www.ncbi.nlm.nih.gov/pubmed/11796077. Accessed May 19, 2013.

Kong, F. Pilot Clinical study on a proprietary elderberry extract: efficacy in addressing influenza symptoms. *Online Journal of Pharmacology and PharmacoKinetics*. 2009;5:32–43. http://omicron-pharma.com/pdfs/elderberryclinicalojpk_published.pdf. Accessed February 15, 2012.

Koyama M, Wachi M, Utsuyama M, et al. Recreational music-making modulates immunological responses and mood states in older adults. *Journal of Medical and Dental Sciences*. 2009 Jun;56(2):79–90.

Krawitz C, Mraheil MA, Stein M, et al. Inhibitory activity of a standardized elderberry liquid extract against clinically-relevant human respiratory bacterial pathogens and influenza A and B viruses. *BMC Complementary and Alternative Medicine*. 2011 Feb 25;11:16.

McElhaney JE, Goel V, Toane B, et al. Efficacy of COLD-fX in the prevention of respiratory symptoms in community-dwelling adults: a randomized, double-blinded, placebo controlled trial. *Journal of Alternative and Complementary Medicine.* 2006;12:153–157.

McElhaney JE, Gravenstein S, Cole SK, et al. A placebo-controlled trial of a proprietary extract of north american ginseng (CVT-E002) to prevent acute respiratory illness in institutionalized older adults. *Journal of the American Geriatric Society.* 2004;52:13–19.

Nantz MP, Rowe CA, Muller CE, Creasy RA, Stanilka JM, Percival SS. Supplementation with aged garlic extract improves both NK and gamma delta T-cell function and reduces the severity of cold and flu symptoms: a randomized, double-blind, placebo-controlled nutrition intervention. *Clinical Nutrition.* 2012 Jun;31(3):337–344. doi: 10.1016/j.clnu.2011.11.019. Epub 2012 Jan 24. www.ncbi.nlm.nih.gov/pubmed/22280901. Accessed May 19, 2013.

Predy GN, Goel V, Lovlin R, et al. Efficacy of an extract of North American ginseng containing poly-furanosyl-pyranosyl-saccharides for preventing upper respiratory tract infections: a randomized controlled trial. *CMAJ (Canadian Medical Association Journal).* 2005;173:1043–1048.

Santibañez S, Fiore AE, Merlin TL, Redd S. A primer on strategies for prevention and control of seasonal and pandemic influenza. *American Journal of Public Health.* 2009;99(Suppl 2):S216–223.

Smiderle FR, Ruthes AC, van Arkel J, et al. Polysaccharides from Agaricus bisporus and Agaricus brasiliensis show similarities in their structures and their immunomodulatory effects on human monocytic THP-1 cells. *BMC Complementary Alternative Medicine.* 2011 Jul 25;11:58. doi: 10.1186/1472-6882-11-58.

Suzuki F, Suzuki C, Shimomura E, Maeda H, Fujii T, Ishida N. Antiviral and interferon-inducing activities of a new peptidomannan, KS-2, extracted from culture mycelia of Lentinus edodes. *Journal of Antibiotics* (Tokyo). 1979 Dec;32(12):1336–1345.

Urashima M, Segawa T, Okazaki M, et al. Randomized trial of vitamin D supplementation to prevent seasonal influenza A in schoolchildren. *American Journal of Clinical Nutrition.* 2010;91:1255–1260.

Viana GS, Vale TG, Pinho RS, Matos FJ. Antinociceptive effect of the essential oil from Cymbopogon citratus in mice. *Journal of Ethnopharmacology.* 2000 Jun;70(3):323–327.

Yang Y, Verkuilen J, Rosengren KS, et al. Effects of a Taiji and Qigong intervention on the antibody response to influenza vaccine in older adults. *American Journal of Chinese Medicine.* 2007;35(4):597–607.

Zakay-Rones Z, Thom E, Wollan T, Wadstein J. Randomized study of the efficacy and safety of oral elderberry extract in the treatment of influenza A and B virus infections. *The Journal of International Medical Research.* 2004;32(2):132–140.

Chapter 46 Insomnia

Buscemi N, Vandermeer B, Hooton N, et al. The efficacy and safety of exogenous melatonin for primary sleep disorders. A meta-analysis. *Journal of General Internal Medicine.* 2005;20:1151–1158.

Chien LW, Cheng SL, Liu CF. The effect of lavender aromatherapy on autonomic nervous system in midlife women with insomnia. *Evidence-based Complementary and Alternative Medicine.* 2012;2012:740813. doi: 10.1155/2012/740813.

Cho MY, Min ES, Hur MH, Lee MS. Effects of aromatherapy on the anxiety, vital signs, and sleep quality of percutaneous coronary intervention patients in intensive care units. *Evidence-Based Complementary and Alternative Medicine.* 2013;2013:381381. doi: 10.1155/2013/381381.

Dhruva A, Miaskowski C, Abrams D, et al. Yoga breathing for cancer chemotherapy-associated symptoms and quality of life: results of a pilot randomized controlled trial. *Journal of Alternative and Complementry Medicine.* 2012 May;18(5):473–479.

Fernández-San-Martín MI, Masa-Font R, Palacios-Soler L, et al. Effectiveness of valerian on insomnia: a meta-analysis of randomized placebo-controlled trials. *Sleep Medicine.* 2010 Jun;11(6):505–511. doi: 10.1016/j.sleep.2009.12.009.

Innes, Kim E., Selfe, Terry Kit. The effects of a gentle yoga program on sleep, mood, and blood pressure in older women with restless legs syndrome (RLS): a preliminary randomized controlled trial. *Evidence-Based Complementary and Alternative Medicine.* 2012;2012:294058. www.ncbi.nlm.nih.gov/pmc/articles/pmc3303621/.

Kolla BP, Auger RR. Jet lag and shift work sleep disorders: how to help reset the internal clock. *Cleveland Clinic Journal of Medicine.* 2011 Oct;78(10):675–684. doi: 10.3949/ccjm.78a.10083. www.ccjm.org/content/78/10/675.long. Accessed May 15, 2013.

Morin CM, Koetter U, Bastien C, et al. Valerian-hops combination and diphenhydramine for treating insomnia: a randomized placebo-controlled clinical trial. *Sleep.* 2005;28:1465–1471.

Muller SF, Klement S. A combination of valerian and lemon balm is effective in the treatment of restlessness and dyssomnia in children. *Phytomedicine.* 2006;13:383–37.

Ngan A, Conduit R. A double-blind, placebo-controlled investigation of the effects of Passiflora incarnata (passionflower) herbal tea on subjective sleep quality. *Phytotherapy Research.* 2011;25:1153–1159.

Peuhkuri K, Sihvola N, Korpela R. Diet promotes sleep duration and quality. *Nutrition Research.* 2012 May;32(5):309–319. doi: 10.1016/j.nutres.2012.03.009.

Sarris J, Byrne GJ. A systematic review of insomnia and complementary medicine. *Sleep Medicine Reviews.* 2011;15:99–106.

Takahashi M. Prioritizing sleep for healthy work schedules. *Journal of Physiologic Anthropology*. 2012 Mar 13;31:6. doi: 10.1186/1880-6805-31-6.

Wood AM, Joseph S, Lloyd J, Atkins S. Gratitude influences sleep through the mechanism of pre-sleep cognitions. *Journal of Psychosomatic Research*. 2009 Jan;66(1):43–48. doi: 10.1016/j.jpsychores.2008.09.002.

Zick SM, Wright BD, Sen A, Arnedt JT. Preliminary examination of the efficacy and safety of a standardized chamomile extract for chronic primary insomnia: a randomized placebo-controlled pilot study. *BMC Complementary and Alternative Medicine*. 2011 Sep 22;11:78. doi: 10.1186/1472-6882-11-78. www.ncbi.nlm.nih.gov/pmc/articles/pmc3198755/. Accessed May 15, 2013.

Chapter 47 Menopause

Afonso RF, Hachul H, Kozasa EH, et al. Yoga decreases insomnia in postmenopausal women: a randomized clinical trial. *Menopause*. 2012 Feb;19(2):186–193. doi: 10.1097/gme.0b013e318228225f.

Auerbach L, Rakus J, Bauer C, et al. Pomegranate seed oil in women with menopausal symptoms: a prospective randomized, placebo-controlled, double-blinded trial. *Menopause*. 2012 Apr;19(4):426–432. doi: 10.1097/gme.0b013e3182345b2f.

Bachman JL, Phelan S, Wing RR, Raynor HA. Eating frequency is higher in weight loss maintainers and normal-weight individuals than in overweight individuals. *Journal of the American Dietetic Associaton*. 2011 Nov;111(11):1730–1734. doi: 10.1016/j.jada.2011.08.006.

Bommer S, Klein P, Suter A. First time proof of sage's tolerability and efficacy in menopausal women with hot flushes. *Advances in Therapy*. 2011;28:490–500.

Cramer H, Lauche R, Langhorst J, Dobos G. Effectiveness of yoga for menopausal symptoms: a systematic review and meta-analysis of randomized controlled trials. *Evidence-Based Complementary and Alternative Medicine*. 2012;2012:863905. doi: 10.1155/2012/863905. www.ncbi.nlm.nih.gov/pmc/articles/pmc3524799/. Accessed May 16, 2013.

Dodin S, Lemay A, Jacques H, et al. The effects of flaxseed dietary supplement on lipid profile, bone mineral density, and symptoms in menopausal women: a randomized, double-blind, wheat germ placebo-controlled clinical trial. *Journal of Clinical Endocrinology and Metabolism*. 2005;90:1390–1397.

Elavsky S, Gonzales JU, Proctor DN, Williams N, Henderson VW. Effects of physical activity on vasomotor symptoms: examination using objective and subjective measures. *Menopause*. 2012 Oct;19(10):1095–1103.

Freeman EW, Sammel MD, Grisso JA, Battistini M, Garcia-Espagna B, Hollander L. Hot flashes in the late reproductive years: risk factors for African American and Caucasian women. *Journal of Women's Health & Gender-Based Medicine*. 2001;10:67–76.

Hyde Riley, E, Inui, TS, Kleinman, K, Connelly, M. Differential association of modifiable health behaviors with hot flashes in perimenopausal and postmenopausal women. *Journal of General Internal Medicine*. 2004 Jul;19(7):740–746.

Lee MS, Shin BC, Yang EJ, Lim HJ, Ernst E. Maca (Lepidium meyenii) for treatment of menopausal symptoms: a systematic review. *Maturitas*. 2011 Nov;70(3):227–233. doi: 10.1016/j.maturitas.2011.07.017.

Lemay A, Dodin S, Kadri N, et al. Flaxseed dietary supplement versus hormone replacement therapy in hypercholesterolemic menopausal women. *Obstetrics and Gynecology*. 2002;100:495–504.

Nappi RE, Malavasi B, Brundu B, Facchinetti F. Efficacy of Cimicifuga racemosa on climacteric complaints: a randomized study versus low-dose transdermal estradiol. *Gynecological Endocrinology*. 2005;20:30–35.

Newton KM, Reed SD, LaCroix AZ, Grothaus LC, Ehrlich K, Guiltinan J. Treatment of vasomotor symptoms of menopause with black cohosh, multibotanicals, soy, hormone therapy, or placebo: a randomized trial. *Annals of Internal Medicine*. 2006 Dec 19;145(12):869–879.

Pachman DR, Jones JM, Loprinzi CL. Management of menopause-associated vasomotor symptoms: current treatment options, challenges and future directions. *International Journal of Women's Health*. 2010 Aug 9;2:123–135. www.ncbi.nlm.nih.gov/pmc/articles/pmc2971731/. Accessed May 16, 2013.

Rossouw JE, Anderson GL, Prentice RL, et al. Risks and benefits of estrogen plus progestin in healthy postmenopausal women: principal results from the Women's Health Initiative randomized controlled trial. *JAMA*. 2002;288(3):321–333.

Schilling, C, Gallicchio L, Miller S, Langenberg P, Zacur H, Flaws, J. Current alcohol use, hormone levels, and hot flashes in midlife women. *Fertility and Sterility*. 2007 Jun;87(6):1483–1486. Published online 2007 February 2. doi: 10.1016/j.fertnstert.2006.11.033.

Setchell KDR, Lydeking-Olsen E. Dietary phytoestrogens and their effect on bone: evidence from in vitro and in vivo, human observational, and dietary intervention studies. *American Journal of Clinical Nutrition*. 2003;78:593S–609S.

Snijder MB, van Dam RM, Visser M, Seidell JC. What aspects of body fat are particularly hazardous and how do we measure them? *International Journal of Epidemiology*. 2006;35:83. http://ije.oxfordjournals.org/content/35/1/83.long. Accessed June 28, 2013.

Sood R, Sood A, Wolf SL, et al. Paced breathing compared with usual breathing for hot flashes. *Menopause*. 2013 Feb;20(2):179–184. doi: 10.1097/gme.0b013e31826934b6.

Welty FK, Lee KS, Lew NS, Nasca M, Zhou JR. The association between soy nut consumption and decreased menopausal symptoms. *Journal of Women's Health* (Larchmont). 2007 Apr;16(3):361–369.

Wuttke W, Seidlova-Wuttke D, Gorkow C. The Cimicifuga preparation BNO 1055 vs. conjugated estrogens in a double-blind placebo-controlled study: effects on menopause symptoms and bone markers. *Maturitas.* 2003;44(Suppl 1):S67–77.

Chung DJ, Kim HY, Park KH, et al. Black cohosh and St. John's wort (GYNO-Plus) for climacteric symptoms. *Yonsei Medical Journal,* 2007;48:289–294.

Chapter 48 Menstrual Cramps

Abdul-Razzak KK, Ayoub NM, Abu-Taleb AA, Obeidat BA. Influence of dietary intake of dairy products on dysmenorrhea. *Journal of Obstetrics and Gynaecology Research.* 2010 Apr;36(2):377–383.

Balbi C, Musone R, Menditto A, et al. Influence of menstrual factors and dietary habits on menstrual pain in adolescence age. *European Journal of Obstetrics, Gynecology and Reproductive Biology.* 2000 Aug;91(2):143–148.

Goldberg RJ, Katz J. A meta-analysis of the analgesic effects of omega-3 polyunsaturated fatty acid supplementation for inflammatory joint pain. *Pain.* 2007;129:210–23.

Guerrera MP, Volpe SL, Mao JJ. Therapeutic uses of magnesium. *American Family Physician.* 2009 Jul 15;80(2):157–162. www.aafp.org/afp/2009/0715/p157.html. Accessed May 16, 2013.

Jun EM, Chang S, Kang DH, Kim S. Effects of acupressure on dysmenorrhea and skin temperature changes in college students: a non-randomized controlled trial. *International Journal of Nursing Studies.* 2007;44:973–981.

Lee EJ, Frazier SK. The efficacy of acupressure for symptom management: a systematic review. *Journal of Pain and Symptom Management.* 2011 Apr 29. [Epub ahead of print]

Nahid K, Fariborz M, Ataolah G, Solokian S. The effect of an Iranian herbal drug on primary dysmenorrhea: a clinical controlled trial. *Journal of Midwifery and Women's Health.* 2009;54:401–404.

Ortiz MI. Primary dysmenorrhea among Mexican university students: prevalence, impact and treatment. *European Journal of Obstetrics, Gynecology, and Reproductive Biology.* 2010 Sep;152(1):73–77.

Ozgoli G, Goli M, Moattar F. Comparison of effects of ginger, mefenamic acid, and ibuprofen on pain in women with primary dysmenorrhea. *Journal of Alternative and Complementary Medicine.* 2009;15:129–132.

Proctor ML, Hing W, Johnson TC, Murphy PA. Spinal manipulation for primary and secondary dysmenorrhoea. Cochrane Database of Systematic Reviews. 2006;3:CD002119.

Rakhshaee Z. Effect of three yoga poses (cobra, cat and fish poses) in women with primary dysmenorrhea: a randomized clinical trial. *Journal of Pediatric and Adolescent Gynecology.* 2011 Aug;24(4):192–196.

Wong CL, Lai KY, Tse HM. Effects of SP6 acupressure on pain and menstrual distress in young women with dysmenorrhea. *Complementary Therapies in Clinical Practice.* 2010 May;16(2):64–69. doi: 10.1016/j.ctcp.2009.10.002.

Chapter 49 Morning Sickness

Borrelli F, Capasso R, Aviello G, Pittler MH, Izzo AA. Effectiveness and safety of ginger in the treatment of pregnancy-induced nausea and vomiting. *Obstetrics and Gynecology.* 2005;105(4):849–856.

Boylan SM, Greenwood DC, Alwan N, et al. Does nausea and vomiting of pregnancy play a role in the association found between maternal caffeine intake and fetal growth restriction? *Maternal and Child Health Journal.* 2013 May;17(4):601–608. doi: 10.1007/s10995-012-1034-7.

Can Gürkan O, Arslan H. Effect of acupressure on nausea and vomiting during pregnancy. *Complementary Therapies in Clinical Practice.* 2008 Feb;14(1):46–52.

Dror DK, Allen LH Interventions with vitamins B_6, B_{12} and C in pregnancy. *Paediatric and Perinatal Epidemiology.* 2012 Jul;26(Suppl 1):55–74. doi: 10.1111/j.1365-3016.2012.01277.x.

Hunt R, Dienemann J, Norton HJ, et al. Aromatherapy as treatment for postoperative nausea: a randomized trial. *Anesthesia and Analgesia.* 2012 Mar 5. [Epub ahead of print]

Mohammadbeigi R, Shahgeibi S, Soufizadeh N, Rezaiie M, Farhadifar F. Comparing the effects of ginger and metoclopramide on the treatment of pregnancy nausea. *Pakistan Journal of Biological Sciences.* 2011 Aug 15;14(16):817–820.

Pongrojpaw D, Somprasit C, Chanthasenanont A. A randomized comparison of ginger and dimenhydrinate in the treatment of nausea and vomiting in pregnancy. *Journal of the Medical Association of Thailand.* 2007 Sep;90(9):1703–1709.

Chapter 50 Musculoskeletal Pain: Arthritis, Joint Pain, Swelling, and Sprains

Bailey SJ, Fulford J, Vanhatalo A, et al. Dietary nitrate supplementation enhances muscle contractile efficiency during knee-extensor exercise in humans. *Journal of Applied Physiology.* 2010 Jul;109(1):135–148. doi: 10.1152/japplphysiol.00046.2010.

Bailey SJ, Winyard P, Vanhatalo A, et al. Dietary nitrate supplementation reduces the O_2 cost of low-intensity exercise and enhances tolerance to high-intensity exercise in humans. *Journal of Applied Physiology.* 2009 Oct;107(4):1144–1155. doi: 10.1152/japplphysiol.00722.2009.

Berman BM, Lao L, Langenberg P, Lee WL, Gilpin AM, Hochberg MC. Effectiveness of acupuncture as adjunctive therapy in osteoarthritis of the knee: a randomized, controlled trial. *Annals of Internal Medicine.* 2004 Dec 21;141(12):901–910.

Bohlooli S, Jastan M, Nakhostin-Roohi B, Mohammadi S, Baghaei Z. A pilot double-blinded, randomized, clinical trial of topical virgin olive oil versus piroxicam gel in osteoarthritis of the knee. *Journal of Clinical Rheumatology*. March 2012;18(2):99–101.

Bronfort G, Haas M, Evans RL, Bouter LM. Efficacy of spinal manipulation and mobilization for low back pain and neck pain: a systematic review and best evidence synthesis. *The Spine Journal: Official Journal of the North American Spine Society*. 2004 May–Jun;4(3):335–356.

Chrubasik S, Weiser W, Beime B. Effectiveness and safety of topical capsaicin cream in the treatment of chronic soft tissue pain. *Phytotherapy Research*. 2010;24:1877–1885.

Connolly DAJ, McHugh MP, Padilla ZakourBr, OI. Efficacy of a tart cherry juice blend in preventing the symptoms of muscle damage. *British Journal of Sports Medicine*. 2006 Aug;40(8):679–683. Published online 2006 June 21. doi: 10.1136/bjsm.2005.025429.

Cymet TC, Sinkov V. Does long-distance running cause osteoarthritis? *Journal of the American Osteopathic Association*. 2006;106(6):342–345.

Davies SJ, Harding LM, Baranowski AP. A novel treatment of postherpetic neuralgia using peppermint oil. *Clinical Journal of Pain*. 2002;18:200–202.

Eccles NK. A critical review of randomized controlled trials of static magnets for pain relief. *Journal of Alternative and Complementary Medicine*. 2005 Jun;11(3):495–509.

Evans S, Moieni M, Lung K, et al. Impact of Iyengar Yoga on quality of life in young women with rheumatoid arthritis. *Clinical Journal of Pain*. 2013 Jan 30. [Epub ahead of print]

Fioravanti A, Iacoponi F, Bellisai B, Cantarini L, Galeazzi M. Short- and long-term effects of spa therapy in knee osteoarthritis. *American Journal of Physical Medicine and Rehabilitation*. 2010 Feb;89(2):125–132. doi: 10.1097/phm.0b013e3181c1eb81.

Fioravanti A, Tenti S, Giannitti C, Fortunati NA, Galeazzi M. Short- and long-term effects of mud-bath treatment on hand osteoarthritis: a randomized clinical trial. *International Journal of Biometeorology*. 2013 Jan 14. [Epub ahead of print]

Fong DT, Chan YY, Mok KM, Yung PSh, Chan KM. Understanding acute ankle ligamentous sprain injury in sports. *Sports Medicine, Arthroscopy, Rehabilitation, Therapy, and Technology*. 2009 Jul 30;1:14. doi: 10.1186/1758-2555-1-14.

Howatson G, McHugh MP, Hill JA, et al. Influence of tart cherry juice on indices of recovery following marathon running. *Scandinavian Journal of Medicine and Science in Sports*. 2010 Dec;20(6):843–852. doi: 10.1111/j.1600-0838.2009.01005.x. http://www.ncbi.nlm.nih.gov/pmc/articles/PMC2724472/. Accessed June 27, 2013.

Jensen GS, Ager DM, Redman KA, Mitzner MA, Benson KF, Schauss AG. Pain reduction and improvement in range of motion after daily consumption of an açai (Euterpe oleracea 'Mart.') pulp–fortified polyphenolic-rich fruit and berry juice blend. *Journal of Medicinal Food*. 2011 Jul;14(7–8):702–711. doi: 10.1089/jmf.2010.0150. www.ncbi.nlm.nih.gov/pmc/articles/pmc3133683/. Accessed June 27, 2013.

Leach MJ, Kumar S. The clinical effectiveness of ginger (Zingiber officinale) in adults with osteoarthritis. *International Journal of Evidence-Based Healthcare*. 2008;6:311–320.

Lee JH, Choi TY, Lee MS, Lee H, Shin BC, Lee H. Acupuncture for acute low back pain: a systematic review. *The Clinical Journal of Pain*. 2013 Feb;29(2):172–185. doi: 10.1097/ajp.0b013e31824909f9.

Lequesne M, Maheu E, Cadet C, Dreiser RL. Structural effect of avocado/soybean unsaponifiables on joint space loss in osteoarthritis of the hip. *Arthritis and Rheumatism*. 2002 Feb;47(1):50–58.

Masson M. [Bromelain in blunt injuries of the locomotor system: a study of observed applications in general practice]. *Fortschritte der Medizin*. 1995;113:303–306.

McAlindon TE, Jacques P, Zhang Y, et al. Do antioxidant micronutrients protect against the development and progression of knee osteoarthritis? *Arthritis and Rheumatism*. 1996;39:648–656.

Najm WI, Reinsch S, Hoehler F, et al. S-adenosyl methionine (SAMe) versus celecoxib for the treatment of osteoarthritis symptoms: a double-blind crossover trial. *BMC Musculoskeletal Disorders*. 2004;5:6.

Sherman KJ, Cherkin DC, Erro J, et al. Comparing yoga, exercise, and a self-care book for chronic low back pain: a randomized, controlled trial. *Annals of Internal Medicine*. 2005;143:849–856.

Terry R, Posadzki P, Watson LK, Ernst E. The use of ginger (Zingiber officinale) for the treatment of pain: a systematic review of clinical trials. *Pain Medicine*. 2011;12:1808–1818.

Towheed TE, Maxwell L, Anastassiades TP, et al. Glucosamine therapy for treating osteoarthritis. Cochrane Database of Systematic Reviews. 2005 Apr 18;(2):CD002946.

Uhlig T. Tai Chi and yoga as complementary therapies in rheumatologic conditions. Best Practice and Research. *Clinical Rheumatology*. 2012 Jun;26(3):387–398. doi: 10.1016/j.berh.2012.05.006.

Walker AF, Bundy R, Hicks SM, Middleton RW. Bromelain reduces mild acute knee pain and improves well-being in a dose-dependent fashion in an open study of otherwise healthy adults. *Phytomedicine*. 2002;9:681–686.

Walsh N. Arthritis: Sun's rays may cut risk in women. MedPage Today. February 4, 2013. www.medpagetoday.com/rheumatology/arthritis/37187. Accessed May 17, 2013.

Wardhana, Surachmanto ES, Datau EA. The role of omega-3 fatty acids contained in olive oil on chronic inflammation. *Acta Medica Indonesiana*. 2011 Apr;43(2):138–143. www.inaactamedica.org/archives/2011/21785178.pdf. Accessed June 27, 2013.

Wigler I, Grotto I, Caspi D, Yaron M. The effects of Zintona EC (a ginger extract) on symptomatic gonarthritis. *Osteoarthritis Cartilage*. 2003;11:783–789.

Winemiller M, Billow R, Laskowski E, Harmsen WS. Effect of magnetic vs sham-magnetic insoles on plantar heel pain: a randomized controlled trial. *The Journal of the American Medical Association*. 2003;290(11):1474–1478. doi:10.1001/jama.290.11.1474. http://jama.jamanetwork.com/article.aspx?articleid=197301. Accessed June 27, 2013.

Yao E, Gerritz PK, Henricson E, et al. Randomized controlled trial comparing acupuncture with placebo acupuncture for the treatment of carpal tunnel syndrome. *PM&R: The Journal of Injury, Function, and Rehabilitation*. 2012 May;4(5):367–173. doi: 10.1016/j.pmrj.2012.01.008.

Zhang Y, Neogi T, Chen C, Chaisson C, Hunter DJ, Choi HK. Cherry consumption and decreased risk of recurrent gout attacks. *Arthritis and Rheumatism*. 2012 Dec;64(12):4004–4011. doi: 10.1002/art.34677.

Chapter 51 Nausea and Vomiting

Ali BH, Blunden G, Tanira MO, Nemmar A. Some phytochemical, pharmacological and toxicological properties of ginger (Zingiber officinale Roscoe): a review of recent research. *Food and Chemical Toxicology*. 2008 Feb;46(2):409–420.

Haniadka R, Saldanha E, Sunita V, Palatty PL, Fayad R, Baliga MS. A review of the gastroprotective effects of ginger (Zingiber officinale Roscoe). *Food and Function*. 2013 Apr 24. [Epub ahead of print]

Hunt R, Dienemann J, Norton HJ, et al. Aromatherapy as treatment for postoperative nausea: a randomized trial. *Anesthesia and Analgesia*. 2012 Mar 5. [Epub ahead of print]

Lane B, Cannella K, Bowen C, et al. Examination of the effectiveness of peppermint aromatherapy on nausea in women post C-section. *Journal of Holistic Nursing*. 2012 Jun;30(2):90–104; quiz 105–106. doi: 10.1177/0898010111423419.

Lua PL, Zakaria NS. A brief review of current scientific evidence involving aromatherapy use for nausea and vomiting. *Journal of Alternative and Complementary Medicine*. 2012 Jun;18(6):534–540.

Marx WM, Teleni L, McCarthy AL, et al. Ginger (Zingiber officinale) and chemotherapy-induced nausea and vomiting: a systematic literature review. *Nutrition Reviews*. 2013 Apr;71(4):245–254. doi: 10.1111/nure.12016.

Pongrojpaw D, Somprasit C, Chanthasenanont A. A randomized comparison of ginger and dimenhydrinate in the treatment of nausea and vomiting in pregnancy. *Journal of the Medical Association of Thailand*. 2007 Sep;90(9):1703–1709.

Tayarani-Najaran Z, Talasaz-Firoozi E, Nasiri R, Jalali N, Hassanzadeh M. Antiemetic activity of volatile oil from Mentha spicata and Mentha × piperita in chemotherapy-induced nausea and vomiting. *Ecancermedicalscience*. 2013;7:290. doi: 10.3332/ecancer.2013.290. www.ncbi.nlm.nih.gov/pmc/articles/pmc3562057/. Accessed May 17, 2013.

Chapter 52 Premenstrual Syndrome

Bertone-Johnson, ER, Chocano-Bedoya PO, Zagarins SE, Micka AE, Ronnenberg AG. Dietary vitamin D intake, 25-hydroxyvitamin D3 levels and premenstrual syndrome in a college-aged population. *The Journal of Steroid Biochemistry and Molecular Biology*. 2010 Jul;121(1–2):434–437. doi: 10.1016/j.jsbmb.2010.03.076.

Bertone-Johnson ER, Hankinson SE, Johnson SR, Manson JE. Cigarette smoking and the development of premenstrual syndrome. *American Journal of Epidemiology*. 2008 Oct 15;168(8):938–945.

Bertone-Johnson ER, Hankinson SE, Willett WC, Johnson SR, Manson JE. Adiposity and the development of premenstrual syndrome. *Journal of Women's Health*. 2010 Nov;19(11):1955–1962.

Chocano-Bedoya PO, Manson JE, Hankinson SE, et al. Dietary B vitamin intake and incident premenstrual syndrome. *The American Journal of Clinical Nutrition*. 2011 May;93(5):1080–1086. doi: 10.3945/ajcn.110.009530.

Cunningham J, Yonkers KA, O'Brien S, Eriksson E. Update on research and treatment of premenstrual dysphoric disorder. *Harvard Review of Psychiatry*. 2009;17(2):120–137.

Dvivedi J, Dvivedi S, Mahajan KK, Mittal S, Singhal A. Effect of '61-points relaxation technique' on stress parameters in premenstrual syndrome. *Indian Journal of Physiology and Pharmacology*. 2008 Jan–Mar;52(1):69–76.

Ghanbari Z, Haghollahi F, Shariat M, Foroshani AR, Ashrafi M. Effects of calcium supplement therapy in women with premenstrual syndrome. *Taiwanese Journal of Obstetrics and Gynecology*. 2009 Jun;48(2):124–129. doi:10.1016/s1028-4559(09)60271-0.

Huang KL, Tsai SJ. St. John's wort (Hypericum perforatum) as a treatment for premenstrual dysphoric disorder: case report. *International Journal of Psychiatry in Medicine*. 2003;33(3):295–297.

Kim SY, Park HJ, Lee H, Lee H. Acupuncture for premenstrual syndrome: a systematic review and meta-analysis of randomised controlled trials. *BJOG*. 2011 Jul;118(8):899–915. doi: 10.1111/j.1471-0528.2011.02994.x.

Low Dog, Tieraona. Premenstrual Syndrome. In Rakel D, ed. *Integrative Medicine*. Philadelphia, PA: Saunders/Elsevier; 2007:601–611.

Prilepskaya VN, Ledina AV, Tagiyeva AV, Revazova FS. Vitex agnus castus: successful treatment of moderate to severe premenstrual syndrome. *Maturitas*. 2006;55(Suppl 1):S55–63.

van Die MD, Bone KM, Burger HG, Reece JE, Teede HJ. Effects of a combination of Hypericum perforatum and Vitex agnus-castus on PMS-like symptoms in late-perimenopausal women: findings from a subpopulation analysis. *Journal of Alternative and Complementary Medicine*. 2009 Sep;15(9):1045–1048.

van Die MD, Burger HG, Teede HJ, Bone KM. Vitex agnus-castus extracts for female reproductive disorders: a systematic review of clinical trials. *Planta Medica*. 2013 May;79(7):562–575. doi: 10.1055/s-0032-1327831.

Chapter 53 Prostate Health

Adhami VM, Siddiqui IA, Syed DN, Lall RK, Mukhtar H. Oral infusion of pomegranate fruit extract inhibits prostate carcinogenesis in the TRAMP model. *Carcinogenesis*. 2012 Mar;33(3):644–651. Epub 2011 Dec 22. doi: 10.1093/carcin/bgr308.

Altavilla D, Bitto A, Polito F, et al. The combination of Serenoa repens, selenium and lycopene is more effective than serenoa repens alone to prevent hormone dependent prostatic growth. *Journal of Urology*. 2011 Oct;186(4):1524–1529.

Cai T, Mazzoli S, Bechi A, et al. Serenoa repens associated with Urtica dioica (ProstaMEV) and curcumin and quercitin (FlogMEV) extracts are able to improve the efficacy of prulifloxacin in bacterial prostatitis patients: results from a prospective randomised study. *International Journal of Antimicrobial Agents*. 2009;33(6):549–553.

Christudoss P, Selvakumar R, Fleming JJ, Gopalakrishnan G. Zinc status of patients with benign prostatic hyperplasia and prostate carcinoma. *Indian Journal of Urology*. 2011 Jan;27(1):14–18. doi: 10.4103/0970-1591.78405.

Davalli P, Rizzi F, Caporali A, et al. Anticancer activity of green tea polyphenols in prostate gland. *Oxidative Medicine and Cellular Longevity*. 2012;2012:984219. doi: 10.1155/2012/984219. www.ncbi.nlm.nih.gov/pmc/articles/pmc3527608/. Accessed May 21, 2013.

Déziel B, MacPhee J, Patel K, et al. American cranberry (Vaccinium macrocarpon) extract affects human prostate cancer cell growth via cell cycle arrest by modulating expression of cell cycle regulators. *Food and Function*. 2012 May;3(5):556–564. doi: 10.1039/c2fo10145a.

Durak I, Yilmaz E, Devrim E, et al. Consumption of aqueous garlic extract leads to significant improvement in patients with benign prostate hyperplasia and prostate cancer. *Nutrition Research*. 2003;23:199–204.

Espinosa G. Nutrition and benign prostatic hyperplasia. *Current Opinion in Urology*. 2013 Jan;23(1):38–41. doi: 10.1097/mou.0b013e32835abd05.

Gupta K, Thakur VS, Bhaskaran N, et al. Green tea polyphenols induce p53-dependent and p53-independent apoptosis in prostate cancer cells through two distinct mechanisms. *PLoS One*. 2012;7(12):e52572. doi: 10.1371/journal.pone.0052572. www.ncbi.nlm.nih.gov/pmc/articles/pmc3527608/. Accessed May 21, 2013.

Hansen J, Lassen CF. Nested case-control study of night shift work and breast cancer risk among women in the Danish military. *Occupational and Environmental Medicine*. 2012 May. doi: 10.1136/oemed-2011-100240.

Hong SH, Choi YS, Cho HJ, et al. Antiproliferative effects of zinc-citrate compound on hormone refractory prostate cancer. *Chinese Journal of Cancer Research*. 2012 Jun;24(2):124–129. doi: 10.1007/s11670-012-0124-9.

Klein EA, Thompson IM Jr, Tangen CM, et al. Vitamin E and the risk of prostate cancer: the Selenium and Vitamin E Cancer Prevention Trial (SELECT). *JAMA*. 2011 Oct 12;306(14):1549–1556. doi: 10.1001/jama.2011.1437.

Kim TH, Lim HJ, Kim MS, Lee MS. Dietary supplements for benign prostatic hyperplasia: an overview of systematic reviews. *Maturitas*. 2012 Nov;73(3):180–185. doi: 10.1016/j.maturitas.2012.07.007.

Kurahashi N, Iwasaki M, Sasazuki S, Otani T, Inoue M, Tsugane S; Japan Public Health Center–based Prospective Study Group. Soy product and isoflavone consumption in relation to prostate cancer in Japanese men. *Cancer Epidemiology, Biomarkers, and Prevention*. 2007 Mar;16(3):538–545.

Kurahashi N, Sasazuki S, Iwasaki M, Inoue M, Tsugane S; Japan Public Health Center–based Study Group. Green tea consumption and prostate cancer risk in Japanese men: a prospective study. *American Journal of Epidemiology*. 2008 Jan 1;167(1):71–77.

Lissoni P, Cazzaniga M, Tancini G, et al. Reversal of clinical resistance to LHRH analogue in metastatic prostate cancer by the pineal hormone melatonin: efficacy of LHRH analogue plus melatonin in patients progressing on LHRH analogue alone. *European Urology*. 1997;31:178–181.

Liu Z, Li M, Chen K, et al. S-allylcysteine induces cell cycle arrest and apoptosis in androgen-independent human prostate cancer cells. *Molecular Medicine Reports*. 2012 Feb;5(2):439–443. doi: 10.3892/mmr.2011.658.

Lopatkin N, Sivkov A, Schläfke S, Funk P, Medvedev A, Engelmann U. Efficacy and safety of a combination of Sabal and Urtica extract in lower urinary tract symptoms—long-term follow-up of a placebo-controlled, double-blind, multicenter trial. *International Urology and Nephrology*. 2007;39(4):1137–1146.

Malik A, Afaq F, Sarfaraz S, Adhami VM, Syed DN, Mukhtar H. Pomegranate fruit juice for chemoprevention and chemotherapy of prostate cancer. *Proceedings of the National Academy of Sciences*. USA. 2005 Oct 11;102(41):14813–14878. Epub 2005 Sep 28.

Moyer VA. Screening for Prostate Cancer: U.S. Preventive Services Task Force Recommendation Statement. *Annals of Internal Medicine*. 2012;157(2):120–134. doi:10.7326/0003-4819-157-2-201207170-00459. http://annals.org/article.aspx?articleid=1216568. Accessed May 21, 2013.

Schwartz GG, Hanchette CL. UV, latitude, and spatial trends in prostate cancer mortality: all sunlight is not the same (United States). *Cancer Causes and Control.* 2006 Oct;17(8):1091–1101.

Shoskes DA, Zeitlin SI, Shahed A, Rajfer J. Quercetin in men with category III chronic prostatitis: a preliminary prospective, double-blind, placebo-controlled trial. *Urology.* 1999;54:960–963.

Sigurdardottir LG, Valdimarsdóttir U, et al. Circadian Disruption, Sleep Loss and Prostate Cancer Risk: A Systematic Review of Epidemiological Studies. *Cancer Epidemiology, Biomarkers, & Prevention.* 2012 May 7. doi: 10.1158/1055-9965.epi-12-0116. [Epub ahead of print]

Vikram A, Jena G, Ramarao P. Insulin-resistance and benign prostatic hyperplasia: the connection. *European Journal of Pharmacology.* 2010 Sep 1;641(2–3):75–81. doi: 10.1016/j.ejphar.2010.05.042.

Wang L, Ho J, Glackin C, Martins-Green M. Specific pomegranate juice components as potential inhibitors of prostate cancer metastasis. *Translational Oncology.* 2012 Oct;5(5):344–355. Epub 2012 Oct 1.

Wilt, T, Ishani A, Mac Donald R. Serenoa repens for benign prostatic hyperplasia. Cochrane Database of Systematic Reviews. 2002;(3):CD001423.

Wilt, T, Ishani A, Mac Donald R, Rutks I, Stark G. Pygeum africanum for benign prostatic hyperplasia. Cochrane Database of Systematic Reviews. 2002;(1):CD001044.

Wilt T, Ishani A, MacDonald R, Stark G, Mulrow C, Lau J. Beta-sitosterols for benign prostatic hyperplasia. Cochrane Database of Systematic Reviews. 2000;(2):CD001043.

Chapter 54 Psoriasis

Choonhakarn C, Busaracome P, Sripanidkulchai B, Sarakarn P. A prospective, randomized clinical trial comparing topical aloe vera with 0.1% triamcinolone acetonide in mild to moderate plaque psoriasis. *Journal of the European Academy of Dermatology and Venereology.* 2010 Feb;24(2):168–172.

Dhabhar FS. Psychological stress and immunoprotection versus immunopathology in the skin. *Clinics in Dermatology.* 2013 Jan–Feb;31(1):18–30. doi: 10.1016/j.clindermatol.2011.11.003.

Ellis CN, Berberian B, Sulica VI, et al. A double-blind evaluation of topical capsaicin in pruritic psoriasis. *Journal of the American Academy of Dermatology.* 1993 Sep;29(3):438–442.

Gulliver WP, Donsky HJ. A report on three recent clinical trials using Mahonia aquifolium 10% topical cream and a review of the worldwide clinical experience with Mahonia aquifolium for the treatment of plaque psoriasis. *American Journal of Therapeutics.* 2005;12:398–406.

Martins MD, Marques MM, Bussadori SK, et al. Comparative analysis between Chamomilla recutita and corticosteroids on wound healing. An in vitro and in vivo study. *Phytotherapy Research.* 2009 Feb;23(2):274–278. doi: 10.1002/ptr.2612.

Pazyar N, Yaghoobi R. Tea tree oil as a novel antipsoriasis weapon. *Skin Pharmacology and Physiology.* 2012;25(3):162–163. doi: 10.1159/000337936.

Stücker M, Memmel U, Hoffmann M, Hartung J, Altmeyer P. Vitamin B12 cream containing avocado oil in the therapy of plaque psoriasis. *Dermatology.* 2001;203(2):141–147.

van de Kerkhof P. Vitamin D and systemic therapy. *Cutis.* 2002 Nov;70(5 Suppl):16–20.

Wolters M. Diet and psoriasis: experimental data and clinical evidence. *British Journal of Dermatology.* 2005 Oct;153(4):706–714.

Zulfakar MH, Edwards M, Heard CM. Is there a role for topically delivered eicosapentaenoic acid in the treatment of psoriasis? *European Journal of Dermatology.* 2007 Jul–Aug;17(4):284–291. www.jle.com/en/revues/medecine/ejd/e-docs/00/04/30/C0/article.phtml. Accessed May 21, 2013.

Chapter 55 Sinusitis

Adappa ND, Wei CC, Palmer JN. Nasal irrigation with or without drugs: the evidence. *Current Opinion in Otolaryngology and Head and Neck Surgery.* 2012 Feb;20(1):53–7.

Ah-See K. Sinusitis (Acute). Clinical Evidence Handbook. *American Family Physician.* 2009 Feb 15;79(4):320–321. www.aafp.org/afp/2009/0215/p320.html. Accessed May 21, 2013.

Cichewicz RH, Thorpe PA. The antimicrobial properties of chile peppers (Capsicum species) and their uses in Mayan medicine. *Journal of Ethnopharmacology.* 1996;52:61–70.

Conrad A, Biehler D, Nobis T, et al. Broad spectrum antibacterial activity of a mixture of isothiocyanates from nasturtium (*Tropaeoli majoris herba*) and horseradish (*Armoraciae rusticanae radix*). *Drug Research* (Stuttgart). 2013 Feb;63(2):65–68. doi: 10.1055/s-0032-1331754.

Garbutt JM, Banister C, Spitznagel E, Piccirillo JF. Amoxicillin for acute rhinosinusitis: a randomized controlled trial. *JAMA.* 2012;307(7):685–692.

Gwaltney JM Jr, Phillips CD, Miller RD, Riker DK. Computed tomographic study of the common cold. *New England Journal of Medicine.* 1994;330:25–30.

Harris JC, Cottrell SL, Plummer S, Lloyd D. Antimicrobial properties of Allium sativum (garlic). *Applied Microbiology and Biotechnology.* 2001 Oct;57(3):282–286.

Hildenbrand T, Weber R, Heubach C, Mösges R. Nasal douching in acute rhinosinusitis. *Laryngorhinootologie.* 2011 Jun;90(6): 346–351.

Inoue T, Sugimoto Y, Masuda H, Kamei C. Antiallergic effect of flavonoid glycosides obtained from Mentha piperita L. *Biological and Pharmaceutical Bulletin.* 2002 Feb;25(2):256–259.

Marz RW, Ismail C, Popp MA. Action profile and efficacy of a herbal combination preparation for the treatment of sinusitis. *Wiener Medizinische Wochenschrift.* 1999;149:202–208.

Mazzone A, Catalani M, Costanzo M, et al. Evaluation of Serratia peptidase in acute or chronic inflammation of otorhinolaryngology pathology: a multicentre, double-blind, randomized trial versus placebo. *Journal of Internal Medicine Research.* 1990;18:379–388.

Meghwal M, Goswami TK. Piper nigrum and piperine: an update. *Phytotherapy Research.* 2013 Apr 29. doi: 10.1002/ptr.4972. [Epub ahead of print]

Nakamura S, Hashimoto Y, Mikami M, et al. Effect of the proteolytic enzyme serrapeptase in patients with chronic airway disease. *Respirology.* 2003;8:316–320.

Neubauer N, Marz RW. Placebo-controlled, randomized, double-blind, clincal trial with Sinupret sugar coated tablets on the basis of a therapy with antibiotics and decongestant nasal drops in acute sinusitis. *Phytomedicine.* 1994;1:177–181.

Purev U, Chung MJ, Oh DH. Individual differences on immunostimulatory activity of raw and black garlic extract in human primary immune cells. *Immunopharmacology and Immunotoxicology.* 2012 Aug;34(4):651–660. doi: 10.3109/08923973.2011.649288.

Timmer A, Günther J, Rücker G, et al. Pelargonium sidoides extract for acute respiratory tract infections. Cochrane Database of Systematic Reviews. 2008;(3):CD006323.

Chapter 56 Sore Throat

Alvarez-Ordóñez A, Carvajal A, Arguello H, Martínez-Lobo FJ, Naharro G, Rubio P. Antibacterial activity and mode of action of a commercial citrus fruit extract. *Journal of Applied Microbiology.* 2013 Apr 12. doi: 10.1111/jam.12216. [Epub ahead of print]

Brinckmann J, Sigwart H, van Houten Taylor L. Safety and efficacy of a traditional herbal medicine (Throat Coat) in symptomatic temporary relief of pain in patients with acute pharyngitis: a multicenter, prospective, randomized, double-blinded, placebo-controlled study. *Journal of Alternative and Complementary Medicine.* 2003 Apr;9(2):285–298. www.health911.com/hoarseness.

Cermelli C, Fabio A, Fabio G, Quaglio P. Effect of eucalyptus essential oil on respiratory bacteria and viruses. *Current Microbiology.* 2008 Jan;56(1):89–92.

Chang JS, Wang KC, Yeh CF, Shieh DE, Chiang LC. Fresh ginger (Zingiber officinale) has anti-viral activity against human respiratory syncytial virus in human respiratory tract cell lines. *Journal of Ethnopharmacology.* 2013 Jan 9;145(1):146–151. doi: 10.1016/j.jep.2012.10.043.

Cichewicz RH, Thorpe PA. The antimicrobial properties of chile peppers (Capsicum species) and their uses in Mayan medicine. *Journal of Ethnopharmacology.* 1996;52:61–70.

Davies SJ, Harding LM, Baranowski AP. A novel treatment of postherpetic neuralgia using peppermint oil. *Clinical Journal of Pain.* 2002;18:200–202.

Dorman HJ, Deans SG. Antimicrobial agents from plants: antibacterial activity of plant volatile oils. *Journal of Applied Microbiology.* 2000;88:308–316.

Duthie GG, Kyle JA, Jenkinson AM, et al. Increased salicylate concentrations in urine of human volunteers after consumption of cranberry juice. *Journal of Agricultural and Food Chemistry.* 2005;53:2897–2900.

Elaissi A, Rouis Z, Salem NA, et al. Chemical composition of 8 eucalyptus species' essential oils and the evaluation of their antibacterial, antifungal and antiviral activities. *BMC Complementary and Alternative Medicine.* 2012 Jun 28;12:81. doi: 10.1186/1472-6882-12-81. www.ncbi.nlm.nih.gov/pmc/articles/pmc3475086/. Accessed April 19, 2013.

Garozzo A, Timpanaro R, Stivala A, Bisignano G, Castro A. Activity of Melaleuca alternifolia (tea tree) oil on Influenza virus A/PR/8: study on the mechanism of action. *Antiviral Research.* 2011 Jan;89(1):83–88. doi: 10.1016/j.antiviral.2010.11.010.

Hemilä H, Chalker E. Vitamin C for preventing and treating the common cold. Cochrane Database of Systematic Reviews. 2013 Jan 31;1:CD000980. doi: 10.1002/14651858.cd000980.pub4.

Iscan G, Kirimer N, Kurkcuoglu M, et al. Antimicrobial screening of Mentha piperita essential oils. *Journal of Agricultural and Food Chemistry.* 2002;50:3943–3946.

Maddocks SE, Lopez MS, Rowlands RS, Cooper RA. Manuka honey inhibits the development of Streptococcus pyogenes biofilms and causes reduced expression of two fibronectin binding proteins. *Microbiology.* 2012 Mar;158(Pt 3):781–790. doi: 10.1099/mic.0.053959-0.

Mason L, Moore RA, Derry S, et al. Systematic review of topical capsaicin for the treatment of chronic pain. *BMJ.* 2004;328:991.

Proestos C, Chorianopoulos N, Nychas GJ, Komaitis M. RP-HPLC analysis of the phenolic compounds of plant extracts. investigation of their antioxidant capacity and antimicrobial activity. *Journal of Agricultural and Food Chemistry.* 2005;53:1190–1195.

Scheier L. Salicylic acid: one more reason to eat your fruits and vegetables. *Journal of American Dietetic Association.* 2001;101:1406–1408.

Tsao N, Kuo CF, Lei HY, Lu SL, Huang KJ. Inhibition of group A streptococcal infection by Melaleuca alternifolia (tea tree) oil concentrate in the murine model. *Journal of Applied Microbiology.* 2010 Mar;108(3):936–944. doi: 10.1111/j.1365-2672.2009.04487.x.

Chapter 57 Stress and Anxiety

Akhondzadeh S, Naghavi HR, Shayeganpour A, et al. Passionflower in the treatment of generalized anxiety: a pilot double-blind randomized controlled trial with oxazepam. *Journal of Clinical Pharmacy and Therapeutics.* 2001;26:363–367.

Amsterdam JD, Li Y, Soeller I, Rockwell K, Mao JJ, Shults J. A randomized, double-blind, placebo-controlled trial of oral Matricaria recutita (chamomile) extract therapy for generalized anxiety disorder. *Journal of Clinical Psychopharmacology.* 2009 Aug;29(4):378–382. doi: 10.1097/jcp.0b013e3181ac935c. www.ncbi.nlm.nih.gov/pmc/articles/pmc3600416/. Accessed May 21, 2013.

Arch J, Ayers C, Baker A, Almklov E, Dean D, Craske M. Randomized clinical trial of adapted mindfulness-based stress reduction versus group cognitive behavioral therapy for heterogeneous anxiety disorders. *Behaviour Research and Therapy.* 2013 May;51(4–5):185–196. doi: 10.1016/j.brat.2013.01.003.

Balaji PA, Varne SR, Ali SS. Physiological effects of yogic practices and transcendental meditation in health and disease. *North American Journal of Medical Sciences.* 2012 Oct;4(10):442–448. doi: 10.4103/1947-2714.101980. www.ncbi.nlm.nih.gov/pmc/articles/pmc3482773/. Accessed May 21, 2013.

Balasubramaniam M, Telles S, Doraiswamy PM. Yoga on our minds: a systematic review of yoga for neuropsychiatric disorders. *Frontiers in Psychiatry.* 2012;3:117. doi: 10.3389/fpsyt.2012.00117. www.ncbi.nlm.nih.gov/pmc/articles/pmc3555015/. Accessed May 21, 2013.

Barr-Anderson DJ, AuYoung M, Whitt-Glover MC, Glenn BA, Yancey AK. Integration of short bouts of physical activity into organizational routine a systematic review of the literature. *American Journal of Preventive Medicine.* 2011 Jan;40(1):76–93. doi: 10.1016/j.amepre.2010.09.033.

Buffart LM, van Uffelen JG, Riphagen II, et al. Physical and psychosocial benefits of yoga in cancer patients and survivors, a systematic review and meta-analysis of randomized controlled trials. *BMC Cancer.* 2012 Nov 27;12:559. doi: 10.1186/1471-2407-12-559. www.ncbi.nlm.nih.gov/pmc/articles/pmc3571972/. Accessed May 21, 2013.

Brand S, Holsboer-Trachsler E, Naranjo JR, Schmidt S. Influence of mindfulness practice on cortisol and sleep in long-term and short-term meditators. *Neuropsychobiology.* 2012 Feb 24;65(3):109–118.

Cardeña E, Svensson C, Hejdström F. Hypnotic tape intervention ameliorates stress: a randomized, control study. *The International Journal of Clinical and Experimental Hypnosis.* 2013 Apr;61(2):125–145. doi: 10.1080/00207144.2013.753820.

Carim-Todd L, Mitchell SH, Oken BS. Mind-body practices: an alternative, drug-free treatment for smoking cessation? A systematic review of the literature. *Drug and Alcohol Dependence.* 2013 May 7. doi:pii: s0376-8716(13)00143-9. 10.1016/j.drugalcdep.2013.04.014. [Epub ahead of print]

Connelly M. More Americans sense a downside to an always plugged-in existence. *The New York Times.* June 6, 2010. www.nytimes.com/2010/06/07/technology/07brainpoll.html. Accessed May 30, 2012.

Cooke M, Holzhauser K, Jones M, Davis C, Finucane J. The effect of aromatherapy massage with music on the stress and anxiety levels of emergency nurses: comparison between summer and winter. *Journal of Clinical Nursing.* 2007 Sep;16(9):1695–1703.

Dhawan K, Kumar S, Sharma A. Anti-anxiety studies on extracts of Passiflora incarnata Linneaus. *Journal of Ethnopharmacology.* 2001;78:165–170.

Dunn C, Sleep J, Collett D. Sensing an improvement: an experimental study to evaluate the use of aromatherapy, massage and periods of rest in an intensive care unit. *Journal of Advanced Nursing.* 1995 Jan;21(1):34–40.

Griffith JM, Hasley JP, Liu H, et al. Qigong stress reduction in hospital staff. *Journal of Alternative and Complementary Medicine.* 2008 Oct;14(8):939–945.

Hanus M, Lafon J, Mathieu M. Double-blind, randomised, placebo-controlled study to evaluate the efficacy and safety of a fixed combination containing two plant extracts (Crataegus oxyacantha and Eschscholtzia californica) and magnesium in mild-to-moderate anxiety disorders. *Current Medical Research and Opinion.* 2004;20:63–71.

Head J, Kivimäki M, Martikainen P, Vahtera J, Ferrie JE, Marmot MG. Influence of change in psychosocial work characteristics on sickness absence: the Whitehall II Study. *Journal of Epidemiology and Community Health.* 2006 Jan;60(1):55–61. www.ncbi.nlm.nih.gov/pmc/articles/pmc2465520/. Accessed May 21, 2013.

Hill C. Is yoga an effective treatment in the management of patients with chronic low back pain compared with other care modalities - a systematic review. *Journal of Complementary and Integrative Medicine.* 2013 May 7;10(1):1–9. doi: 10.1515/jcim 2012-0007.

Lee YL, Wu Y, Tsang HW, Leung AY, Cheung WM. A systematic review on the anxiolytic effects of aromatherapy in people with anxiety symptoms. *Journal of Alternative and Complementary Medicine.* 2011 Feb;17(2):101–108. doi: 10.1089/acm.2009.0277.

Liu L, Luo Y, Zhang R, Guo J. Effects of ginsenosides on hypothalamic-pituitary-adrenal function and brain-derived neurotrophic factor in rats exposed to chronic unpredictable mild stress. *Zhongguo Zhong yao za zhi.* 2011 May;36(10):1342–1347.

Michalsen A, Grossman P, Acil A, et al. Rapid stress reduction and anxiolysis among distressed women as a consequence of a three-month intensive yoga program. *Medical Science Monitor.* 2005 Dec;11(12):CR555–561.

Moljord IE, Moksnes UK, Eriksen L, Espnes GA. Stress and happiness among adolescents with varying frequency of physical activity. *Perceptual and Motor Skills.* 2011 Oct;113(2):631–646.

Nogawa M, Yamakoshi T, Ikarashi A, Tanaka S, Yamakoshi K. Assessment of slow-breathing relaxation technique in acute stressful tasks using a multipurpose non-invasive beat-by-beat cardiovascular monitoring system. *Conference Proceedings IEEE Engineering in Medicine and Biology Society*. 2007;2007:5323–5325.

Olsson EM, von Schéele B, Panossian AG. A randomised, double-blind, placebo-controlled, parallel-group study of the standardised extract shr-5 of the roots of Rhodiola rosea in the treatment of subjects with stress-related fatigue. *Planta Medica*. 2009 Feb;75(2):105–112.

Panossian A, Wikman G, Sarris J. Rosenroot (Rhodiola rosea): traditional use, chemical composition, pharmacology and clinical efficacy. *Phytomedicine*. 2010 Jun;17(7):481–493.

Perry R, Terry R, Watson LK, Ernst E. Is lavender an anxiolytic drug? A systematic review of randomised clinical trials. *Phytomedicine*. 2012 Jun 15;19(8–9):825–835. doi: 10.1016/j.phymed.2012.02.013.

Rai D, Bhatia G, Palit G, Pal R, Singh S, Singh HK. Adaptogenic effect of Bacopa monniera (Brahmi). *Pharmacology, Biochemistry, and Behavior*. 2003 Jul;75(4):823–830.

Rai D, Bhatia G, Sen T, Palit G. Anti-stress effects of Ginkgo biloba and Panax ginseng: a comparative study. *Journal of Pharmacological Sciences*. 2003 Dec;93(4):458–464.

Sarris J, Stough C, Teschke R, et al. Kava for the treatment of generalized anxiety disorder RCT: analysis of adverse reactions, liver function, addiction, and sexual effects. *Phytotherapy Research*. 2013 Jan 24. doi: 10.1002/ptr.4916. [Epub ahead of print]

Taylor SE, Klein LC, Lewis BP, Gruenewald TL, Gurung RA, Updegraff JA. Biobehavioral responses to stress in females: tend-and-befriend, not fight-or-flight. *Psychological Review*. 2000 Jul;107(3):411–429.

Toth M, Wolsko PM, Foreman J, et al. A pilot study for a randomized, controlled trial on the effect of guided imagery in hospitalized medical patients. *Journal of Alternative and Complementary Medicine*. 2007;13:194–197.

Vancampfort D, De Hert M, Knapen J, et al. Effects of progressive muscle relaxation on state anxiety and subjective well-being in people with schizophrenia: a randomized controlled trial. *Clinical Rehabilitation*. 2011 Jun;25(6):567–575. doi: 10.1177/0269215510395633. Epub 2011 Mar 14. www.ncbi.nlm.nih.gov/pubmed/21402653, Accessed May 23, 2013.

Wang C, Bannuru R, Ramel J, Kupelnick B, Scott T, Schmid CH. Tai chi on psychological well-being: systematic review and meta-analysis. *BMC Complementary and Alternative Medicine*. 2010 May 21;10:23.

Ward L, Stebbings S, Cherkin D, Baxter GD. Yoga for functional ability, pain and psychosocial outcomes in musculoskeletal conditions: a systematic review and meta-analysis. *Musculoskeletal Care*. 2013 Jan 9. doi: 10.1002/msc.1042. [Epub ahead of print]

Xu Y, Ku B, Tie L, et al. Curcumin reverses the effects of chronic stress on behavior, the HPA axis, BDNF expression and phosphorylation of CREB. *Brain Research*. 2006 Nov 29;1122(1):56–64.

Chapter 58 Ulcers

Amagase K, Nakamura E, Endo T, et al. New frontiers in gut nutrient sensor research: prophylactic effect of glutamine against Helicobacter pylori-induced gastric diseases in Mongolian gerbils. *Journal of Pharmacological Sciences*. 2010;112(1):25–32.

Babaee N, Zabihi E, Mohseni S, Moghadamnia AA. Evaluation of the therapeutic effects of Aloe vera gel on minor recurrent aphthous stomatitis. *Dental Research Journal* (Isfahan). 2012 Jul;9(4):381–385. www.ncbi.nlm.nih.gov/pmc/articles/pmc3491322/. Accessed May 22, 2013.

Bdioui F, Melki W, Ben Mansour W, et al. [Duodenal ulcer disease and Ramadan]. *Presse Medicale*. 2012 Sep;41(9 Pt 1):807–812. doi: 10.1016/j.lpm.2012.05.007.

Bhalang K, Thunyakitpisal P, Rungsirisatean N. Acemannan, a polysaccharide extracted from Aloe vera, is effective in the treatment of oral aphthous ulceration. *Journal of Alternative and Complementary Medicine*. 2013 May;19(5):429–434. doi: 10.1089/acm.2012.0164.

Birt D, From L, Main J. Diagnosis and management of long-standing benign oral ulceration. *Laryngoscope*. 1980 May;90(5 Pt 1):758–768.

Boye B, Lundin KE, Jantschek G, et al. INSPIRE study: does stress management improve the course of inflammatory bowel disease and disease-specific quality of life in distressed patients with ulcerative colitis or Crohn's disease? A randomized controlled trial. *Inflammatory Bowel Disease*. 2011 Sep;17(9):1863–1873. doi: 10.1002/ibd.21575. Epub 2011 Feb 1.

Buckley MJM, O'Morain CA. Helicobacter biology—discovery. *British Medical Bulletin*. 1988;54(1):7–16. http://bmb.oxfordjournals.org/content/54/1/7.full.pdf. Accessed May 22, 2013.

Cheney G, Waxler SH, Miller IJ. Vitamin U therapy of peptic ulcer; experience at San Quentin Prison. *California Medicine*. 1956 Jan;84(1):39–42. www.ncbi.nlm.nih.gov/pmc/articles/pmc1532869/. Accessed May 22, 2013.

Correia M, Michel V, Matos AA, et al. Docosahexaenoic acid inhibits Helicobacter pylori growth in vitro and mice gastric mucosa colonization. *PLoS One*. 2012;7(4):e35072. doi: 10.1371/journal.pone.0035072. http://www.ncbi.nlm.nih.gov/pmc/articles/pmc3328494/. Accessed June 27, 2013.

Cwikla C, Schmidt K, Matthias A, Bone KM, Lehmann R, Tiralongo E. Investigations into the antibacterial activities of phytotherapeutics against Helicobacter pylori and Campylobacter jejuni. *Phytotherapy Research*. 2010 May;24(5):649–656. doi: 10.1002/ptr.2933.

Das SK, Das V, Gulati AK, Singh VP. Deglycyrrhizinated liquorice in aphthous ulcers. *Journal of the Association of Physicians of India*. 1989 Oct;37(10):647.

Gaus K, Huang Y, Israel DA, Pendland SL, Adeniyi BA, Mahady GB. Standardized ginger (Zingiber officinale) extract reduces bacterial load and suppresses acute and chronic inflammation in Mongolian gerbils infected with cagAHelicobacter pylori. *Pharmaceutical Biology*. 2009;47(1):92–98.

Han KS. The effect of an integrated stress management program on the psychologic and physiologic stress reactions of peptic ulcer in Korea. *International Journal of Nursing Studies*. 2002 Jul;39(5):539–548.

Hwang SW, Kim N, Kim JM, et al. Probiotic suppression of the H. pylori-induced responses by conjugated linoleic acids in a gastric epithelial cell line. *Prostaglandins, Leukotrienes, and Essential Fatty Acids*. 2012 Jun;86(6):225–231. doi: 10.1016/j.plefa.2012.04.002.

Langmead L, Feakins RM, Goldthorpe S, et al. Randomized, double-blind, placebo-controlled trial of oral aloe vera gel for active ulcerative colitis. *Alimentary Pharmacology and Therapeutics*. 2004;19:739–747.

Marone P, Bono L, Leone E, Bona S, Carretto E, Perversi L. Bactericidal activity of Pistacia lentiscus mastic gum against Helicobacter pylori. *Journal of Chemotherapy*. 2001 Dec;13(6):611–614.

Miron A, Hancianu M, Aprotosoaie AC, Gacea O, Stanescu U. Contributions to chemical study of the raw polysaccharide isolated from the fresh pressed juice of white cabbage leaves. *Revista medico-chirurgicala a Societatii de Medici si Naturalisti din Iasi*. 2006 Oct–Dec;110(4):1020–1026.

Morgan AG, Pacsoo C, McAdam WAF. Maintenance therapy: a two year comparison between Caved-S and cimetidine treatment in the prevention of symptomatic gastric ulcer recurrence. *Gut*. 1985 Jun;26(6):599–602. www.ncbi.nlm.nih.gov/pmc/articles/pmc1432764/pdf/gut00379-0067.pdf.

Nanjundaiah SM, Annaiah HN, Dharmesh SM. Gastroprotective effect of ginger rhizome (Zingiber officinale) extract: role of gallic acid and cinnamic acid in H(+), K(+)-ATPase/H. pylori inhibition and anti-oxidative mechanism. *Evidence-Based Complementary and Alternative Medicine*. 2011;2011:249487. Epub 2011 Jun 23. doi: 10.1093/ecam/nep060.

Peters HP, De Vries WR, Vanberge-Henegouwen GP, Akkermans LM. Potential benefits and hazards of physical activity and exercise on the gastrointestinal tract. *Gut*. 2001 Mar;48(3):435–439. www.ncbi.nlm.nih.gov/pmc/articles/pmc1760153/. Accessed May 22, 2013.

Preeti L, Magesh KT, Rajkumar K, Karthik R. Recurrent aphthous stomatitis. *Journal of Oral and Maxillofacial Pathology*. 2011 Sep–Dec;15(3):252–256. doi: 10.4103/0973-029x.86669. www.ncbi.nlm.nih.gov/pmc/articles/pmc3227248/.

Rosenstock S, Jørgensen T, Bonnevie O, Andersen L. Risk factors for peptic ulcer disease: a population based prospective cohort study comprising 2416 Danish adults. *Gut*. 2003 Feb;52(2):186–193. www.ncbi.nlm.nih.gov/pmc/articles/pmc1774958/. Accessed May 22, 2013.

Shikov AN, Pozharitskaya ON, Makarov VG, Kvetnaya AS. Antibacterial activity of Chamomilla recutita oil extract against Helicobacter pylori. *Phytotherapy Research*. 2008 Feb;22(2):252–253.

Tang Y, Preuss F, Turek FW, Jakate S, Keshavarzian A. Sleep deprivation worsens inflammation and delays recovery in a mouse model of colitis. *Sleep Medicine*. 2009 Jun;10(6):597–603. doi: 10.1016/j.sleep.2008.12.009. www.ncbi.nlm.nih.gov/pmc/articles/pmc3509796/. Accessed May 22, 2013.

Chapter 59 Vaginal Yeast Infections

Abad CL, Safdar N.The role of lactobacillus probiotics in the treatment or prevention of urogenital infections--a systematic review. *Journal of Chemotherapy*. 2009 Jun;21(3):243–252.

Abdelmonem AM, Rasheed SM, Mohamed AS. Bee-honey and yogurt: a novel mixture for treating patients with vulvovaginal candidiasis during pregnancy. *Archives of Gynecology and Obstetrics*. 2012 Feb 8.

Bozin B, Mimica-Dukic N, Samojlik I, Jovin E. Antimicrobial and antioxidant properties of rosemary and sage (Rosmarinus officinalis L. and Salvia officinalis L., Lamiaceae) essential oils. *Journal of Agricultural and Food Chemistry*. 2007 Sep 19;55(19):7879–7885.

Carson CF, Hammer KA, Riley TV. Melaleuca alternifolia (Tea Tree) oil: a review of antimicrobial and other medicinal properties. *Clinical Microbiology Reviews*. 2006 Jan;19(1):50–62. www.ncbi.nlm.nih.gov/pmc/articles/pmc1360273/?tool=pubmed. Accessed August 29, 2011.

Iavazzo C, Gkegkes ID, Zarkada IM, Falagas ME. Boric acid for recurrent vulvovaginal candidiasis: the clinical evidence. *Journal of Women's Health*. 2011 Aug;20(8):1245–1255. www.ncbi.nlm.nih.gov/pmc/articles/pmC1784796/pdf/9812253.pdf.

Mårdh PA, Rodrigues AG, Genç M, Novikova N, Martinez-de-Oliveira J, Guaschino S. Facts and myths on recurrent vulvovaginal candidosis—a review on epidemiology, clinical manifestations, diagnosis, pathogenesis and therapy. *International Journal of STD & AIDS*. 2002 Aug;13(8):522–539.

Martino JL, Vermund SH. Vaginal douching: evidence for risks or benefits to women's health. *Epidemiologic Reviews*. 2002;24(2):109–124. www.ncbi.nlm.nih.gov/pmc/articles/pmc2567125/. Accessed May 22, 2013.

Pena EF. Melaleuca alternifolia oil. Its use for trichomonal vaginitis and other vaginal infections. *Obstetrics and Gynecology*. 1962 Jun;19:793–795.

Murina F, Graziottin A, Felice R, Radici GL, Di Francesco S. The recurrent vulvovaginal candidiasis: proposal of a personalized therapeutic protocol. *ISRN Obstetrics and Gynecology.* 2011;2011:806065. doi: 10.5402/2011/806065. www.ncbi.nlm.nih.gov/pmc/articles/pmc3153925/. Accessed May 22, 2013.

Reid G, Dols J, Miller W. Targeting the vaginal microbiota with probiotics as a means to counteract infections. *Current Opinion in Clinical Nutrition and Metabolic Care.* 2009 Nov;12(6):583–587.

Shalev E, Battino S, Weiner E, et al. Ingestion of yogurt containing Lactobacillus acidophilus compared with pasteurized yogurt as prophylaxis for recurrent candidal vaginitis and bacterial vaginosis. *Archives of Family Medicine.* 1996;5:593–596.

Spence D. Candidiasis (vulvovaginal). *Clinical Evidence* (Online). 2010;2010: 0815. www.ncbi.nlm.nih.gov/pmc/articles/pmc2907618/. Accessed May 22, 2013.

Turchetti B, Pinelli P, Buzzini P, et al. In vitro antimycotic activity of some plant extracts towards yeast and yeast-like strains. *Phytotherapy Research.* 2005 Jan;19(1):44–49.

Zárate G, Nader-Macias ME. Influence of probiotic vaginal lactobacilli on in vitro adhesion of urogenital pathogens to vaginal epithelial cells. *Letters in Applied Microbiology.* 2006 Aug;43(2):174–180.

Chapter 60 Weight Management

Aggarwal BB. Targeting inflammation-induced obesity and metabolic diseases by curcumin and other nutraceuticals. *Annual Review of Nutrition.* 2010 Aug 21;30:173–199. doi: 10.1146/annurev.nutr.012809.104755. www.ncbi.nlm.nih.gov/pmc/articles/pmc3144156/. Accessed April 8, 2013.

Alappat L, Awad AB. Curcumin and obesity: evidence and mechanisms. *Nutrition Reviews.* 2010 Dec;68(12):729–738. doi: 10.1111/j.1753-4887.2010.00341.x.

Appel LJ, Clark JM, Yeh H-C, et al. Comparative effectiveness of weight-loss interventions in clinical practice. *New England Journal of Medicine.* 2011;365;21:1959–1968.

Bradford PG. Curcumin and obesity. *Biofactors.* 2013 Jan–Feb;39(1):78–87. doi: 10.1002/biof.1074.

Buijsse B, Feskens EJ, Schulze MB, et al. Fruit and vegetable intakes and subsequent changes in body weight in European populations: results from the project on diet, obesity, and genes (DiOGenes). *American Journal of Clinical Nutrition.* 2009 Jul;90(1):202–209.

Clegg ME, Golsorkhi M, Henry CJ. Combined medium-chain triglyceride and chilli feeding increases diet-induced thermogenesis in normal-weight humans. *European Journal of Nutrition.* 2012 Nov 20. Abstract available at www.ncbi.nlm.nih.gov/pubmed/23179202. [Epub ahead of print]

Conceição de Oliveira M, Sichieri R, Sanchez Moura A. Weight loss associated with a daily intake of three apples or three pears among overweight women. *Nutrition.* 2003;19:253–256.

de Bock M, Derraik JG, Brennan CM, et al. Psyllium supplementation in adolescents improves fat distribution & lipid profile: a randomized, participant-blinded, placebo-controlled, crossover trial. *PLoS One.* 2012;7(7):e41735. doi: 10.1371/journal.pone.0041735. www.ncbi.nlm.nih.gov/pmc/articles/pmc3407232/. Accessed April 8, 2013.

De Coster S, van Larebeke N. Endocrine-disrupting chemicals: associated disorders and mechanisms of action. *Journal of Environmental and Public Health.* 2012;2012:713696. www.ncbi.nlm.nih.gov/pmc/articles/pmc3443608/. Accessed April 8, 2013.

Haines J, Neumark-Sztainer D, Wall M, Story M. Personal, behavioral, and environmental risk and protective factors for adolescent overweight. *Obesity* (Silver Spring). 2007 Nov;15(11):2748–2760.

DiBaise JK, Zhang H, Crowell MD, Krajmalnik-Brown R, Decker GA, Rittmann BE. Gut microbiota and its possible relationship with obesity. *Mayo Clinic Proceedings.* 2008;83(4):460–469. doi: 10.4065/83.4.460. www.mayoclinicproceedings.com/content/83/4/460.long. Accessed June 25, 2011.

Duffey KJ, Gordon-Larsen P, Steffen LM, Jacobs DR Jr, Popkin BM. Regular consumption from fast food establishments relative to other restaurants is differentially associated with metabolic outcomes in young adults. *Journal of Nutrition.* 2009 Nov;139(11):2113–2118.

Epel E, Lapidus R, McEwen B, Brownell K. Stress may add bite to appetite in women: a laboratory study of stress-induced cortisol and eating behavior. *Psychoneuroendocrinology.* 2001 Jan;26(1):37–49.

Harris KM, Perreira KM, Lee D. Obesity in the transition to adulthood: predictions across race/ethnicity, immigrant generation, and sex. *Archives of Pediatric and Adolescent Medicine.* 2009;163:1022–1028.

Hill AL, Rand DG, Nowak MA, Christakis NA. Infectious disease modeling of social contagion in networks. *PLoS Computational Biology.* 2010 Nov 4;6(11):e1000968.

Ibrügger S, Kristensen M, Mikkelsen MS, Astrup A. Flaxseed dietary fiber supplements for suppression of appetite and food intake. *Appetite.* 2012;58:490–495.

Kershaw EE, Flier JS. Adipose tissue as an endocrine organ. *Journal of Clinical Endocrinology & Metabolism.* 89(6):2548–2556. doi: 10.1210/jc.2004-0395. http://jcem.endojournals.org/content/89/6/2548.full.pdf+html. Accessed April 8, 2013.

Leong SL, Madden C, Gray A, Waters D, Horwath C. Faster self-reported speed of eating is related to higher body mass index in a national survey of middle-aged women. *Journal of the American Dietetic Association.* 2011;111(8):1192–1197.

McCaffery JM, Papandonatos GD, Bond DS, Lyons MJ, Wing RR. Gene X environment interaction of vigorous exercise and body mass index among male Vietnam-era twins. *American Journal of Clinical Nutrition.* 2009 Apr;89(4):1011–1018.

Mattes RD, Kris-Etherton PM, Foster GD. Impact of peanuts and tree nuts on body weight and healthy weight loss in adults. *Journal of Nutrition.* 2008 Sep;138(9):1741S–1745S.

Mozaffarian D, Hao T, Rimm EB, Willett WC, Hu FB. Changes in diet and lifestyle and long-term weight gain in women and men. *New England Journal of Medicine.* 2011;364:2392–2404.

Ogden CL, Lamb MM, Carroll MD, Flegal KM. Obesity and socioeconomic status in children and adolescents: United States, 2005–2008. NCHS Data Brief. 2010;51:1–8.

Piehowski KE, Preston AG, Miller DL, Nickols-Richardson SM. A reduced-calorie dietary pattern including a daily sweet snack promotes body weight reduction and body composition improvements in premenopausal women who are overweight and obese: a pilot study. *Journal of the American Dietetic Association.* 2011 Aug;111(8):1198–1203.

Tilg H. Obesity, metabolic syndrome, and microbiota: multiple interactions. *Journal of Clinical Gastroenterology.* 2010 Sep;44(Suppl 1):S16–18.

Wardle J, Chida Y, Gibson EL, Whitaker KL, Steptoe A. Stress and adiposity: a meta-analysis of longitudinal studies. *Obesity* (Silver Spring). 2011 Apr;19(4):771–778.

Whiting S, Derbyshire E, Tiwari BK. Capsaicinoids and capsinoids. A potential role for weight management? A systematic review of the evidence. *Appetite.* 2012 Oct;59(2):341–348. doi: 10.1016/j.appet.2012.05.015.

Acknowledgments

Linda B. White: I'd like to acknowledge Mindy Green, Brigitte Mars, Rosemary Gladstar, and Shelley Torgove for sharing their wisdom about herbal medicine; the American Botanical Council and the Natural Medicines Comprehensive Database for their invaluable and credible information about plant medicines; my yoga teachers for keeping me mentally and physically flexible; my colleagues and students at Metropolitan State University of Denver for teaching me so much about humanity and healing; my wonderful coauthors Barbara Brownell Grogan and Barbara Seeber; Cara Connors and Iris Bass for their careful editing; and Barney, Alex, and Darcy White for many years of sampling my kitchen medicine.

Barbara H. Seeber: I would like to thank my coauthors, Linda White and Barbara Brownell Grogan, for their unfailing good sense, good humor, and good will along with their expertise and creative command of the subject matter. Thank you to Cara Connors for her careful editing and respect for our wishes and efforts. And thanks to my husband, Allen, for his able and indefatigable support in testing recipes.

Barbara Brownell Grogan: I would like to thank my coauthors Linda White and Barbara Seeber for their enthusiasm, dedication, and depth of knowledge as well as for their lovely and energetic writing styles, camaraderie, and senses of humor. I thank my friends, family members, and colleagues for sharing recipes, stories, and lifestyle tips that will enhance the lives of our readers. Thank you to Cara Connors for guiding us through the editing process. Much gratitude goes to Kevin Mulroy for proposing the project to us. Finally, thank you to my incomparable husband, Dan, and stepdaughters, Meredith and Caroline, for their patience, support, and dedicated recipe testing.

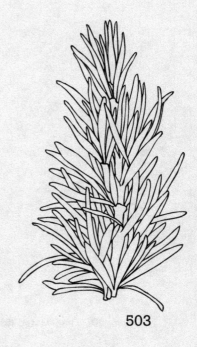

About the Authors

Linda B. White, MD, is the author of *The Grandparent Book* and *Health Now: An Integrative Approach to Personal Health,* and coauthor of *The Herbal Drugstore* and *Kids, Herbs, and Health.* The author of many magazine articles, she has served as a medical adviser and contributor to *The National Geographic Guide to Medicinal Herbs.* Since 2004, she has taught in the integrative therapies program at Metropolitan State University of Denver.

Barbara H. Seeber is a *National Geographic* writer and editor, award-winning feature writer, and thirty-year veteran of the publishing world. She has helped launch a number of titles in *National Geographic*'s line of health books.

Barbara Brownell Grogan, former editor in chief at *National Geographic* Books, is a graduate of the Institute for Integrative Nutrition, in New York City. At *National Geographic* she grew the health line of publications, including *Body: The Complete Human, Brainworks,* and *Guide to Medicinal Herbs,* and has worked with health and well-being experts, including Joe and Terry Graedon of *The People's Pharmacy* and author of *The People's Pharmacy: Quick and Handy Home Remedies;* Dan Buettner, author of *The Blue Zones;* and Tieraona Low Dog, MD, of the University of Arizona Center for Integrative Medicine and author of *Life is Your Best Medicine.*

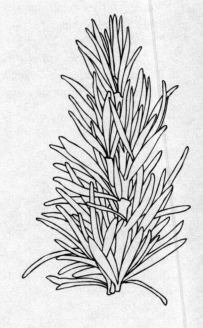

index

CPSIA information can be obtained
at www.ICGtesting.com
Printed in the USA
LVHW06s0241220718
584417LV00018B/33/P

9 781592 335756